ROUTLEDGE HANDBOOK OF COMMUNICATION DISORDERS

The *Routledge Handbook of Communication Disorders* provides an update on key issues and research in the clinical application of the speech, language and hearing sciences in both children and adults.

Focusing on areas of cutting-edge research, this handbook showcases what we know about communication disorders, and their assessment and treatment. It emphasizes the application of theory to clinical practice throughout, and is arranged by the four key bases of communication impairments:

- Genetic, Neurobiological and Neurophysiological Bases
- Perceptual-Motor Bases
- Cognitive and Linguistic-Discourse Bases
- Social Interactional Bases.

The handbook ends with an integrative section, which looks at innovative ways of working across domains to arrive at novel assessment and treatment ideas. It is an important reference work for researchers, students and practitioners working in the communication sciences and speech and language therapy.

Ruth Huntley Bahr is Professor of Communication Sciences and Disorders with a Courtesy appointment in Psychology at the University of South Florida, USA. She is a Fellow of the American Speech–Language–Hearing Association (ASHA), a Fellow of the International Society of Phonetic Sciences (ISPhS), and was awarded the Svend Smith Award for Practical Applications of Phonetics. Her areas of specialization include clinical phonology, voice production, dialectal variations, and prosody. Recent research involves the spelling abilities of typically developing children and dialectal/second language influences on literacy. She is currently serving as the President of ISPhS and Executive Secretary of the International Association of Forensic Phonetics and Acoustics and was past Editor of *Language, Speech, and Hearing Services in Schools*.

Elaine R. Silliman is Professor Emeritus of Communication Sciences and Disorders and Courtesy Professor of Psychology at the University of South Florida, a Fellow of the American Speech–

Language–Hearing Association (ASHA), a recipient of the ASHA Honors for her significant scholarly contributions, and a Fellow of the International Association of Research on Learning Disabilities. Her research interests and publications focus on academic language proficiency in children and adolescents who are struggling with reading, writing, and spelling, including monolingual English-speaking children with social dialect variations and bilingual (Spanish–English) children. She is the author or co-author of numerous journal articles and chapters, and a co-editor of eight books, including the *Routledge Handbook of Communication Disorders*.

ROUTLEDGE HANDBOOK OF COMMUNICATION DISORDERS

Edited by Ruth Huntley Bahr and Elaine R. Silliman

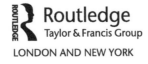

Routledge
Taylor & Francis Group

LONDON AND NEW YORK

First published 2015
by Routledge
2 Park Square, Milton Park, Abingdon, Oxon OX14 4RN

and by Routledge
711 Third Avenue, New York, NY 10017

First issued in paperback 2017

Routledge is an imprint of the Taylor & Francis Group, an informa business

British Library Cataloguing in Publication Data
A catalogue record for this book is available from the British Library

Library of Congress Cataloging in Publication Data
Routledge handbook of communication disorders / edited by Ruth Huntley Bahr and Elaine R. Silliman.
p. ; cm.
Handbook of communication disorders
Includes bibliographical references.
I. Bahr, Ruth Huntley, editor. II. Silliman, Elaine R., editor. III. Title: Handbook of communication disorders.
[DNLM: 1. Communication Disorders--diagnosis. 2. Communication Disorders--therapy. WL 340.2]
RC423
616.85'5--dc23
2014041820

ISBN 13: 978-1-138-55194-7 (pbk)
ISBN 13: 978-0-415-82102-5 (hbk)

Typeset in Bembo
by Saxon Graphics Ltd, Derby

CONTENTS

Dedication

For my children, Coleman and Alyssa, who brighten every day with their laughter, love and support.

For my husband, Paul, who has always been the shining light across the years; our daughter, Dawn Woods, and son, Scott Silliman, who are the diamonds in the crown; and our grandchildren, Ryan, Michael, and Jenna Woods and Lauren and Julia Silliman, who are the rubies of our lives.

AUTHOR BIOGRAPHIES

Elena Babatsouli

Elena Babatsouli was born and raised in Greece. She has a BA in English (Honours) from Royal Holloway, University of London, a MA in European Languages and Business from London South Bank University and a PhD in Linguistics from the University of Crete. Her doctoral thesis was on her daughter's Greek/English bilingual phonological development. Her research interests are in the acquisition and use of monolingual and bilingual speech, in children and adults, normal and disordered. Currently, she is Director of the Institute of Monolingual and Bilingual Speech in Chania, Greece.

Steven M. Barlow

Steven M. Barlow is the Corwin Moore Professor of Special Education and Communication Disorders, Department of Biological Systems Engineering, and the Center for Brain, Biology and Behavior. His team studies the neurobiology and plasticity of orofacial and hand sensorimotor systems across the lifespan. A recent NIH-funded project led to a new FDA-approved therapy using pulsed somatosensory stimulation to facilitate oral feeding skills and brain development in preterm infants. A variant of this approach using dynamic somatosensory fields is being implemented to map (fNIRS, fMRI, MEG, EEG) the brain for velocity encoding, with neurotherapeutic applications in stroke and traumatic brain injury.

Deryk Beal

Deryk Beal is Assistant Professor in the Department of Communication Sciences and Disorders and the Executive Director of the Institute for Stuttering Treatment and Research in the Faculty of Rehabilitation Medicine at the University of Alberta. He is also a member of the Neuroscience and Mental Health Institute. Dr. Beal's research focuses on combining neuroimaging and genetics to understand how genes influence the development of the brain network for speech motor control and its related pathologies.

Virginia W. Berninger

Virginia W. Berninger, PhD, Psychology (Johns Hopkins University), is Professor of Learning Sciences and Human Development, University of Washington, a licensed clinical psychologist, and former teacher who is Principal Investigator for the University of Washington NICHD-funded Interdisciplinary Learning Disabilities Center on Defining and Treating Specific Learning Disabilities. She is author of *Interdisciplinary Frameworks for Schools: Best Professional Practices for Serving the Needs of All Students* (American Psychological Association) and co-editor of Arfé, Dockrell, and Berninger, *Writing Development in Children with Hearing Loss, Dyslexia, or Oral Language Problems: Implications for Assessment and Instruction* (Oxford University Press), and McCardle and Berninger, *Narrowing the Achievement Gap for Native American Students: Paying the Educational Debt* (Routledge).

Marcelo L. Berthier

Marcelo L. Berthier is Professor of Neurology and Director of the Cognitive Neurology and Aphasia Unit at the University of Malaga, Spain. His current research involves cognitive and neuroimaging studies on aphasia mainly focusing on the development of interventions combining cognitive enhancing drugs and aphasia therapy. He is also involved in research dealing with the neural basis of language repetition and in examining the benefits provided by repetition-imitation in speech production deficits among aphasic patients.

Alexis Bosseler

Alexis Bosseler is a cognitive neuroscientist with a PhD in Speech and Hearing Sciences. Her research, which utilizes behavioral measures and neurophysiological methods (event-related potentials/electroencephalography and magnetoencephalography), focuses on the development of language processing systems in infants. She has also conducted research on the speech processing skills of children with autism.

Bonnie Brinton

Bonnie Brinton is Professor of Communication Disorders at Brigham Young University (BYU), Provo, Utah. Her work focuses on assessment and intervention with children who experience difficulty with social communication. She has served as Associate Professor at the University of Nevada, Research Scientist at the Schiefelbusch Institute for Lifespan Studies at the University of Kansas, Associate Dean, McKay School of Education at BYU, and Dean of Graduate Studies at BYU. She has been an Associate Editor for the journal *Language, Speech, and Hearing Services in Schools*. She is a Fellow of the American Speech–Language–Hearing Association.

Megan C. Brown

Megan C. Brown earned her PhD in Experimental Psychology from the University of Wisconsin–Madison. Her research interests include the influence of dialect variation on language and literacy skills for adults and children.

Lindsey J. Byom

Lindsey J. Byom, PhD, is a postdoctoral Fellow at the Center for Women's Health Research at the University of Wisconsin–Madison. Her research focuses on links between social cognition and social communication outcomes in adults with traumatic brain injury.

Kate Cain

Kate Cain is Professor of Language and Literacy in the Department of Psychology at Lancaster University. Her research focuses on how language skills and cognitive resources influence reading and listening comprehension development and how weaknesses in these contribute to reading comprehension problems. Her books include *Understanding and Teaching Reading*

Comprehension: A Handbook (Routledge) and *Reading Development and Difficulties* (Wiley-Blackwell). She is the Editor of *Scientific Studies of Reading*.

Giselle D. Carnaby

Giselle D. Carnaby, MPH, PhD, SLP-CCC, FASHA, is speech pathologist, public health epidemiologist and Co-director of the Swallowing Research Laboratory at the University of Florida. Since 2000, she has been on faculty at the University of Florida and held appointments in the Departments of Communicative Disorders, Behavioral Science-Public Health and Psychiatry. She teaches and specializes in research methodology and biostatistics. She is a well-recognized researcher in dysphagia with over 30 years' experience in the evaluation and management of swallowing disorders. She specializes in the areas of stroke and head/neck cancer, and has a strong track record of research funding and publication.

Barbara T. Conboy

Barbara Conboy is a developmental psycholinguist and a certified speech–language pathologist with specialized training and professional experience in bilingualism and child language disorders. She studies language and cognitive processing and development in infants and children from monolingual and bilingual backgrounds where English, Spanish, or both are spoken. Her research, which utilizes behavioral measures and neurophysiological methods (event-related potentials/electroencephalography), focuses on the experiential factors that shape young children's processing systems and lead to variations in typical and atypical development.

Michael A. Crary

Michael A. Crary, PhD, is Professor of Speech–Language Pathology and Director of the Swallowing Research Laboratory at the University of Florida. His current clinical and research interests focus on disorders of swallowing in adults. Current research includes screening methods for dysphagia in at risk populations, characteristics of dysphagia and related morbidities in stroke patients, outcomes of dysphagia treatment in patients with head/neck cancer, and application of exercise-based therapy for dysphagia in adults. He has published over 80 refereed papers and five books. He has a long history as a practicing clinician and is an ASHA Fellow.

Madeline Cruice

Madeline Cruice, PhD is a speech pathologist and Senior Lecturer at City University London, UK, specializing in quality of life and stroke rehabilitation for people with aphasia. Her core research focuses on understanding the relationships between communication impairment, activity and participation (WHO ICF) with well-being and quality of life in individuals who live with aphasia, so that treatment is best targeted for maximum effect. She investigates the use of self-report questionnaires, goal setting, treatment planning, and integrated interventions; is actively involved in teaching undergraduate and postgraduate students, and supervises practising clinicians undertaking research in the workplace.

Robin L. Danzak

Robin L. Danzak is an Assistant Professor of Speech–Language Pathology at Sacred Heart University in Fairfield, Connecticut. Her research focus is on the language and literacy of bilingual students, particularly adolescents. Areas of interest include bilingual/translingual writing, critical literacy, and writing instruction through authentic and multimedia text composition. She values a collaborative, sociocultural framework in which classroom research aligns with engaging instruction and assessment. She is a recipient of a Fulbright Junior Research

Grant to investigate linguistic and cognitive contributions to the bilingual writing of Italian adolescents learning English as an additional language.

Guadalupe Dávila

Guadalupe Dávila is Associate Professor of Psychobiology and staff member of the Cognitive Neurology and Aphasia Unit at the University of Malaga, Spain. Her current research deals with the cognitive-behavioral assessment and treatment of attentional deficits in chronic patients with post-stroke aphasia. She also participates in the study of the neural basis of attention and speech production deficits (accent) as well as in development of new speech-language therapies for Spanish-speaking aphasic patients. She is the principal investigator of a trial combining two drugs with intensive rehabilitation in patients with aphasia.

Luc De Nil

Luc De Nil is Professor in the Department of Speech-Language Pathology at the University of Toronto and Vice-Dean of Students in the School of Graduate Studies. His research focuses on investigating the behavioral and neural characteristics of developmental and acquired neurogenic fluency disorders. In addition to his university appointment, he is an affiliated scientist at the Toronto Western Research Institute and a visiting Professor at the University of Leuven in Belgium. He is a Fellow of the American Speech–Language–Hearing Association and Editor-in-Chief of the *Journal of Communication Disorders*.

Roxana Del Campo

Roxana Del Campo is a PhD candidate in Learning Sciences and Human Development at the University of Washington. She has a BA in Neuroscience and Latin American Studies from the Johns Hopkins University and a MA in Urban Education Policy from Brown University. Her research interests are in phonological/phonemic skill, pitch/rhythmic discrimination skills and musical skills in students with and without dyslexia. She is also interested in brain and language and the use of novel methodological tools for educational data analysis, research, and measurement.

Melissa C. Duff

Melissa C. Duff, PhD, is an Assistant Professor of Communication Sciences and Disorders and Neurology and a faculty member of the Interdisciplinary Neuroscience Program at the University of Iowa. Her research focuses on the contributions of hippocampal declarative memory to language use and social interaction and the characterization of preserved and impaired memory and learning abilities in individuals with acquired brain damage.

Laurie S. Eisenberg

Laurie S. Eisenberg, PhD, CCC-A, is Professor of Research Otolaryngology at the Keck School of Medicine of the University of Southern California. She began her career as an audiologist working with the "Father of Neurotology", William F. House, MD, on first generation cochlear implants and auditory brainstem implants at the House Ear Institute. For the past 38 years she has conducted clinical research on sensory devices, new test development, and communication outcomes in children who are deaf and hard of hearing. Her research is funded by the National Institutes of Health.

Julia L. Evans

Julia L. Evans is Professor in the School of Behavioral and Brain Sciences at the University of Texas at Dallas and Research Scientist at the University of California, San Diego. She works in the fields of child language disorders, child language development, cognitive neuroscience, and human memory and learning. The goal of her research is to develop more effective intervention strategies for children with Specific Language Impairment (SLI). To this end, her research focuses on the neurobiology of SLI, in particular the brain structure and functions that support learning and memory in these children.

Lynda Feenaughty

Lynda Feenaughty is a doctoral candidate working in the Motor Speech Disorders Laboratory at the University at Buffalo. She received her master's degree in communicative disorders from the State University of New York at Geneseo. Her research interests include investigating acoustic and linguistic characteristics of speech to determine how cognition influences motor speech behavior and perceived speech adequacy in adults. She has presented at speech motor control conferences that resulted in publications in *Clinical Linguistics and Phonetics*.

Lizbeth H. Finestack

Lizbeth H. Finestack, PhD, CCC-SLP is an Assistant Professor in the Department of Speech–Language–Hearing Sciences at the University of Minnesota, Twin Cities. Her research is focused on identifying effective and efficient language interventions for children with language impairment, including children with specific language impairment (SLI), Down syndrome, and fragile X syndrome. She is particularly interested in better understanding the grammatical and narrative language profiles of children with developmental disabilities to inform intervention services.

Eileen M. Finnegan

Eileen M. Finnegan is Associate Professor in the Department of Communication Sciences and Disorders at the University of Iowa. Her initial research focused on understanding how respiratory and laryngeal systems coordinate activity to control fundamental aspects of phonation, including pitch, loudness, voicing, and register. Her current research deals with the assessment and treatment of persons with laryngeal movement disorders, such as vocal tremor and spasmodic dysphonia. In addition, she has contributed to a NIH-funded project examining the aeroacoustics of voice and the biomechanics of the ventricular folds.

Martin Fujiki

Martin Fujiki is Professor of Communication Disorders at BYU, Provo, Utah. He has authored numerous publications in the area of social and emotional competence in children with language impairment. He has been an Assistant Professor at the University of Nevada and a Research Scientist at the Schiefelbusch Institute for Lifespan Studies, University of Kansas. He has served as an Associate Editor for the *Journal of Speech, Language, and Hearing Research, Language Speech and Hearing Services in Schools*, and the *American Journal of Speech Language Pathology*. He is a Fellow of the American Speech–Language–Hearing Association.

Amanda Garcia

Amanda Garcia is a doctoral student in the Department of Clinical and Health Psychology at the University of Florida. She received her bachelor's degrees in Psychology and Linguistics from the University of Florida in 2011. Amanda is currently interested in brain imaging technologies to understand the neurocorrelates of language in healthy and pathological aging.

Diane J. German

Diane J. German is Professor at National-Louis University, Chicago, Illinois. She is holder of the Ryan Endowed Chair in Special Education created to support her work in Word Finding. She is an ASHA 2008 Fellow and a Fellow in the International Academy for Research in Learning Disabilities. She has published/presented many articles and technical papers, and has conducted numerous seminars in Child Word Finding. She has authored the *Test of Word Finding,* Third Edition; the *Test of Adolescent/Adult Word Finding*; and the *Test of Word Finding in Discourse.* She is also author of the *Word Finding Intervention Program,* Second Edition.

Ronald B. Gillam

Ronald B. Gillam is the Raymond and Eloise Lillywhite Endowed Chair of Speech-Language Pathology at Utah State University. His research primarily concerns information processing, diagnostic markers of language impairment and language intervention. He has published two books, three clinical tests, and more than 100 articles and book chapters. Ron has received numerous teaching and research awards, including ASHA Fellow, the Haydn Williams Fellow at Curtin University in Western Australia, the Editor's Award for the Article of Highest Merit in the *Journal of Speech, Language, and Hearing Research* (twice) and the Robins Award for the Outstanding Researcher at Utah State University.

Allison Gladfelter

Allison Gladfelter, PhD, CCC-SLP, is Assistant Professor of Speech–Language Pathology at Northern Illinois University. Her research explores multidimensional aspects of language acquisition in children with autism spectrum disorder, SLI, and typical language development. Recently, she has focused on factors that influence how children learn words, specifically in the areas of phonological aspects of words, prosodic patterns, and the semantic richness of the learning context. Her overall goal is to develop more effective interventions for these populations by improving our understanding of specific semantic and phonological cues that facilitate word learning in children with autism and SLI.

Lisa Goffman

Lisa Goffman is Professor in the Department of Speech, Language, and Hearing Sciences at Purdue University. The major objective of her research program is to provide an empirical foundation for understanding developmental language disorders, one that incorporates findings about shared language and motor substrates. Children with developmental language disorders, such as SLI and autism, have well documented motor difficulties. Her laboratory uses a combination of approaches from psychology, linguistics, motor control and physiology to assess how language and motor domains interact over the course of language learning.

Mira Goral

Mira Goral, PhD, CCC-SLP, is a Professor of Speech–Language–Hearing Sciences at Lehman College and the Graduate Center of The City University of New York. She also holds an appointment at the Aphasia Research Center of the Boston University School of Medicine. She completed her BA in Linguistics at Tel Aviv University and her PhD in Neurolinguistics at the Graduate Center of the City University of New York. She has published in the areas of bilingualism, multilingualism, aphasia, language attrtition, and language and cognition in aging.

Elena L. Grigorenko

Elena L. Grigorenko received her PhD in general psychology from Moscow State University, Russia and her PhD in developmental psychology and genetics from Yale University, USA. Currently, she is the Emily Fraser Beede Professor of Developmental Disabilities, Child Studies, Psychology, and Epidemiology and Public Health at Yale (USA), Adjunct Senior Research Scientist at Moscow City University for Psychology (Russia), and Education and Lead Scientist at St. Petersburg State University (Russia).

Nancy J. Haak

Nancy Jeanne Haak, PhD, CCC-SLP is an Associate Professor and the current Chair of the Department of Communication Disorders at Auburn University. Over the past 25 years, she has taught undergraduate and graduate courses in medical aspects of speech-language pathology including dysphagia, motor speech disorders, aphasia, cognitive/linguistic disorders, and neuroanatomy. Her primary research interests lie within the realm of cognitive disorders, including mild cognitive impairment, dementia of the Alzheimer's type, caregiver interaction and in practice patterns associated with dysphagia.

Roy Hamilton

Roy Hamilton is Assistant Professor in the Departments of Neurology and Physical Medicine and Rehabilitation at the University of Pennsylvania, where he also directs the Laboratory for Cognition and Neural Stimulation. The central thrust of his research is to use noninvasive electrical and magnetic brain stimulation to determine the characteristics and limits of functional plasticity in the intact and injured human brain. His work also explores the therapeutic use of brain stimulation in patients with aphasia. his research has been supported by grants from the NIH, American Academy of Neurology, Robert Wood Johnson Foundation, and Dana Foundation.

Dianne Hammes Ganguly

Dianne Hammes Ganguly, MA, CCC-SLP, is Adjunct Assistant Professor of Clinical Otolaryngology at the Keck School of Medicine of the University of Southern California (USC) and a speech–language pathologist for the USC Center for Childhood Communication. She has nearly 20 years of clinical experience working with children who have hearing loss and their families. In both clinical and research roles, she evaluates children's speech, language, and literacy skills. She has published on outcomes and communication development following cochlear implantation.

Barry Heselwood

Barry Heselwood, PhD, is Honorary Senior Lecturer in Phonetics at the University of Leeds, UK. He has researched and published in the areas of phonetic transcription, speech perception, atypical speech, the phonetics and phonology of English, Persian, Punjabi, Arabic, and Modern South Arabian languages.

Sara Howard

Sara Howard, PhD, is Professor of Clinical Phonetics in the Department of Human Communication Sciences at the University of Sheffield, UK. Her academic background spans linguistics and speech and language pathology. Her research focuses on the phonetic and phonological analysis of developmental speech disorders and the phonetics of conversation in individuals with atypical speech. Sara is Past President of the International Clinical Phonetics and Linguistics Association (ICPLA) and her most recent books are *Handbook of Clinical Linguistics* (co-edited with M. Ball, M. Perkins and N. Müller, Wiley-Blackwell, 2008) and *Cleft Palate Speech* (co-edited with A. Lohmander, Wiley-Blackwell, 2011).

Tiffany L. Hutchins

Tiffany L. Hutchins is Assistant Professor at the University of Vermont in the Department of Communication Sciences and Disorders. She has researched the relationships from mother–child interaction strategies to social cognition, as well as child cognitive and language development. She has developed and validated new measures of theory of mind and is currently investigating the efficacy of story-based interventions to remediate the core deficits of Autism Spectrum Disorders (ASD). With the use of eye-tracking technology, she has also established a program of research to examine how individuals with ASD allocate visual attention when viewing face stimuli.

David Ingram

David Ingram is a Professor in the Department of Speech and Hearing Science at Arizona State University. He received his BS from Georgetown University and his PhD in Linguistics from Stanford University. His research interests are in language acquisition in typically developing children and children with language disorders, with a cross-linguistic focus. The language areas of interest are phonological, morphological, and syntactic acquisition. He is the author of *Phonological Disability in Children* (1976), *Procedures for the Phonological Analysis of Children's Language* (1981), and *First Language Acquisition* (1989). His most recent work has focused on whole word measures of phonological acquisition.

Karen C. Johnson

Karen C. Johnson, PhD, is Associate Professor of Clinical Otolaryngology at the University of Southern California. A pediatric audiologist with over 30 years of experience in the assessment of young children with hearing loss, she has directed pediatric audiology programs at children's hospitals in Houston, Chicago, and Louisville. In 2002, she joined the Childhood Development after Cochlear Implantation (CDaCI) Investigational Team, assisting in the development and implementation of the study's speech recognition assessment protocol. She has published in the areas of pediatric audiologic assessment, outcomes in children with hearing loss, and cochlear implants in special populations.

Kathryn Kohnert

Kathryn Kohnert is Professor Emeritus in Speech–Language–Hearing Sciences at the University of Minnesota. She received her PhD from the joint doctoral program in Language and Communicative Disorders at San Diego State University and the University of California, San Diego. Her research and publications are focused on language and cognition in diverse populations, including bilingual children and adults with and without language impairment. She is a Fellow of the American Speech–Language–Hearing Association and has received numerous awards for teaching, research and professional service. She is also a nationally certified bilingual speech–language pathologist.

Jennifer Lam

Jennifer Lam is a doctoral student in the Department of Communicative Disorders and Sciences at the University of Buffalo. She received her MA in Communicative Disorders and Sciences at the University at Buffalo. Her research interests are in the areas of speech acoustics, speech perception and motor speech disorders.

Julie Longard

Julie Longard is completing her PhD in Clinical Psychology at Dalhousie University under the co-supervision of Chris Moore and Susan Bryson. Her research interests include the socio-emotional development of typically developing children and children with Autism Spectrum Disorders (ASD). Her dissertation is focusing on the development of prosocial behavior in early childhood. She is also completing a project on early language trajectories in children with ASD. She has recently published peer-reviewed research on various areas of early social cognition in typically developing children, as well as research on positive affect in children with ASD.

Ben A. M. Maassen

Ben A. M. Maassen (Professor of Dyslexia and Clinical Neuropsychologist) has a background in cognitive neuropsychology and speech–language pathology. His previous affiliations include: Max Planck Institute for Psycholinguistics and Department of Child Neurology at Radboud University Medical Center, Nijmegen. His main research areas are dyslexia and neurocognitive precursors; neurogenic speech disorders, in particular childhood apraxia of speech; perception-production modeling in speech development; and speech-related cognitive dysfunctions. He has served as Chair of the International Conference on Speech Motor Control (Nijmegen 2001, 2006; Groningen 2011), and Chair of the Motor Speech Disorders Committee of the Ingternational Association of Logopedics and Phoniatrics (IALP).

Aarthi Madhavan

Aarthi Madhavan, MA, CCC-SLP, is an ASHA member and fourth year doctoral student in the Swallowing Research Laboratory at the University of Florida. Prior to pursuing her PhD, she obtained her master's degree from Case Western Reserve University and worked as an acute care speech pathologist for three years. Her research interests include assessment and treatment methods in an adult dysphagic population. Currently, her research is focused on patients with head and neck cancer and community dwelling elderly adults.

Amy S. Martinez

Amy S. Martinez, MA, CCC-A, is Assistant Professor of Clinical Otolaryngology at the University of Southern California (USC), and Clinical Research Coordinator at the USC Center for Childhood Communication. With over 30 years of experience as a research audiologist, she has been engaged in studies investigating auditory perception and speech recognition abilities in adults and children with hearing loss. She has conducted longitudinal studies of auditory development in children identified with hearing loss in early infancy, and helped to develop new speech perception tests for infants, toddlers, and preschool children.

Nathan D. Maxfield

Nathan D. Maxfield is Associate Professor in Communication Sciences and Disorders at the University of South Florida's (USF) Tampa campus. His research emphasis is in cognitive neuroscience investigations of speech/language/hearing, and his clinical emphasis is in stuttering. Nathan's research in stuttering has focused on brain electrophysiological correlates of real-time language and cognitive processing in people who stutter, both supported by funding from the National Institute of Deafness and other Communication Disorders (NIH-NIDCD) and the USF Seckel-West Fluency Scholarship. He is a member of the National Stuttering Association's

Research Committee, and directs an intensive treatment program for stuttering (Program for the Advanced Treatment of Stuttering, PATS, formerly directed by Pat Sacco).

Erica L. Middleton

Erica L. Middleton is an Institute Scientist at Moss Rehabilitation Research Institute and directs the Language and Learning Laboratory. Her research is dedicated to characterizing the representation of lexical knowledge and how learning through language use affects changes in lexical processing. Her work is also dedicated to the development of efficacious treatments of naming impairments in acquired aphasia that draw on best practices provided by basic research on learning and memory. Her research has been supported by grants from the National Institutes of Health (NIH) and Albert Einstein Healthcare Network.

James W. Montgomery

James W. Montgomery, PhD, is Professor in Communication Sciences and Disorders and Director of the Developmental Psycholinguistics Laboratory at Ohio University. His research has centered on the intersection of cognition and sentence processing/comprehension in children with SLI. He has focused on the influence of memory, storage, retrieval, and attention on the offline and online sentence processing/comprehension of children with SLI. Current research efforts are directed at building cognitively-based models of sentence comprehension.

Chris Moore

Chris Moore received his PhD from the University of Cambridge and moved to Canada in 1985. Apart from a two-year stop at the University of Toronto, where he was a Canada Research Chair in Social Cognitive Development, he has been Professor of Psychology at Dalhousie University since 1988. His long-standing research focus has been the development of children's social understanding, including joint attention and theory of mind. He has published over 100 papers in peer-reviewed journals and edited five books and journal special issues. His authored book, *The Development of Commonsense Psychology* was published in 2006.

Bilge Mutlu

Bilge Mutlu, PhD, is Assistant Professor of Computer Science, Psychology, and Industrial Engineering at the University of Wisconsin–Madison where he directs a research program on designing social robots and their applications in education, health and well-being, and collaborative work. He also uses social robots as experimental tools to study communicative disorders, particularly in populations with traumatic brain injury and autism, developing diagnostic and therapeutic applications.

Stephen E. Nadeau

Stephen E. Nadeau was educated at the Massachusetts Institute of Technology and the University of Florida College of Medicine. He trained in neurology at the University of Florida/Shands Hospital and pursued a fellowship in behavioral neurology with Kenneth Heilman. He is presently Associate Chief of Staff for Research at the Malcom Randall VA Medical Center and Medical Director for the VA Rehabilitation Research and Development funded Brain Rehabilitation Research Center of Excellence. His major research interests are in the neural basis of cognitive functions, particularly language, connectionist approaches to brain function, neuroplasticity, and neurorehabilitation.

Patricia A. Prelock

Patricia A. Prelock, PhD, CCC-SLP, BCS-CL, is Dean of the College of Nursing and Health Sciences and Professor of Communication Sciences and Disorders at the University of Vermont. She coordinates parent training programs designed for caregivers of children with Autism Spectrum Disorder (ASD) and has been awarded more than 11 million dollars as PI or Co-PI in university, state and federal funding to develop innovations in interdisciplinary training supporting children and youth with neurodevelopmental disabilities and their families, facilitate training in speech–language pathology, and support her intervention work in ASD. She has more than 145 publications and 455 peer-reviewed and invited presentations.

Natalia Rakhlin

Natalia Rakhlin is Associate Professor in the Department of Communication Sciences and Disorders at Wayne State University. Her research focuses on child language acquisition, in typical development and under conditions of developmental pathology. She is interested in how children's ability to represent linguistic structure and carry out grammatical computation interacts with extra-linguistic cognitive capacities (working memory, executive control, and social cognition) during language development and how compromises in various parts of the system lead to heterogeneous outcomes found across neurodevelopmental disorders with impaired language. She is also interested in how the social and physical environment interact with child-internal characteristics shaping his or her development.

Jamie Reilly

Jamie Reilly joined the Eleanor M. Saffran Center for Cognitive Neuroscience at Temple University as an Assistant Professor in January 2014. Jamie is an academic researcher and also a clinically licensed speech pathologist specializing in dementia and progressive aphasia. He completed doctoral and postdoctoral training in cognitive neuroscience at Temple University and the University of Pennsylvania. His research addresses the organization of human semantic memory and its disruption in neurodegenerative conditions, such as Alzheimer's Disease and Frontotemporal Degeneration. He currently serves as the Director of the Memory, Concepts, and Cognition Laboratory (www.reilly-coglab.com).

Austin Oder Rosner

Austin Oder Rosner is a PhD candidate in Human Sciences, with a specialization in Communication Disorders and Neuroscience, at the University of Nebraska–Lincoln. She previously received her BA in Speech–Language–Hearing: Sciences and Disorders, with a minor in Linguistics, from the University of Kansas. Her primary research interests include the development of oromotor coordination, sensorimotor integration in healthy and disordered populations, and the role of sensory influence on neuroprotection, neuroplasticity, and brain maturation. Her doctoral research examines the cortical hemodynamics associated with somatosensory and motor experiences across the lifespan using functional near-infrared spectroscopy (fNIRS).

Meredith Saletta

Meredith Saletta is an Assistant Professor in the Department of Communication Sciences and Disorders at the University of Iowa in Iowa City, Iowa. She explores the multifaceted interaction between language and speech, balance, and other motor skills. She uses production-based methodologies, including language transcription, phonetic transcription, articulatory kinematics, and analyses of postural stability and timing, to investigate the fundamental mechanisms of human communication and learning. She has studied these issues in children and adults with typical language skills, as well as in individuals with specific language impairment (SLI), Parkinson's disease, or dyslexia.

Myrna F. Schwartz

Myrna F. Schwartz is the Associate Director of Moss Rehabilitation Research Institute (MRRI) and Research Professor of Rehabilitation Medicine at Thomas Jefferson University. She directs MRRI's Language and Aphasia Lab, which conducts basic and applied research on language processing impairments in stroke, including behavioral, computational, and neuroimaging investigations of word retrieval impairments. She is also co-founder and Research Director of the Moss Aphasia Center, which since 1998 has provided community-based clinical, educational, psychosocial and research services to families living with aphasia. Her research is supported by the National Institute on Deafness and Other Communication Disorders, National Institutes of Health.

Willy Serniclaes

Willy Serniclaes is Senior Scientist at the National Center for Scientific Research (CNRS)-Paris Descartes University and Honorary Professor at the Brussels Free University. His main research interest is on speech perception, with a special emphasis on perceptual models and developmental disorders (mainly dyslexia and cochlear implants). He is currently working on the applications of the "allophonic" theory of dyslexia for remediation.

Robert J. Shprintzen

Robert J. Shprintzen, PhD, ASHA Fellow, was awarded ASHA's Honors of the Association in 2013. He is Past President of the Society for Ear, Nose, and Throat Advances in Children and received their Robert Ruben Award for Excellence in Science. He was President of the Society of Craniofacial Genetics and Editor of the *Cleft Palate-Craniofacial Journal*. He has published 210 journal articles, 43 chapters, and 7 books. He is credited for discovering four genetic syndromes. His specialty spanning 40 years is genetic and craniofacial disorders. He is President and Chairman of the Board of the Virtual Center for Velo-Cardio-Facial Syndrome.

Liliane Sprenger-Charolles

From 1990, Liliane Sprenger-Charolles has been working as a Senior Researcher (first in Paris Descartes, then in Aix Marseille University). Her research focuses on the establishment of written-word recognition mechanisms in typical development, their dysfunctions in dyslexia and the origin (at behavioral and brain levels) of these dysfunctions. She has also investigated the relationships between these mechanisms and reading comprehension, especially in dyslexia compared to specific language impairment (SLI). She has also developed tools, such as tests to assess reading and statistics on French grapheme–phoneme and phoneme–grapheme correspondences. She is (and has been) a consultant for French ministries (Education, Health), international institutes (World–Bank, UNESCO) and private industries (Leapfrog), among others.

C. Addison Stone

C. Addison Stone, PhD, is Professor Emeritus, School of Education, University of Michigan. He served previously as Professor and Head of the Learning Disabilities Program, Department of Communication Sciences and Disorders, Northwestern University. His research interests center on the social contexts of typical and atypical language, cognitive, and social development, with a particular interest in children with learning disabilities and language disorders. He has published extensively in both the developmental psychology and special education fields. He is past Editor of *Learning Disabilities: Research and Practice*, co-Editor of a book series for Guilford Press on *Challenges in Language and Literacy Development*, and Fellow of the International Academy for Research in Learning Disabilities.

Adrienne Stuckey

Adrienne Stuckey is a former high school teacher and current doctoral student in Special Education (Learning Disabilities) at Georgia State University. Her research interests include teacher–student verbal interactions and development of general educator and special educator co-teaching skills in urban and suburban high schools.

Nicole Patton Terry

Nicole Patton Terry is an Associate Professor at Georgia State University in the Department of Educational Psychology, Special Education, and Communication Disorders. She is the Director of the Urban Child Study Center in the College of Education. Her research interests concern young children with and without learning disabilities who struggle to acquire language and literacy skills, particularly children from culturally and linguistically diverse backgrounds in preschool through third grade who speak nonmainstream dialects of American English, live in low-income households, and attend urban schools. She completed her graduate studies at Northwestern University.

Kris Tjaden

Kris Tjaden is Professor in the Department of Communicative Disorders and Sciences and Director of the Motor Speech Disorders Laboratory at the University at Buffalo. Her research focuses on the acoustic and perceptual consequences of dysarthria.

María José Torres-Prioris

María José Torres-Prioris is a student at the Cognitive Neurology and Aphasia Unit at the University of Malaga, Spain. She graduated in Clinical Psychology. Her BA thesis focused on the effect of cholinergic modulation in visual attention and naming in aphasic patients, obtaining the maximum grade with honors. She is particularly interested in research and clinical application of neuroscientifically-based approaches to aphasia rehabilitation and its associated cognitive deficits.

Lyn S. Turkstra

Lyn S. Turkstra, PhD, is a Professor of Communication Disorders and Sciences and Trauma Surgery and a faculty member in the Neuroscience Training Program at the University of Wisconsin–Madison. Her research focuses on effects of cognitive impairments on communication ability in adolescents and adults with acquired neurologic disorders.

Janet Vuolo

Janet Vuolo is a speech–language pathologist and doctoral student in Speech, Language, and Hearing Sciences at Purdue University. The overarching goal of her research is to improve treatment outcomes for children with speech and language disorders. Her research focuses on understanding the relationship between speech, language, and motor skills in children with specific language impairment (SLI) and childhood apraxia of speech. She utilizes kinematic, acoustic, and transcription measures to investigate these relationships.

Nae-Yuh Wang

Nae-Yuh Wang is Associate Professor of Medicine at the Johns Hopkins University. He earned his PhD in Biostatistics from the Bloomberg School of Public Health, and joined the Faculty of Medicine upon graduation. He is a core member of the Welch Center for Prevention, Epidemiology and Clinical Research, and holds joint appointments in Biostatistics and Epidemiology. He has published more than 100 peer-reviewed research articles, of which a significant portion focused on longitudinal outcomes after pediatric cochlear implantation. He is the Principal Investigator of the Data Coordinating Center for the Childhood Development after Cochlear Implantation Study.

Louise C. Wilkinson

Louise C. Wilkinson is the Distinguished Professor of Education, Psychology, and Communication Sciences at Syracuse University. She studies children's language and literacy learning and has published 151 articles, chapters and volumes. She served on the editorial boards of and/or as guest Editor of: the *British Journal of Education Studies; American Education Research Journal; Linguistics and Education; Discourse Processes;* the *Journal of Mathematics Behavior;* and *Language, Speech and Hearing Sciences in Schools.* She is Fellow of the American Psychological Association, the Association for Psychological Science, the American Education Research Association, and the American Association of Applied and Preventative Psychology.

Kerri Wingert

Kerri Wingert is a doctoral student at the University of Washington. As a former language teacher, she is interested in the ways teachers create opportunities so that each student – with their unique profile of skills and needs – can engage in rich and meaningful language learning in schools. Currently she is investigating how certain teacher practices afford opportunities for students to develop language skills in the context of science instruction.

INTRODUCTION

Rethinking the accepted wisdom in communication disorders

Ruth Huntley Bahr and Elaine R. Silliman[1]

Many decades ago, Albert Einstein in surveying the state of scientific progress at that time observed "We can't solve problems by using the same kind of thinking we used when we created them." Einstein's challenge is still pertinent today. Little question exists that the advent of improved imaging tools and more efficacious behavioral measures has resulted in international advances in the understanding of typical communication processes and disorders across the lifespan. Moreover, the incorporation of sociocognitive and sociocultural factors into research has uncovered the relevance of individual differences in explaining the communication profiles of children and adults who struggle with their speech, voice, or language abilities. Hence, our understanding of the complex systems affecting communication has expanded at an exponential rate. A consequence is that the very breadth of communication sciences and disorders makes it difficult for either scientists or practitioners in particular areas of the field to appreciate how scientific advances in one aspect of communication may affect another facet of communication.

The purpose of the *Routledge Handbook of Communication Disorders* is to provide readers with an overview of this multilayered discipline by highlighting contemporary developments over the lifespan in at least four fundamental aspects of typical and impaired communication. These aspects are captured by the systems complexity of communication and include: 1) genetic, neurobiological, and neurophysiological systems; 2) perceptual-motor systems; 3) cognitive and linguistic-discourse systems; and 4) social interactional systems. Each of these systems constitutes a thematic section of the book. The final section presents a blueprint for theory integration in advocating the concept of systems interdependence through synergistic interactions that include the sociocognitive and sociocultural contexts of communication. The notion of systems interdependence, which is proposed as the primary mechanism that motivates systems interactions, offers two rich opportunities to advance the knowledge bases in communication sciences and disorders. First, it creates a new frontier for research and clinical practices and, second, it serves as a bridge for enhanced cross-fertilization of ideas across the many disciplines involved with communication and its impairments. Systems interdependence is explored further in the next section.

From systems independence to systems interdependence: Reaching towards new frontiers and cross-fertilization

The nature of Einstein's challenge within communication disorders

The field of communication disorders faces the multifaceted quandary reflected in the Einstein quotation. In the United States, as with many other disciplines from psychology to engineering, the teacher-researcher is typically prepared at the doctoral level in a localized area of expertise within communication disorders, e.g., aphasia, dysphagia, autism spectrum disorders (ASD), speech sound disorder (SSD), oral language impairment, vocal disorders, stuttering. Individuals tend to collaborate primarily with others inside their expertise area, generate data within particular subsystems of the expertise area, and publish in journals specific to their sub-discipline. In sum, we tend to spend professional careers in like communities with like epistemologies (Bower, 2013).

As shown in Figure 0.1, the dashed circle indicates that those in the sub-areas of language, speech, or hearing tend to maintain a microscopic eye primarily within their own research milieu, which does not necessarily take into account how interactions among the four subsystems influence communicative functioning as a whole. If the social contexts of communication are considered, they are often treated as "add-ons," not as central to understanding individual patterns of communication performance.

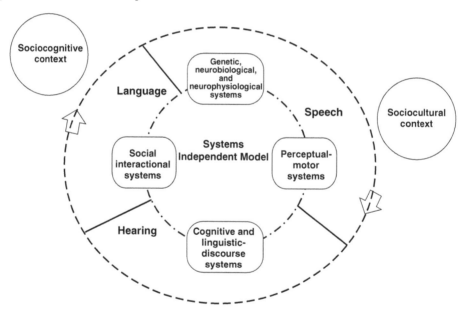

Figure 0.1 The systems independent model. This inner circle of the model depicts four basic systems of the communication process, which research and practice frequently regard as four separate subsystems. The broken dotted line represents inadequate consideration of synergistic interconnections among the systems. The outer dashed circle represents the tendency for research and clinical practice within each of the subsystems to be approached primarily within the domain of expertise. The external circles, depicting sociocognitive and sociocultural contexts of communication, are acknowledged occasionally in research and clinical practice as influences on how subsystems perform, but not as major contributors to variations in subsystem functioning.

A similar kind of fractionation in psychology has led to a reframing of Einstein's admonition. For example, Mischel (2009) refers to "the *toothbrush problem* (author's italics): Psychologists treat other peoples' theories like toothbrushes – no self-respecting person wants to use anyone else's" (p. 1). Others (e.g., Bower, 2013) argue that outcomes of this culture are professional isolationism and closed thinking that leads to disorganized theories. In fact, the narrowness or broadness of epistemological orientations to the work of science influence what phenomena are relevant to attend to; the hypotheses generated; the elements of adequate explanations; and the nature of related practices (Medin and Bang, 2014).The "toothbrush" culture is one that scholars in communication disorders should be aware of because of at least two pernicious effects for realizing models of systems interdependence as discussed next.

Two possible reasons for an insular perspective in communication disorders

One likely basis for a restricted perspective is that, unlike psychology or engineering, communication disorders is a highly amalgamated field as described in Duchan's (2011) history. In the nineteenth century United States, the original "practitioners" were educators, physicians, and elocutionists; in Europe, physicians or "speech doctors" offered apprenticeships. By the mid-twentieth century, areas of expertise were beginning to crystallize: neuro-psychiatrists (and psychoanalysts) interested in aphasia or stuttering; laryngologists who focused on voice problems; and a small, but emerging, cadre of graduates in communication disorders concerned with stuttering and, to a lesser extent, developmental problems in language and speech. With the psycholinguistic revolution of the 1970s under the tutelage of developmental psychologists, language separated from speech[2] in research and practice. This partition then culminated in a wide expansion of the discipline and profession into sub-areas of knowledge in both domains, including demarcation into child and adult focuses. In the United States, from the late 1970s until now, federal policies further fueled the child–adult demarcation through the funding of basic research in a variety of communication disorders and in the support of special education (for review, see Silliman and Wilkinson, 2014) and health services. We can only presume that the rapid rate of the technological revolution in the past 25 years combined with federal government research and service initiatives in the United States has further heightened the insularity of expertise within the language and speech areas.

A second possibility accounting for insularity is that early researchers in communication disorders, regardless of the type of disorder, increasingly concentrated on tests and practices, e.g., the development of normative data (Duchan, 2011). This attention to practice, including evidence-based practices, still appears ascendant, which is apparent from a new emphasis on implementation science within the discipline (Embry, 2014). Without question, attention to practices is vital for professional continuance. However, in today's scientific world, comprehensive understanding of the intricacies of the human communication system and the multiple ways that its disruption can affect structure and functions often requires expertise that transcends the discipline. Because the crossing of disciplinary boundaries is not common, with some notable exceptions in language impairment, SSD, ASD, aphasia, and hearing impairment (see Dunham, 2014), the door has opened for a wide variety of researchers from disciplines outside of communication disorders to take a lead in investigating mechanisms underlying the four systems identified in Figure 0.1.

In sum, new research questions and strands do continue to develop in the sub-domains of language and speech, for example, as stimulated by the advent of the neurosciences and neuroimaging. However, despite these developments, Einstein's challenge for the communication disorders discipline has not been adequately considered until recently (e.g., Prelock, 2014).

Rethinking traditional wisdom through a model of systems interdependence

An integrated model of research and practice would have characteristics similar to that shown in Figure 0.2. As in Figure 0.1, the subsystem foundation remains the same. However, this model explicitly recognizes that, because of interactions among subsystems in their functional contexts, the whole contributes to possible explanations of variations in the subsystems. As just one brief example, comprehensive understanding of a communication disorder, such as childhood apraxia of speech (CAS), entails consideration of: 1) the integrity of neurophysiological functions; 2) how and in what ways this integrity influences speech perception and oral motor systems; 3) the impact of these disruptions on cognitive, oral language, and literacy development; and 4) the ways in which home and school socialization experiences may differ among individual children, which then affects how the other systems evolve. Clearly, no one researcher possesses the necessary levels of expertise about the four subsystems and their dynamic interactions to resolve the multiple manifestations of CAS. However, to shift to a systems interdependent model, we will likely need to consider three issues: transdisciplinary thinking, the impact of poverty, and population health.

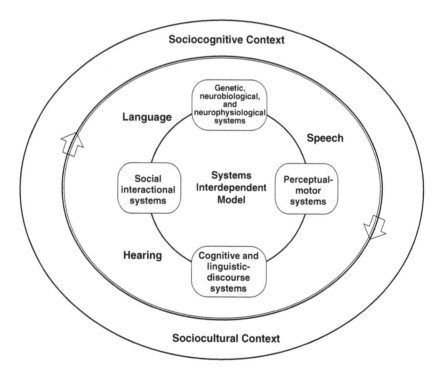

Figure 0.2 The systems interdependent model. This model illustrates that communication simultaneously incorporates interconnections among language, speech, and hearing and that the social contexts of communication are equally paramount for understanding both typical and atypical communication.

Transdisciplinary thinking

Meeting the Einstein (or toothbrush; Mischel, 2009) challenge head-on requires more explicit and shared awareness that the fabric of human communication is multilayered in its complexity within and across societies and cultures. Although no consensus exists on the differences between interdisciplinary and transdisciplinary research, the latter designation appears to best capture Einstein's call for new perspectives in scientific problem solving. A transdisciplinary approach also appears suited to generating a systems interdependent model as displayed in Figure 0.2.

The definition of the Harvard Transdisciplinary Research in Energetics and Cancer Center (n.d.) is pertinent here for creating organized theories of systems interdependence. In addressing a common problem, transdisciplinary research brings together scientists from different fields to create innovations (conceptual, theoretical, methodological, and translational) that go beyond existing discipline-specific frameworks. The emphasis on the *transformation of knowledge* into a new way of scientific thinking and practice distinguishes transdisciplinary research from interdisciplinary research, which stresses the *integration of knowledge* from different disciplines. In fact, the notion of knowledge transformation is consistent with Kuhn's (1970) still relevant description of the reconstruction of scientific paradigms.

> The transition from a paradigm in crisis to a new one from which a new tradition of normal science can emerge is far from a cumulative process.... Rather it is a reconstruction of the field from new fundamentals, a reconstruction that changes some of the field's most elementary theoretical generalizations as well as many of its paradigm methods and applications.... When the transition is complete, the profession will have changed its view of the field, its methods, and its goals.
>
> *(Kuhn, 1970, pp. 84–85)*

Restructuring existing paradigms in communication disorders to build parsimonious models of systems interdependence will likely require us to forge transdisciplinary partnerships. As Prelock (2014) observes, we can draw on and merge the talents of many disciplines to achieve the reconstruction of traditional wisdoms, from public health to anthropology to mental health as well as medicine, psychology, education, and epidemiology.

The impact of poverty

We do well to remember that communication disorders are especially damaging for children of poverty in the developing world where "fragile health care systems" (Olusanya *et al.*, 2006, p. 442), and much less supportive educational and/or rehabilitation systems, are the rule. Just in the United States alone, twice as many Americans with disabilities (approximately 28 percent) live in poverty as those without disabilities, a percentage that transcends racial/ethnic categories living in poverty (U.S. Senate Committee on Health, Education, Labor, and Pensions, 2014).

Thus, world-wide, the economic and social consequences of disabilities, which includes communication disorders, are staggering, especially when we consider that many communication disorders are not readily apparent (e.g., a language learning disability or word finding difficulties associated with early Alzheimer's disease or traumatic brain injury). Even worse, in many developing countries communication disorders are often unreported (Olusanya *et al.*, 2006). Thus, in reconsidering traditional wisdom, an essential aspect is how to "scale-up" obtaining epidemiological data internationally on a host of child and adult communication disorders in order to build meaningful service networks appropriate to national and cultural traditions (Olusanya *et al.*, 2006).

The idea of population health

An emerging idea is population health. Kindig (2007) describes this notion as a conceptual framework for considering both individual and group health as a human resource for everyday living. The population health framework encompasses three intertwined facets of prevention: 1) consideration of health disparities among individuals and populations; 2) appreciation of health outcomes, including how outcomes are distributed at individual and group levels; and 3) impacts of external influences on health outcomes, such as social, economic, and physical environments, early childhood development, and availability of health services. All three aspects of prevention influence governmental policies, research agendas, and resource allocations that stem from the population health framework (Kindig, 2007). Hence, despite some disagreement as to what "population health" means, consensus exists that its focus is the improvement of health outcomes by "reducing disparities and inequalities" (Stoto, 2013, p. 2) in health status and health care delivery systems.[3]

The population health construct has potential to serve as a catalyst for forming transdisciplinary teams because it requires the researcher to look beyond his or her immediate investigative focus. In effect, as displayed in Figure 0.2, the communication disorders researcher as a transdisciplinary team member must attend to the inclusion of sociocognitive and sociocultural contexts in research agendas in ways equal to the attention given to neurobiological and mental systems. Similarly, a sole research focus on the social contexts of communication without incorporating the neurobiological and mental contexts into theory making and hypothesis testing (however defined) can also result in the kind of insularity discussed earlier. Embedding the "disorder in contexts" at both the individual and group levels means that creating partnerships with other disciplines is essential to frame meaningful research questions about systems interdependence and to develop more evidence-based and utilitarian practices through implementation science (Embry, 2014).

Conclusion

Transdisciplinary research can potentially transform traditional wisdoms into new epistemological orientations and engender new disciplinary interactions at a deep level that may now only be accessible on a superficial level. In this way, we can begin to address Einstein's challenge through a vibrant shift in paradigms, from a focus on narrow aspects of disrupted communication to creative modeling of systems interdependence in typical and atypical communication. Our anticipation is that this volume is a step in encouraging a paradigm shift.

Notes

1 Alphabetical order indicates shared authorship.
2 The *Handbook* does not include a hearing science/audiology section. This decision was based on the current depth and breadth of the many sub-disciplines in language and speech and the fact that, in many countries, speech-language pathology and audiology are credentialed as separate professions.
3 To some extent, the population health perspective serves as one of the bases for the Affordable Care Act, implemented in 2013 in the United States (Stoto, 2013).

References

Bower, B. (2013), "Closed thinking: Without scientific competition and open debate, much psychology research goes nowhere", *Science News*, Vol. 183, No. 11, pp. 26–29.

Duchan, J. F. (2011), "A history of speech-language pathology", available at: www.acsu.buffalo.edu/~duchan/new_history/overview.html (accessed September 24, 2014).

Dunham, G. (2014), "Rewarding research", *ASHA Leader*, Vol. 19, No. 10, pp. 32–45.

Embry, D.D. (2014), *Paradigm Shift: Rethinking Research in the Context of Healthcare and Education Reform*, Presented at the Implementation Science Summit of the American Speech-Language-Hearing Foundation, Rockville, MD. www.ashfoundation.org/news/Implementation-Science-Summit--Session-Descriptions (accessed September 24, 2014).

Harvard Transdisciplinary Research in Energetics and Cancer Center (n.d.), "Definitions", available at: www.hsph.harvard.edu/trec/about–us/definitions (accessed September 24, 2014).

Kindig, D.A. (2007), "Understanding population health terminology", *Millbank Quarterly*, Vol. 85, pp. 139–161.

Kuhn, T.S. (1970), *The Structure of Scientific Revolutions*, 2nd ed., University of Chicago Press, Chicago, IL, US.

Medin, D.L. and Bang, M. (2014), "The cultural side of science communication", *Proceedings of the National Academy of Sciences,* Vol. 111 (suppl. 4), pp. 13621–13626.

Mischel, W. (2009), "The toothbrush problem", *Association for Psychological Science Observer*, Vol. 21, No. 11, p. 1.

Olusanya, B.O., Ruben, R.J. and Parving, A. (2006), "Reducing the burden of communication disorders in the developing world: An opportunity for the millennium development project", *Journal of the American Medical Association*, Vol. 29, No. 4, pp. 441–444.

Prelock, P. (2014), *Our Envisioned Future: Where Does Implementation Science Fit?* Presented at the Implementation Science Summit of the American Speech-Language-Hearing Foundation, Rockville, MD, US. www.ashfoundation.org/news/Implementation-Science-Summit--Session-Descriptions (accessed September 24, 2014).

Silliman, E.R. and Wilkinson, L.C. (2014), "Policy and practice issues for students at risk in language and literacy learning: Back to the future", in Stone, C.A., Silliman, E.R., Ehren, B.J. and Wallach, G.P. (Eds.), *Handbook of Language and Literacy: Development and Disorders,* Guilford Press, New York, NY, pp. 105–126.

Stoto, M.A. (2013), *Population Health in the Affordable Care Act Era* available at: www.academyhealth.org/files/AH2013pophealth.pdf (accessed September 24, 2014).

United States Senate Committee on Health, Education, Labor and Pensions, Majority Committee Staff Report (2014), September 18, 2014. *Fulfilling the promise: Overcoming persistent barriers to economic self-sufficiency for people with disabilities.* www.help.senate.gov/imo/media/doc/HELP%20Committee%20Disability%20and%20Poverty%20Report.pdf (accessed September 24, 2014).

SECTION I

Genetic, neurobiological, and neurophysiological systems of communication impairments

1

(A)TYPICAL LANGUAGE DEVELOPMENT

Genetic and environmental influences

Natalia Rakhlin and Elena L. Grigorenko

A key insight from twentieth century cognitive science is that the scientific study of language is best understood not solely as a cultural or social phenomenon but as an epiphenomenon of human neurobiology. As such, the human genome underwrites language development during early childhood (Chomsky, 1965; Lenneberg, 1967). The extent of the role played by "nature" in typical language development is still a subject of intense debate, which cannot be resolved without evidence from genetics/genomics. In this chapter, we review the literature that addresses the role of the genome in language development and developmental language disorder (henceforth DLD). As defined by DSM-5, DLD: 1) represents difficulties in the acquisition and use of language; 2) is manifested in comprehension or production; 3) is not attributable to sensory impairment, motor dysfunction, or another medical condition; and 4) is not better explained by intellectual disability or global developmental delay. We first explain three behavior-genetic approaches and then discuss some observations on complex genetic traits followed by accounts of the genetic bases of DLD. We conclude with research implications and directions.

Behavior-genetic approaches

Behavioral genetic investigations include family aggregation, adoption, and twin studies. This approach seeks to establish the involvement of genes in a behavioral trait through statistical inference, without establishing an explicit connection between specific (sets of) genes and the trait in question.

Familial aggregation studies

Familial aggregation studies are important for determining genetic risk of a disorder. The frequency of a disorder within families of affected individuals (probands) is compared to that in the general population (i.e., it is estimated whether the frequency of the condition is higher in probands' families than would be expected by chance alone).

If the disorder is found to cluster in families, however, it may be due to genetic or shared environmental exposure and follow-up studies are needed to disentangle the role of genes and environment in increasing susceptibility to the disorder. DLD indeed clusters in families

(Stromswold, 1998); however, rates of affected first-degree relatives for language-impaired probands vary from 24–32 percent (Barry, Yasin, and Bishop, 2007) to over 70 percent (Tallal, Ross, and Curtiss, 1989).

Adoption studies

The adoption design is another behavioral genetic method used to disentangle "nature" and "nurture." It compares language characteristics of children with a biological risk of DLD (e.g., children of an affected biological parent reared by unaffected adoptive parents) and those without such risk (children of unaffected biological parents reared by affected adoptive parents). One such study (Felsenfeld and Plomin, 1997) reported that while 25 percent of the children with a genetic background of speech disorder displayed degraded speech, language, or fluency skills at age 7, only 9 percent of the children with no known genetic history did so. Furthermore, positive biological DLD history was the best predictor of children's affected status. Such studies contribute additional evidence for the genetic transmission of DLD risk. They do not, however, provide a formal estimate of the respective roles of genetic versus environmental influences on language outcomes.

Heritability estimates

Behavior-genetic modeling studies aim to disentangle the respective roles of additive genetic influences, shared environmental (e.g., exposure to toxins, maternal health, and family characteristics) and non-shared environmental effects (e.g., injuries, illnesses, and aspects of the physical and social environment unique to each child) in individual phenotypic differences. These studies do not look at genetic or environmental effects directly, but partition observed phenotypic variance (i.e., observable traits) into components reflecting assumed genetic and environmental effects. Heritability estimates are not estimates of the total genetic contribution to a trait, but an estimate of the extent to which phenotypic variance can be explained by genetic variance. Heritability estimates are determined by comparing phenotypic concordance across individuals of different degrees of genetic identity. For example, identical twins have full identity (100 percent) and dizygotic twins or siblings (and parents and offspring) have the mean identity of 50 percent.

One common technique here is to compare concordance rates in monozygotic (MZ) to dizygotic (DZ) twins for a particular trait (e.g., language disorder diagnosis, phonological short-term memory score, a verb inflexion index, or another categorical or continuous language measure). A significantly higher concordance rate in MZ compared to DZ twins is taken as an indication of a substantial genetic contribution to the phenotype. A formula is used to derive heritability estimates, values of which lie between 1 (no environmental influences on phenotypic variance) and 0 (no genetic influences on phenotypic variance). The similarity in MZ twins that cannot be accounted for by genetic effects is attributed to shared environmental effects, and remaining differences between MZ twins are attributed to non-shared environmental effects and measurement error (DeThorne *et al.*, 2012).

Behavior-genetic studies of DLD have yielded heritability estimates ranging between 0.5 and 0.75 for school-aged children (Bishop, 2006), reaching 1 in some studies (Grigorenko, 2009; Stromswold, 2001). They tend to be lower in normative samples, i.e., 0.34 to 0.39 (Colledge *et al.*, 2002; Hayiou-Thomas, 2008), with higher estimates in middle childhood in comparison with early childhood (Hayiou-Thomas *et al.*, 2012). Studies also investigated the extent to which genetic sources of variation in one trait (e.g., vocabulary) are linked with those of another trait (e.g., grammar), to evaluate the extent to which both traits share the same genetic etiology. These investigations yielded similar estimates for lexical and grammatical, as well as other language (e.g., articulation and verbal memory) skills (Kovas *et al.*, 2005) and language and other cognitive abilities (Colledge *et al.*, 2002). Finally, studies compared heritability at the low end of the performance distribution and within the normal range of variation. Results have been inconclusive, with some studies showing higher heritability in low performing samples (Spinath *et al.*, 2004), while others show a similar pattern for both (Kovas *et al.*, 2005).

An important caveat for interpreting behavior-genetic results is that they cannot be straightforwardly interpreted as a measure of how important the contribution of genes to language is, how susceptible language development is to the effects of the environment, or whether various aspects of language share the same genetic etiology. As mentioned above, these estimates only explain what accounts for variability in the studied phenotypes. Thus, if there exists a non-varying genetic component involved in the universal aspects of normative language development, it would not account for observable variations in phenotypes (and would be impossible to detect in the absence of measurable corresponding phenotypic and genotypic variation). This, however, does not mean that such a constant genetic factor is unimportant in determining outcomes (Stromswold, 2001). Likewise, if variability in the environment in the sample is reduced (e.g., if access to quality early childhood education were to become universal), heritability estimates of normal language development would likely increase.

Another caveat is that heritability is a population parameter that depends on population-specific factors and does not necessarily predict the value of heritability in other populations or even at different time points in the same population. Thus, behavior-genetic studies have limitations, and molecular-genetic studies are necessary for identifying the genetic/genomic bases of language and DLD.

Observations about the genetic bases of complex traits

The genetic complexity and heterogeneity of complex behavioral traits

Molecular-genetic studies attempt to identify the genomic architecture of (a)typical language development by finding specific genetic markers associated with phenotypic language variability. It has become clear that such a complex cognitive function as language, requiring the analysis and synthesis of elements at multiple levels of structure in real time and utilizing complex neural architecture with multiple brain areas (Poeppel *et al.*, 2012), could not be dependent on a single gene (i.e., does not follow Mendelian patterns of inheritance). Instead, as with other complex traits, multiple genes appear to be in control (Plomin *et al.*, 2009). Furthermore, the relationship between genes and traits is frequently non-linear and involves complex interactions between genes, as well as between genes and environmental factors. Moreover, individual genes can have multiple functions (be pleiotropic). For example: 1) a mutation in a single gene can lead to a complex disorder phenotype; 2) the same gene product may be used for different chemical purposes in different tissues or for the same purpose in multiple pathways; or 3) the same gene product may be engaged in multiple chemical activities in support of a common biological function.

Polygenic inheritance and pleiotropy are not the only layers of complexity in the genome that obscure the connection between the observed phenotype and its genetic bases. In complex disorders, such as DLD, with much phenotypic diversity (Conti-Ramsden *et al.*, 1997) and likely polygenic inheritance (Plomin *et al.*, 2009), the overall genomic architecture is immensely complex. For example, unrelated affected individuals with the same clinical manifestations may carry mutations in different genes or different mutations in the same gene. One level of complexity is that genetic variation among individuals occurs on multiple scales, ranging from changes in single nucleotide polymorphisms (SNPs) to large-scale alterations in the human karyotype (i.e., the number and appearance of chromosomes in the nucleus of a eukaryotic cell). A broad landscape of genetic variation, uncovered by the Human Genome Project, was followed by genome sequences from 1000 individuals. As a result, in addition to studying the effects of structural variations in a DNA sequence (base substitutions), studies of other types of structural variation have become possible (insertions, deletions, and translocations).

Furthermore, gene mutations can vary in penetrance (i.e., the rate at which a given genotype gives rise to the expected phenotype) and expressivity (the level of genotype expression in a given phenotype). The reason for this is other genes and/or the environment acting as modifiers or suppressors. Such heterogeneity is a key feature of complex disorders rather than simply "genetic noise" (Heng *et al.*, 2011). The magnitude of potential genetic heterogeneity is astounding because the acquisition and processing of a complex trait like language involves multiple brain structures and possibly hundreds (if not thousands) of genes significant for their development (given that 76 percent of all human genes are expressed in the brain, with approximately 44 percent differentially regulated) (Johnson *et al.*, 2009).

DLD may be best construed as a spectrum of disorder subtypes with similar, partially overlapping, or even non-overlapping behavioral phenotypes. The genetic bases of DLD are likely to be a constellation of diverse genetic "events," with cases in which DLD is associated with only one or multiple loci. If a mutation causes a substantial change in a gene product that plays a fundamental role in a given pathway, damage to a single gene could be sufficient to be manifested as DLD. If multiple mutations each alter a protein structure only slightly, or if the resulting alterations affect neurogenesis only in subtle ways, each may make only a modest contribution to the phenotype, with an accumulation of multiple such mutations being required to result in DLD. In cases of common polygenic disorders (i.e., those that occur in at least 1 percent of the population), including DLD, individual genes are expected to contribute only a small-to-moderate increase in susceptibility to the disorder—hard to detect without large samples. Rare variants of large effect, on the other hand, are easier to detect, but, by definition, they are rare and only explain a small percentage of cases in the general population.

Sources of genetic complexity beyond structural variations in the DNA sequence

In addition to structural genetic complexity (or "horizontal"—i.e., associated with inherited or *de novo* variations in the DNA sequence), there exists considerable functional complexity (or "vertical"—i.e., arising through functional modifications of coding components in the DNA sequence). These layers of complexity greatly obscure the relationship between genotypes and phenotypes and make the search for the genetic bases of complex traits dauntingly complicated. These mechanisms include: 1) gene-by-gene interactions (effects of one gene modified synergistically or antagonistically by the presence of another gene); 2) genetic variation interacting with environment; 3) complex molecular machinery that controls gene expression, including variation in gene regulation by non-coding parts of the genome; and 4) modifications of the genome functioning through epigenetic mechanisms—changes in gene expression not based on changes in the DNA sequence and referred to as the epigenome.

The epigenome

The epigenome modifies gene expression levels at precise points in development and in certain locations, such that genes become more and less active (or completely inactive) in response to genetically preprogrammed or environmentally induced stimuli (Borrelli *et al.*, 2008). One epigenetic mechanism involves bio-chemical tags, methyl groups, attaching to certain genes in certain cells to modulate gene activity (i.e., increasing, decreasing, or completely stopping the processes of gene transcription and translation thus affecting protein synthesis).

Gene methylation may occur as a response to environmental conditions (positive ones, such as education or social enrichment, or negative ones, such as stress, social isolation, or toxins). This is an example of a biological mechanism that converts our experiences (social and somatic) into our basic biology, altering (possibly permanently) the state of our genomes. These modifications can be heritable, providing a plausible biological basis for events such as the occurrence of intergenerational transmission of trauma, documented, for example, in adult offspring of Holocaust survivors or the invisible transfer of class privilege (Yehuda *et al.*, 2001). Differential gene methylation patterns across the whole genome have been documented in children raised in socially depriving institutions in comparison with children raised by biological parents (Naumova *et al.*, 2012). This mechanism may potentially provide a biological explanation for the well-documented phenomenon of SES-dependent differences in language development (Hoff, 2006).

Thus, nature and nurture appear not to be completely autonomous influences, but to be intimately intertwined. One implication of this discovery is to challenge the misconception of equating "genetic basis" with immutability of the trait and environmental influences with changeability. Disorders with identifiable genetic markers are not necessarily harder to remediate than disorders that have a clear environmental basis. Providing timely high quality treatment can substantially improve functioning of children with genetically based developmental disorders. On the other hand, environmental effects, e.g., severe deprivation or maltreatment early in life, may leave permanent damage, including at the biological level.

The unraveling of the role of epigenetics in the development of the brain, cognitive functioning, and neurodevelopmental psychopathology has only just begun. It is already revealing, however, that the development of a complex multicellular organism, let alone the human brain, is a product of a process that involves much more than the DNA sequence. This process involves a complex tissue-specific orchestration of gene activity by mechanisms regulating gene expression, including those that involve environmental triggers.

Genetic bases of DLD

Mendelian DLD

There has been one notable success story in identifying a monogenetically transmitted DLD. It is the much publicized case of the KE family, members who were identified as suffering from a rare form of a developmental communication disorder, albeit distinct from the common form of DLD. It involved deficits in various grammatical aspects of language, with additional, extra-linguistic deficits, such as verbal apraxia and in some cases lowered IQ (Vargha-Khadem *et al.*, 1995). The gene, a mutation identified as causal in the etiology of the disorder, was *FOXP2*, a gene that regulates the expression of other genes. The single base-pair mutation found in the affected members of the KE family resulted in a modification of the *FOXP2* protein—a substitution of one nucleotide with another, introducing an incorrect amino acid into the protein sequence and impairing its functioning. The outcome was an imbalance in the genetic networks regulated by the *FOXP2* protein (Fisher *et al.*, 1998).

Can *FOXP2* be considered a "language gene"? First, cases of DLD caused by a mutation of *FOXP2* are rare and not representative of the common type of DLD (Fisher and Ridley, 2013). Second, it is expressed not only in multiple brain areas (e.g., thalamus, cerebellum, striatum, inferior olivary complex, and deep cortical layers), but also in other organs, such as the lung, the gut, and the heart (Marcus and Fisher, 2003). Furthermore, it is evolutionarily conserved, i.e., largely unchanged throughout evolution and found across a variety of species, including songbirds and even mice. Studies using animal models demonstrated the *FOXP2* role in multiple aspects of neurogenesis, including neurite growth and branching, motor learning, and vocal learning, suggesting similarity across species in its phenotypic effect. It should be noted that there is some evidence for differential patterns of *FOXP2* expression (Konopka *et al.*, 2009) and in *FOXP2* protein structures (Enard *et al.*, 2002) in humans and chimpanzees. Thus, it is neither a "new" gene nor a gene that selectively underpins the properties of human language thought to be "uniquely human" (e.g., combinatorial grammar). Indeed, it has been argued that the genetic evolution of *FOXP2* might have been driven by human cultural innovations, not the other way around (Fisher and Ridley, 2013). However, in modern humans it is clearly part of a large genetic network relevant to language development, which includes multiple genes targeted by *FOXP2* (whose protein products are influenced by the *FOXP2* gene product) and their own targets (genes whose expression levels they regulate or with which they interact). Thus, a disruption of normal functioning at any point in this complex network may have a measurable effect on the functioning of other parts of the network, setting off cascading effects of varying magnitudes at different points of the system.

Whole-genome and candidate-gene studies of language

For a number of years, the primary method of mapping genetic loci for inherited conditions were linkage studies, which identify regions of the genome likely to contain genetic markers for certain phenotypes by observing families of probands and analyzing the co-segregation of genetic loci and phenotypes in these pedigrees.

Linkage studies of DLD have identified several chromosomal regions associated with the disorder. Thus, loci on the chromosomal region 16q24 (SLI1) and 19q13 (SLI2) were identified using indicators of spoken language skills—e.g., pseudoword repetition and the expressive language composite from a standardized test of language development, as well as literacy measures, such as decoding, spelling, and reading comprehension (Falcaro *et al.*, 2008; Newbury *et al.*, 2004). Significant linkage to 13q21 and 2p22 (Bartlett *et al.*, 2002) was also found using both the oral language and reading measures. Finally, linkage regions on chromosome 7 were identified in an isolated Chilean population of the Robinson Crusoe Island, who exhibited an increased frequency of DLD when assessed using a spoken language battery (Villanueva *et al.*, 2011). Linkage studies do not result in the identification of genes, but merely in chromosomal loci likely to contain genes involved in the phenotype of interest.

Follow-up studies of the regions of interest identified in linkage studies are aimed at finding candidate genes, mutations of which may be causally connected to DLD. Such studies have identified a number of candidate genes. For example, in one study, SNPs in two genes in the 16q24 region, *CMIP* and *ATP2C2*, were related (each independently and both additively) to pseudoword repetition scores with the combined effect equal to a decrease in accuracy of 1 SD (Newbury *et al.*, 2009). Further studies showed that *CMIP* was associated with reading disability (Scerri *et al.*, 2011), while *ATP2C2* was associated with DLD (Newbury *et al.*, 2011). *CMIP* and *ATP2C2* are both expressed in the brain and might be involved in neuronal migration and synaptic formation and plasticity through a complex molecular network. However, the role of these genes in language development has been detected only in populations with impairment (not in typical development), exerting only a modest effect, which is unlikely to be sufficient for causing DLD without additional, yet unknown, influences.

A study that looked at another region of interest, 7q31 (i.e., the SPCH1 locus containing *FOXP2*), in families with DLD did not find any association between a DLD phenotype (namely, pseudoword repetition scores) with SNP variants located in *FOXP2,* but with a gene down-regulated by *FOXP2, CNTNAP2.* This gene has been linked to spoken language development at the age of two years in a representative sample from the general population (Whitehouse *et al.*, 2011), as well as with distinct patterns of neural activation on Event Related Potential language tasks in healthy adults (Kos *et al.*, 2012) and fMRI (Whalley *et al.*, 2011). *CNTNAP2* is highly expressed in the brain, including language-related brain areas, and codes for a neuronal trans-membrane protein involved in cell-to-cell communication. However, *CNTNAP2* is not specific to DLD. Various *CNTNAP2* polymorphisms are associated with other neurodevelopmental or psychiatric disorders, such as autism, intellectual disability, schizophrenia, and epilepsy (e.g., Alarcon *et al.*, 2008; Friedman *et al.*, 2010).

Recently, genome-wide association (GWA) has become a leading method of genetic analyses. Strategically preselected genetic markers (SNPs) across the genome of large samples of unrelated individuals with and without the phenotype of interest are scanned in search of significant associations between particular SNPs and the presence of a given phenotype (Hirschhorn and Daly, 2005).

In summary, at the time of writing this chapter, with over 1000 GWA studies published, only a few focused on spoken language (Eicher *et al.*, 2013; Luciano *et al.*, 2013; Nudel *et al.*, 2014). Neither the first two studies of population-based samples, nor the third study of families of DLD probands revealed any significant associations.

Conclusions

The present review suggests three conclusions. First, although the search for "language genes" has resulted in some spectacular successes, it seems fair to say that observed familiality (clustering within biological families) and heritability of DLD have not easily translated into abundant discoveries of susceptibility genes as had been hoped. Furthermore, as GWA studies of complex disorders have demonstrated, identified genetic variants are not consistently replicated and can explain only a small fraction of the increased risk associated with the additive contribution of genes. These problems are not unique for the study of language, but are common in studies of complex phenotypes (e.g., general intelligence) and complex diseases (e.g., psychiatric disorders, Type 2 diabetes).

Second, the phenotypes used to identify language-related genes involve simple quantitative measures of linguistic performance (e.g., pseudoword repetition, past tense marking) or coarse measures of general language development based on performance on standardized language tests. In many cases, the same loci and candidate genes are related to both spoken language and reading measures.

Third, it appears that the language-related genes identified to date do not exhibit a high level of specialization. As an example, one can look at a frequent finding in the field of the genetic bases of higher cognitive functions, specifically an association between working memory and a common variant of the *COMT* gene (val158met polymorphism), which is an important regulator of dopamine in the brain expressed in the prefrontal cortex. In particular, the low-activity *met* allele has been found to be associated with better performance on cognitive tasks with a substantial working memory component (e.g., Bruder *et al.*, 2005). However, this finding was not replicated in a recent large population-based study (Wardle *et al.*, 2013), nor in a meta-analysis (Barnett *et al.*, 2008). This underscores the problem of trying to relate complex cognitive traits to individual genes. Furthermore, the same gene has been implicated in a wide array of other phenotypes, from alcoholism, aggressive personality traits, personality traits associated with being a successful Wall Street trader, to lung cancer. Thus, *COMT* is not likely to be a "gene for working memory," although it may be one of the significant genes influencing working memory.

What are the implications of the realization that *COMT* is not a "specialist gene" for working memory? Moreover, what if a gene or group of genes that code specifically for the human capacity to hold a string of phonological segments in memory cannot be found, even though genes that contribute to individual differences in working memory are identified? This realization does not dictate that we discard the notion of working memory as a discrete cognitive function or its sub-specialization for the input of a particular type, if these constructs are well supported by carefully designed behavioral experiments. Likewise, individual "language" genes may be "generalist" rather than "specialist," pleiotropic rather than single-effect, and interact with other genes and the environment rather than exerting a simple linear effect on language-related traits. But this, in and of itself, should not impose restrictions on a theory of language development because an immense wealth of information that shapes development must exist between the proximate genotypic level and the ultimate phenotypic level (Panksepp and Panksepp, 2001).

In sum, genes are rarely related to phenotypes in a straightforward linear way. In the era preceding the current advances in genomics, philosophers of science debated whether "genes code for traits" (Wheeler, 2003). This is no longer an open question. The function of genes is to provide information for the synthesis of proteins or for producing non-coding RNA, which play various roles in cell functioning (Brown, 2002). Complex behavioral phenotypes arise from an intricate and finely tuned interplay between multiple components of the system, which consists of massively distributed networks and include the genome, the machinery for gene expression regulation, and the epigenome. The genome is a source of genetic stability and the epigenome of genetic plasticity, partly in response to changing environments. Genes, in many cases are pleiotropic, organized in gene networks characterized by complex patterns of interactions between the members of each network, as well as between the networks and the environment in determining phenotypes. At least in the majority of common cases, complex disease phenotypes, such as DLD, are likely polygenic and include not only protein-coding, but also regulatory regions. Normal development of complex cognitive functions, such as language, must depend on all members of the system working in concert, as a disruption or change in one part of the network may have far-reaching cascading effects in multiple other parts. We are still far from unraveling the inner workings of any language-related gene network, particularly linking it to specific causal molecular mechanisms. However, some interesting conjectures have been made. One notable proposal is Growth Signaling Disruption by Rice (2012), which posits (via regulatory genes such as *FOXP2* and epigenetic mechanisms) a disruption in the sequence of chemical signals that are normally precisely timed and insure cellular functioning underwriting developmental plasticity and bringing about the developmental cascades characterizing normal language growth. According to this idea, disrupted timing leads to a developmental trajectory, whereby the delayed onset (with essentially unchanged mechanisms and growth curves) leads to a cascade of delays across the linguistic system. The maturation of these systems depends on the maturation of earlier developing components, with a deceleration of growth at later stages.

The child who starts late essentially "runs out of time" and never reaches the end-state of language development. To test this proposal, animal models would be needed, which, of course, in the case of language research present a challenge, since human language has no analogs in the animal kingdom.

Acknowledgments

Preparation of this article was supported in part by grant HD070594 (PI: E. L. Grigorenko) from the National Institutes of Health (NIH). Grantees undertaking such projects are encouraged to express their professional judgment freely; therefore, this article does not necessarily reflect NIH position or policies, and no official endorsement should be inferred. We are grateful to the editors for their comments and to Ms. Mei Tan for her editorial support.

References

Alarcon, M., Abrahams, B.S., Stone, J.L., Duvall, J.A., Perederiy, J.V., Bomar, J.M., *et al.* (2008), "Linkage, association, and gene-expression analyses identify CNTNAP2 as an autism-susceptibility gene", *American Journal of Human Genetics,* Vol. 82, pp. 150–159.

Barnett, J.H., Scoriels, L. and Munafo, M.R. (2008), "Meta-analysis of the cognitive effects of the catechol-O-methyltransferase gene Val158/108Met polymorphism", *Biological Psychiatry,* Vol. 64, pp. 137–144.

Barry, J.G., Yasin, I. and Bishop, D.V.M. (2007), "Heritable risk factors associated with language impairments", *Genes, Brain and Behavior,* Vol. 5, No. 1, pp. 66–76.

Bartlett, C.W., Flax, J.F., Logue, M.W., Vieland, V.J., Bassett, A.S., Tallal, P. and Brzustowicz, L.M. (2002), "A major susceptibility locus for specific language impairment is located on 13q21", *American Journal of Human Genetics,* Vol. 71, No. 1, pp. 45–55.

Bishop, D.V.M. (2006), "What causes specific language impairment in children?", *Current Directions in Psychological Science,* Vol. 15, No. 5, pp. 217–221.

Borrelli, E., Nestler, E.J., Allis, C.D. and Sassone-Corsi, P. (2008), "Decoding the epigenetic language of neuronal plasticity", *Neuron,* Vol. 60, No. 6, pp. 961–974.

Brown, T.A. (2002), *Genomes, 2nd Edition.* Oxford, UK: Wiley-Liss; Available from: www.ncbi.nlm.nih.gov/books/NBK21128/

Bruder, G.E., Keilp, J.G., Xu, H., Shikhman, M., Schori, E., Gorman, J.M., *et al.* (2005), "Catechol-O-methyltransferase (COMT) genotypes and working memory: Associations with differing cognitive operations", *Biological Psychiatry,* Vol. 58, No. 11, pp. 901–907.

Chomsky, N. (1965), *Aspects of the Theory of Syntax.* Cambridge, MA, US: The MIT press.

Colledge, E., Bishop, D.V.M., Koeppen-Schomerus, G., Price, T.S., Happe, F.G.E., Eley, T.C., *et al.* (2002), "The structure of language abilities at 4 years: a twin study", *Developmental Psychology,* Vol. 38, No. 5, pp. 749–757.

Conti-Ramsden, G., Crutchley, A. and Botting, N. (1997), "The extent to which psychometric tests differentiate subgroups of children with SLI", *Journal of Speech, Language and Hearing Research,* Vol. 40, No. 4, pp. 765–777.

DeThorne, L.S., Harlaar, N., Petrill, S.A. and Deater-Deckard, K. (2012), "Longitudinal stability in genetic effects on children's conversational language productivity", *Journal of Speech, Language and Hearing Research,* Vol. 55, No. 3, pp. 739–753.

Eicher, J.D., Powers, N.R., Miller, L.L., Akshoomoff, N., Amaral, D.G., Bloss, C.S., *et al.* (2013), "Genome-wide association study of shared components of reading disability and language impairment", *Genes, Brain and Behavior,* Vol. 12, No. 8, pp. 792–801.

Enard, W., Przeworski, M., Fisher, S.E., Lai, C.S.L., Wiebe, V., Kitano, T., *et al.* (2002), "Molecular evolution of FOXP2, a gene involved in speech and language", *Nature,* Vol. 418, No. 6900, pp. 869–872.

Falcaro, M., Pickles, A., Newbury, D.F., Addis, L., Banfield, E., Fisher, S.E., *et al.* (2008), "Genetic and phenotypic effects of phonological short-term memory and grammatical morphology in specific language impairment", *Genes, Brain and Behavior,* Vol. 7, No. 4, pp. 393–402.

Felsenfeld, S. and Plomin, R. (1997), "Epidemiological and offspring analyses of developmental speech disorders using data from the Colorado Adoption Project", *Journal of Speech, Language, and Hearing Research*, Vol. 40, No. 4, pp. 778–791.

Fisher, S.E. and Ridley, M. (2013), "Culture, genes, and the human revolution", *Science*, Vol. 340, No. 6135, pp. 929–930.

Fisher, S.E., Vargha-Khadem, F., Watkins, K.E., Monaco, A.P. and Pembrey, M.E. (1998), "Localisation of a gene implicated in a severe speech and language disorder", *Nature Genetics*, Vol. 18, No. 2, pp. 168–170.

Friedman, J.I., Vrijenhoek, T., Markx, S., Janssen, I.M., van der Vliet, W.A., Faas, B.H.W., *et al.* (2010), "CNTNAP2 gene dosage variation is associated with schizophrenia and epilepsy", *Molecular Psychiatry*, Vol. 15, No. 11, p. 1121.

Grigorenko, E.L. (2009), "Speaking genes or genes for speaking? Deciphering the genetics of speech and language", *Journal of Child Psychology and Psychiatry*, Vol. 50, No. 1–2, pp. 116–125.

Hayiou-Thomas, M.E. (2008), "Genetic and environmental influences on early speech, language and literacy development", *Journal of Communication Disorders*, Vol. 41, No. 5, pp. 397–408.

Hayiou-Thomas, M.E., Dale, P.S. and Plomin, R. (2012), "The etiology of variation in language skills changes with development: A longitudinal twin study of language from 2 to 12 years", *Developmental Science*, Vol. 15, No. 2, pp. 233–249.

Heng, H.H., Liu, G., Stevens, J.B., Bremer, S.W., Ye, K.J., Abdallah, B.Y., *et al.* (2011), "Decoding the genome beyond sequencing: The new phase of genomic research", *Genomics*, Vol. 98, No. 4, pp. 242–252.

Hirschhorn, J.N. and Daly, M.J. (2005), "Genome-wide association studies for common diseases and complex traits", *Nature Reviews Genetics*, Vol. 6, No. 2, pp. 95–108.

Hoff, E. (2006), "How social contexts support and shape language development", *Developmental Review*, Vol. 26, No. 1, pp. 55–88.

Johnson, M.B., Kawasawa, Y.I., Mason, C.E., Krsnik, Z., Coppola, G., Bogdanovic, D., *et al.* (2009), "Functional and evolutionary insights into human brain development through global transcriptome analysis", *Neuron*, Vol. 62, No. 4, pp. 494–509.

Konopka, G., Bomar, J.M., Winden, K., Coppola, G., Jonsson, Z.O., Gao, F.Y., *et al.* (2009), "Human-specific transcriptional regulation of CNS development genes by *FOXP2*", *Nature*, Vol. 462, No. 7270, pp. 213–217.

Kos, M., van den Brink, D., Snijders, T.M., Rijpkema, M., Franke, B., Fernandez, G., *et al.* (2012), "*CNTNAP2* and language processing in healthy individuals as measured with ERPs", *Plos One*, Vol. 7, No. 10: e46995.

Kovas, Y., Hayiou-Thomas, M.E., Oliver, B., Dale, P.S., Bishop, D.V.M. and Plomin, R. (2005), "Genetic influences in different aspects of language development: The etiology of language skills in 4.5-year-old twins", *Child Development*, Vol. 76, No. 3, pp. 632–651.

Lenneberg, E.H. (1967), *Biological foundations of language*. Oxford, England: Wiley.

Luciano, M., Evans, D.M., Hansell, N.K., Medland, S.E., Montgomery, G.W., Martin, N.G., *et al.* (2013), "A genome-wide association study for reading and language abilities in two population cohorts", *Genes, Brain and Behavior*, Vol. 12, No. 6, pp. 645–652.

Marcus, G.F. and Fisher, S.E. (2003), "*FOXP2* in focus: What can genes tell us about speech and language?", *Trends in Cognitive Science*, Vol. 7, No. 6, pp. 257–262.

Naumova, O.Y., Lee, M., Koposov, R., Szyf, M., Dozier, M. and Grigorenko, E.L. (2012), "Differential patterns of whole-genome DNA methylation in institutionalized children and children raised by their biological parents", *Development and Psychopathology*, Vol. 24, pp. 143–155.

Newbury, D.F., Cleak, J.D., Banfield, E., Marlow, A.J., Fisher, S.E., Monaco, A.P. *et al.* (2004), "Highly significant linkage to the *SLI1* locus in an expanded sample of individuals affected by specific language impairment", *American Journal of Human Genetics*, Vol. 74, No. 6, pp. 1225–1238.

Newbury, D.F., Paracchini, S., Scerri, T.S., Winchester, L., Addis, L., Richardson, A.J., *et al.* (2011), "Investigation of Dyslexia and SLI risk variants in reading- and language-impaired subjects", *Behavior Genetics*, Vol. 41, No. 1, pp. 90–104.

Newbury, D.F., Winchester, L., Addis, L., Paracchini, S., Buckingham, L.L., Clark, A., *et al.* (2009), "*CMIP* and *ATP2C2* modulate phonological short-term memory in Language Impairment", *American Journal of Human Genetics*, Vol. 85, No. 2, pp. 264–272.

Nudel, R., Simpson, N.H., Baird, G., O'Hare, A., Conti-Ramsden, G., Bolton, P.F., *et al.* (2014), "Genome-wide association analyses of child genotype effects and parent-of-origin effects in specific language impairment", *Genes, Brain and Behavior*, Vol. 13, No. 4, pp. 418–429.

Panksepp, J. and Panksepp, J.B. (2001), "A continuing critique of evolutionary psychology: Seven sins for seven sinners, plus or minus two", *Evolution and Cognition*, Vol. 7, pp. 56–80.

Plomin, R., Haworth, C.M.A. and Davis, O.S.P. (2009), "Common disorders are quantitative traits", *Nature Reviews Genetics*, Vol. 10, No. 12, pp. 872–878.

Poeppel, D., Emmorey, K., Hickok, G. and Pylkkanen, L. (2012), "Towards a new neurobiology of language", *Journal of Neuroscience*, Vol. 32, No. 41, pp. 14125–14131.

Rice, M.L. (2012), "Toward epigenetic and gene regulation models of specific language impairment: Looking for links among growth, genes, and impairments", *Journal of Neurodevelopmental Disorders*, Vol. 4, No. 1, p. 27.

Scerri, T.S., Morris, A.P., Buckingham, L.L., Newbury, D.F., Miller, L.L., Monaco, A.P., *et al.* (2011), "*DCDC2, KIAA0319* and *CMIP* are associated with reading-related traits", *Biological Psychiatry*, Vol. 70, No. 3, pp. 237–245.

Spinath, F.M., Price, T.S., Dale, P.S. and Plomin, R. (2004), "The genetic and environmental origins of language disability and ability", *Child Development*, Vol. 75, No. 2, pp. 445–454.

Stromswold, K. (1998), "Genetics of spoken language disorders", *Human Biology*, Vol. 70, No. 2, pp. 297–324.

Stromswold, K. (2001), "The heritability of language: A review and meta-analysis of twin, adoption, and linkage studies", *Language*, Vol. 77, No. 4, pp. 647–723.

Tallal, P., Ross, R. and Curtiss, S. (1989), "Familial aggregation in specific language impairment", *Journal of Speech and Hearing Disorders*, Vol. 54, No. 2, pp. 167–173.

Vargha-Khadem, F., Watkins, K., Alcock, K., Fletcher, P. and Passingham, R. (1995), "Praxic and nonverbal cognitive deficits in a large family with a genetically transmitted speech and language disorder", *Proceedings of the National Academy of Sciences of the United States of America*, Vol. 92, No. 3, pp. 930–933.

Villanueva, P., Newbury, D.F., Jara, L., De Barbieri, Z., Mirza, G., Palomino, H.M., *et al.* (2011), "Genome-wide analysis of genetic susceptibility to language impairment in an isolated Chilean population", *European Journal of Human Genetics*, Vol. 19, No. 6, pp. 687–695.

Wardle, M.C., de Wit, H., Penton-Voak, I., Lewis, G. and Munafo, M.R. (2013), "Lack of association between *COMT* and working memory in a population-based cohort of healthy young adults", *Neuropsychopharmacology*, Vol. 38, No. 7, pp. 1253–1263.

Whalley, H.C., O'Connell, G., Sussmann, J.E., Peel, A., Stanfield, A.C., Hayiou-Thomas, M.E., *et al.* (2011), "Genetic variation in *CNTNAP2* alters brain function during linguistic processing in healthy individuals", *American Journal of Medical Genetics Part B-Neuropsychiatric Genetics*, Vol. 156B, No. 8, pp. 941–948.

Wheeler, M. (2003), *Do Genes Code for Traits?* Dortrecht, The Netherlands: Kluwer.

Whitehouse, A.J.O., Bishop, D.V.M., Ang, Q.W., Pennell, C.E. and Fisher, S.E. (2011), "*CNTNAP2* variants affect early language development in the general population", *Genes, Brain and Behavior*, Vol. 10, No. 4, pp. 451–456.

Yehuda, R., Halligan, S.L. and Grossman, R. (2001), "Childhood trauma and risk for PTSD: relationship to intergenerational effects of trauma, parental PTSD, and cortisol excretion", *Development and Psychopathology*, Vol. 13, No. 3, pp. 733–753.

2

NEURAL NETWORK MECHANISMS OF ADULT LANGUAGE

Stephen E. Nadeau

Despite enormous progress made by linguists, psycholinguists, cognitive neuropsychologists, and behavioral neurologists over the past 75 years in understanding the cerebral basis for language function, a fundamental question has remained unanswered: how biological tissue made up of tens of billions of neurons densely interconnected with each other in neural networks (1,000–10,000 connections per cortical neuron), and operating on the basis of electrochemical principles, could possibly support the substantially symbolic processes involved in language function. In 1986, in an epochal work, McClelland *et al.* (1986) elaborated an essential insight: representations in the brain are population encoded (distributed), that is, instantiated as patterns of activity involving very large numbers of relatively simple units (plausibly corresponding to neurons or cortical micro-columns). Computer simulations have demonstrated that such networks have very characteristic behavioral properties; these properties are highly germane to understanding how the brain supports language function; and networks incorporating population-encoded representations have a remarkable capacity to emulate the behavior of normal and brain-injured human subjects.

Most of this chapter will involve an overview of language systems that takes into account the fundamental neurobiological principle of population encoding of representations (for further detail, see Nadeau, 2001, 2012; Roth *et al.*, 2006). This conceptualization will define features of aphasia and applications to aphasia therapy, the topics of the final section of the chapter. Although the population encoding of representations has long been well established (Rolls and Deco, 2002; Rolls and Treves, 1998), any particular model, including that discussed here, represents but a hypothesis, to be tested and refined through further empirical work.

Language function

Core functions: Phonology, semantics, and lexical-semantics

The topography of the Wernicke–Lichtheim model (Roth *et al.*, 2006) is presented in Figure 2.1. Each oval signifies a very large number of individual units. Every unit in a given oval is connected to every unit in the adjacent ovals. All connections are two-way, thereby emulating what we see in the brain. Information is represented in the model as the strength of connections between units (in analogy to synapses in the brain). The activity of units is defined as a nonlinear function of their input (in many simulations as a sigmoid (∫) function over the range of 0–1). The output of units is another nonlinear function. The units in hidden unit domains support representations that cannot be defined in behavioral terms. These domains, coupled with nonlinear unit functions, are essential to the computational capabilities of the network and endow the network with the capacity for supporting discrete entities (e.g., symbols); translating representations in one domain into substantially unrelated (orthogonal) representations, e.g., concept representations (semantics/word meanings) into phonological representations (word sounds); and representing sequence knowledge. The small circles appended to the three major linguistic domains signify that every unit within a domain is connected to every other unit in that domain. This endows these domains with an auto-associator property: the propensity for the activity pattern within the domain to settle into a state—an attractor basin—that represents an optimal response to the pattern of input. Input to the network leads to spreading activation throughout the network, such that, in the course of repeated bottom-up/top-down interactions, the entire network eventually settles into an optimal state, which defines output. Figure 2.1 also shows how this network might be plausibly mapped onto the brain surface and it captures the fact that, although language is predominantly supported by the left hemisphere in right handers and most left handers, there is some redundant representation of language knowledge in the right hemisphere (see Nadeau, 2012 for detail).

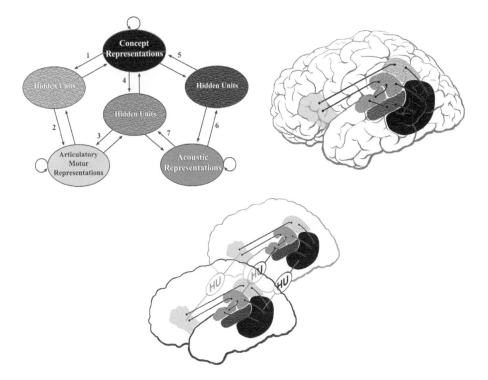

Figure 2.1 Parallel distributed processing model of language (upper left) with plausible mapping to the brain (upper right). There is abundant evidence that there is substantial redundant language knowledge in the right hemisphere (lower). Domains are shaded similarly in each figure. HU = hidden units. (From Roth *et al.*, 2006).

Concept representations: Semantics

I will begin with the domain of concept representations because its function provides the most insight into the meaning of a population encoded representation. The operation of this domain can be best illustrated by a model developed by Rumelhart *et al.* (1986). This "rooms in a house" model was comprised of 40 "feature" units, each corresponding to an article typically found in particular rooms or an aspect of particular rooms. Connection strengths were defined by the likelihood that any two features might appear in conjunction in a typical house. When one or more units was clamped into the "on" state, activation spread throughout the model and the model eventually settled into a steady state that implicitly defined a particular room in a house. Thus, clamping "oven" ultimately resulted in activation of all the items one would expect to find in a kitchen and thereby *implicitly* defined, via a *distributed or population encoded representation*, the concept of a kitchen. No kitchen unit *per se* was turned on. Rather, kitchen was defined by the pattern of feature units that were activated. The network contained the knowledge, in the totality of its connections, that enabled this representation to be generated. The model could also generate distributed representations of other rooms in a house (e.g., bathroom, bedroom, living room, study) and blends of rooms that were not anticipated in the programming of the model (e.g., clamping both bed and sofa led to a distributed representation of a large, fancy bedroom replete with a fireplace, television, and sofa). This auto-associator model, simple though it is, has the essential attributes of a network that might instantiate semantic knowledge and be capable of generating distributed representations corresponding to concepts.

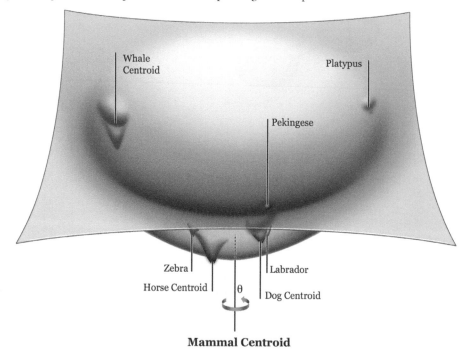

Figure 2.2 The topography of the semantic network activity function in the vicinity of the mammal attractor basin. Each point corresponds to an activity level of all features in a N-dimensional feature hyperspace. The point of maximal typicality is represented by the centroid of a basin/sub-basin. Distance from the centroid reflects degree of atypicality. The value of θ defines the manner in which atypicality is defined. For example, whales and platypuses are both atypical but in very different ways. (From Nadeau, 2012).

Let us now scale this up to a concepts network that could plausibly support the knowledge in the human brain. The activity pattern of this much larger concepts domain would be defined by a function in a N-dimensional feature hyperspace. By taking a three-dimensional "slab" of this network activity function, for example, a slab in the vicinity of mammal knowledge (Figure 2.2), we can achieve some insight into the order in the patterns of activity. The central, lowest energy point—the "centroid" of mammal knowledge—corresponds to the representation of a creature that best defines our sense of "mammalness". Within the mammal basin, there are innumerable attractor sub-basins corresponding to specific mammals. Very close to the centroid are sub-basins corresponding to mammals likely to be very close to the centroid representation, e.g., dogs, cats, cows, and horses. Distance from the centroid is defined by the degree of atypicality, which is defined by feature and feature combination frequency within the mammal domain. Highly atypical animals, such as whales and platypuses, are represented near the periphery. Within any given sub-basin, there may be sub-sub-basins, for example, corresponding to types of dogs. The depth of the mammal basin and its sub-basins (the z-axis in Figure 2.2) is determined by the strength of encoding of knowledge in neural connectivity. This in turn is determined by the degree to which a given exemplar shares features with other exemplars in the domain, the frequency of the exemplar, and age of acquisition. The depth of a basin relative to that of its sub-basins reflects the degree to which features are shared by the sub-basins within that basin. The network's settled activity state is most strongly influenced by the specific input features, which in most circumstances will absolutely define the sub-basin or sub-sub-basin into which the network settles (its position in state space), all the other factors exerting their major influence either on response latencies or the occasional errors. Errors will consist of slips into nearby sub-basins. This settling in response to input features instantiates *content addressable memory*. This capacity for content addressable memory, which is intrinsic to auto-associator networks supporting distributed representations, automatically accounts for the fact that with exposure to but scant features of a memory, we can instantly realize the full memory.

The effect of lesions (focal or diffuse) will be to produce *graceful degradation* of network performance. Network function does not simply cease. Instead, it becomes less reliable and more errorful, even as it continues to reflect the statistical regularities of remaining knowledge encoded in the network. Graceful degradation is another intrinsic property of population encoded representations. With network damage, deep basins will become shallower and sub-basins, particularly those that are shallower and more distant from the centroid—corresponding to more atypical exemplars—will disappear. As sub-basins become shallow or disappear, responses will reflect the settling of the network into surviving neighbors located nearer the centroid—neighbors of higher typicality (yielding coordinate errors, e.g., horse in lieu of donkey), the parent basin (yielding superordinate errors, e.g., animal in lieu of donkey), or failure to settle at all, yielding omission errors. This is precisely what has been observed in semantic dementia.

There is good evidence that in the brain, the meaning of a given word is distributed not over one network, as we have been discussing, but over a number of networks. This idea, which owes to Lissauer (1988) and Wernicke (as cited in Eggert, 1977), has recently been resurrected as the Embodied Cognition Framework (Buxbaum and Kalénine, 2010). In this conceptualization, the distributed representation of the concept "dog" has major components in the visual association cortices (incorporating knowledge of the visual appearance of dogs in general, as well as particular dogs); auditory association cortices (sounds that dogs characteristically make); the limbic system (one's feelings about dogs); somatosensory cortex; olfactory cortex; frontal cortex (supporting a predicative component corresponding to our knowledge of what dogs do—a component of the semantic representation of a verb [see below]); and perisylvian language cortex, which enables us to translate the semantic representation of dog into an articulatory motor representation. The multiple component representation of concepts provides the basis for category specific naming and recognition deficits (Forde and Humphreys, 1999).

Phonology

We return now to Figure 2.1 to consider the acoustic representations–articulatory motor representations pathway. This is referred to as a pattern associator network because it translates representations in one form into corresponding representations in a different form. Acoustic and articulatory motor representations correspond to the acoustic and articulatory forms of phonemes, respectively. As conceptualized in the Wernicke–Lichtheim model, this is the pathway that supports repetition. In addition, because this network has acquired, through language experience, knowledge of the systematic relationships between acoustic and articulatory sequences, it has learned the statistical sound *sequence* regularities of the language: the phonemic sequences of joint phonemes (e.g., st, str), rhymes, syllables, affixes, morphemes and words characteristic of the language (Nadeau, 2001). I will use a reading model to illustrate the process (Plaut *et al.*, 1996; Seidenberg and McClelland, 1989). It fundamentally recapitulates the acoustic–articulatory motor pathway of Figure 2.1, the major difference (inconsequential to this discussion) being that in place of acoustic representations, it employed orthographic representations. The three-layer pattern associator network was equipped with a learning algorithm and it was trained by presenting the orthographic representations of 3000 English single syllable words and their corresponding phonologic forms.

One of the most striking things about the trained model was that it also was able to produce correct pronunciations of plausible English nonwords (i.e., orthographic sequences it had never encountered before). This was possible because the model had learned the statistical relationships between *sequences* of graphemes and *sequences* of phonemes that are characteristic of the English language. To the extent that there is a limited repertoire of sequence types, the model was able to learn it and apply it. Certain sequences, those most commonly found in English single syllable words, were more thoroughly etched in network connectivity. Thus, it was very fast with high frequency words. It was also very fast with words with an absolutely consistent orthographic–phonologic sequence relationship, for example, words ending in "ust," which are always pronounced /ʌst/ (must, bust, trust, lust, crust, etc.). The model encountered difficulty (reflected in prolonged reading latency) only with low frequency words, and only to the extent that it had learned different, competing pronunciations of the same orthographic sequence. Thus, it was slow to read *pint* because in every case but *pint*, the sequence "int" is pronounced /ɪnt/ (e.g., mint, tint, flint, lint). It also was very slow with words that are unique in their orthographic–phonologic sequence relationship (e.g., *aisle, guide* and *fugue*). These behaviors precisely recapitulate the behavior of normal human subjects given reading tasks. The model was equipped to acquire the very limited set of sequences involving syllabic onset, nucleus, and coda. However, it provided proof of the principle that sequence knowledge in general can be acquired by a simply pattern associator neural network employing a hidden unit domain and units with nonlinear functions.

Lexicons: Lexical-semantic knowledge

The phonologic input lexicon is represented as the connections between the substrate for acoustic representations and the substrate for concept representations (Figure 2.1: pathway 6–5). The phonologic output lexicon is represented as the two pathways between the substrate for concept representations and articulatory motor representations (pathways 1–2 and 4–3). Evidence of the existence pathway 1–2 derives from patients with repetition conduction aphasia who demonstrate the ability to repeat by the semantic route but have no capacity for repeating nonwords (Nadeau, 2001). Evidence of the existence of pathway 4–3 comes from normal subjects, who make phonologic slips of the tongue, and from patients with reproduction conduction aphasia, who make phonemic paraphasic errors in both repetition and naming.

Attractor basins, attractor trenches, and quasi-regular domains

Implicit in the discussion thus far is an explanation of the mechanism by which regularities encoded in neural networks support language (Figure 2.3). In the final section of this chapter, it will become clear how this mechanism also constrains the generalizability of language therapies. In our discussion of concept representations, we considered a mathematical activity function in N-dimensional hyperspace that, depending on the particular pattern of input, would yield a distributed representation of any entity we know about. The mammal attractor basin (Figure 2.2) is the product of a thought experiment in which we took a three-dimensional slice through the N-dimensional activity function in the vicinity of mammal knowledge. The shape of this complex surface reflects the strength of regularities wired into neural connectivity and shared, to varying degree, by all mammals. The mammal attractor basin corresponds in psychological terms to a quasi-regular domain. It is regular to the extent that all mammals share a set of common features. However, it is quasi-regular because no two mammals are exactly alike.

The same concept can be applied to sequence knowledge in pattern associator networks, e.g., acoustic–articulatory or orthographic-articulatory. Because pattern associator networks support a pathway from one representation to another, the regularities encoded in their neural connectivity support activity patterns that I have termed attractor trenches. These attractor trenches also correspond to psychological quasi-regular domains. The neural activity patterns generated by phonologic sequence knowledge supporting words with the rhyme "int" correspond to one such domain, this one containing two sub-trenches, one corresponding to

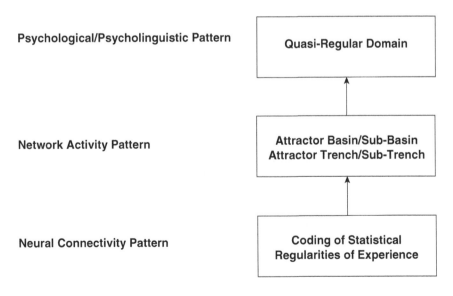

Psychological/Psycholinguistic Pattern — Quasi-Regular Domain

Network Activity Pattern — Attractor Basin/Sub-Basin / Attractor Trench/Sub-Trench

Neural Connectivity Pattern — Coding of Statistical Regularities of Experience

Figure 2.3 The relationship between neural network connectivity, attractor basins and trenches, and patterns of behaviour. (From Nadeau, 2012).

lint, mint, stint, and *tint,* and one corresponding to *pint.* Figure 2.3 illustrates the fundamental principle that knowledge is represented in patterns of neural connectivity, these patterns define the shapes of attractor basins and attractor trenches, and these basins and trenches correspond to the psychological form of quasi-regular domains.

Grammatic sequence knowledge

Grammatic sequence knowledge is evident at two levels: 1) grammatic morphology, which subsumes roots, grammatic inflections (e.g., affixes), and phrase structure rules; and 2) sentence level sequence, that is, syntax. I have discussed the potential for a simple pattern associator network (e.g., Plaut *et al.,* 1996; Seidenberg and McClelland, 1989), to acquire sequence knowledge. Models with intrinsically greater power to capture sequence knowledge have been developed, e.g., the simple recurrent network. In training such a network, a series of consecutive forms (e.g., morphemes comprising a word, words comprising a sentence) is presented, one at a time, to the input layer. Each form generates a pattern of activity in the hidden units and the output layer. However, an additional domain, termed context units, represents the pattern of activity of the hidden units generated in response to one or more prior forms. Equipped with a standard training algorithm, the network has the capability for learning the sequential relationships between the forms. The work of Joanisse and Seidenberg (2003) is exemplary. They reported a simulation involving a phonology-hidden units-context units semantics network in which, during training, connection strengths were adjusted on the basis of present input, target output, and data reflecting up to ten previous inputs, thereby potentially instantiating implicit knowledge of sequence regularities involving much longer sentences. The network, through its experience with the statistical regularities of the dataset, was able to acquire implicit knowledge of rules governing verb argument structure, subcategorization rules, preposition choice, and pronoun anaphora.

For over half a century, linguists have sought a deterministic account for language function and for nearly as long, psycholinguists and cognitive neuropsychologists have sought to explain grammatic breakdown in aphasia in terms of a defect in one or more components of such a mechanism. Here we offer a far simpler explanation: neural networks supporting population encoded representations and endowed with learning mechanisms, while capable of learning unique knowledge (e.g., *aisle, guide,* and *fugue,* as discussed above), have a particular facility for acquiring knowledge of statistical regularities, including sequence regularities, from experience. Furthermore, by virtue of the intrinsic properties of these networks, performance breakdown is characterized by graceful degradation.

The work of Thompson and colleagues (2003) is illustrative. They reported a syntactic treatment experiment that, although motivated by linguistic theory, enables us to relate the results of the Joanisse and Seidenberg (2003) simulation in a rather direct way to human acquisition of syntactic skills and to put this within the more general context of neural network support of language function. They trained four subjects with Broca's aphasia to produce three sentence types, starting from active NP–V–NP (NP = noun phrase; V = verb) sentences (e.g., The thief chased the artist). The sentence types were: WH questions (Who has the thief chased?), object-clefts (It was the artist who the thief chased), and object relatives (The man saw the artist who the thief chased). The two participants trained to produce object relative sentences showed generalization to the production of object-cleft sentences and WH questions. The two participants trained to produce the WH questions showed no generalization to the other forms. These results supported the "complexity account," in which treatment focused on more complex forms results in generalization to less complex forms requiring the same type of movement (Thompson *et al.*, 2003). However, an alternative explanation is that Thompson *et al.* were retraining an attractor trench supported by a recurrent pattern associator network with a sequence knowledge acquisition capacity similar to that of the network employed by Joanisse and Seidenberg and representing the general class of sequences expressed by the sentence types they studied. This network learned variations on a particular theme of sequential concept manipulation (a quasi-regular sequence domain) that could enable production of the correct sequence of words. Training the pattern associator with atypical ("complex") exemplars retrained network connections that could support both the atypical sequence exemplars (e.g., object relatives) and exemplars close to the centroid of the attractor trench (e.g., WH questions). Retraining WH questions succeeded in retraining connections that could support sequences near the centroid but did little to tune connections that would support atypical exemplars more distant from the centroid.

Verbs

Although the function of verbs is traditionally conceptualized as predominantly grammatical, the population encoded neural network model conceptualizes their function largely in semantic terms. Consider this sentence:

"The old man shot the burglar."

It is a simple matter to conceptualize "old man" and "burglar," but what about "shot"? Shot can be represented as a *modification* of the "old man" and "burglar" distributed concept representations but not as its own discrete concept representation. "Old man" becomes "shooter old man," and thus acquires the property of agency (a specific thematic role) and a "flavor," that of a shooter rather than a sleeper or a raconteur. Correspondingly, burglar also acquires the property (thematic role) of patient and a flavor (e.g., lying prostrate bleeding). The verb here emerges as a peculiar sort of adjective. Although verbs, in and of themselves, do not correspond to distributed concept representations, they nonetheless have a distributed representation comprised of nominative, thematic, flavor, and implementational components.

The nominative component is defined by the connectivity between substrates for verb and noun representations. There is good evidence that these connections are extensive, as a given verb primes the nouns it is commonly associated with (Ferretti *et al.*, 2001) and vice versa (McRae *et al.*, 2005).

In theory, the thematic component should be represented in prefrontal cortex because prefrontal cortex supports the volitional formulation of plans precisely tailored to the demands of the situation (Nadeau and Heilman, 2007) and intention requires a role to be associated with the action taken. If you are planning, or are engaged in the plans of the actors you are thinking about, then you are imputing agency and consequence. Prefrontal cortex also provides the substrate for dynamic time sense. Extensive empirical studies demonstrating differential impairment in verb production with frontal lesions/Broca's aphasia provide strong validation of this hypothesis.

The flavor component is supplied variously by manner, path, and limbic representations. The manner/path distinction is illustrated by the following:

The bird flew into the wind. (flew confers manner)
The bird flew over the house. (flew confers path)

Manner is instantiated in nuances of verb meaning, e.g., *walk, amble, stroll, saunter, strut, sashay, march,* and *hasten.* In manner incorporating languages (e.g., English, German, Russian, Swedish, Chinese), it is incorporated directly in the verb, whereas in path incorporating languages (e.g., Greek, Spanish, Japanese, Turkish, Hindi), it is incorporated in a prepositional phrase. The manner component of action verbs would logically be supported by cerebral cortex supporting movement perception, particularly visual—that is, in the vicinity of the posterior inferior temporal gyrus. Deficits in movement perception, action recognition, and action naming have been observed with lesions in this region. Functional imaging studies have also confirmed this hypothesis (Kemmerer *et al.*, 2008). The path component would logically be represented in parietal cortex because it involves movement across space. Functional imaging studies provide some support for this hypothesis as well (Wu *et al.*, 2008). Any verb might have a limbic component to its representation but this is most obviously the case for emotion verbs.

There is abundant evidence that the implementational component of action verb meaning is represented in motor cortex. Reading sentence segments involving movement is slowed when the motion conveyed conflicts with concurrently performed movement. The implementational component is markedly attenuated when the meaning of a verb is changed from ongoing to complete action (i.e., from progressive to perfect aspect). Patients with Parkinson's disease exhibit robust masked priming of both nouns and verbs in the on-condition (when motor cortex function is optimized, e.g., by the administration of dopaminergic drugs), but prime only nouns in the off-condition.

Application of the model to aphasia

The following is a brief sketch of the mechanisms of aphasia viewed through the lens of this model. The signature linguistic manifestation of Broca's aphasia, simplification of syntax to the point of simple declarative sentences or single words, can be substantially related to attenuation of sentence level sequence knowledge attractor trenches, such that neural connectivity is no longer sufficient to support atypical sequences. Impairments in grammatic morphology differ from language to language. In heavily inflected languages (i.e., substantially, all the major languages of the world except English and Chinese), there is evidence of sufficient redundant grammatic morphologic sequence knowledge in the non-dominant hemisphere that grammatic morphemes are infrequently omitted but are susceptible to substitution (grammatic morphologic paraphasic errors) (reviewed in Nadeau, 2012). It is the poverty and inconsistency of English grammatic morphology, reflective of poor encoding of regularities in neural connectivity, that sets the stage for widespread omission of grammatic morphemes. We have already noted the consequences of the loss of the thematic component of verb representations. Many features of Broca's aphasia, most notably the limited ability to modify distributed concept representations with serial adjectives and the particular difficulties with two- and three-argument verbs, can be attributed to impairment in working memory.

All perisylvian aphasias (Broca's, conduction, Wernicke's) are characterized by disorders of phonologic sequence. With anterior lesions, these reflect attenuation of phonemic sequence attractor trenches, which predisposes to near-miss phonemic slips that tend to be less marked (represented nearer the centroid). With more posterior lesions, paraphasic errors are substantially influenced by disruption of phonemic neighborhoods by damage to connections between semantic and phonologic substrates (i.e., loss of lexical–semantic knowledge), leading to larger substitutions that may share both semantic and phonologic relationships to the target, or no apparent relationship at all, as is often the case in neologistic jargon aphasia.

Posterior perisylvian aphasias (Wernicke's and, to some degree, conduction) are characterized by anomia, reflecting in part disconnection of semantic and phonologic substrates by the ischemic lesion, but also degradation of phonologic and/or semantic substrates (see Treatment, below). Wernicke's aphasia is additionally associated with damage to the substrate for the phonologic input lexicon, hence problems with comprehension.

Transcortical sensory aphasia likely reflects the consequences of semantic–phonologic disconnection in the context of preserved phonologic, morphologic, and sentence level sequence knowledge. Language may be fluent and characterized by complex syntax but it is substantially devoid of major lexical items.

Treatment

This model has strong implications for aphasia treatment, and most particularly, for generalization of treatment effects to untrained items and everyday verbal communication. Consider first the treatment of anomia, the single most common and disabling feature of aphasia. From the foregoing, it is apparent that because the relationship between word meaning (semantics) and word form (phonology) is largely arbitrary (except for onomatopoeic and derivational forms), there are very few regularities in the pattern associator networks linking the substrates for semantics and phonology—regularities that might be further developed through therapy, thereby deepening attractor trenches and re-establishing sub-trenches. If you have trained a patient to name 30 words, the knowledge gained is of no value in naming the thirty-first. This theoretically motivated prediction finds strong support in the results of a recent meta-analysis, which indeed demonstrated no generalization of commonly used treatments for anomia (Wisenburn and Mahoney, 2009). However, to the extent that damage to substrates for phonologic sequence knowledge or semantics contribute to anomia, training of these networks, which do contain extensive regularities, could potentially improve lexical access to untrained exemplars.

Kendall and colleagues (2008, 2015) have just reported the results of a trial of phonologic sequence therapy, a derivative of the Lindamood Phonemic Sequencing Program (LiPS) (Lindamood and Lindamood, 1998), in 26 subjects. The first phase of treatment consisted of developing the neural substrate for linked distributed representations of individual phonemes (see Figure 2.1). For example, at the end of completely successful training, insertion of the acoustic form of /b/ into the acoustic domain (by saying /b/ to the subject) would instantly lead to generation of distributed representations of the articulatory form of /b/, a concept of /b/, the sound of /b/, and an orthographic representation corresponding to the letter b. The concept of /b/ is formed in a variety of ways: labeling it as a "lip-popper," the tactile feel of the patient's larynx during phonation, a picture of a sagittal section through the head with mouth and oropharynx positioned for production of /b/, and the patient's recalled image of her own mouth, reflected in a mirror, as she produces the phoneme. The second phase of treatment trains the regularities of English phonological sequences by inserting 1–3 syllable nonwords and some real words. Three months after completing training, participants demonstrated an absolute gain in *untrained* real word naming of 5.28 percent ($p = 0.002$, d = 0.70) and an even greater gain in *untrained* nonword repetition.

Other treatment studies have provided evidence of broad generalization of treatment effects for semantic (Edmonds *et al.*, 2009) and syntactic therapies (Thompson *et al.*, 2003). In addition, syntactic therapies are intrinsically generalizing to the extent that successfully acquired sequence knowledge (e.g., how to produce an object relative sentence) applies to all concepts and words in the language.

Generalization is traditionally conceptualized as the process of translating treatment effects to daily verbal communication. However, it can also provide a useful therapeutic tool. Plaut (1996) demonstrated, in a computer simulation of "rehabilitation" of a damaged lexical-semantic network, that training with atypical exemplars was preferable to training with typical exemplars. Training atypical exemplars instantiates both knowledge of features unique to atypicals and knowledge shared with typicals, but not the other way around. Subsequently, Kiran and Thompson (2003) confirmed these results in a study of semantic treatment of human subjects with aphasia, and in their syntactic treatment (Thompson *et al.*, 2003). In the phonologic sequence therapy tested by Kendall *et al.* (2015), only atypical phonological sequences were trained with a view to reducing therapy time and there was robust generalization to untrained sequences.

Conclusion

In this brief review, we have seen how a multi-component neural network supporting population encoded semantic, acoustic and articulatory motor representations, and pattern associator networks supporting the lexical–semantic knowledge instantiating the phonologic lexicons and phonologic, morphologic, and sentence level sequence knowledge, can provide a plausible account for language function. The operation of this network is constrained by regularities encoded in neural network connectivity on the basis of the statistics of language experience. These regularities define a neural activation landscape consisting of attractor basins and attractor trenches, which in turn support quasi-regular knowledge domains. Aphasia, whether due to focal brain injury (e.g., stroke) or degenerative disease (e.g., semantic dementia) reflects graceful degradation of knowledge that corresponds to loss of depth and breadth of basins and trenches. Rehabilitation of aphasia that generalizes to untrained exemplars and daily verbal communication corresponds to further development of residual regularities in neural connectivity such that basins and trenches are deepened and sub-basins and sub-trenches redeveloped. Generalization cannot be achieved by therapies directed at networks (e.g., lexical–semantic) that do not support substantial regularities. The neural network model discussed here provides the potential for rekindling the dialectic between neuroanatomy and neurophysiology on the one hand and language function and rehabilitation on the other.

References

Buxbaum, L.J. and Kalénine, S. (2010), "Action knowledge, visuomotor activation, and embodiment in the two action systems", *Annals of the New York Academy of Science*, Vol. 1191, pp. 201–218.

Edmonds, L.A., Nadeau, S.E. and Kiran, S. (2009), "Effect of verb network strengthening treatment (VNeST) on lexical retrieval of content words in sentences in persons with aphasia," *Aphasiology,* Vol. 23, pp. 402–424.

Eggert, G.H. (1977), *Wernicke's Works in Aphasia: A Sourcebook and Review. Volume 1*, The Hague, Netherlands: Mouton.

Ferretti, T.R., McCrae, K. and Hatherell, A. (2001), "Integrating verbs, situation schemas, and thematic role concepts", *Journal of Memory and Language,* Vol. 44, pp. 516–547.

Forde, E.M.E. and Humphreys, G.W. (1999), "Category specific recognition impairments: A review of important case studies and influential theories", *Aphasiology,* Vol. 13, pp. 169–193.

Joanisse, M.F. and Seidenberg, M.S. (2003), "Phonology and syntax in specific language impairment: Evidence from a connectionist model", *Brain and Language,* Vol. 86, pp. 40–56.

Kemmerer, D., Gonzalez Castillo, J., Talavage, T., Patterson, S. and Wiley, C. (2008), "Neuronanatomical distribution of five semantic components of verbs: Evidence from fMRI", *Brain and Language,* Vol. 107, pp. 16–43.

Kendall, D.L., Oelke, M., Brookshire, C.E. and Nadeau, S.E. (2015), "The influence of phonomotor treatment on word retrieval abilities in 26 patients with chronic aphasia: An open trial", *Journal of Speech, Language, and Hearing Research*, in press.

Kendall, D.L., Rosenbek, J.C., Heilman, K.M., Conway, T.W., Klenberg, K., Gonzalez Rothi, L.J. and Nadeau, S.E. (2008), "Phoneme-based rehabilitation of anomia in aphasia", *Brain and Language*, Vol. 105, pp. 1–17.

Kiran, S. and Thompson, C.K. (2003), "The role of semantic complexity in treatment of naming deficits: Training semantic categories in fluent aphasia by controlling exemplar typicality", *Journal of Speech, Language and Hearing Research*, Vol. 46, pp. 773–787.

Lindamood, P.C. and Lindamood, P.D. (1998), *The Lindamood Phoneme Sequencing Program for Reading, Spelling and Speech*, Austin, TX, US: PRO-ED Publishing.

Lissauer, H. (1988), "Ein fall von seelenblindheit nebst einem beitrag sur theorie derselven", *Cognitive Neuropsychology*, Vol. 5, pp. 157–192.

McClelland, J.L., Rumelhart, D.E. and the PDP Research Group (1986), *Parallel Distributed Processing*, Cambridge, MA, US: MIT Press.

McRae, K., Hare, M., Elman, J.L. and Ferretti, T.R. (2005), "A basis for generating expectancies for verbs from nouns", *Memory and Cognition*, Vol. 33, pp. 1174–1184.

Nadeau, S.E. (2001), "Phonology: A review and proposals from a connectionist perspective", *Brain and Language*, Vol. 79, pp. 511–579.

Nadeau, S.E. (2012), *The Neural Architecture of Grammar*, Cambridge, MA, US: MIT Press.

Nadeau, S.E. and Heilman, K.M. (2007), "Frontal mysteries revealed", *Neurology*, Vol. 68, pp. 1450–1453.

Plaut, D.C. (1996), "Relearning after damage in connectionist networks: Toward a theory of rehabilitation", *Brain and Language*, Vol. 52, pp. 25–82.

Plaut, D.C., McClelland, J.L., Seidenberg, M.S. and Patterson, K. (1996), "Understanding normal and impaired word reading: Computational principles in quasi-regular domains", *Psychological Review*, Vol. 103, pp. 56–115.

Rolls, E.T. and Deco, G. (2002), *Computational Neuroscience of Vision*, Oxford, UK: Oxford University Press.

Rolls, E.T. and Treves, A. (1998), *Neural Networks and Brain Function*, New York, NY: Oxford University Press.

Roth, H.L., Nadeau, S.E., Hollingsworth, A.L., Cimino-Knight, A.M. and Heilman, K.M. (2006), "Naming concepts: Evidence of two routes", *Neurocase*, Vol. 12, pp. 61–70.

Rumelhart, D.E., Smolensky, P., McClelland, J.L. and Hinton, G.E. (1986), "Schemata and sequential thought processes in PDP models", in McClelland, J. L., Rumelhart, D. E. and the PDP Research Group (eds.) *Parallel Distributed Processing*, Vol. 2, Cambridge, MA, US: MIT Press. pp. 7–57.

Seidenberg, M.S. and McClelland, J.L. (1989), "A distributed, developmental model of word recognition and naming", *Psychological Review*, Vol. 96, pp. 523–568.

Thompson, C.K., Shapiro, L.P., Kiran, S. and Sobecks, J. (2003), "The role of syntactic complexity in treatment of sentence deficits in agrammatic aphasia: The complexity account of treatment efficacy (CATE)", *Journal of Speech, Language, and Hearing Research*, Vol. 46, pp. 591–607.

Wisenburn, B. and Mahoney, K. (2009), "A meta-analysis of word-finding treatments for aphasia", *Aphasiology*, Vol. 23, pp. 1338–1352.

Wu, D.H., Morganti, A. and Chatterjee, A. (2008), "Neural substrates of processing path and manner information of a moving event", *Neuropsychologia*, Vol. 46, pp. 704–713.

3

READING IMPAIRMENT

From behavior to brain

Willy Serniclaes and Liliane Sprenger-Charolles

Reading impairment: From behavior to brain

Studies on the language impairments in children cover a wide range of different topics and they have given rise to various theoretical accounts. Here we focus on specific reading impairments (dyslexia), and we relate them to different cognitive deficits. We first explain speech perception using phonemic units, which have vital importance for learning to read and are the end-product of a long-standing developmental process. Then we review the three basic competencies that are necessary for typical reading acquisition (phonemic speech perception, grapho-phonemic associations, and visual perception of graphemic units) explaining how a deficit in one of these three competencies may be at the root of dyslexia. Finally, some clinical implications of the current knowledge are provided and suggestions for remediation are offered.

Speech in the linguistic framework

An understanding of the complex processes involved in speech communication is crucial for identifying and remediating various language and cognitive impairments. The main vector of speech communication is an acoustic signal produced by a human vocal tract. Due to the fairly continuous movements of the vocal organs, the speech signal does not contain discrete phonemic segments comparable to the letters in alphabetic writings (Liberman *et al.*, 1967). How can we then perceive phonemes? Phonemic perception is mediated by complex processes that result from the adaptation, during early development, of universal acoustic–auditory features, hereafter "allophonic" features, to language-specific features, hereafter "phonological" features. For example, a child less than six months old, whatever his or her native language, can perceive the contrast between voiced and devoiced stop consonants, although this contrast is phonemic only in some languages (e.g., in Thai) and allophonic in other languages (e.g. in English and French; Hoonhorst *et al.*, 2009). After the child has acquired these phonological features, he/she still has to learn to combine features into phonological segments, i.e. phonemes. The perception of phonemic segments is the end-product of a developmental process that starts before one year of age and lasts up to the adolescence years (for a review, Hoonhorst *et al.*, 2011). As complex as it may be, the perception of speech as phonemic units is naturally acquired during typical development. In alphabetic writings, phonemic perception has crucial importance for typical reading acquisition and is significantly impaired in children with severe and specific reading impairment.

Skilled reading and typical reading acquisition in alphabetic writings

It is not possible to understand dyslexia, which is the result of an atypical development, without knowing what happens in skilled reading and in typical reading acquisition. To correctly understand a written utterance, it is necessary to have automated access to written words; that is, the ability to read words rapidly and precisely (Perfetti, 2007). This automated access to written words, which allows proficient readers to allocate a large part of their processing capacities to reading comprehension, depends on three main factors: the perception of speech sounds with phonemic units, the mastering of grapho-phonemic correspondences, and the direct perception of words with graphemic units.

Phonemic perception

To be able to use grapheme–phoneme correspondences (GPCs), a child should be able to "crack" the spoken code at the phonemic level, a skill named "phonemic awareness" (Liberman *et al.*, 1974). Children do not perform well on phonemic awareness tasks before reading acquisition (Liberman *et al.*, 1974). Indeed, a high phonemic awareness level is mainly observed after reading acquisition for children (Ziegler and Goswami, 2005) or in ex-illiterate versus illiterate adults (Morais *et al.*, 1979), thus suggesting that phonemic awareness results from having learned to read in alphabetic writings. Nevertheless, among pre-reading skills, early phonemic awareness is the best predictor of future reading skills (Melby-Lervåg *et al.*, 2012). To be able to use GPCs, it is also necessary to perceive speech with phonemic units, a competence that is spontaneously acquired during typical development but raises serious problems for children with reading impairments.

Grapho-phonemic correspondences

Following the seminal studies of Shaywitz and collaborators in the US (e.g., Shaywitz *et al.*, 2002), neuroimaging investigations with speakers of the Dutch language, which has a fairly transparent orthography, have identified areas in the temporal cortex that are sensitive to letter–speech sound associations (Blomert, 2011). These temporal areas (Superior Temporal Sulcus and Gyrus: STS and STG) responded to both letters and speech sounds and, most interestingly, showed an enhanced sensitivity to congruent letter–sound pairs compared to incongruent pairs (van Atteveldt *et al.*, 2004). However, unlike natural audiovisual speech, it is only when a letter and a sound are presented simultaneously that feedback is sent to the auditory part of the STG (van Atteveldt *et al.*, 2007) and this is typical of arbitrary (learned) associations between visual and auditory stimuli (Blomert and Froyen, 2010). Also, fast visual processing of letters is done in a specific part of the occipital cortex, the "visual word form area" (VWFA: Cohen *et al.*, 2000), a process that occurs later in the course of reading acquisition and might be dependent on the initial learning of correspondences between letters (or graphemes) and speech sounds (or phonemes). In sum, these studies not only confirm that integrating graphemes and phonemes is the starting point of reading acquisition but they also suggest that letter–sound integration is performed by a specific neural network and that it affects both auditory and visual perception. A cultural factor that considerably impacts the automation of written-word processing is the consistency of GPCs in the writing system. If each grapheme is always pronounced the same way, then the orthography is considered shallow. This is almost the case for Spanish orthography, but not for English orthography (Share, 2008). French orthography is somewhere in between (Sprenger-Charolles *et al.*, 2006). Different studies suggest that reading acquisition is easier in orthographies in which GPCs are highly consistent (Ziegler and Goswami, 2005; Sprenger-Charolles *et al.*, 2006). Qualitative differences are also observed. For instance, the more transparent the orthography is, the more children rely on the same procedure (based on GPCs) to read words and pseudowords.

Graphemic perception

During reading acquisition, occipital brain areas also become gradually specialized for graphemic perception. Using magneto-encephalography, the perception of words has been compared to the perception of strings of geometric shapes in beginning readers (first-graders) and skilled readers (adults) of Finnish (a language with a shallow orthography; Parviainen *et al.*, 2006). In children, as in adults, activations reflecting geometric-shapes perception were observed bilaterally in the occipital cortex, whereas those reflecting written-word perception occurred only in the left occipito-temporal cortex (in the VWFA; Cohen and Dehaene, 2004). Bilateral activation was observed about 100 milliseconds (ms) after the onset of the geometric shapes in both children and adults. In sharp contrast, the left activations observed for words appeared almost as quickly as those observed for geometric shapes in adults, but not in children for whom the activations for words appeared later than those for geometric shapes. This indicates that the VWFA becomes progressively specialized for visual-word perception. In addition, during reading acquisition, the VWFA becomes more strongly activated by reading tasks and less by non-reading tasks in ex-illiterate adults (Dehaene *et al.*, 2010a). Finally, new connections are progressively established during reading acquisition between the VWFA and some left temporal area involved in the processing of spoken language (Dehaene and Cohen, 2011).

The VWFA is part of two neural reading pathways used to process written words, a sublexical one and a lexical one: A dorsal (sublexical) pathway connects the VWFA to temporo-parietal regions, themselves connected to Broca's area. A ventral (lexical) pathway directly connects the VWFA and Broca's area. The sublexical pathway predominates first, with the ventral circuit developing later (Cohen *et al.*, 2008). The effects of learning on the neural networks involved in reading were assessed in studies in which adults who just learned to read were compared to adults who were illiterate (e.g. Carreiras *et al.*, 2009; Dehaene *et al.*, 2010b). These studies showed that learning to read increased connectivity in the dorsal pathway between the occipito-temporal area and the supra-marginal gyrus. Furthermore, activations in an area specifically involved in spoken language processing (planum temporale) were more significant in ex-illiterates than in individuals who were illiterate (Dehaene *et al.*, 2010b). These findings suggest that the left occipito-temporal cortex (Figure 3.1) appears as the endpoint of a developmental reading process that starts with the integration of phonological and visual representations.

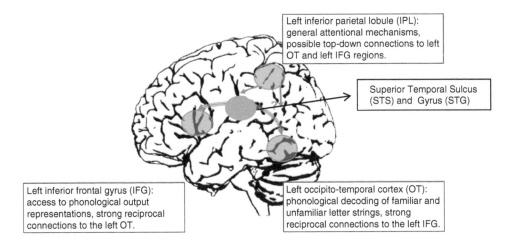

Left inferior parietal lobule (IPL): general attentional mechanisms, possible top-down connections to left OT and left IFG regions.

Superior Temporal Sulcus (STS) and Gyrus (STG)

Left inferior frontal gyrus (IFG): access to phonological output representations, strong reciprocal connections to the left OT.

Left occipito-temporal cortex (OT): phonological decoding of familiar and unfamiliar letter strings, strong reciprocal connections to the left IFG.

Figure 3.1 Left-hemisphere reading pathways. Adapted from Richlan, 2012 (Fig. 1).

Developmental dyslexia

Definition and basic facts

According to Lyon *et al.* (2003), developmental dyslexia is defined as "a specific learning disability that is neurological in origin [...] characterized by difficulties with accurate and/or fluent word recognition, and by poor spelling and decoding abilities" (p. 104) (Research definition used by the National Institute of Health: www.dys-add.com/define.html). This specific learning disability affects about 7 percent of the population (Peterson and Pennington, 2012). The core criterion for diagnosing dyslexia in English is accuracy scores in word and pseudoword reading. Alternatively, the core criterion for the same diagnosis in languages with a shallower orthography (for instance, Spanish, German, Dutch, and French) is word and pseudoword reading speed since deficits in accuracy are frequently compensated in such orthographies (Richlan, 2012; Sprenger-Charolles *et al.*, 2011).

Core deficits in dyslexia

As discussed, the ability to associate graphic symbols (graphemes) with speech sounds (phonemes) has crucial importance for learning to read. Children with dyslexia present an early deficit in learning GPCs and show a persistent lack of automation when they eventually acquire such associations (Blomert and Vaessen, 2009). Most of these children can eventually read after a long instructional period, often with the help of phonics remediation, but they read slowly and painfully, with a much greater allocation of metabolic resources (i.e., a greater physiological energy cost) than typical reading children (Wimmer and Mayringer, 2002).

The severe and persistent grapho-phonemic deficit that characterizes dyslexia is not necessarily the core deficit, as it can also be a proxy for remote audio-phonological or visuo-graphemic impairments. Most of the children with dyslexia have a phonological deficit and some of them have a graphemic deficit. However, there are no clear indications on the prevalence of these three possible core deficits (grapho-phonemic, audio-phonological and visuo-graphemic), primarily because of the heterogeneity of dyslexia due to genetic variations.

Phonological deficit

A classical argument in support of a deficit in phonemic representations is that individuals with dyslexia have serious difficulties in consciously extracting phonemes from the speech signal, as evidenced in tasks involving the manipulation of phonemic segments within words or pseudowords. A deficit in phonemic awareness has been shown to be one of the most consistent manifestations of dyslexia which, together with phonological short-term memory (STM) impairment, remain the most popular indexes of phonological impairment in the present-day literature on dyslexia (Melby-Lervåg *et al.*, 2012).

As regards phonological STM, meta-analysis shows that variability in the size of a pseudoword repetition deficit is mostly due to differences in oral language skills (Melby-Lervåg and Lervåg, 2012). The inferior frontal gyrus (IFG), a fronto-cortical area that is part of the dorsal stream that links acoustic speech signals to articulatory networks (Hickok and Poeppel, 2007), is associated with phonological recoding during reading (Sandak *et al.*, 2004). Impaired activation has been noted in the IFG for readers with dyslexia during processing of unfamiliar letter strings (for a review: Richlan, 2012).

Other studies have been aimed at demonstrating speech perception deficits in dyslexia (Mody *et al.*, 1997). As we have seen, phonemic representations are the end-product of a long-standing developmental process with two major stages: the integration of universal allophonic features into language-specific phonological features that occurs before age one year, and the combination of phonological features into phonemic segments, which occurs much later, between ages five and six years (Hoonhorst *et al.*, 2009, 2011). Allophonic theory claims that people affected by dyslexia do not integrate allophonic features into phonological features during the development of speech perception and, consequently, they perceive speech in allophonic rather than phonemic units (Serniclaes, 2011). Allophonic perception has obvious implications for reading acquisition because it interferes with relationships between speech and print, so that even completely transparent writing systems become radically opaque (Figure 3.2).

Different studies have shown that individuals with dyslexia perceive the differences between allophonic variants of the same phoneme, whereas typical reading controls do not discriminate such allophonic distinctions (Bogliotti *et al.*, 2008; Noordenbos *et al.*, 2012a, 2012b, 2013; Serniclaes *et al.*, 2004). Those with dyslexia do not always exhibit allophonic perception (e.g. Messaoud-Galusi *et al.*, 2011) and this is probably due to neural inhibition in specific brain areas. Indeed, studies in Dutch with children at risk for dyslexia and with adults with dyslexia showed that, even when behavioral data did not show allophonic perception, it was nevertheless present in neural recordings (Noordenbos *et al.*, 2012b, 2013; see Figure 3.3). The fact that the allophonic contrast elicited an increase in neural activity despite the absence of behavioral response suggests that inhibitory processes are at work in the brains of individuals with dyslexia. According to a PET scan study with French adults with dyslexia, such processes might take place in the frontal cortex, close to Broca's area (Dufor *et al.*, 2009). The inhibition of allophonic percepts mobilizes metabolic resources that are also needed for reading. This might explain the slow and laborious reading performances of people with dyslexia (Shaywitz and Shaywitz, 2005; Sprenger-Charolles *et al.*, 2011).

Allophonic perception also has implications for segmenting the speech signal into phonemes. The temporal threshold for perceiving a vowel within a consonant cluster is shorter for children with dyslexia when compared to chronological age and reading level controls, suggesting that they better perceive the relatively short allophonic segments within the cluster (Serniclaes and Seck, 2013). The enhanced perception of allophonic segments might be related to a better fine-grained segmentation of the speech signal by high-frequency neural oscillatory networks (Goswami, 2011).

PHONEMES	da	ta	ti
LETTERS	*da*	*ta*	*ti*

ALLOPHONES	da	ta	tʰi
LETTERS	*da*	*ʔa*	*ti*

Figure 3.2 Allophones vs. phonemes. With a completely transparent orthography, each letter corresponds to a single speech sound with phonemic decoding (left, e.g., the /d/ and /t/ phonemes), but it corresponds to different speech sounds with allophonic decoding (right, e.g., /d/ and two allophones of /t/, depending on the vocalic context).

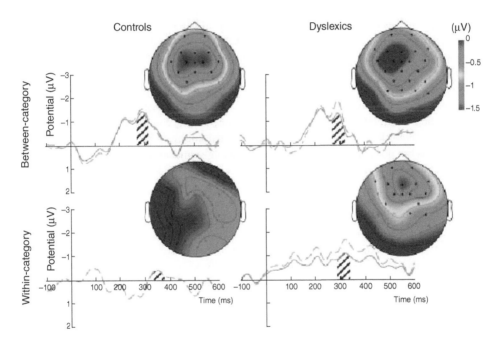

Figure 3.3 Neural response (MMN) to a phonemic contrast in both adults with dyslexia and controls (above) and to an allophonic contrast in adults with dyslexia (below, right). From Noordenbos *et al.*, 2013 (Fig. 3). © 2013, Elsevier.

Grapho-phonemic deficit

Blomert (2011) argues that the cause of dyslexia resides in a dysfunction of the mechanisms that normally generate fluent letter–sound associations. A Mismatch Negativity (MMN) study (Froyen *et al.*, 2011) showed that the mechanisms for letter–sound integration were impaired in children with dyslexia compared to chronological age controls with the same four years of reading instruction. This could be a bottleneck that prevents children with dyslexia from acquiring fluent reading, keeping in mind that associating graphemes with phonemes has crucial importance for reading acquisition (Share, 1995).

As explained above, a cultural factor that impacts the automation of written-word processing is the consistency of the GPCs in the writing system, and this is not limited to early reading acquisition. Indeed, it also emerges in adults, as indicated in a study with English, French and Italian participants (Paulesu *et al.*, 2001) in which typical readers and those with dyslexia read regular words and pseudowords. Response times indicated that the deeper the orthography, the more severe the dyslexia. However, regardless of the depth of the orthography, the dyslexia deficit was more pronounced for pseudowords than for word reading (i.e., when readers have to use GPCs without the help of their lexical knowledge).

Graphemic deficit

Remember that, after the set-up of pairings between isolated letters (or graphemes) and speech sounds (or phonemes) in the STG–STS, sequences of speech sounds characterizing whole words are connected to letter strings in the fusiform gyrus. This broader parieto-temporal network modifies the functioning of a specific area of the fusiform gyrus, the VWFA, which becomes progressively specialized for the recognition of letter strings (Cohen *et al.*, 2000). A specific problem in the development of the VWFA might also be responsible for dyslexia. Suppose you have well-formed letter–sound pairs but you cannot assemble them in the right way for obtaining the correct representation of the visual word; then you will obviously have a serious problem for reading. One study showed that 11-year-old children with dyslexia presented the same activation of the VWFA as chronological age controls, but unlike the controls, did not exhibit differential activation of printed letters compared to false fonts (van der Mark *et al.*, 2009). In addition, the VWFA is activated during spoken language processing in literate adults but not in illiterates, suggesting that letter–sound associations induce a top-down effect of phonology on VWFA functioning (Blomert, 2011; Dehaene and Cohen, 2011; Dehaene *et al.*, 2010a).

Genetic bases

In summary, three different core deficits are possibly at the origin of dyslexia and each is associated with a different neural dysfunction in the left hemisphere. These are: (1) a phonological deficit in regions of the frontal cortex, close to "Broca's area," that contributes to the phonological processing of speech sounds (Dufor *et al.*, 2009; Sandak *et al.*, 2004); (2) a grapho-phonemic deficit in a heteromodal area located in the temporal cortex that reacts both to visual and auditory inputs (Blomert, 2011); and (3) a graphemic deficit in a visual area located in the occipito-temporal cortex (van der Mark *et al.*, 2009).

Genetic variations contribute to the presence of these three different possible core deficits in dyslexia (phonological, grapho-phonemic, and graphemic). The genes contributing to dyslexia have been progressively identified and a preliminary account of the genetic bases of the different deficits associated with dyslexia is now possible, although much remains to be done. Eicher and Gruen (2013) present a general view of the relationships among genetic variants, brain areas, and reading impairments. These authors summarize the outcomes of these imaging-genetic studies by brain region. Broca's area, the left IFG, and a left temporo-parietal region are associated with three different genes (DYX2 on chromosome 6, FOXP2 and CNTNAP2 on chromosome 7). As Broca's area and the IFG are part of the phonological network of speech perception, these genes presumably contribute to the speech perception deficits noted in dyslexia. The fronto-parietal reading circuitry is responsible for the propagation of action potentials that might in turn contribute to the building of grapho-phonemic relationships. Finally, the loss of asymmetry between the left and right hemispheres in the brains of individuals with dyslexia is associated with a fourth gene (KIAA0319 on chromosome 6).

In sum, current research suggests that the main genetic variants that are responsible for dyslexia affect brain regions related to phonological speech perception, phoneme–grapheme relationships, and brain asymmetry (Eicher and Gruen, 2013). However, as different genes interact during neural development, a single genetic variant does not necessarily result in dyslexia, but can also produce other language and cognitive impairments (Plomin and McGuffin, 2003).

Dyslexia vs. other developmental impairments

Dyslexia overlaps with several other developmental impairments, mainly "Specific Language Impairment" (SLI) and Attention Deficit Hyperactivity Disorder (ADHD). Such comorbidity arises from the complex genotypes that are associated with each of these impairments. Some children with dyslexia exhibit language deficits that are not only of a phonological nature but also of a syntactic–semantic nature characteristic of SLI (Bishop and Snowling, 2004; for a somewhat different perspective, see the chapter by Montgomery, Gillam, and Evans, this volume). Another portion of the population with dyslexia exhibits a broader ADHD deficit (DuPaul *et al.*, 2013). Such comorbidity between dyslexia and other developmental impairments gives rise to a large variety of children with severe reading impairments.

Conclusion and implications for remediation

Reading acquisition basically depends on the construction of a neural network that links phoneme representations (frontal cortex) to grapheme representations (occipital cortex), via grapheme–phoneme associations (temporal cortex). Dyslexia can thus arise from three possible causes: a phonemic deficit arising from an atypical development of speech perception, a graphemic deficit due to a failure to acquire visual-word representations, and a grapho-phonemic deficit. The prevalence of these deficits depends on genetic variations and it is possible that each is present in a child with dyslexia. Considering the high degree of interconnectivity of brain circuitry, one of these core deficits might in turn give rise to the other deficits. Finally, these deficits can take more severe forms when severe reading impairments are associated with other cognitive dysfunctions (e.g. oral language deficits in children with SLI).

The available methods for the remediation of reading impairments follow two main directions: those tapping into high-level cognitive processes and those tapping into low-level perceptual processes. Low-level remediation methods using perceptual tools might provide therapies for dyslexia. However, the use of modified speech (Tallal *et al.*, 1996) remains inconclusive on meta-analytic grounds (e.g., Strong *et al.*, 2011). Enhancing letter spacing offers spontaneous improvement of reading accuracy and speed in both Italian and French children with dyslexia (Zorzi *et al.*, 2012). However, as made clear in a subsequent study with Spanish children, the reading speed that children with dyslexia attain remains lower than that of typical readers (Perea *et al.*, 2012). Nevertheless, these results are impressive and further improvements should be sought using combinations of letters modifications and perceptual training of phonemic distinctions. In this regard, a study using discrimination training of a phonological boundary resulted in remediation of allophonic perception in children with SLI and had positive effects on phoneme awareness (Collet *et al.*, 2012), although the effects of such training on reading performances are still unknown.

Alternatively, high-level remediation has proven to be successful with some limitations. Indeed, the results of two meta-analyses indicate that: (1) early training on phonemic awareness helps reading acquisition, especially for children at risk for reading and when letters are used in such training (Ehri *et al.*, 2001a); and that (2) systematic phonics instruction (compared to unsystematic or no-phonics instruction) also helps reading acquisition, especially when that training begins early (Ehri *et al.*, 2001b). In addition, according to training studies with randomized controlled trials, phonics instruction is the only treatment approach whose efficacy on reading in children and adolescents with reading disabilities is statistically confirmed (Galuschka *et al.*, 2014). Furthermore, phonological interventions, using training in both GPCs and phonemic awareness, induce changes of activity in the left hemisphere reading network (Démonet *et al.*, 2004), including the VWFA (Brem *et al.* 2010). However, gains after phonological interventions are only retained by about 50 percent of the children trained and those who retain their gains do not reach the fluent reading competencies of typical reading children (Gabrieli, 2009).

In conclusion, the major determinants of dyslexia are: the perception of speech sounds with allophonic units, the failure to associate graphical symbols with phonological units, and the construction of graphical word representations. Each of these factors can disrupt the emergence of a neural reading network that links phoneme to grapheme representations. The prevalence of these deficits depends on genetic variations and they can take more severe forms when dyslexia is associated with other cognitive dysfunctions.

Acknowledgment

This work was supported by a public grant overseen by the French National Research Agency (ANR) as part of the "Investissements d'Avenir" program (reference: ANR-10-LABX-0083).

References

Bishop, D.V.M. and Snowling, M.J. (2004), "Developmental dyslexia and specific language impairment: Same or different?", *Psychological Bulletin*, Vol. 130, pp. 858–886.

Blomert, L. (2011), "The neural signature of orthographic-phonological binding in successful and failing reading development", *NeuroImage*, Vol. 57, pp. 695–703.

Blomert, L. and Froyen, D. (2010), "Multi-sensory learning and learning to read", *International Journal of Psychophysiology*, Vol. 77, pp. 186–194.

Blomert, L. and Vaessen, A. (2009), *3DM Differentiaal Diagnose Voordyslexie: Cognitieve Analyse Van Lezen En Spelling* [3DM Differential Diagnostics For Dyslexia: Cognitive Analysis Of Reading And Spelling], Boom Test Publishers, Amsterdam.

Bogliotti, C., Serniclaes, W., Messaoud-Galusi, S. and Sprenger-Charolles, L. (2008), "Discrimination of speech sounds by dyslexic children: Comparisons with chronological age and reading level controls", *Journal of Experimental Child Psychology*, Vol. 101, pp. 137–175.

Brem, S., Bach, S., Kucian, K., Guttorm, T.K., Martin, E., *et al.* (2010), "Brain sensitivity to print emerges when children learn letter-speech sound correspondences", *Proceedings of the National Academy of Sciences*, Vol. 107, pp. 7939–7944.

Carreiras, M., Seghier, M.L., Baquero, S., Estevez, A., Lozano, A., *et al.* (2009), "An anatomical signature for literacy", *Nature*, Vol. 461, pp. 983–986.

Collet, G., Colin, C., Serniclaes, W., Hoonhorst, I., Markessis, E., *et al.* (2012), "Effect of phonological training in French children with SLI: Perspectives on voicing identification, discrimination and categorical perception", *Research in Developmental Disabilities*, Vol. 33, pp. 1805–1818.

Cohen, L. and Dehaene, S. (2004), "Specialization in the ventral stream: The case for the visual word form area", *Neuroimage*, Vol. 22, pp. 466–476.

Cohen, L., Dehaene, S., Vinckier, F., Jobert, A. and Montavont, A. (2008), "Reading normal and degraded words: Contribution of the dorsal and ventral visual pathways", *NeuroImage*, Vol. 40, pp. 353–366.

Cohen, L., Dehaene, S., Naccache, L., Lehericy, S., Dehaene-Lambertz, *et al.* (2000), "The visual word form area: Spatial and temporal characterization of an initial stage of reading in normal subjects and posterior split-brain patients", *Brain*, Vol. 123, pp. 291–307.

Dehaene, S. and Cohen, L. (2011), "The unique role of the visual word form area in reading", *Trends in Cognitive Sciences*, Vol. 15, pp. 254–262.

Dehaene, S., Pegado, F., Braga, L.W., Ventura, P., Nunes-Filho, G., *et al.* (2010a), "How learning to read changes the cortical networks for vision and language", *Science*, Vol. 330, pp. 1359–1364.

Dehaene, S., Nakamura, K., Jobert, A. Kuroki, C., Ogawa, S., *et al.* (2010b), "Why do children make mirror errors in reading? Neural correlates of mirror invariance in the visual word form area", *Neuroimage*, Vol. 49, pp. 1837–1848.

Démonet, J.-F., Taylor, M.J. and Chaix, Y. (2004), "Developmental dyslexia", *The Lancet*, Vol. 363, pp. 1451–1460.

Dufor, O., Serniclaes, W., Sprenger-Charolles, L. and Démonet, J.-F. (2009), "Left pre-motor cortex and allophonic speech perception in dyslexia: A PET study", *NeuroImage*, Vol. 46, pp. 241–248.

DuPaul, G.J., Gormley, M.J. and Laracy, S.D. (2013), "Comorbidity of LD and ADHD: Implications of DSM-5 for assessment and treatment", *Journal of Learning Disabilities*, Vol. 46, pp. 43–51.

Ehri, L.C., Nunes, S.R., Willows, D., Schuster, B.V., Yaghoub-Zadeh, Z., *et al.* (2001a), "Phonemic awareness instruction helps children learn to read: Evidence from the National Reading Panel's meta-analysis", *Reading Research Quarterly*, Vol. 36, pp. 250–283.

Ehri, L.C., Nunes, S.R., Stahl, S.A. and Willows, D.M. (2001b), "Systematic phonics instruction helps students learn to read: Evidence from the National Reading Panel's meta-analysis", *Review of Educational Research*, Vol. 71, pp. 393–447.

Eicher, J.D. and Gruen, J.R. (2013), "Imaging-genetics in dyslexia: Connecting risk genetic variants to brain neuroimaging and ultimately to reading impairments", *Molecular Genetics and Metabolism*, Vol. 110, pp. 201–212.

Froyen, D., Willems, G. and Blomert, L. (2011), "Evidence for a specific cross-modal association deficit in dyslexia: An electrophysiological study of letter-speech sound processing", *Developmental Science*, Vol. 14, pp. 635–648.

Gabrieli, J.D.E. (2009), "Dyslexia: A new synergy between education and cognitive neuroscience", *Science*, Vol. 325, pp. 280–283. 10.1126/science.1171999.

Galuschka, K., Ise, E., Krick, K. and Schulte-Körne, G. (2014), "Effectiveness of treatment approaches for children and adolescents with reading abilities: A meta-analysis of randomized control trials", *Plos One*, Vol. 9, e89900.

Goswami, U. (2011), "A temporal sampling framework for developmental dyslexia", *Trends in Cognitive Sciences*, Vol. 15, pp. 1–10.

Hickok, G. and Poeppel, D. (2007), "The cortical organization of speech processing", *Nature Reviews Neuroscience*, Vol. 8, pp. 393–402.

Hoonhorst, I., Colin, C., Markessis, E., Radeau, M., Deltenre, P., *et al.* (2009), "French native speakers in the making: From language-general to language-specific voicing boundaries", *Journal of Experimental Child Psychology*, Vol. 104, pp. 353–366.

Hoonhorst, I., Medina, V., Colin, C., Markessis, E., Radeau, M., *et al.* (2011), "The development of categorical perception: Comparisons between voicing, colors and facial expressions", *Speech Communication*, Vol. 53, pp. 417–430.

Liberman, A.M., Cooper, F.S., Shankweiler, D.P. and Studdert-Kennedy, M. (1967), "Perception of the speech code", *Psychological Review*, Vol. 74, pp. 431–461.

Liberman, I.Y., Shankweiler, D., Fisher, W.F. and Carter, B. (1974), "Explicit syllable and phoneme segmentation in the young child", *Journal of Experimental Child Psychology*, Vol. 18, pp. 201–212.

Lyon, G.R., Shaywitz, S.E. and Shaywitz, B.A. (2003), "A definition of dyslexia", *Annals of Dyslexia*, Vol. 53, pp. 1–14.

Melby-Lervåg, M. and Lervåg, A. (2012), "Oral language skills moderate nonword repetition skills in children with dyslexia: A meta-analysis of the role of nonword repetition skills in dyslexia", *Scientific Studies of Reading*, Vol. 16, pp. 1–34.

Melby-Lervåg, M., Lyster, S.A.H. and Hulme, C. (2012), "Phonological skills and their role in learning to read: A meta-analytic review", *Psychological Bulletin*, Vol. 138, pp. 322–352.

Messaoud-Galusi, S., Hazan, V. and Rosen, S. (2011), "Investigating speech perception in children with dyslexia: Is there evidence of a consistent deficit in individuals?", *Journal of Speech, Language, and Hearing Research*, Vol. 54, pp. 1682–1701.

Mody, M., Studdert-Kennedy, M. and Brady, S. (1997), "Speech perception deficits in poor readers: Auditory processing or phonological coding?", *Journal of Experimental Child Psychology,* Vol. 64, pp. 199–231.

Morais, J., Cary, L., Alegria, J. and Bertelson, P. (1979), "Does awareness of speech as a sequence of phones arise spontaneously?", *Cognition,* Vol. 7, pp. 323–331.

Noordenbos, M., Segers, E., Serniclaes, W., Mitterer, H. and Verhoeven, L. (2012a), "Allophonic mode of speech perception in children at-risk for dyslexia: A longitudinal study", *Research in Developmental Disabilities,* Vol. 33, pp. 1469–1483.

Noordenbos, M., Segers, E., Serniclaes, W., Mitterer, H. and Verhoeven, L. (2012b), "Neural evidence of allophonic perception in children at risk for dyslexia", *Neuropsychologia,* Vol. 50, pp. 2010–2017.

Noordenbos, M.W., Segers, E., Serniclaes, W. and Verhoeven, L. (2013), "Neural evidence of the allophonic mode of speech perception in adults with dyslexia", *Clinical Neurophysiology,* Vol. 124, pp. 1151–1162.

Parviainen, T., Helenius, P. Niemi, P. and Salmelin, R. (2006), "Cortical sequence of word perception in beginning readers", *Journal of Neuroscience,* Vol. 26, pp. 6052–6061.

Paulesu, E., Démonet, J.F., Fazio, F., McCrory, E., Chanoine, V., *et al.* (2001), "Dyslexia: Cultural diversity and biological unity", *Science,* Vol. 291, pp. 2165–2167.

Perea, M., Panadero, V., Moret-Tatay, C. and Pablo Gómez, P. (2012), "The effects of inter-letter spacing in visual-word recognition: Evidence with young normal readers and developmental dyslexics", *Learning and Instruction,* Vol. 22, pp. 420–430.

Perfetti, C. (2007), "Reading ability: Lexical quality to comprehension", *Scientific Studies of Reading,* Vol. 11, pp. 357–383.

Peterson, R.L. and Pennington, B.F. (2012), "Developmental dyslexia", *Lancet,* Vol. 379, pp. 1997–2007.

Plomin, R. and McGuffin, P. (2003), "Psychopathology in the postgenomic era", *Annual Review of Psychology,* Vol. 54, pp. 205–228.

Richlan, F. (2012), "Developmental dyslexia: Dysfunction of a left hemisphere reading network", *Frontiers in Human Neuroscience,* Vol. 6, pp. 120. doi:10.3389/fnhum.2012.0012

Sandak, R., Menckl, W.E., Frost, S.J. and Pugh, K.R. (2004), "The neurobiological basis of skilled and impaired reading: Recent findings and new directions", *Scientific Studies of Reading,* Vol. 8, pp. 273–292.

Serniclaes, W. (2011), "Percepción alofónica en la dislexia: Una revisión". (Allophonic Perception in dyslexia: An overview). In W. Serniclaes and J.L. Luque (Eds.), *Avances En La Investigación Sobre La Dislexia Evolutiva. Escritos De Psicología,* Vol. 4, pp. 25–34. www.escritosdepsicologia.es/descargas/revistas/vol4num2/i_vol4num2_4.pdf

Serniclaes, W. and Seck, M. (2013), "Perception of subphonemic segments: A new instance of allophonic perception in dyslexia", *Scientific Studies of Reading (SSRC) Conference,* July 10–13, 2013, Hong Kong.

Serniclaes, W., Van Heghe, S., Mousty, Ph., Carré, R. and Sprenger-Charolles, L. (2004), "Allophonic mode of speech perception in dyslexia", *Journal of Experimental Child Psychology,* Vol. 87, pp. 336–361.

Share, D.L. (1995), "Phonological recoding and self-teaching: Sine-qua-non of reading acquisition", *Cognition,* Vol. 55, pp. 151–218.

Share, D.L. (2008), "Orthographic learning, phonological recoding, and self-teaching", *Advances in Child Development and Behavior,* Vol. 36, pp. 31–82.

Shaywitz, B.A., Shaywitz, B.E., Pugh, K.R., Mencl, W.E., Fulbright, R.K., *et al.* (2002), "Disruption of posterior brain systems for reading in children with developmental dyslexia", *Biological Psychiatry,* Vol. 52, pp. 101–110.

Shaywitz, S.E. and Shaywitz, B.A. (2005), *Dyslexia (specific reading disability). Biological Psychiatry,* Vol. 57, pp. 1301–1309.

Sprenger-Charolles, L., Colé, P. and Serniclaes, W. (2006), *Reading Acquisition And Developmental Dyslexia.* Psychology Press, Hove, UK, and New York, USA.

Sprenger-Charolles, L., Siegel, L.S., Jiménez, J.E. and Ziegler, J.C. (2011), "Prevalence and reliability of phonological, surface, and mixed profiles in dyslexia: A review of studies conducted in languages varying in orthographic depth", *Scientific Studies of Reading,* Vol. 15, pp. 498–521.

Strong, G.K., Torgerson, C.J., Torgerson, D. and Hulme, C. (2011), "A systematic meta-analytic review of evidence for the effectiveness of the 'Fast ForWord' language intervention program", *Journal of Child Psychology and Psychiatry,* Vol. 52, pp. 224–235.

Tallal, P., Miller, S., Bedi, G., Wang, X., Nagarajan, S.S., *et al.* (1996), "Language comprehension in language-learning impaired children improved with acoustically modified speech", *Science,* Vol. 271, pp. 81–84.

Van Atteveldt, N., Formisano, E., Goebel, R. and Blomert, L. (2004), "Integration of letters and speech sounds in the human brain", *Neuron*, Vol. 43, pp. 1–12.

Van Atteveldt, N., Formisano, E., Goebel, R. and Blomert, L. (2007), "Top-down task effects overrule automatic multisensory responses to letter-sound pairs in auditory association cortex", *Neuroimage*, Vol. 36, pp. 1345–1360.

van der Mark, S., Bucher, K., Marer, U., Schulz, E., Brem, S., *et al.* (2009), "Children with dyslexia lack multiple specializations along the visual word-form (VWF) system", *Neuroimage*, Vol. 47, pp. 1940–1949.

Wimmer, H. and Mayringer, H. (2002), "Dysfluent reading in the absence of spelling difficulties: A specific disability in regular orthographies", *Journal of Educational Psychology*, Vol. 94, pp. 272–277.

Ziegler, J.C. and Goswami, U. (2005), "Reading acquisition, developmental dyslexia, and skilled reading across languages: A psycholinguistic grain size theory", *Psychological Bulletin*, Vol. 131, pp. 3–29.

Zorzi, M., Barbiero, C., Facoetti, A., Lonciari, I., Carrozzi, M., *et al.* (2012), "Extra-large letter spacing improves reading in dyslexia", *Proceedings of the National Academy of Sciences*, Vol. 109, pp. 11455–11459.

4

BRAIN IMAGING STUDIES OF DEVELOPMENTAL STUTTERING

A review

Luc De Nil and Deryk Beal

The core characteristics of developmental stuttering are typically described as involuntary sound or part-word repetitions, prolongations and audible or inaudible blockages of speech (Bloodstein and Bernstein-Ratner, 2008). Children with developmental stuttering usually start showing the first signs of speech fluency disruptions between the ages of two and six years. Approximately 60 to 80 percent of children will recover from stuttering within two years after onset, but others will go on to develop chronic stuttering, which can be difficult to treat (Yairi and Ambrose, 1999) often because children may very quickly develop struggle, secondary coping behaviors, speech anxiety and other emotional reactions.

The etiology of developmental stuttering is not completely understood but research to date points toward a multifactorial model as the best explanatory approach. There is clear evidence for the role of genetic factors in the onset, development and recovery from stuttering (Yairi and Ambrose, 2013). Children who stutter also have been found to show language deficits (Sasisekaran and Byrd, 2013) and differences in temperamental characteristics (Eggers, *et al.*, 2010). Behavioral, electrophysiological and brain imaging research has pointed to deficits in sensorimotor integration processes during speech (Beal, *et al.*, 2010, 2011; Loucks and De Nil, 2012). Recent brain imaging studies of developmental stuttering have highlighted the central role of speech-related brain processing abnormalities in stuttering. In this chapter, we will review brain imaging research aimed at investigating the functional and neuroanatomical components of that system. We will conclude by providing an overall synthesis and interpretation of the brain imaging data and some directions for future research.

Functional imaging of developmental stuttering

Since the first publication by Wood, *et al.* (1980), who reported atypical left cerebral blood flow in two adults who stutter, scientists and clinicians have gained significant insights into possible cortical and subcortical neural deficiencies that may lead to the development, maintenance and recovery of stuttering. Brown and colleagues (2005) identified what they called the three neural signatures of developmental stuttering in adults: (1) overactivation of cortical and subcortical motor areas; (2) atypical right hemisphere lateralization of activation in the frontal operculum, Rolandic operculum, and anterior insula; and (3) deactivation of auditory cortex during typical (habitual) speech. Subsequent research has confirmed some of these conclusions, qualified others and added additional potential signatures of developmental stuttering. Moreover, researchers increasingly are finding appropriate paradigms to study neural activation in younger children who stutter (see Beal, *et al.*, 2011, 2013; Chang, *et al.*, 2008; Chang and Zhu, 2013). In the following sections, we will review some of the main functional imaging findings reported in the literature.

Increased neural activation in people who stutter

Overactivation of various brain areas compared to that seen in typically fluent speakers was among the earliest observations reported in adults who stutter. For instance, Fox, *et al.* (1996) reported on a positron emission tomography (PET) study of adult speakers who stutter that showed significant overactivation in the supplementary motor area, premotor and motor cortex and cerebellum, regions that are important for speech production. Most of the overactivation was seen primarily in the right hemisphere. Similar PET findings were reported by Braun, *et al.* (1997) during an oral reading task, and by De Nil, *et al.* (2000, 2003) who scanned participants prior to an intensive treatment program. Recent functional magnetic resonance imaging (fMRI) studies have also reported increased cortical activation in people who stutter. For instance, Lu, *et al.* (2010) reported that adults with normal fluency showed more widespread activation in the left than in the right hemisphere during a picture-naming task, while the participants who stutter showed a reversed pattern (right more widespread than left). Similarly, Loucks, *et al.* (2011) reported that while increased activation in adults who stutter was present bilaterally during an oral naming task, it was present in more cortical regions in the right than in the left hemisphere.

In keeping with previous findings, Chang, *et al.* (2009) reported increased activation in left premotor and primary motor regions, including the putamen subcortically, and bilateral auditory regions in adults who stutter. Importantly, these researchers found that these differences in activation patterns were present not only during speech tasks but also during non-verbal oral motor tasks. Ingham, *et al.* (2012) reported on a PET study in which participants engaged in oral reading and a monologue, as well as an eyes closed rest condition. Participants who stutter showed a trend toward higher levels of activation in the supplementary motor area and precentral gyrus. Control participants showed increased activation in the insula, basal ganglia and cerebellum, but only for the oral reading task. These researchers observed a positive correlation between stuttering severity and activation in the cortico-striatal-thalamic loop and a negative correlation with activation in the cerebellum.

Interpretation of increased activation

The reason for the increased activation in people who stutter seen in most studies is not yet clear. Chang, *et al.* (2009) suggested that "many previously reported differences involving right hemisphere and subcortical activity in speakers who stutter likely reflect altered functional responses to deficient connectivity of the left premotor/motor areas" (p. 2516). Similarly, Kell, *et al.* (2009) suggested that the increased activations may point to compensatory speech mechanisms rather than some underlying inherent deficiency. De Nil and colleagues (De Nil, 1999; De Nil, *et al.*, 2008) have argued that people who stutter have an unstable speech motor system, easily disrupted by internal and external triggers, which may lead to increased effort as the person who stutters attempts to exert greater voluntary control over speech production.

The important role of effort in understanding observed brain differences has been highlighted in a number of other studies investigating stuttering (Brown, *et al.*, 2005; Chang, *et al.*, 2009; Kell, *et al.*, 2009), simulated stuttering (De Nil, *et al.*, 2008), as well as a number of explanatory models (De Nil, 2004; Packman, Code and Onslow, 2007). One of the characteristics of this unstable motor system may be a difficulty with the smooth integration of sensory and motor processes. Indirect support for this interpretation has come from reports of atypical neural activations in areas that have an important role in such integration, including the Operculum Parietale (Chang, *et al.*, 2009) and the cerebellum (Brown, *et al.*, 2005; De Nil, Kroll and Houle, 2001; Lu, *et al.*, 2010; Watkins, *et al.*, 2008). Whether differences in activation that are observed more globally during speech tasks can be extended to single moments of stuttering is still an outstanding question. Some early attempts at this question have resulted in ambiguous answers (Sowman, *et al.*, 2012; Wymbs, *et al.*, 2013).

Resting state brain activity

The question whether differences in brain activation reflect compensatory vs. innate processes can be addressed through the study of resting state brain activity. It is generally believed that such differences are more likely to reflect innate differences in brain activity (Ingham, *et al.*, 1996; but see Kell, 2012). In one such study, Xuan, *et al.* (2012) reported systematic differences between adults who do and do not stutter in amplitude of low frequency fluctuation (ALFF) involving many of the cortical areas previously identified as showing atypical activation in persons who stutter, as well as differences in functional connectivity between several of these regions, especially in the left hemisphere. They concluded that persons who stutter show a deficit in multiple speech-related functional systems and their interconnections.

Brain imaging in children

Other researchers have used the approach of studying functional and structural brain scans of school-age children in order to investigate causal brain activation closer to the onset of stuttering (Beal, *et al.*, 2011, 2013; Chang, *et al.*, 2008; Chang and Zhu, 2013). While similarities and differences were found with adults, there remains a not insignificant time lapse between the typical age of onset of stuttering and the age at which the children's brain scans were obtained, leaving plenty of time for experience or maturation-based functional and structural changes to take place (Taubert, Villringer and Ragert, 2012).

Reduced activation in auditory cortex

In contrast to observations of overactivation, studies have reported reduced activation in the auditory cortex of persons who stutter during habitual speech. In an early study, Watson, *et al.* (1992) reported that participants who stutter and displayed relative blood flow asymmetry lower than the normal median value in both the left superior and middle temporal regions, also demonstrated significantly longer laryngeal reaction times compared to those with above-normal median relative flow. A few years later, Fox, *et al.* (1996) also reported reduced temporal activation, a finding that has been confirmed in a number of follow-up studies (for review, see De Nil, 2004), although there is some evidence that the level of activation may differ between hemispheres (Chang, *et al.*, 2009; Lu, *et al.*, 2010). While reduced auditory activation has been observed repeatedly in individuals who stutter, the reason for this finding is not clear although a number of possible explanations have been proposed. According to Brown, *et al.* (2005), it may be the result of increased auditory inhibition originating in the motor cortex, but this was not confirmed by Beal and colleagues (2010, 2011), who observed similar auditory inhibition in adults and children who do or do not stutter during perception and production tasks. They did, however, observe differences in the timing of the auditory processing, suggesting that the observed auditory deactivation seen in those who stutter may partially reflect a timing deficiency in sensory-motor integration, rather than auditory inhibition (Beal, *et al.*, 2011).

A related but alternative hypothesis regarding reduced auditory activation in speakers who stutter, proposed by Brown, *et al.* (2005), was that auditory deactivation could result from repeated productions of the initial phonemes of a word. However, when asking adults who stutter to produce words while repeating the initial sound several times, De Nil, *et al.* (2008) did not find an increase in inhibition as predicted by Brown, *et al.* (2005). Also, if auditory inhibition is a direct result of stuttering, it is hard to understand why such inhibition has been observed repeatedly in studies where the participants who stutter were essentially fluent.

Effects of fluency treatment

Fluency enhancing conditions have been found to lead to greater normalization of brain activation in individuals who stutter (Fox, *et al.*, 1996; Toyomura, Fujii and Kuriki, 2011). More traditional fluency treatment has also been found to affect brain activation. De Nil, *et al.* (2003) investigated short- and long-term treatment effects on cortical and subcortical activation in adults who stutter during silent and oral reading of single words. Immediately post-treatment, there was increased left cortical and subcortical activation as a result of greater self-monitoring during speech production. After a one-year maintenance treatment phase, the participants who stutter showed a general reduction in overactivation, especially in the motor cortex, which the researchers attributed to increased automatization and decreased self-monitoring during speech. Similarly, Neumann, *et al.* (2003) reported that immediately following therapy, differential activations were even more distributed and left-sided. Two years later, these overactivations were observed to be reduced and more right-sided. Because the observed left frontal deactivations remained relatively stable over the two years of the study, Neumann and colleagues speculated that such deactivation may be one of the core neural characteristics of stuttering. In contrast, activations that were correlated with stuttering severity were suggested to be indicative of compensatory strategies used by the individuals who stutter.

An interesting study was published by Kell, *et al.* (2009) who investigated unassisted recovery from stuttering. They reported that persistent stuttering was associated with activation in contralateral brain regions, while recovery from stuttering was associated with activation of the left BA 47/12. These regions were adjacent to a region in which white matter anomalies were observed to be associated with persistent but not recovered stuttering. However, it needs to be noted that the directionality of the fractional anisotropy (FA) data in this case was reversed compared to previous studies (Chang, *et al.*, 2008; Sommer, *et al.*, 2002; Watkins, *et al.*, 2008); a finding that needs further clarification.

Neuroanatomical abnormalities associated with developmental stuttering

The literature addressing neuroanatomical abnormalities in developmental stuttering is small relative to that detailing anomalies in brain function during speech production. However, a picture is emerging of structural abnormalities that are present in as early as school-age children with persistent stuttering and continue into adulthood. The data are indicative of an altered trajectory of development in both grey and white matter throughout the neural network for speech production in people who stutter across the lifespan.

Grey vs. white matter differences

The neuroanatomical abnormalities associated with stuttering appear to be defined by regional differences in grey and white matter relative to fluently speaking controls, even though the total brain volume does not differ between groups. Children who stutter have less grey matter volume than controls in a number of regions throughout the neural network for speech production (Beal, *et al.*, 2013; Chang, *et al.*, 2008). Conversely, adults who stutter have more grey matter volume than controls in the left inferior frontal gyrus, right cerebellum and bilateral superior temporal gyri (Beal, *et al.*, 2007). This contradictory finding may seem problematic, but it does not need to be when the developmental trajectories of frontal region cortical architecture are considered. Normally, development of grey matter volume in the inferior frontal gyrus follows a course that sees this measure gradually increase in value over the early childhood years, peaking in the late school-aged years, and then gradually lessening and leveling off in early adulthood (Raznahan, *et al.*, 2011). The fact that children who stutter present with less grey matter volume in the left inferior frontal gyrus is suggestive of abnormal or delayed growth in this region, possibly affecting their ability to establish the motor representations required for stable and fluent speech sound production, and leading to decreased efficiency in the complex brain network that drives speech production resulting in persistent stuttered speech.

White matter pathways

One of the most robust findings in the literature is the reduction of FA values in the white matter pathways underlying the left inferior frontal gyrus in both children and adults who stutter (Cai, *et al.*, 2014; Chang, *et al.*, 2008; Cykowski, *et al.*, 2010; Lu, *et al.*, 2010; Sommer, *et al.*, 2002; Watkins, *et al.*, 2008). Low FA values suggest poor myelination and reduced connectivity of the brain's white matter. The data indicate that the left superior longitudinal fasciculus, which underlies the inferior frontal gyrus and links it to other brain regions in the neural network for speech production, is not as well myelinated in both children and adults who stutter. Less efficient myelination may result in a lack of connectivity of the left inferior frontal gyrus to other regions leading to an inefficient and slow system for speech production characterized by timing deficiencies and manifesting itself as stuttering.

If the left inferior frontal gyrus and its underlying white matter connections are deficient in both children and adults who stutter, periods of fluent speech may be achieved via compensatory support from the right hemisphere homologues of these structures. Although children who stutter have also been shown to have reduced grey matter volume of the right inferior frontal gyrus relative to controls, there was a strong negative association with this measure and stuttering severity (Beal, *et al.*, 2013). Children with mild severity had more grey matter volume in this region than children who were severe. It may be the case that successful reduction of stuttering severity is dependent on more typical neural growth and maturation in this region in the right hemisphere. Adults who stutter have been shown to have increased white matter connectivity in the right superior longitudinal fasciculus (Chang, *et al.*, 2011) as well as more white matter volume underlying critical speech regions in the right hemisphere (Jäncke, Hänggi and Steinmetz, 2004).

Some insight into the question of right hemisphere homologue recruitment can be had from studies that have examined the corpus callosum, known as an important pathway between the two hemispheres, in people who stutter. Children who stutter have been found to have lesser white matter volume bilaterally in the forceps minor of the corpus callosum (Beal, *et al.*, 2013).

However, Choo, *et al.* (2012) reported no differences in white matter volume of the corpus callosum in children who stutter. There is some evidence that white matter abnormalities identified in the corpus callosum of children who stutter continue into adulthood as both Cai, *et al.* (2014) and Cykowski, *et al.* (2010) found lesser FA in the forceps minor and callosal body in adults who stutter relative to controls. It is unclear just how the corpus callosum differs in people who stutter relative to controls, as the directionality of the differences across studies is not consistent.

Structural anatomy of auditory cortex

The structural integrity of auditory regions has also been investigated in people who stutter. In healthy individuals, the planum temporale is commonly asymmetrical in volume with the left having greater volume than the right. As a group, adults who stutter have been shown to have atypical right greater than left asymmetry of the planum temporale (Foundas, *et al.*, 2004). Subgroups of adults who stutter were identified by the degree of asymmetry. The adults who stutter and who had atypical asymmetry were found to be more severe than those with symmetrical or typical asymmetric planum temporale volumes. Adults who stutter have also been shown to have more grey matter volume in the bilateral superior temporal gyri than controls (Beal, *et al.*, 2007). It may be that adults who stutter rely on a more frequent and detailed monitoring of their own speech and that this behavior has resulted in overdevelopment of these auditory brain regions.

Integration and conclusion

Neuroimaging studies to date have provided strong support for both functional and structural differences between children and adults who do and do not stutter. The reasons behind these differences and their significance with respect to the onset and development of stuttering are still emerging. As proposed in previous writing, one interpretation, based on existing imaging as well as behavioral data (De Nil, 1999, 2004; De Nil, *et al.*, 2008; Smits-Bandstra and De Nil, 2007), is that the observed functional differences point to an unstable speech motor system. This overactivation would result from efforts to control and maintain stability within the system during speech production. The fact that similar overactivations can be triggered in adults with typical fluency during speech tasks that require more voluntary control of speech supports this interpretation. The relative lack of sensorimotor stability also is thought to lead to reduced speech motor skill learning in children during speech development, a period during which stuttering is most likely to start.

Furthermore, we believe that this unstable speech motor system results, at least in part, from observed structural deficits. These structural data are best summarized as showing altered developmental trajectories of grey matter development especially in the inferior frontal gyri accompanied by reductions in connectivity of the white matter pathways underlying this region with other parts of the speech network. This lack of connectivity with other speech regions may contribute to impairment in the integration and timing of information from sensory feedback with articulation during speech production, resulting in a failure to form the stable neural representations required for speech production early in development. Such an unstable neural system may be especially susceptible to internal and external stressors. In addition, one cannot exclude the possibility, indeed supported by some of the data, that regional differences in grey and white matter may reflect compensatory neural reorganization during brain development, quite probably also influenced by treatment history as well as behavioral strategies employed by the person who stutters. Of particular importance here is the potential role of the basal ganglia, known to have a critical role in motor timing, control and learning (Alm, 2004; Giraud, *et al.*, 2008; Smits-Bandstra and De Nil, 2007; Theys, *et al.*, 2012). Alm (2004) has argued that the core dysfunction of stuttering may be found in an impaired ability of the basal ganglia to produce the timing cues necessary for fluent speech. Giraud, *et al.* (2008) also reported a positive correlation between stuttering severity and basal ganglia activation. Together, these findings suggest that investigating the specific role of basal ganglia in stuttering is a much needed and promising direction for future research.

Which of the observed functional and structural differences are causal in nature remains unanswered at present. It is highly unlikely that the use of neuroimaging methodologies alone will lead us to an answer, and multidimensional approaches combining imaging and hypothesis-driven observational behavior studies will be required. Indeed, several such studies are currently under way (Olander *et al.*, 2010; Smith, *et al.*, 2012). Equally important is the question of the clinical significance of the brain imaging findings. Any neuroanatomic and functional abnormalities in people who stutter are subtle and, currently, only detectable at the group level. Brain imaging is, of course, also currently beyond routine clinical use for the treatment of stuttering. As a result, individual diagnostics using structural and functional neuroimaging for developmental stuttering at this point is not feasible. However, increased understanding of neuroplasticity (Cramer, *et al.*, 2011), as well as how behavioral intervention can actively influence such plasticity, offers much promise in developing greater insight into factors that affect speech fluency enhancement and post-treatment maintenance of treatment gains. Equally, if not more important, is a greater understanding of neural signatures that may be correlated with recovery from stuttering in childhood and post-treatment relapse of stuttering (De Nil, *et al.*, 2003; Kell, *et al.*, 2009). A promising avenue for research also is offered by recent methodologies in health informatics, such as imaging-genetics, that allow for integrated analyses of large datasets (Bohland *et al.*, 2013; Meyer-Lindenberg and Weinberger, 2006). Such approaches might shed light on how genetics influences structural brain development and the deviations from normal development that lead to stuttering in some populations.

Acknowledgement

The preparation of this chapter was supported by grants from the Natural Sciences and Engineering Research Council (#72036056) and the Canadian Institutes of Health Research (#143926).

References

Alm, P. (2004), "Stuttering and the basal ganglia circuits: A critical review of possible relations", *Journal of Communication Disorders*, Vol. 37, pp. 325–369.

Beal, D., Gracco, V., Lafaille, S. and De Nil, L. (2007), "Voxel-based morphometry of auditory and speech-related cortex in stutterers", *Neuroreport*, Vol. 18, pp. 1257–1260.

Beal, D., Cheyne, D., Gracco, V., Quraan, M., Taylor, M. and De Nil, L. (2010), "Auditory evoked fields to vocalization during passive listening and active generation in adults who stutter", *NeuroImage*, Vol. 52 , pp. 1645–1653.

Beal, D., Quraan, M., Cheyne, D., Taylor, M., Gracco, V. and De Nil, L. (2011), "Speech-induced suppression of evoked auditory fields in children who stutter", *NeuroImage*, Vol. 54, pp. 2994–3003.

Beal, D., Gracco, V., Brettschneider, J., Kroll, R. and De Nil, L. (2013), "A voxel-based morphometry (VBM) analysis of regional grey and white matter volume abnormalities within the speech production network of children who stutter", *Cortex*, Vol. 49, pp. 2151–2161.

Bloodstein, O. and Bernstein-Ratner, N. (2008), *A Handbook on Stuttering (6th edn.)*, Clifton Park, NY, US: Delmar.

Bohland, J., Myers, E. and Kim, E. (2013), "An informatics approach to integrating genetic and neurological data in speech and language neuroscience", *Neuroinformatic*, Vol. 12, pp. 39–62.

Braun, A., Varga, M., Stager, S., Schulz, G., Selbie, S., Maisog, J., *et al.* (1997), "Altered patterns of cerebral activity during speech and language production in developmental stuttering: An H215O positron emission tomography study", *Brain*, Vol. 120, pp. 761–784.

Brown, S., Ingham, R., Ingham, J., Laird, A. and Fox, P. (2005), "Stuttered and fluent speech production: An ALE meta-analysis of functional neuroimaging studies", *Human Brain Mapping*, Vol. 25, pp. 105–117.

Cai, S., Tourville, J., Beal, D., Perkell, J., Guenther, F. and Ghosh, S. (2014), "Diffusion imaging of cerebral white matter in persons who stutter: Evidence for network-level anomalies", *Frontiers in Human Neuroscience*, Vol. 8, p. 54. doi:10.3389/fnhum.2014.00054.

Chang, S. and Zhu, D. (2013), "Neural network connectivity differences in children who stutter", *Brain*, Vol. 136, pp. 3709–3726.

Chang, S., Erickson, K.I., Ambrose, N.G., Hasegawa-Johnson, M.A. and Ludlow, C.L. (2008), "Brain anatomy differences in childhood stuttering", *NeuroImage*, Vol. 39, pp. 1333–1344.

Chang, S., Kenney, M., Loucks, T. and Ludlow, C. (2009), "Brain activation abnormalities during speech and non-speech in stuttering speakers", *NeuroImage*, Vol. 46 1, pp. 201–212.

Chang, S., Horwitz, B., Ostuni, J., Reynolds, R. and Ludlow, C. (2011), "Evidence of left inferior frontal-premotor structural and functional connectivity deficits in adults who stutter", *Cerebral Cortex*, Vol. 21, pp. 2507–2518.

Choo, A., Chang, S., Zengin-Bolatkale, H., Ambrose, N. and Loucks, T. (2012), "Corpus callosum morphology in children who stutter", *Journal of Communication Disorders*, Vol. 45, pp. 279–289.

Cramer, S., Sur, M., Dobkin, B., O'Brien, C., Sanger, T., Trojanowski, J., *et al.* (2011), "Harnessing neuroplasticity for clinical applications", *Brain*, Vol. 134, pp. 1591–1609.

Cykowski, M., Fox, P., Ingham, R., Ingham, J. and Robin, D. (2010), "A study of the reproducibility and etiology of diffusion anisotropy differences in developmental stuttering: A potential role for impaired myelination", *NeuroImage*, Vol. 52, pp. 1495–1504.

De Nil, L. (1999), "Stuttering: A neurophysiological perspective", In Bernstein-Ratner, N. and Healey, C. (Eds.), *Stuttering Research and Practice: Bridging the Gap*. Mahwah, NJ, US: Erlbaum, pp. 85–102.

De Nil, L. (2004), "Recent developments in brain imaging research in stuttering", In Maassen, B., Peters, H. and Kent, R. (Eds.), *Speech Motor Control in Normal and Disordered Speech*. Proceedings of the Fourth International Speech Motor Conference. Oxford, UK: Oxford University Press, pp. 113–138.

De Nil, L., Kroll, R., Kapur, S. and Houle, S. (2000), "A positron emission tomography study of silent and oral single word reading in stuttering and nonstuttering adults", *Journal of Speech, Language, and Hearing Research*, Vol. 43, pp. 1038–1053.

De Nil, L., Kroll, R. and Houle, S. (2001), "Functional neuroimaging of cerebellar activation during single word reading and verb generation in stuttering and nonstuttering adults", *Neuroscience Letters*, Vol. 302, pp. 77–80.

De Nil, L., Kroll, R., Lafaille, S. and Houle, S. (2003), "A positron emission tomography study of short- and long-term treatment effects on functional brain activation in adults who stutter", *Journal of Fluency Disorders*, Vol. 28, pp. 357–380.

De Nil, L., Beal, D., Lafaille, S., Kroll, R., Crawley, A. and Gracco, V. (2008), "The effects of simulated stuttering and prolonged speech on the neural activation patterns of stuttering and nonstuttering adults", *Brain and Language*, Vol. 107, pp. 114–123.

Eggers, K., De Nil, L. and Vandenbergh, B. (2010), "Temperament dimensions in stuttering and typically developing children", *Journal of Fluency Disorders*, Vol. 35, pp. 355–372.

Foundas, A., Bollich, A., Feldman, J., Corey, D., Hurley, M., Lemen, L. and Heilman, K. (2004), "Aberrant auditory processing and atypical planum temporale in developmental stuttering", *Neurology*, Vol. 63, pp. 1640–1646.

Fox, P., Ingham, R., Ingham, J., Hirsch, T., Downs, J., Martin, C., *et al.* (1996), "A PET study of the neural systems of stuttering", *Nature*, Vol. 382, pp. 158–162.

Giraud, A., Neumann, K., Bachoud-Levi, A., Von Gudenberg, A., Euler, H., Lanfermann, H., *et al.* (2008), "Severity of dysfluency correlates with basal ganglia activity in persistent developmental stuttering", *Brain and Language*, Vol. 104, pp. 190–199.

Ingham, R., Fox, P., Ingham, J., Zamarripa, F., Martin, C., Jerabek, P. and Cotton, J. (1996), "Functional-lesion investigation of developmental stuttering with positron emission tomography", *Journal of Speech, Language, and Hearing Research*, Vol. 39, pp. 1208–1227.

Ingham, R., Grafton, S., Bothe, A. and Ingham, J. (2012), "Brain activity in adults who stutter: Similarities across speaking tasks and correlations with stuttering frequency and speaking rate", *Brain and Language*, Vol. 122, pp. 11–24.

Jäncke, L., Hänggi, J. and Steinmetz, H. (2004), "Morphological brain differences between adult stutterers and non-stutterers", *BMC Neurology*, Vol. 4, pp. 1–8.

Kell, C. (2012), "Resting-state MRI: A peek through the keyhole on therapy for stuttering", *Neurology*, Vol. 79, pp. 614–615.

Kell, C., Neumann, K., Von Kriegstein, K., Posenenske, C., Von Gudenberg, A., Euler, H., *et al.* (2009), "How the brain repairs stuttering", *Brain*, Vol. 132, pp. 2747–2760.

Loucks, T. and De Nil, L. (2012), "Oral sensorimotor integration in adults who stutter", *Folia Phoniatrica et Logopaedica*, Vol. 64, pp. 116–121.

Loucks, T., Kraft, S., Choo, A.L., Sharma, H. and Ambrose, N. (2011), "Functional brain activation differences in stuttering identified with a rapid fMRI sequence", *Journal of Fluency Disorders*, Vol. 36, pp. 302–307.

Lu, C., Chen, C., Ning, N., Ding, G., Guo, T., Peng, D., *et al.* (2010), "The neural substrates for atypical planning and execution of word production in stuttering", *Experimental Neurology*, Vol. 221, pp. 146–156.

Meyer-Lindenberg, A. and Weinberger, D. (2006), "Intermediate phenotypes and genetic mechanisms of psychiatric disorders", *Nature Reviews Neuroscience*, Vol. 7, pp. 818–827.

Neumann, K., Euler, H., Von Gudenberg, A., Giraud, A., Lanfermann, H., Gall, V., *et al.* (2003), "The nature and treatment of stuttering as revealed by fMRI – A within- and between-group comparison", *Journal of Fluency Disorders*, Vol. 28, pp. 381–410.

Olander, L., Smith, A. and Zelaznik, H. (2010), "Evidence that a motor timing deficit is a factor in the development of stuttering", *Journal of Speech, Language, and Hearing Research*, Vol. 53, pp. 876–886.

Packman, A., Code, C. and Onslow, M. (2007), "On the cause of stuttering: Integrating theory with brain and behavioral research", *Journal of Neurolinguistics*, Vol. 20, pp. 353–362.

Raznahan, A., Shaw, P., Lalonde, F., Stockman, M., Wallace, G., Greenstein, D., *et al.* (2011), How does your cortex grow?, *Journal of Neuroscience*, Vol. 31, pp. 7174–7177.

Sasisekaran, J. and Byrd, C. (2013), "Nonword repetition and phoneme elision skills in school-age children who do and do not stutter", *International Journal of Language and Communication Disorders*, Vol. 48, pp. 625–639.

Smith, A., Goffman, L., Sasisekaran, J. and Weber-Fox, C. (2012), "Language and motor abilities of preschool children who stutter: Evidence from behavioral and kinematic indices of nonword repetition performance", *Journal of Fluency Disorders*, Vol. 37, pp. 344–358.

Smits-Bandstra, S. and De Nil, L. (2007), "Sequence skill learning in persons who stutter: Implications for cortico-striato-thalamo-cortical dysfunction", *Journal of Fluency Disorders*, Vol. 32, pp. 251–278.

Sommer, M., Koch, M., Paulus, W., Weiller, C. and Büchel, C. (2002), "Disconnection of speech-relevant brain areas in persistent developmental stuttering", *Lancet*, Vol. 360, pp. 380–383.

Sowman, P., Crain, S., Harrison, E. and Johnson, B. (2012), "Reduced activation of left orbitofrontal cortex precedes blocked vocalization: A magnetoencephalographic study", *Journal of Fluency Disorders*, Vol. 37, pp. 359–365.

Taubert, M., Villringer, A. and Ragert, P. (2012), "Learning-related gray and white matter changes in humans: An update", *Neuroscientist*, Vol. 18, pp. 320–325.

Theys, C., De Nil, L., Thijs, V., Van Wieringen, A. and Sunaert, S. (2012), "A crucial role for the cortico-striato-cortical loop in the pathogenesis of stroke-related neurogenic stuttering", *Human Brain Mapping*, Vol. 34, pp. 2103–2112.

Toyomura, A., Fujii, T. and Kuriki, S. (2011), "Effect of external auditory pacing on the neural activity of stuttering speakers", *NeuroImage*, Vol. 57, pp. 1507–1516.

Watkins, K., Smith, S., Davis, S. and Howell, P. (2008), "Structural and functional abnormalities of the motor system in developmental stuttering", *Brain*, Vol. 131, pp. 50–59.

Watson, B., Pool, K., Devous, M. and Freeman, F. (1992), "Brain blood flow related to acoustic laryngeal reaction time in adult developmental stutterers", *Journal of Speech and Hearing Research*, Vol. 35, pp. 555–561.

Wood, F., Stump, D., Mckeehan, A., Sheldon, S. and Proctor, J. (1980), "Patterns of regional cerebral blood flow during attempted reading aloud by stutterers both on and off haloperidol medication: Evidence for inadequate left frontal activation during stuttering", *Brain and Language*, Vol. 9, pp. 141–144.

Wymbs, N., Ingham, R., Ingham, J., Paolini, K. and Grafton, S. (2013), "Individual differences in neural regions functionally related to real and imagined stuttering", *Brain and Language*, Vol. 124, pp. 153–164.

Xuan, Y., Meng, C., Yang, Y., Zhu, C., Wang, L., Yan, Q., *et al.* (2012), "Resting-state brain activity in adult males who stutter", *PLoS ONE*, Vol. 7, p. e30570.

Yairi, E. and Ambrose, N. (1999), "Early childhood stuttering I: Persistency and recovery rates", *Journal of Speech, Language, and Hearing Research*, Vol. 42, pp. 1097–1112.

Yairi, E. and Ambrose, N. (2013), "Epidemiology of stuttering: 21st century advances", *Journal of Fluency Disorders*, Vol. 38, pp. 66–87.

5

SPEECH AND LANGUAGE DISORDERS IN CHILDREN WITH CRANIOFACIAL MALFORMATIONS

Robert J. Shprintzen

Craniofacial anomalies are among the most common of congenital disorders in humans. Although there have been a number of studies sponsored by the World Health Organization, various national health agencies, and independent researchers, the true frequency of craniofacial anomalies remains elusive. One of the reasons for the difficulty in pinning down the frequency of such anomalies is that there are a large number of malformations that can affect the craniofacial complex and many of them are features in multiple anomaly syndromes. As an example, Apert syndrome, a well-recognized genetic disorder, has cleft palate, maxillary deficiency, dental malocclusion, wide-spaced eyes, shallow orbits, and premature fusion of the cranial sutures. Therefore, specific numbers of anomalies may be difficult to estimate accurately, but we do know that estimates show that craniofacial anomalies are among the most frequent congenital abnormalities.

It is very likely that nearly all speech–language pathologists (SLPs) and audiologists encounter children who are affected. The frequency of cleft palate with or without cleft lip is generally estimated to be about 1 per 600 living individuals. This does not include submucous cleft palate that has been reported to be as frequent as 1 per 30 people in the general population, although often asymptomatic (Shprintzen *et al.*, 1985). There are also hundreds of rare genetic mutations that cause craniofacial malformations. Although each of these rare disorders affect small numbers of people, in total there are hundreds of thousands of children with these rare complex disorders added to the population annually. Because speech, language, and hearing are all completely dependent on the structures of the head and neck, a very high percentage of these cases require the services of communication disorders specialists.

Almost all children with craniofacial anomalies, including those that cause major functional problems in children, attend public schools because of the availability of special services within most school systems. Moreover, many states currently have mandated early intervention services for children with multiple anomaly syndromes, speech and language disorders, and hearing impairment. Therefore, a very large percentage of SLPs will have children with craniofacial anomalies in their caseload. This chapter will attempt to add to the reader's knowledge of craniofacial disorders by approaching the problems in relation to how congenital anomalies can lead to specific speech symptoms, what causes these anomalies, and how the primary etiologies for the anomalies can affect treatment outcomes. Evaluation techniques will be discussed within this framework, as will treatment protocols, including emphasis on those treatments that are known to be effective and those that are known to have no known benefit.

The literature and accepted clinical practice demonstrate a problem

A review of the literature over the past decade clearly demonstrates a problem within the communication sciences in terms of providing information about the most core element of what its clinicians do. Reviewing the major literature search engines and databases for studies that directly relate to cleft palate, craniofacial anomalies, and communication disorders shows an astonishing lack of scientific publications describing therapeutic techniques (new or old) and treatment outcome studies. There were nearly 1250 articles cited in PubMed or Medline relating to craniofacial disorders and communication issues. Most are related to cleft palate, focusing on surgical outcomes from operations such as palate repair, surgery for velopharyngeal insufficiency (VPI), maxillofacial and craniofacial reconstruction, tongue surgery, and mandibular surgery. In total, there were fewer than 20 publications, approximately 0.01 percent, describing speech–language therapy procedures or reporting therapy outcomes.

Speech–language therapy techniques are more typically discussed in textbooks, but what is lacking are outcome data that substantiate the efficacy of such techniques. Since many training programs do not offer specific coursework in this area, this chapter will discuss craniofacial disorders within the framework of the communication impairments likely to be associated with the various types of anomalies commonly seen in clinical settings by SLPs.

Craniofacial disorders and communicative impairment

The craniofacial complex is comprised of a number of separate yet interrelated segments: the calvarium (or calvaria) which is the upper portion of the skull covering the brain; the skull base (basicranium); the orbitonasal complex and maxilla (including the palate); and the mandible (including the tongue). When integrated together, these components constitute the skull and face along with all of its functions that include eating, speaking, hearing, seeing, and our cognitive and behavioral traits. It is obvious that congenital anomalies of the eyes, the nose, or the shape of the calvarium will be unlikely to directly impact speech production, language acquisition, or hearing, but it is often true that anomalies of any of the structures of the craniofacial complex will signal the presence of an overall abnormality of craniofacial embryogenesis that has implications for communication impairment. Therefore, it is important for clinicians to be aware that the presence of an anomaly, such as cleft palate, does not predict specific symptoms or indicate a specific treatment if other anomalies are also present. The presence of multiple anomalies in a single individual most often signals the presence of a syndrome. The interaction of the multiple anomalies in syndromes can create a specific profile, or phenotypic spectrum, of communicative impairments, as well as a pattern of the expression of communicative impairments over time, known as the natural history of the syndrome (Shprintzen, 1997). Syndromes also often have a predictable prognosis (Shprintzen, 1997) that may limit the treatment options if the outcome is predictably poor. An example may help to clarify the issue of isolated versus syndromic anomalies.

Clinicians associate cleft palate with hypernasal speech and possible secondary articulation impairment referred to as compensatory articulation disorder (Golding-Kushner, 2001). If a child presents with hypernasal speech, clinicians are likely to find a history of overt or submucous cleft palate, although the majority of children who have had overt palatal clefts repaired, and most children with submucous cleft palate do not have velopharyngeal insufficiency (VPI). The success rate with palate repair in overt clefts is typically cited at approximately 70 to 90 percent (Sullivan *et al.*, 2009), while it has been reported that most children with submucous clefts are not hypernasal (Shprintzen *et al.*, 1985). Therefore, when a child presents with hypernasality, it is important to avoid assumptions and determine the cause of the problem based on what is known about the total picture of the child.

If the child has no other anomalies that can be gleaned from history, observation, and review of past records, then a beginning assumption prior to any instrumental assessments of VPI is that the problem is one of palatal structure. However, if there is a history of multiple anomalies, or the clinician's observation is that there are abnormalities that go beyond the cleft, then the reason for the symptom and the potential treatments may be quite different. For example, VPI is a common finding in many multiple anomaly syndromes, including velo-cardio-facial syndrome (VCFS), Prader-Willi syndrome, and oculo-auriculo-vertebral spectrum (OAVS) (Shprintzen, 2000b). The cause for the VPI and recommended management for each syndrome can be quite different because of the associated anomalies. VCFS has multiple anomalies that impact velopharyngeal closure, including structural anomalies of the velum, hypotonia of the pharynx, a deep pharynx, and asymmetry of the palate and pharynx. In Prader-Willi, cleft palate is not a feature and VPI is related to severe hypotonia that resolves with age (Shprintzen, 2000b). In OAVS, clefting is common, but so is severe asymmetry of the pharyngeal and palatal movement and structure, often the root of VPI (Shprintzen *et al.*, 1980; Shprintzen, 2000b). The treatment of VPI in VCFS has been shown to be different than for isolated clefting (Shprintzen and Golding-Kushner, 2008), often requiring very wide pharyngeal flaps rather than other reconstructive procedures. In Prader-Willi syndrome, VPI is related only to severe hypotonia, and it resolves with age, therefore not requiring surgical management at all (Kleppe *et al.*, 1990; Shprintzen, 2000b). In OAVS, VPI is almost always asymmetric so that gaps are rarely located centrally and surgical procedures designed to close a central gap typically fail (Shprintzen *et al.*, 1980). Therefore, although hypernasal speech secondary to VPI is present in all three syndromes, the direct cause and treatment are different. Clinicians should conclude that each case must have a careful review of a detailed history with special attention to the physical and developmental issues considered to be outside of the range of normal.

Clinician observations: Being on the lookout

It should be standard practice for clinicians to request any and all medical records for review, especially if there are known problems that have required tertiary assessments, such as visits to a specialist beyond the primary care physician. Requests for growth charts (height, weight, and head circumference), developmental milestones, and the results of any radiographic procedures, standardized cognitive assessments, or other specialty assessments should also be obtained. The reason for referral should be made very clear to the clinician so it can be seen within the context of any historical information obtained. Included in the reason for referral should be a detailed description from the parent/caregiver of the nature of the problem. This author's experience is that a careful analysis of history narrows the search for a clinical diagnosis, focusing the clinician's evaluation on likely scenarios.

Craniofacial anatomy is typically easily observable by clinicians during the course of any type of evaluation, including speech, language, cognitive, and hearing assessments. Clinicians should be able to note observations about a child's appearance and behavior and ask questions of the parents or caregivers about these observations when appropriate. Besides the standard oral examination, clinicians can observe properties of the skull, eyes, ears, nose, mouth, maxilla, mandible, and the intraoral structures. These will be described below.

Skull shape, size and symmetry

Abnormalities of skull shape, size and symmetry can be related to three possible causes: craniosynostosis (premature fusion of the cranial sutures), underlying abnormalities of brain shape and/or size, and positional molding. Craniosynostosis occurs both as an isolated and syndromic finding. As an isolated finding, craniosynostosis results in variations of cranial shape, but does not typically result in abnormalities of development or cognition. In syndromes with craniosynostosis, associated findings often include speech, language, cognitive, and hearing disorders (Shprintzen, 2000a). Cleft palate occurs in association with several of these syndromes and another common association is abnormalities of the limbs. A comprehensive listing of syndromes with craniosynostosis and their communicative impairments are available in compendium form (Shprintzen, 2000b) while a general listing of craniosynostosis syndromes can be found online at OMIM (2014), a free access resource.

When skull size is above the ninety-eighth percentile or below the second percentile, it is considered abnormal. In both cases, the problem can be either the bones of the skull or the brain. If the brain is too large, the result is a large head circumference known as macrencephaly, whereas if the large size is related to skull thickness or hydrocephalus, it is referred to as macrocephaly. Similarly, small head circumference can be classified as micrencephaly or microcephaly, although many clinicians refer to small brain size resulting in reduced head circumference as primary microcephaly, while small head size related to bone abnormalities (including caniosynostosis) is referred to as secondary microcephaly. In the cases of both large and small head circumferences, there is the frequent association of cognitive and language abnormalities and potential motor speech impairment because of the brain's direct control over these functions. Syndromes associated with head size abnormalities can also be found in compendium form (Shprintzen, 2000b) and on OMIM (2014).

Symmetry of the cranium is often caused by positional molding, often called posterior positional plagiocephaly (PPP). PPP has increased in frequency since the American Academy of Pediatrics (AAP) recommended in 1992 that babies be positioned on their backs during sleep to reduce the risk of Sudden Infant Death Syndrome (AAP, 2013). If infants get into a persistent favored position with the left or right posterior cranium persistently pressed against the mattress, the external force will mold the cranium so that the skull adopts a parallelogram shape with the forehead more anterior on one side and the opposite side of the posterior cranium more flattened. PPP by itself does not impact on speech, language, or cognition, but if the PPP is related to low muscle tone or excessive muscle tone that reduces movement of the head during sleep, then the PPP is secondary to a possible abnormality of brain function that could also result in communicative impairment.

Position, structure and symmetry of the eyes

Because the position of the eyes is dictated in large part by the structure of the cranium, noticing differences in eye placement can be an important observation relative to the presence of a multiple anomaly disorder. When the eyes are at a different vertical or horizontal placement, the anomaly is known as dystopia. Dystopia can be related to underlying brain anomalies, but positional molding can also result in a different position of the cranial bones in which case the brain is more likely to be normal.

When eyes are positioned more laterally than normal so that the eyes are further apart than normal, the condition is known as hypertelorism. Hypertelorism is associated with a large number of craniofacial syndromes, many of which have speech, language, and cognitive impairments as a feature. Hypertelorism can be caused by underlying thickening of the cranial bones, or underlying abnormalities of the brain including hydrocephalus or macrencephaly. In cases where the brain is involved, there is a high likelihood of speech and language impairment. Many of these syndromes also have cleft palate as a feature. When thickening of the bones is the cause, as in craniometaphyseal dysplasia or craniodiaphyseal dysplasia, hyponasality is common because the bony overgrowth may also cause obstruction of the nasal cavity (Shprintzen, 2000b).

If the eyes are more medially displaced than normal, the result is eyes that are too close together, known as hypotelorism. Hypotelorism is more frequently associated with underlying brain anomalies than hypertelorism. This is because the two primary causes of hypotelorism are microcephaly/micrencephaly and midline abnormalities of the brain. Hypotelorism is a strong indicator of possible underlying deficiency of neural tissue, primarily in brain parts derived from the prosencephalon. The frontal lobes and the prefrontal cortex, so vital to cognitive development, are typically smaller than normal in cases of hypotelorism. Although some cases of hypotelorism can be related to positional molding of the skull (prenatal or postnatal) or synostosis of the median suture in the frontal bone, most cases are related to brain development.

Eye structure

Observations of eye color, shape of the pupils, or the presence of any abnormal structures in or on the eye should be noted. One of the more noticeable anomalies is a coloboma, or cleft, of the iris making the iris and pupil look like a keyhole rather than two concentric circles. Iris colobomas often accompany underlying abnormalities of the optic nerve and brain indicating a developmental anomaly of the central nervous system that might cause developmental, language and speech disorders.

Position, structure and symmetry of the ears

Ear position, like eye position, is also affected by underlying abnormalities of skull shape. Ear structure should generally be symmetric, and differences between ear size and structure can be associated with a number of multiple anomaly syndromes that have a high association of speech, language, and cognitive disorders. Cleft palate is also a commonly associated finding with anomalous ears.

Size, structure, and position of the nose

The nose is one of the most variable of structures in humans. There are substantial ethnic and racial variations in nose anatomy, and the nose also is highly responsive to growth and change during puberty. Therefore, minor variations in nasal structure and position are probably not very informative based on casual observation, but there are certain minor variations that may be of interest. The glabella (the place where the nasal bridge meets the forehead) can be unusual in appearance in a number of syndromes, such as the "Greek helmet" appearance of the nasal bridge and eyes in Wolf-Hirschhorn syndrome or the nasal bridge that extends directly from the frontal bone in Treacher Collins syndrome. The placement of the nose on the face in OAVS can be asymmetric. However, it is rare that a diagnosis can be confirmed or rejected based on nasal anatomy alone.

Size and symmetry of the mouth

Mouth size and shape is also highly variable and is dependent on the underlying skeletal structure of the maxilla and mandible. Very small or very large mouth size can be a clinical finding of importance. A number of genetic disorders have microstomia (a small mouth) while several others have macrostomia (a large mouth). Microstomia is usually reported when the corners of the mouth do not extend beyond the outermost rim of the nostrils on each side of the nose. Macrostomia is more of a judgment call made on a mouth that simply appears very large. Syndromes with micro- or macrostomia can be found in Shprintzen (2000b) and OMIM (2014).

Oral symmetry is a clinical finding in a number of disorders that can also be predictive of associated anomalies that can affect speech and language. Asymmetric animation of the oral musculature is frequent in a number of common syndromes, including OAVS and VCFS among others. Often attributed to an abnormality of the facial nerve, especially in the lower third of the face, the finding is more cosmetic than functional, rarely resulting in articulation or oral resonance abnormalities.

Besides clefting anomalies, the structure of the lips can also be informative. The term "coarse facies" often refers to children with overly prominent lips, as seen in Williams syndrome, Hunter syndrome (and other lysosomal storage diseases) and Costello syndrome. The presence of macrostomia often accompanies large lips.

Size, position and symmetry of the maxilla

The maxilla constitutes most of the midface from the bone containing the upper teeth to the base of the orbits. Abnormalities of the maxilla are present in many multiple anomaly disorders that have communicative impairment, and when the position of the maxilla relative to the mandible results in a severe malocclusion, articulation will very often be impaired by obligatory errors related to difficulties with tongue placement. Articulation errors could be related to a deep maxillary overbite, a severely retruded maxilla, an anterior open-bite, or asymmetric structure. Any sound requiring movement of or contact with the tongue, teeth, and lips could be affected by an abnormal relationship between the upper and lower jaws or abnormal movements of the tongue and lower jaw in relation to the maxilla. Micorognathia, prognathism, and other maxillary and mandibular anomalies are listed in compendium form in relation to communication impairment (Shprintzen, 2000b) and in relation to general findings (OMIM, 2014).

Size, position and symmetry of the mandible

Mandibular anomalies are common and can be caused by disorders of embryogenesis (such as genetic or teratogenic influence) as well as positional problems, specifically compression of the fetal lower jaw secondary to intrauterine crowding or oligohydramnios (Shprintzen, 1997). Unlike the maxilla which is stationary, the mandible is a moving structure making anomalies both structural and functional. Abnormalities of the mandible can include abnormally small size (micrognathia), abnormally large size (macrognathia, more commonly referred to as mandibular prognathism), asymmetry, and limited range of motion. All of these problems can cause speech disorders. Mandibular abnormalities are frequently part of multiple anomaly syndrome findings and most of these syndromes have disorders of communication and many have disorders of cognition and language development.

Asymmetry of the mandible by itself may not cause many communication problems, but is likely to be a sign of an underlying syndromic diagnosis that has broader implications for communication because of accompanying findings, such as abnormalities of the upper airway, asymmetric movement of the velum resulting in VPI, and asymmetric movement of the tongue. OAVS is one example of these problems, but asymmetry is found in a number of other disorders as well (Shprintzen, 2000b).

Intraoral structures

The tongue

Congenital anomalies of the tongue are not common. Tongue size tends to vary with mandibular size. People with small mandibles (micrognathia) tend to have small tongues; people with prognathism tend to have large tongues. There are a number of multiple anomaly disorders that feature tongue anomalies including hypoplastic tongue, hyperplastic tongue, and cleft or lobulated tongue. A high percentage of these disorders also have cognitive impairment that contributes to communicative impairment, and in some, anomalies of the tongue may be contributory, but in most cases, the contribution of the tongue is minimal. To date there is no well-controlled data to suggest that tongue reconstruction, tongue reduction, or other surgical procedures have a positive impact on speech in people with tongue anomalies.

The teeth

Dentition can play a role in speech impairment when anomalous, although abnormal dentition is also often accompanied by jaw malformations as well as neurologic disorders in some cases. Occlusal disorders, like anterior open-bites, are typically related to jaw relationships, not dental problems, except in cases of severe thumb-sucking or prolonged pacifier use. Other dental anomalies include absent teeth, small teeth, large teeth, but these disorders rarely result in significant speech disorders.

The palate

The palate consists of the anterior portion, the hard palate, and posteriorly, the soft palate, or velum. Clefts of the palate vary in severity, ranging from overt clefts of the entire palate from the incisive foramen through the uvula, to submucous clefts (Figure 5.1). Overt clefts will certainly affect speech if unrepaired because of the lack of separation of the oral and nasal cavities. Once surgically repaired, the majority of children go on to develop normal resonance without additional surgery. In some cases, secondary surgery is necessary if the child has residual VPI. If the cleft involves only the muscles of the velum, but the overlying mucous membrane is intact (submucous cleft palate), VPI occurs in less than half of these individuals. Observable VPI and abnormal nasal resonance has been reported in about 20 percent of cases (Shprintzen *et al.*, 1985). Submucous cleft palate is usually recognized by the presence of a bifid uvula and, in obvious cases, a thin membranous area, known as a zona pellucida, can be seen in the midline of the velum (Figure 5.1) and a notch in the posterior border of the hard palate can be palpated.

An under-recognized abnormality of the palate is known as the occult submucous cleft (Croft *et al.*, 1978). First described by Kaplan (1975) based on surgical dissection of the velum, the disorder was eventually defined by nasopharyngoscopic findings of absence of the musculus uvulae on the nasal surface of the velum (Shprintzen, 1982, 2005). On oral examination, an occult submucous cleft palate cannot be differentiated from a normal palate (Figure 5.1). There is no bifid uvula or zona pellucida. This is because the defect is isolated to the muscles of the velum, and all of the muscles are arranged on the nasal surface of the velum. The oral side of

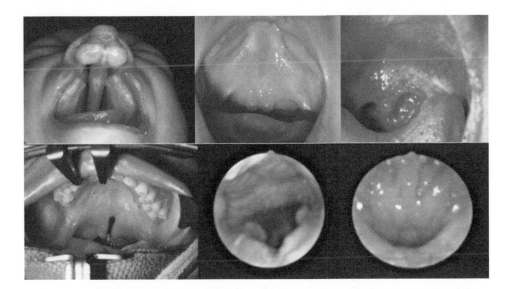

Figure 5.1 Upper left, overt bilateral cleft of the lip and palate; lower left, cleft of the soft palate only; upper center, submucous cleft of the soft palate; lower center, nasopharyngoscopic appearance of the velum in that case showing a deep midline groove where the musculus uvulae is absent and the muscles are separated; top right, occult submucous cleft velum showing a normal appearing soft palate; bottom right, nasopharyngoscopy in that case showing absence of the musculus uvulae and a concave nasal surface of the velum.

the velum is comprised of a sheet of ligamentous tissue, the aponeurosis, covered by mucous membrane. Occult submucous cleft palate is a strong biomarker for VCFS, but the anomaly can also be present in otherwise normal people and in other syndromes.

Velopharyngeal closure and VPI

Velopharyngeal closure, which cannot be seen directly without instrumentation such as fluoroscopy and endoscopy, is a learned motor task and requires the articulation of the velum to the surrounding pharyngeal walls (lateral and posterior). Both the completeness of closure and the timing of the movements of the velum and pharyngeal walls are critical to the development of normal oral pressure during the production of pressure consonants.

In most people, when the velopharyngeal valve closes during the normal production of non-nasal speech, there is an airtight seal that separates the oral cavity from the nasal cavity. In some cases, there can be a small leak of air from the oropharynx into the nasopharynx that is either inaudible or not distracting enough to be labeled as abnormal. In cases where an air leak is significant enough to be audible, several direct symptoms may be evident: abnormal nasal resonance of sound, persistent audible nasal airflow, or occasional bursts of nasal air that have a "snort like" quality. None of these findings are mutually exclusive, but all are caused by an abnormal opening in the velopharyngeal valve. When this problem is consistent and present for all oral speech sounds, there is a strong likelihood that its cause is structural or neurological, and in nearly all cases, remediation of abnormal nasality is not possible using speech therapy techniques (Golding-Kushner, 2001; Golding-Kushner and Shprintzen, 2010). The causes for consistent VPI include structural anomalies of the velum, central nervous system disorders, and a number of neuromuscular diseases including muscular dystrophies and progressive myopathies. It is important to understand that in cases where VPI is related to neurologic problems, there may be concomitant effects on speech including disorders of rate, fluency, and motor movements.

Nasal fricatives

Inconsistent nasal emission of air during normally oral sound production is usually a learned error and most often occurs on fricative and sibilant sounds. Often referred to as "nasal fricatives," (Witzel, 1995) or sound-specific VPI, these substitutions occur as frequently in children who do not have cleft palate as they occur in children with cleft palate and often occur in children with hypertrophic tonsils. Because nasal fricatives are learned errors, correct production of the sound can be taught in speech therapy. A nasal fricative is produced by pushing air through the nose creating a "hissing" sound that qualifies as a fricative. Nasal fricative substitutions are often seen for the sounds /s/, /z/, /f/, /v/, and occasionally for affricates.

It is also possible for some children to learn to produce other sounds by directing air out of the nose, but in all of these cases, the problem can be corrected by teaching the child to redirect airflow through the mouth. This can be done by using nasal occlusion, while in other cases the correct manner of production is taught by using a phoneme that is produced correctly and has a similar placement or mode of production. For example, if there is nasal escape on /s/, but a voiceless /th/ is produced correctly, simply request a prolonged production of the voiceless /th/ and then instruct the child to retract the tongue behind the teeth while still making the /th/. This will result in the production of /s/. Another strategy is to have a normal /t/ produced while placing a coffee stirrer or thin straw along the midline of the tongue and press down on it while a forceful /t/ is produced. This will also result in the correct production of /s/. Once the sound is obtained, it should be produced over and over again in a rapid drill and demonstrated for parents so they can reinforce it at home (Golding-Kushner, 2001). The child can be taught to recognize the difference between oral and nasal emission of air during sound production using nasal occlusion. Therapy for this type of articulation substitution is typically rapid, sometimes resolved within a very small number of sessions. It is important to remember that this is not VPI, but rather a different way of producing frication that is nothing more than an articulation error.

Consistent VPI

When hypernasality or nasal air escape is detected across all sounds, there is no technique of speech therapy that will resolve the problem with one exception. If the child has developed a compensatory articulation pattern (glottal stops, pharyngeal stops, pharyngeal fricatives, etc.) from the onset of speech, it is common for the velopharyngeal mechanism to show no movement during non-nasal speech production (Henningsson and Isberg, 1986). This is because the production of glottal stops cuts off airflow at the level of the vocal folds. With the airflow effectively modified at that lower level, there is no reason for the valves above the glottis to function during speech. This includes the palate and pharyngeal walls, the tongue, lips, and teeth. It is typical in cases with ubiquitous glottal stop substitutions for articulatory movements to be absent during productions of oral consonants except for /m/, /n/, and /ŋ/. It has been found that if correct production of orally produced pressure consonants is established, improved movement can be seen in the velum and pharynx (Henningsson and Isberg, 1986; Golding-Kushner, 2001). In some cases, eliminating glottal stops can improve movement in the velopharyngeal valve so much that VPI and hypernasality can be eliminated or improved to the point where surgical management is no longer necessary (Golding-Kushner, 2001). It is therefore typically recommended in cases with VPI and gross glottal stop substitutions that surgical management be delayed until it is determined if improvement in oral articulation can also improve velopharyngeal valving. These therapy procedures must be focused on eliminating abnormal compensations (i.e., glottal stop) rather than the teaching of oral placement (Golding-Kushner, 1995; Golding-Kushner, 2001; Golding-Kushner and Shprintzen, 2010).

Assessment of VPI

The assessment of VPI is critical for determining its cause, consistency, and the need for surgical intervention. Although there are many indirect procedures for assessing hypernasality, such as nasometry, the best instrument for determining abnormality of resonance is the ear of an experienced clinician. Following that, if VPI is suspected or confirmed by listening, two instrumental tests are considered to be indispensable: multi-view videofluoroscopy and nasopharyngoscopy (Golding-Kushner *et al.*, 1990; Shprintzen, 1995). A protocol for reporting the results of these examinations has been suggested by using a ratio scale developed by an international working group (Golding-Kushner *et al.*, 1990). Experience has shown it to be very useful for defining velopharyngeal gaps in terms of their location and relative size. Indirect procedures, such as nasometry, may be able to reliably compute the degree of nasal resonance, but the technique does not provide any information about the nature of the VPI or what causes it.

Summary

Unlike the rest of our anatomy, the craniofacial complex is uniquely relevant to the process of communication. Whether it is speech production, cognition, language, or hearing, all of these functions reside in the craniofacial structures. Craniofacial anomalies are common and directly impact speech and language and it is therefore likely that many children seen by SLPs will have associated anomalies of craniofacial structure and function. In this chapter, the complexity and interrelationship of the structures and functions of our craniofacial features has been discussed to present a broad base of thinking that demonstrates that focusing on a single symptom is too narrow an approach to the successful diagnosis and treatment of communication disorders.

References

American Academy of Pediatrics (2013), "AAP Expands Guidelines for Infant Sleep Safety and SIDS Risk Reduction", at www.aap.org/en-us/about-the-aap/aap-press-room/pages/AAP-Expands-Guidelines-for-Infant-Sleep-Safety-and-SIDS-Risk-Reduction.aspx, (accessed 10/29/13).

Croft, C.B., Shprintzen, R.J., Daniller, A.I. and Lewin, M.L. (1978), "The occult submucous cleft palate and the musculus uvuli", *Cleft Palate Journal*, Vol. 15, p. 1504.

Golding-Kushner, K.J. (1995), "Treatment of articulation and resonance disorders associated with cleft palate and VPI", in Shprintzen R.J. and Bardach, J. (Eds.), *Cleft Palate Speech Management*, Mosby, St. Louis, MO, US, pp. 327–351.

Golding-Kushner K.J. (2001), *Therapy Techniques for Cleft Palate Speech and Related Disorders*, Singular Publishing, San Diego, CA, US.

Golding-Kushner, K.J. and Shprintzen, R.J. (2010), *Velo-Cardio-Facial Syndrome, Volume II*, Plural Publishing, San Diego, CA, US.

Golding-Kushner, K.J., Argamaso, R.V., Cotton, R.T., Grames, L.M., Henningsson, G., Jones, *et al.*, (1990), "Standardization for the reporting of nasopharyngoscopy and multi-view videofluoroscopy: A report from an international working group", *Cleft Palate Journal*, Vol. 27, pp. 337–347.

Henningsson, G. and Isberg, A. (1986), "Velopharyngeal movement patterns in patients alternating between oral and glottal articulation: A clinical and cineradiographical study", *Cleft Palate Journal*, Vol. 23, pp. 1–9.

Kaplan, E.N. (1975), "The occult submucous cleft palate", *Cleft Palate Journal*, Vol. 12, pp. 356–368.

Kleppe, S.A., Katayama, K.M., Shipley, K.G. and Foushee, D.R. (1990), "The speech and language characteristics of children with Prader-Willi syndrome", *Journal of Speech and Hearing Disorders*, Vol. 55, pp. 300–309.

OMIM (2014), *Online Mendelian Inheritance in Man*, (authored and edited at the McKusick-Nathans Institute of Genetic Medicine, Johns Hopkins University School of Medicine, under the direction of Dr. Ada Hamosh) at www.ncbi.nlm.nih.gov/omim/ (accessed 10/29/13).

Shprintzen, R.J. (1982), "Palatal and pharyngeal anomalies in craniofacial syndromes", *Birth Defects Original Article Series*, Vol. 18, No. 1, p. 5378.

Shprintzen, R.J. (1995), "Instrumental assessment of velopharyngeal valving", in Shprintzen R.J. and Bardach, J. (Eds.), *Cleft Palate Speech Management*, Mosby, St. Louis, MO, US, pp. 221–256.

Shprintzen, R.J. (1997), *Genetics, Syndromes, and Communication Disorders*, Singular Publishing, San Diego, US, pp. 4–6.

Shprintzen, R.J. (2000a), "Speech and language disorders in syndromes of craniosynostosis", in Cohen, M.M. Jr. and MacLean, R.E. (Eds.), *Craniosynostosis*. Oxford University Press, New York, NY, pp. 197–203.

Shprintzen, R.J. (2000b), *Syndrome Identification for Speech-Language Pathology: Illustrated Pocket Guide*, Singular Publishing, San Diego, CA, US.

Shprintzen, R.J. (2005), "Velo-cardio-facial syndrome", *Progress in Pediatric Cardiology*, Vol. 20, pp. 187–193.

Shprintzen R.J. and Golding-Kushner, K.J. (2008), *Velo-Cardio-Facial Syndrome, Volume I*, Plural Publishing, San Diego, CA.

Shprintzen, R.J., Croft, C.B., Berkman, M.D. and Rakoff, S.J. (1980), "Velopharyngeal insufficiency in the facioauriculovertebral malformation complex", *Cleft Palate Journal*, Vol. 17, p. 1327.

Shprintzen, R.J., Schwartz, R., Daniller, A. and Hoch, L. (1985), "The morphologic significance of bifid uvula", *Pediatrics*, Vol. 75, p. 55361.

Sullivan, S.R., Marrinan, E.M., LaBrie, R.A., Rogers, G.F. and Mulliken, J.B. (2009), "Palatoplasty outcomes in nonsyndromic patients with cleft palate: A 29 year assessment of one surgeon's experience", *Journal of Craniofacial Surgery*, Vol. 20, pp. 1629–1630.

Witzel, M.A. (1995), "Communication impairment associated with clefting", in Shprintzen, R.J. and Bardach, J. (Eds.), *Cleft Palate Speech Management*, Mosby, St. Louis, MO, pp. 137–175.

6

NEUROPHYSIOLOGY AND VOICE PRODUCTION

Eileen M. Finnegan

A deeper knowledge of laryngeal anatomy and physiology contributes to a better understanding of symptoms experienced by patients with vocal disorders, the nature of the underlying etiology, and enables more flexible thinking about intervention strategies. The significance of this knowledge is reflected in the fact that the larynx serves an important role in vital reflexive and voluntary functions, such as respiration, airway protection, swallowing, and phonation. The emphasis of this chapter, which is presented in three parts, is on the phonatory role of the larynx. First, a discussion of the larynx, its sensory receptors, and intrinsic muscles is presented. Then, the cortical structures and motor pathways that control movement of the larynx are described. Finally, how laryngeal muscles coordinate activity to control aspects of phonation (pitch, register, loudness, and voicing) is discussed.

Laryngeal neuroanatomy

Clinicians who practice in the area of voice treat patients who have some disruption or dysfunction of their sensory-motor system. This can be most clearly appreciated in the case of clients with movement disorders, such as vocal fold paralysis, paresis, vocal tremor, and spasmodic dysphonia. However, in many cases, vocal fold lesions or functional voice disorders result from habituation of an ineffective motor pattern. Although we generally think of voice disorders in terms of muscle activity, the motor system does not operate independently of the sensory system; they function as an integrated system. Therefore, it is useful to review what is known about sensory as well as motor innervation of the larynx.

Sensory innervation

Voice therapists are aware that pain is experienced by patients with posterior (cartilaginous) lesions, like contact ulcer, but not by those with anterior (membranous) lesions, such as vocal nodules. This clinical finding may be related to what is known about the distribution of sensory endings in the larynx. For example, Konig and von Leden (1961) reported that the posterior vocal folds are more richly innervated than the anterior vocal folds. In the cartilaginous vocal folds, there is a continuous network of sensory fiber endings, while the membranous vocal folds contain only isolated neurofibrils and few free nerve endings. The paucity of sensory endings in the membranous vocal folds has the practical effect of depriving patients with anterior vocal fold lesions of the pain sensation that might otherwise motivate them to decrease voice use or change their vocal habits. Therefore, patients with membranous lesions must rely on voice quality, rather than pain, to signal the health of their vocal fold tissue. Alternatively, higher sensitivity in the posterior aspect of the larynx may be necessary for airway protection. The posterior vocal folds separate much more widely than the anterior, therefore the risk for penetration is greater posteriorly.

There are differences in the distribution of sensory nerve endings in the supra- and subglottic regions of the larynx, which may also be related to airway protection. Sensory endings are most frequently observed on the laryngeal surface of the epiglottis, with a relatively large number also located in the arytenoid region, the aryepiglottic folds, and the false vocal folds (Konig and von Leden, 1961). In the subglottic region, sensory receptors are most prevalent on the inferior aspects of the vocal folds, with diminished density toward the trachea. Differences in cough function are noted with stimulation of sensory ending in each laryngeal area. A cough provoked by the perception of a foreign substance in the supraglottic region triggers reflex glottic closure and is designed to prevent substance entry into the trachea. While a cough stimulated by a substance in the trachea causes a brief reflexive opening of the vocal folds in order to expel the item.

Laryngeal muscles

Anatomical studies indicate that most laryngeal muscles can be viewed as a combination of subunits with differing functions. The posterior cricoarytenoid (PCA) muscle, an abductor, is composed of vertical, oblique, and horizontal compartments that differ in fiber orientation (Sanders et al., 1993a). It is speculated that the vertical compartment stabilizes the vocal processes during phonation, the oblique compartment is active in rapid breathing, and the horizontal compartment operates during normal inspiration. The interarytenoid (IA) is composed of the transverse interarytenoid, which contracts to close the posterior glottis, and the oblique interarytenoids, which are a continuation of the aryepiglottic musculature and may contribute to "purse-string" closure during swallowing (Mu et al., 1994). The lateral cricoarytenoid (LCA) muscle is comprised of a single compartment (Sanders et al., 1993b) that contracts to approximate the vocal processes. The thyroarytenoid (TA) muscle consists of the lateral muscularis that activates for reflex glottal closure and the medial vocalis, which activates to cause medial bulging of the membranous vocal folds. The vocalis muscle can be further divided into the superior vocalis and medial inferior vocalis, which may act as separate masses during vibration (Han et al., 1999). Finally, the cricothyroid (CT) muscle is composed of three bellies (rectus, oblique and horizontal) (Mu and Sanders, 2009). The rectus belly may contribute to fast changes in pitch, while the oblique affects slow changes in tension.

Interestingly, histologic studies have found distinct regional differences in the distributions of muscle fiber types within the laryngeal muscles that appear consistent with the proposed function of sub-compartments. For example, the lateral oblique belly of the PCA (active in rapid breathing) has faster fibers than the horizontal belly of the muscle (active in normal breathing). Table 6.1 provides information about the approximate distribution of fiber types in intrinsic laryngeal muscles. Slow fibers (type I) have an oxidative metabolism, generate sustained contractions, and are slow to fatigue, while fast fibers (type II) have an anaerobic metabolism, generate more powerful contractions, and fatigue more rapidly. Fast fibers have been further differentiated based on their power and speed of contraction (Type IIa < IIx < IIb). Hybrid fibers that express two or more fiber types also have been identified. The purpose of these fibers is unclear but they may be transitioning from one fiber type to another (i.e., fibers grow and change to match properties of neural input) or they may be combining to provide a greater range of contractile properties (Korfage *et al.*, 2005). These researchers found a relatively high number of hybrid fibers in the lateral TA muscle.

The finding of laryngeal muscle sub-compartments with differential fiber type composition may be relevant in the interpretation of nasendoscopy findings. For example, vocal fold bowing in elderly patients may be related to muscle atrophy or reduced neural drive secondary to Parkinson's disease. However, when bowing is seen in a healthy larynx, a more likely diagnosis may be muscle tension dysphonia. In this vocal disorder, the likelihood of a paresis that affects only the vocalis sub-compartment of the TA muscle would be relatively low. Instead, it may be that the patient has developed a motor pattern of reduced TA muscle activation during speech that presents as bowing.

Sensorymotor system

The structures involved in voice production are innervated with a highly integrated sensory-motor system. This sensory innervation is provided by the two branches of the vagus nerve: (a) the internal branch of the superior laryngeal branch (SLN), which innervates the supraglottic

Table 6.1 Distribution of fiber types in intrinsic laryngeal muscles* (Wu *et al.*, 2000a, 2000b; Shiotani *et al.*, 1999).

Intrinsic Laryngeal Muscle	Muscle Subunit	Subunit Function	Muscle Fiber Types				Comments
			slow fibers	IIa	IIx	hybrid	
PCA	vertical	stablizer					more fast fibers (hybrids are a combination of fast fibers)
	oblique	rapid breathing	40%	15%	5%	40%	
	horizontal	normal breathing	70%	20%		10%	more slow fibers
IA	transverse	adduct post glottis	20%	60%	20%		information for IA as a whole
	oblique						
LCA		adduct vocal processes	20%	70%	10%		
TA	lateral	reflex glottic closure	20%	20%	5%	55%	more fast fibers compared to medial TA
	medial (superior) medial (inferior)	adduction/ vibration	30%	30%	5%	35%	
CT	rectus	fast pitch changes	40%	55%		5%	
	oblique	slow change in tension	35%	55%		10%	
	horizontal		45%	40%		15%	

*The intrinsic laryngeal muscles include: PCA = posterior cricoarytenoid; IA = interarytenoid; LCA = lateral cricoarytenoid; TA = thyroarytenoid; CT = cricothyroid.

larynx (Sanders and Mu, 1998); and (b) the recurrent laryngeal nerve (RLN), which innervates the subglottic larynx. Motor innervation of the intrinsic laryngeal muscles is provided by; (a) the external branch of the SLN, which innervates the CT muscle; (b) the RLN, which innervates the TA, LCA, and PCA ipsilaterally and the IA muscle bilaterally; and (c) the internal branches of SLN, which also innervate the IA muscle bilaterally, although the purpose of the internal branch SLN innervation to the IA is not clear (Mu *et al.*, 1994; Sanders and Mu, 1998).

Voice clinicians are aware of the importance of sensory information to developing new motor programs. As sensory information is projected to, and motor information is projected from, the cortex, there is thought to be interaction of sensory and motor information at all levels of the pathway. The sensory pathway begins with the sensory fibers of the vagus nerve that project centrally to brainstem nuclei (i.e., the nucleus tractus solitarius and/or parabrachial nucleus), then to the thalamus (i.e. the ventral posteromedial nucleus) and on to the lateral post-central cortex (Larson *et al.*, 1993). In addition, there is some limited knowledge regarding anatomical connections between the sensory and motor systems. For example, there are direct projections from the nucleus tractus solitarius and the parabrachial nucleus to the nucleus ambiguus, which is the brainstem motor nucleus containing the neuronal cell bodies that project to laryngeal muscles (Larson *et al.*, 1993). These motor pathways are detailed in the next section.

Two motor systems involved in vocalization

There are two motor systems involved in the production of speech: one phonatory and one responsible for fine motor control, the articulatory pathway (Holstege and Ehling, 1996). An illustration of these pathways is provided in Figure 6.1. The phonatory pathway, which has been referred to as the cingulo-periaqueductal pathway (Jürgens, 2009), is a pathway that we share with other animals. Although other animals do not have the ability to speak, they do have the ability to phonate, and they often use this ability to express a variety of emotions. Likewise, this pathway may assist in the expression of emotion in humans as well. On the other hand, the ability to mold vocalization into speech is the result of activation of the articulatory pathway or the corticobulbar tract carries motor information from the cortex to the brain stem. Jürgens (2009) suggests that the two pathways converge at the level of the premotor areas in the reticulatory formations in the pons and medulla (as shown with dotted line in Figure 6.1). Information from the two separate pathways comes together in a well integrated manner for normal speech production.

The phonatory pathway

The phonatory pathway originates in the limbic system. Electrical stimulation of the anterior cingulate cortex, hypothalamus, and amygdala has been found to elicit vocalization in a monkey (Price, 1996). These limbic system structures project to the periaqueductal grey (PAG) in the brain stem. Stimulation of the PAG results in normal sounding vocalization, eliciting a coordinated response of the respiratory, laryngeal, and articulatory muscles. Ablation of the PAG results in a change in vocal acoustics or mutism. Because stimulation of the limbic system structures does not elicit vocalization if the PAG is substantially damaged (Jürgens and Pratt, 1979), it appears that these cortical structures may not contain the neural mechanisms for vocalization. Instead, these structures may provide emotional modulation or excitation to a brain stem vocalization network located in the PAG (Raichle *et al.*, 1994).

The PAG projects to the premotor areas of the lower brain stem, primarily areas of the pontine and medullary reticular formations. These premotor areas appear to be involved in the

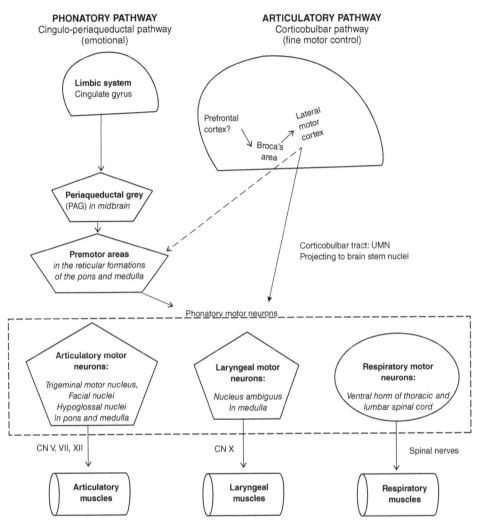

Figure 6.1 Two pathways involved in speech production: the phonatory pathway (left side) and the articulatory pathway (right side). Starting from the top of the figure, the semi-circle shapes indicate brain structures; trapezoids – brain stem structures; ovals – spinal cord structures; cylinders – muscles; the dotted arrow – possible convergence of the two pathways. For the sake of simplicity, sensory structures and other CNS structures such as the basal ganglia, cerebellum, and thalamus, which are known to contribute to speech motor control, are not included. (UMN – upper motor neuron.)

integration of respiratory, laryngeal, and articulatory muscles involved in phonation. Lesions to these areas cause profound changes in the acoustic structures of vocalizations in monkeys (Kirzinger and Jürgens, 1985). The premotor areas then connect to the motor nuclei that project to respiratory, laryngeal and oral musculature. Motor neurons in the trigeminal motor nucleus, facial nucleus, and the hypoglossal nucleus project to the articulatory muscles of the lips, tongue, jaw, and velum via cranial nerves V, VII, and XII. Motor neurons in the nucleus ambiguus project to the intrinsic laryngeal muscles via the vagus (CN X). Finally, motor neurons in the ventral horn of the thoracic and lumbar spinal cord project to respiratory muscles via spinal nerves.

The phonatory pathway appears to be well protected in humans. Although, as speech language pathologists, we frequently encounter patients who have a speech disorder as a result of a cerebral vascular accident or trauma to the brain, it is rare to observe a patient who has completely lost their ability to vocalize. Mutism is generally seen only in patients who have suffered widespread damage to the brain, such as in the case of encephalitis.

The articulatory pathway

The corticobulbar pathway is responsible for the fine motor control of the articulatory and laryngeal muscles needed for speech. It is a two neuron chain composed of an upper motor neuron (UMN) and a lower motor neuron (LMN). This neuron chain originates in the lateral motor cortex, just above the Sylvian fissure. The UMNs project to the motor nuclei in the brain stem and the LMNs project from the brain stem motor nuclei to the articulatory and laryngeal muscles via the cranial nerves. Kuypers (1958a, 1958b) found that the motor cortex projects to the nucleus ambiguus directly or with a few connections in both humans and chimpanzees. Jaffe *et al.* (1996) found stimulation of the motor cortex in a dog elicited laryngeal activity, but not vocalization because there was no coordinated activation of the respiratory system to produce sound. These results are consistent with the idea that the corticobulbar pathway provides a means for rapid, fine control of laryngeal muscles, but that it is not the primary pathway for vocalization.

The limbic system and emotional expression

The idea that the limbic system, which is responsible for display of emotion, plays an essential role in speech production makes sense in terms of our everyday experiences. Most persons are capable of hearing a stranger's voice on the phone and rapidly making a judgment about that person's emotional state. In this example, there is no information aside from the sound of the voice and the content of the message. Interestingly, when the content of the message appears to be contradicted by the quality of the voice, more credence is generally given to the emotion perceived in the voice rather than to the words spoken. Most persons also have had an experience in which the two pathways appear to be in conflict. For instance, when someone is trying to talk in a highly emotional situation, the phonatory pathway may receive the stronger excitation, as illustrated by speech interruptions with uncontrolled crying or laughing. At other times, the more voluntary articulatory pathway is able to maintain a higher degree of control. Even in situations that are less emotionally charged, speakers are generally not very good at successfully controlling the tone of their voice. An appreciation of this close link between the emotional motor system and speech may be fundamental to understanding the physiology of primary muscle tension dysphonia and the idea that emotional stress may manifest in a disordered voice.

There has been considerable interest in the relationship between personality, emotion, and dysphonia. The trait theory of voice disorders (Roy and Bless, 2000), suggests that certain personality traits predispose speakers to certain types of voice disorders. For example, neurotic introverts may be at risk for developing muscle tension dysphonia, while neurotic extroverts may be at risk for developing vocal nodules. The relationship between stress reaction, limbic activity, and other cortical areas involved in phonation has been examined using functional MRI. Dietrich *et al.* (2012) found that participants with high stress reaction scores, which would be associated with neuroticism, exhibited greater activation of the prefrontal and limbic areas during sentence reading in comparison to participants with low stress reaction scores. Continued investigation of central nervous system control of voice and speech is needed to more fully understand the interesting interplay between who we are, how we feel, and how we sound.

Coordinated activity of laryngeal muscles

Although we frequently think of laryngeal muscles in terms of the effect they have when contracted in isolation, this is rarely, if ever, the case. Generally, several muscles are active to variable degrees and the activation is typically bilateral. Laryngeal muscle activity has been measured to determine how fundamental aspects of phonation (pitch, register, vocal intensity, and voicing) are controlled.

Pitch

The perception of pitch is related to the frequency of vocal fold vibration, which is determined by the mass and stiffness of the vibrating tissue. However, only a portion of the vocal fold is involved in vibration. As such, the vocal folds have been modeled as consisting of two layers, a cover (the epithelium and the superficial and intermediate lamina propria) and a body (the deep lamina propria and the thyroarytenoid muscle), each with different mechanical properties (Hirano, 1974). It is primarily the cover that vibrates during phonation. Therefore, pitch is largely determined by the stiffness of the cover. Altering vocal fold stiffness involves contracting the CT muscle to increase the passive stress on the non-contractile tissue of the cover and contracting the TA muscle to increase the active stress of the body of the vocal fold. These muscles are antagonists and it is their joint activity, combined with the biomechanics of the larynx, which determines the resultant stress on the vibrating tissue and, consequently, the frequency of vocal fold tissue vibration (Titze *et al.*, 1988; Titze, 2011).

Vocal fold elongation is one strategy for controlling pitch and it is achieved by muscle activity. There have been numerous descriptive electromyographic (EMG) studies of laryngeal muscle activity and pitch (Gay *et al.*, 1972; Hillel, 2001; Hirano, 1987; Löfqvist *et al.*, 1984; Martin *et al.*, 1990), as well as some quantitative studies (McCulloch *et al.*, 1996; Shipp and McGlone, 1971). The findings here indicate that, as a person alters pitch during an ascending pitch glide, the intrinsic laryngeal muscles activate in a coordinated fashion. In order to maintain closure of the posterior glottis during the glide, the PCA muscle activity is relatively low and stable, while IA muscle activity is moderate and stable or slightly increasing. To gradually elongate the vocal folds, CT and TA muscle activity increases, although CT activity increases to a greater extent than TA activity. Finally, to adjust the vocal process gap, LCA muscle activity increases but not as consistently; this may be related to register control (as discussed below). In the end, CT muscle activity is most strongly and consistently correlated with alteration in pitch (Atkinson, 1978).

Although vocal fold elongation appears to be an important strategy for pitch control during modal (chest) register, other less well understood strategies may contribute to pitch control during falsetto register. One possible mechanism could be a progressive reduction in the effective mass of the vocal fold involved in vibration, as pitch increases at the top of the pitch range in falsetto register (Titze, personal communication). The vocal folds are not at maximum extension at the top of the pitch range, because greater elongation is seen during vocal fold abduction. However, the stiffness of the vocal fold is high due to co-activation of the CT and TA muscles. The stiffness may be relatively greater at the anterior and posterior ends of the vocal fold due to the presence of the anterior and posterior macula flava. As these areas stiffen, the effective vibrating area may be reduced.

Register

Vocal registers are defined as a phonation frequency range in which all tones are perceived as being produced in a similar way and possessing a similar quality (Garcia, 1982, originally published in 1841). It is somewhat difficult to separate pitch from register. In general, low pitches are produced in modal register and high pitches in falsetto. However, pitches in the middle range can be produced in multiple registers (van den Berg, 1963). It is, in part, manipulation of register over that portion of the pitch range that distinguishes musical theatre belters, from pop artists, from opera singers (Kochis-Jennings *et al.*, 2012). Classically trained singers tend to shift to a lighter register lower in their pitch range in comparison to most pop singers, while belters produce a greater proportion of notes in modal voice before shifting to a lighter register.

There are multiple complementary theories about how singers control register. According to van den Berg (1963), the vocal ligaments play an important role in register control. During modal voice, the vocal ligaments are short, lax, and adducted, allowing for a wide amplitude of vocal fold vibration. In falsetto, they are elongated, tense, abducted, and allow for only small amplitudes of vibration. A second theory proposed by Titze (1988) also emphasized that the degree of vocal fold abduction and amplitude of vibration play a role in register control. He suggests that, when the vocal folds are fully adducted and the amplitude of vibration is greater, modal voice occurs, while when they are abducted and the amplitude of vibration is smaller, falsetto occurs. A third theory advocated by Vilkman *et al.* (1995) is that there must be sufficient collision along the horizontal and vertical planes of the vocal folds for production of modal register. During production of a sustained pitch, it is possible to shift register from falsetto to modal by increasing: (a) LCA activation to adduct the vocal processes; (b) TA activation to create a more rectangular shaped medial edge; or (c) tracheal pressure to increase the amplitude of vibration. These adjustments affect the amount of vocal fold tissue involved in collision.

As a singer shifts from modal to falsetto register while maintaining the same pitch, activity in all intrinsic laryngeal muscles decreases (Gay *et al.*, 1972; Hirano, 1987). This is consistent with the theory that falsetto tones are produced with less adduction, reduced amplitude of vibration, and/or less collision between the membranous vocal folds. In order to maintain a heavier register as pitch is increased, singers have been shown to exhibit: (a) a smaller vocal process gap, which is presumably due to increased LCA muscle activity; and (b) greater TA muscle activity (Kochis-Jennings *et al.*, 2012). The latter finding is consistent with the theories of pitch change described above.

Clinically, patients who present with an asthenic (weak) voice quality, due to paresis or a functional voice disorder, may appear to speak in a lighter (head) register rather than in the modal register typically used during normal speech production. Based on what is understood about registers, a clinician could hypothesize that there is not adequate collision between the vocal folds to produce modal phonation. This could be remedied by training voice production incorporating greater approximation of the vocal processes, increased medial bulging of the membranous vocal folds for a more rectangular shaped medial edge, and greater subglottal pressure to increase the amplitude of vibration for greater collision.

Vocal intensity

Vocal intensity, which is related to the amplitude of vocal fold vibration and the speed of vocal fold closure, is positively related to tracheal pressure. Comfortable phonation is produced with approximately 0.6 kPa of tracheal pressure, in comparison to soft (0.3 kPa) and loud (1.0 kPa) phonation. Normal speakers modulate tracheal pressure to change overall loudness or add emphatic stress primarily by altering lung pressure (Finnegan *et al.*, 2000). However, the level of laryngeal muscle activity does not change with increased intensity during sustained phonation. Studies indicated that, when pitch was controlled, TA and CT muscle activity were relatively stable or only slightly increased with loudness (Gay *et al.*, 1972; Titze *et al.*, 1989).

Laryngeal muscle activity can play a role in reducing vocal intensity in the disordered voice. For example, vocal intensity can be reduced by 4–7 dB due to less than normal (hypofunction) or greater than normal adduction (hyperfunction) (Titze, 1988). In addition, aphonia may result when the vocal folds are not adequately adducted/tensed for flow-induced phonation.

Phonation onset and offset

During sentence production, speakers alternate between voiced and voiceless sounds and manipulate the degree of aspiration by fine control of the tension and position of the vocal folds. Adjustment of glottal width is associated with the reciprocal activation of the posterior PCA and IA muscles (Hirose and Gay, 1972; Hirose, 1976; Löfqvist and Yoshioka, 1981; Sawashima *et al.*, 1978). There is limited information regarding the contribution of other laryngeal muscles to vocal fold adduction. However, there is some evidence that the TA (and perhaps the LCA) activates in concert with the IA to achieve adduction (Hirose 1987; Löfqvist *et al.*, 1984). Finally, the CT muscle appears to assist with voice offset in some speakers (Löfqvist *et al.*, 1989), suggesting that stiffening of the vocal fold also diminishes the amplitude of vocal fold vibration (Titze and Talkin, 1979).

Conclusion

As illustrated by this brief review, many decades of research have contributed to a growing understanding of the structures involved in phonation, their connections, and the muscle activation patterns that allow speakers to control voicing. It is equally clear that more research is needed for a complete picture to emerge. Although we have a basic understanding of the effects of laryngeal muscle contraction, further research is needed to explore to what extent the nervous system activates muscle sub-compartments differentially to accomplish different tasks. A more detailed picture of laryngeal activity is needed to aid clinicians in their quest to continually develop and refine diagnostic procedures and intervention strategies for treatment of persons with vocal disorders.

References

Atkinson, J.E. (1978), "Correlation analysis of the physiological factors controlling fundamental voice frequency", *Journal of the Acoustical Society of America*, Vol. 63, pp. 211–222.

Dietrich, M., Andreatta, R.D., Jiang, Y., Joshi, A. and Stemple, J.C. (2012), "Preliminary findings on the relation between the personality trait of stress reaction and the central neural control of human vocalization", *International Journal of Speech-Language Pathology*, Vol. 14, pp. 377–389.

Finnegan, E.M., Luschei, E.S. and Hoffman, H.T. (2000), "Modulations in respiratory and laryngeal activity associated with changes in vocal intensity during speech", *Journal of Speech, Language, and Hearing Research*, Vol. 43, pp. 934–950.

Garcia, M. (1982), *A Complete Treatise on the Art of Singing: Part 1*, (Paschke, D. V., Ed. and Trans.), New York, NY: Da Capo Press, Inc. (Original work published in 1841).

Gay, T., Hirose, H., Strome, M. and Sawashima, M. (1972), "Electromyography of the intrinsic laryngeal muscles during phonation", *Annals of Otology, Rhinology, and Laryngology*, Vol. 81, pp. 401–409.

Han, Y., Wang, J., Fischman, D.A., Biller, H.F. and Sanders, I. (1999), "Slow tonic muscle fibers in the thyroarytenoid muscles of human vocal folds; A possible specialization for speech", *The Anatomical Record*, Vol. 256, pp. 146–157.

Hillel, A.D. (2001), "The study of laryngeal muscle activity in normal human subjects and in patients with laryngeal dystonia using multiple fine–wire electromyography", *The Laryngoscope*, Vol. 111 (S97), pp. 1–47.

Hirano, M. (1974), "Morphological structure of the vocal cord as a vibrator and its variations", *Folia Phoniatrica et Logopaedica*, Vol. 26, pp. 89–94.

Hirano, M. (1987), "The laryngeal muscles in singing", in Hirano, M., Kirchner, J.A. and Bless, D.M. (Eds.), *Neurolaryngology: Recent Advances*, San Diego, California, US: College-Hill Publication, pp. 209–230

Hirose, H. (1976), "Posterior cricoarytenoid as a speech muscle", *Annals of Otology, Rhinology and Laryngology*, Vol. 85, pp. 334–342.

Hirose, H. (1987), "Laryngeal articulatory adjustments in terms of EMG", in Hirano, M., Kirchner J.A. and Bless, D.M. (Eds.), *Neurolaryngology: Recent Advances*. Boston, Massachussetts, US: College-Hill. pp. 200–208.

Hirose, H. and Gay, T. (1972), "The activity of the intrinsic laryngeal muscles in voicing control – An electromyographic study", *Phonetica*, Vol. 25, pp. 140–164.

Holstege, G. and Ehling, T. (1996), "Two motor systems involved in the production of speech", in Davis, P.H. and Fletcher, N.H. (Eds.), *Vocal Fold Physiology: Controlling Complexity and Chaos*. San Diego, California, US: Singular Publishing, pp. 153–169.

Jaffe, D.M., Solomon, N.P. and Luschei, E.S. (1996), "Activation of laryngeal muscle by electrical stimulation of the canine motor cortex", in Davis, P.H. and Fletcher, N.H, (Eds.), *Vocal Fold Physiology: Controlling Complexity and Chaos*. San Diego, CA, US: Singular Publishing, pp. 187–200.

Jürgens, U. (2009), "The neural control of vocalization in mammals: A review", *Journal of Voice*, Vol. 23, pp. 1–10.

Jürgens, U. and Pratt, R. (1979), "Role of the periaqueductal grey in vocal expression of emotion", *Brain Research*, Vol. 167, pp. 367–378.

Kirzinger, A. and Jürgens, U. (1985), "The effects of brainstem lesions on vocalization in the squirrel monkey", *Brain Research*, Vol. 358, pp. 150–162.

Kochis-Jennings, K.A., Finnegan, E.M., Hoffman, H.T. and Jaiswal, S. (2012), "Laryngeal muscle activity and vocal fold adduction during chest, chestmix, headmix, and head registers in females", *Journal of Voice*, Vol. 26, pp. 182–193.

Konig, W.F. and von Leden, H. (1961), "The peripheral nervous system of the human larynx: Part I. The mucous membrane", *Archives of Otolaryngology*, Vol. 73, pp. 1–14.

Korfage, J.A.M., Koolstra, J.H., Langenbach, G.E.J. and Van Eijden, T.M.G.J. (2005), "Fiber-type composition of the human jaw muscles—(Part 2) Role of hybrid fibers and factors responsible for inter-individual variation", *Journal of Dental Research*, Vol. 84, pp. 784–793.

Kuypers, H.G. (1958a), "An anatomical analysis of cortico-bulbar connexions to the pons and lower brain stem in the cat", *Journal of Anatomy*, Vol. 92 (Pt. 2), p. 198.

Kuypers, H.G. (1958b), "Corticobulbar connexions to the pons and lower brain-stem in man", *Brain*, Vol. 81, pp. 364–388.

Larson, C., Yoshida, Y. and Sessle, B.J. (1993), "Higher level motor and sensory organization", in Titze I.R. (Ed.), *Vocal Fold Physiology: Frontiers in Basic Science*. San Diego, California, US: Singular Publishing, pp. 227–258

Löfqvist, A. and Yoshioka, H. (1981), "Interrarticulator programming in obstruent production", *Phonetica*, Vol. 38, pp. 21–34.

Löfqvist, A., McGarr, N.S. and Honda, K. (1984), "Laryngeal muscles and articulatory control", *The Journal of the Acoustical Society of America*, Vol. 76, pp. 951–954.

Löfqvist, A., Baer, T., McGarr, N.S. and Story, R.S. (1989), "The cricothyroid muscle in voicing control", *The Journal of the Acoustical Society of America*, Vol. 85, pp. 1314–1321.

McCulloch, T.M., Perlman, A.L., Palmer, P.M. and Van Daele, D.J. (1996), "Laryngeal activity during swallow, phonation, and the Valsalva maneuver: An electromyographic analysis", *The Laryngoscope*, Vol. 106, pp. 1351–1358.

Martin, F., Thumfart, W.F., Jolk, A. and Klingholz, F. (1990), "The electromyographic activity of the posterior cricoarytenoid muscle during singing", *Journal of Voice*, Vol. 4, pp. 25–29.

Mu, L. and Sanders, I. (2009), "The human cricothyroid muscle: Three muscle bellies and their innervation patterns", *Journal of Voice*, Vol. 23, pp. 21–28.

Mu, L., Sanders, I., Wu, B.L. and Biller, H.F. (1994), "The intramuscular innervation of the human interarytenoid muscle", *The Laryngoscope*, Vol. 104, pp. 33–39.

Price, J.L. (1996), "Vocalization and the orbital and medial prefrontal cortex", in Davis, P.H. and Fletcher, N.H. (Eds.), *Vocal Fold Physiology: Controlling Complexity and Chaos*. San Diego, California, US: Singular Publishing, pp. 171–185.

Raichle, M.E., Fiez, J.A., Videen, T.A., MacLeod, A.M.K., Pardo, J.V., Fox, P.T. and Petersen, S.E. (1994), "Practice-related changes in human brain functional anatomy during nonmotor learning", *Cerebral Cortex*, Vol. 4, pp. 8–26.

Roy, N. and Bless, D.M. (2000), "Personality traits and psychological factors in voice pathology: A foundation for future research", *Journal of Speech, Language, and Hearing Research*, Vol. 43, pp. 737–748.

Sanders, I. and Mu, L. (1998), "Anatomy of the human internal superior laryngeal nerve", *The Anatomical Record*, Vol. 252, pp. 646–656.

Sanders, I., Jacobs, I., Wu, B.L. and Biller, H.E. (1993a), "The three bellies of the canine posterior cricoarytenoid muscle: Implications for understanding laryngeal function", *The Laryngoscope*, Vol. 103, pp. 171–177.

Sanders, I., Mu, L., Wu, B.L. and Biller, H.F. (1993b), "The intramuscular nerve supply of the human lateral cricoarytenoid muscle", *Acta Oto-Laryngologica*, Vol. 113, pp. 679–682.

Sawashima, M., Hirose, H. and Yoshioka, H. (1978), "Abductor (PCA) and adductor (INT) muscles of the larynx in voiceless sound production", *Annual Bulletin Research Institute of Logopedics and Phoniatrics, University of Tokyo*, Vol. 12, pp. 53–60.

Shipp, T. and McGlone, R.E. (1971), "Laryngeal dynamics associated with voice frequency change", *Journal of Speech and Hearing Research*, Vol. 14, pp. 761–768.

Titze, I.R. (1988), "A framework for the study of vocal registers", *Journal of Voice*. Vol. 2, No. 4, pp. 1–12.

Titze, I.R. (2011), "Vocal fold mass is not a useful quantity for describing F0 in vocalization", *Journal of Speech, Language, and Hearing Research*, Vol. 54, pp. 520–522.

Titze, I.R., Jiang, J. and Drucker, D.G. (1988), "Preliminaries to the body-cover theory of pitch control", *Journal of Voice*, Vol. 1, No. 4, pp. 314–319.

Titze I.R., Luschei E.S. and Hirano, M. (1989), "Role of the thyroarytenoid muscle in regulation of fundamental frequency", *Journal of Voice*, Vol. 3, pp. 213–224.

Titze, I.R. and Talkin, D.T. (1979), "A theoretical study of the effects of various laryngeal configurations on the acoustics of phonation", *The Journal of the Acoustical Society of America*, Vol. 66, pp. 60–74.

Van den Berg, J. (1963), "Vocal ligaments versus registers", *The National Association of Teachers of Singing Bulletin*, December, pp. 16–21.

Vilkman, E., Alku, P. and Laukkanen, A.A. (1995), "Vocal-fold collision mass as a differentiator between registers in the low pitch range", *Journal of Voice*, Vol. 9, pp. 66–73.

7

NEURAL CONTROL OF SWALLOWING AND TREATMENT OF MOTOR IMPAIRMENTS IN DYSPHAGIA

Aarthi Madhavan, Nancy J. Haak, Giselle D. Carnaby and Michael A. Crary

Human swallowing is a complex, adaptable phenomenon, essential to human existence on many levels. It is susceptible to impairment from a multitude of diseases and health status changes, but is responsive to active rehabilitation efforts. The key thesis of this chapter is that swallowing is movement, and to understand both normal and disordered swallowing, control of movement within the swallowing mechanism must be emphasized. The evidence base for treatment strategies employed in dysphagia management will be reviewed, specifically in reference to their impact on critical aspects of movement required for adequate swallowing.

Stages of human swallowing

Human swallowing is best depicted as a 'pressure-flow' phenomenon, in which pressures are applied at different levels to facilitate flow of swallowed materials through the swallowing mechanism. Human swallowing is typically discussed in three stages: oral, pharyngeal, and esophageal. The primary functions of the oral component of swallowing are to process foods to support adequate swallowing and to transit oral contents to the pharynx. Evidence from swallowing impairment following cortical/hemisphere deficits suggests a voluntary, cortical control over the oral components of swallowing (Groher and Crary, 2010). Complex oral processing is highly dependent on sensory input (Steele, 2010), adequate motor control of multiple muscle groups, systematic introduction of saliva to lubricate drier materials (Chen, 2009), and taste and smell. The tongue plays a primary role in containing and moving liquids and solid foods within the mouth to facilitate mastication and to mix foods with saliva for lubrication (Hiiemae and Palmer, 1999).

The general function of the pharynx is the appropriate transit and direction of swallowed material into the esophagus. This highly complex pharyngeal activity is accomplished within a safe and efficient timeframe by pressures applied to swallowed materials by paired pharyngeal constrictor muscles in conjunction with airway closure and opening of the upper esophageal sphincter (UES). The UES is opened by a combination of neural relaxation (from the brainstem swallowing center) and mechanical stretch responses resulting from the upward/forward excursion of the larynx (Miller *et al.*, 2013) allowing swallowed materials to pass into the esophagus. In adults, this complex pharyngeal pattern is considered more automatic/reflexive, or more accurately a learned sensorimotor pattern governed by a brainstem 'central pattern generator' (Jean, 2001).

The esophagus is a distensible tube (i.e., 'closed' at rest) between the pharynx and stomach and is the final component of the upper aerodigestive tract for swallowing in humans. Once swallowing has occurred, effective clearance of swallowed material occurs via coordinated, sequential wave-like muscular contractions (peristalsis) through the esophagus and the lower esophageal sphincter (LES).

Neurologic control of swallowing functions

As implicated from the diverse components of human swallowing, the neurologic infrastructure is widespread and complex. Ultimately, swallowing depends on movement. From this perspective, significant overlap exists in the neural control of swallowing and non-swallowing movements in the upper aerodigestive tract. From an oversimplified point of view, swallowing neural controls can be separated into brainstem and hemisphere functions. In the rostral brainstem, a 'central pattern generator' (Jean, 2001) includes the nucleus tractus solitarius (NTS) and the nucleus ambiguous (NA). Sensory information from various components of the swallow mechanism (oral, pharyngeal, esophageal) provides input to the NTS, which communicates at the brainstem level with the NA to modulate swallowing related movements. One basic demonstration of this brainstem control is seen in the automatic process of 'bolus accommodation' in which oral and pharyngeal motor functions of swallowing are involuntarily changed in response to sensory signals provided by different swallowed materials (Buchholz, Bosma, and Donner, 1985; Kendall, Leonard, and Mckenzie, 2001). In adults, this automatic, brainstem governed process permits ingestion of a wide variety of materials without conscious, voluntary participation during eating. A second aspect of brainstem swallowing control is reflected in spontaneous swallowing. Spontaneous swallowing is considered an airway protection mechanism. Individuals swallow 'reflexively' in response to secretions or other residuals within the pharynx (Dua *et al.*, 2011). Though the motoric pattern of spontaneous swallows is essentially the same as 'voluntary swallowing' during food/liquid ingestion, the trigger for the spontaneous swallow is brainstem mediated via the 'swallowing center' in the rostral brainstem. This brainstem swallowing center not only modulates oropharyngeal swallowing, it also coordinates swallow activity with respiratory activity. Brainstem damage, especially to this central pattern generator (NTS and NA) typically results in severe dysphagia, which is often accompanied by respiratory impairments. Brainstem swallowing controls include this swallowing center and a two-way conduit between the peripheral neuromuscular system and hemisphere control centers.

The brainstem also functions as a 'junction box' between hemisphere neural control and peripheral sensorimotor components of swallowing (Groher and Crary, 2010). Unlike the focal control of swallowing noted within brainstem structures, cortical swallowing controls are thought to be bilateral and diffuse (Malandraki *et al.*, 2009; Michou and Hamdy, 2009; Mihai, Und Halbach, and Lotze, 2013). Investigators using various brain imaging approaches (transcranial magnetic stimulation, functional magnetic imaging, functional near-infrared spectroscopy) conclude that swallowing function is diffusely represented in both hemispheres and not related to neural control for speech or handedness (Hamdy *et al.*, 1996; Malandraki *et al.*, 2009; Michou and Hamdy, 2009; Mihai *et al.*, 2013). This diffuse 'cortical organization' of swallowing function likely underlies a degree of neuroplasticity in which a contralateral homologue area can 'assume' neural control if the primary neural control area is damaged. For example, Hamdy and colleagues (Hamdy *et al.*, 1996; 2000) have demonstrated that swallowing motor functions are bilaterally represented, with one hemisphere being dominant for swallowing function. If the dominant hemisphere is impaired, the contralateral hemisphere demonstrates increased activity corresponding to recovery of swallowing functions. To further emphasize this point, patients with bilateral hemisphere damage (e.g., bilateral strokes) demonstrate the most severe and persistent swallowing difficulties (Ickenstein *et al.*, 2003).

Not surprisingly, a large portion of frontal cortex has been implicated in swallowing motor control. Areas including the primary motor and sensory cortical areas, inferior frontal lobule, and insula have been implicated. The apparent contribution of motor control centers of the hemispheres may be related to the basic movement components inherent in swallowing (recall that swallowing depends on movements within the upper aerodigestive tract). Investigators have tried to 'dissect' cortical control of swallowing from non-swallow movements of the same structures. Results from these studies report overlap between swallow and non-swallow functions, but indicate that swallowing has a distinct pattern of cortical control (Malandraki *et al.*, 2009; Martin *et al.*, 2004). Moreover, swallowing different materials (liquids, pudding, masticated foods) has been shown to result in different patterns of cortical activation (Shibamoto *et al.*, 2007; Soros *et al.*, 2009). Finally, hemisphere swallowing control mechanisms seem to adjust with increasing age, presumably in response to age-related changes in basic sensorimotor processing that occurs with healthy aging. fMRI studies comparing activation patterns during swallowing in healthy young vs. elderly adults reported a wider distribution of cortical activation in older adults (Malandraki *et al.*, 2009; 2011). Furthermore, one fMRI study indicated that older adults had expected patterns of motor cortex activation, but diminished sensory and sensorimotor integration activation patterns (Malandraki *et al.*, 2011). Though the current state of knowledge on hemisphere control of swallowing function is vastly incomplete, the emerging picture is that of a neural network that is flexible to the motoric demands required to swallow various materials, adjustable in response to sensorimotor changes associated with aging, and plastic when impacted by damage to one component of central neural control.

Dysphagia from neurological deficit

As might be expected from the above description of neural control of swallowing functions, damage to different neural components will result in different patterns of swallowing impairment. The overt contribution of motor deficits will often be the hallmark of dysphagia associated with different neurologic impairments. For example, damage to the upper motor neuron system (anywhere from cortex to brainstem) will result in a spastic motor performance resulting in weakness, slowness, and restricted range of movement (and possibly more). These movement deficits will translate into difficulties transporting swallowed materials through the swallowing mechanism; resulting in residue within the mouth, pharynx, and/or reduced esophageal clearance. Misdirection of swallowed material may also contribute to airway compromise, noted as aspiration of materials into the respiratory tract. Yet, each of these 'dysphagia signs' (residue, aspiration, poor clearance) results directly from movement impairments related to specific aspects of the neurological deficit. Table 7.1 summarizes some of the more salient movement deficits noted in dysphagia associated with neurologic deficits at various levels of the nervous system.

Table 7.1 Descriptions of dysphagia resulting from characteristic cortical, subcortical, brainstem, and lower motor neuron (LMN) lesions.

Disorder	Neurologic Deficit/Lesion	Salient Dysphagia (Motor) Deficits
Cortical Lesions		
Stroke/CVA	Focal lesion to various areas of the CNS – motor and sensory deficits may be widespread (dependent on location, size, and if unilateral vs. bilateral)	• Delayed triggering of pharyngeal swallow • Uncoordinated oral movements • Increased pharyngeal transit duration • Reduced pharyngeal constriction • Aspiration • UES dysfunction
TBI	Diffuse neurologic deficits, greater motor deficits in the acute phase	• Diffuse motor deficits in balance, coordination, gross and fine motor skills, strength, and endurance – affecting oral and pharyngeal phases of swallowing equally • Frequent aspiration, impaired cough observed in acute phase (Terre and Mearin, 2007)
Dementia	Progressively worsening, diffuse lesions	• Impaired voluntary oral control • Slow oral movements • Slow/delayed pharyngeal response • Overall slow swallowing duration
Subcortical Lesions		
Parkinson's Disease	Impaired basal ganglia functioning from depletion of dopamine – progressively worsening execution of motor functions	• Overall slowness in all stages of swallowing • Involuntary movements (e.g. tremor) results in loss of movement control during swallowing • Poor bolus control • Oral and pharyngeal residue • Esophageal dysmotility • Aspiration in later stages of disease (Ali *et al.*, 1996)
Brainstem Lesions		

Brainstem lesions can include – stroke, trauma, neoplasms, and pressure effects e.g. hydrocephalus	Lesions in this 'junction box' result in sensory deficits to the head and neck region, and motor deficits from UMN and LMN damage i.e. can be spastic or flaccid weakness along with associated impairments	• Severe dysphagia is often associated with lesions that affect multiple CNs
		• Generalized respiratory incoordination
		• Characteristics of an 'incomplete swallow'
		• Delayed or absent pharyngeal response
		• Reductions in
		    Hyolaryngeal elevation
		    Laryngeal closure
		    UES opening

Table 7.1 continued

Disorder	Neurologic Deficit/Lesion	Salient Dysphagia (Motor) Deficits
Lower Motor Neuron (LMN) Lesions		
Myasthenia Gravis	Myoneural junction disruption – depletion of neurotransmitter with use Muscles fatigue into flaccid weakness	• Fatigue with use; recovery with rest • From mouth to esophagus
Amyotrophic Lateral Sclerosis (ALS)	Rapidly progressive neurodegenerative disease • Mixture of spastic and flaccid weakness (Wijesekera and Leigh, 2009) • CNS structures also involved	Mixed pattern of weakness (spastic and flaccid) resulting in: • Reduced oral control of bolus • Reduced oral transport • Reduced pharyngeal constriction • Oral and pharyngeal residue • Ineffective airway clearance (laryngeal and/or respiratory muscle weakness)

In addition to movement deficits associated with neurologic insult, motor aspects of swallowing may also be impacted by 'disuse'. Neurologic impairments, such as stroke, are acute and leave patients in a weakened state in which oral intake may not be possible for a variable time period. This absence of oral intake can contribute to disuse weakness (Kortebein *et al.*, 2007), which may be related to another movement deficit associated with reduced functional activity, 'learned non-use' (Taub *et al.*, 2006). Disuse weakness is meant to reflect a peripheral muscle weakness related to reduced workload, whereas learned nonuse is thought to be a cortical response to the same reduced workload and/or maladaptive neuroplasticity. Both of these phenomena can compound the basic motor deficits associated with neurologic deficit, complicating and prolonging swallowing difficulties in patients.

Management of neurogenic swallowing disorders

As noted above, dysphagia, especially neurogenic dysphagia, typically involves deficits in motor control of swallowing structures. From this perspective, attempts to improve swallowing performance in patients with dysphagia should incorporate strategies to improve motor control of swallowing. That said, some acutely ill patients are not appropriate candidates for therapy to improve motor control. In these cases, strategies to facilitate 'safe swallowing' (e.g., swallowing without aspiration of material into the airway) might be appropriate. Thus, dysphagia treatment can incorporate compensatory strategies (short-term strategies to maintain safe swallowing) or rehabilitation strategies (interventions to improve motor control/performance of swallowing). Table 7.2 describes common strategies that are employed in the management of dysphagia with consideration for the motor 'impact' of each technique.

Table 7.2 Common compensatory and rehabilitative strategies employed in dysphagia management.

Technique		Description	Suggested Use/ Motor Impact on Swallowing Mechanism
Compensation: Postural Adjustments	Head extension	Raised chin: widens oropharynx, uses gravity – may help in transport of bolus from mouth to pharynx	Oral/ Lingual deficits like glossectomy, oral resection, reconstruction, lingual paralysis
			Increases intraluminal pressure and decreases relaxation duration of the UES; changing the coordination between pharyngeal and UES swallow pressures
			May also result in defective laryngeal closure
	Chin tuck	Chin down: widens vallecular, displaces base of tongue (BOT) and epiglottis posteriorly	Delayed pharyngeal response, reduced posterior BOT motion
			Weakens pharyngeal constriction
			Interferes with swallow/respiratory coordination
	Head rotation	Rotate head to affected side: closes damaged side from bolus path, reduces LES pressure, increases true vocal cord adduction	Unilateral pharyngeal weakness
			Relaxes contralateral UES pressure during swallow
	Side lying	Maximizes residual pharyngeal function and reduces bolus speed due to reduction of gravity	Difference in pharyngeal function between right and left sides
			Possible increase in pharyngeal muscle contraction (untested)
Rehabilitation: Strengthening Exercises	Various lingual resistance exercises	Increasing tongue push against palate: progressive strengthening of lingual musculature	Increases strength of lingual-palatal contact to improve initial driving force on swallowed material
	Head Lift	Head raises while lying supine: strengthens weakened suprahyoid muscle groups	Strengthen suprahyoid musculature to increase and prolong impaired UES opening
	EMST*	Forced expiration through a one-way resistance programmable valve	Progressively strengthen expiratory respiratory muscles to increase cough strength
			Increased motor unit recruitment of subnental muscles
			Limited evidence on improved swallowing (some reduction in aspiration events)
	Pharyngocise	Prophylactic exercise program performing falsetto, tongue press, hard swallow, and jaw stretching	Less structural deterioration in muscles of swallowing
			Maintenance of swallow function, dietary intake, taste and smell, salivation, nutritional status
	MDTP**	Swallowing foods and liquids of different physical properties • Progressive strengthening program • Challenges the weakened swallowing system	Strengthen oral and pharyngeal components of swallowing; resulting in increased lingual-palatal pressures, hyolaryngeal excursion, pharyngeal clearance, improved swallow timing, and pharyngeal pressures

* EMST – Expiratory Muscle Strength Training
** MDTP – McNeill Dysphagia Therapy Program

Compensatory strategies

The focus of compensatory strategies is 'safe swallowing', meaning the ability to swallow food and liquid without entry into the airway. Compensatory strategies are intended to be short term and are not expected to have a major impact on the motor system subserving swallowing function. However, some compensatory strategies may have a positive or negative impact on motor functions subserving swallowing performance. Commonly used compensatory strategies are typically directed at food properties or patient positioning.

Modified diets/liquids

Allowing patients to continue receiving oral intake, even of modified foods and liquids, rather than non-oral alternatives is deemed a more acceptable and emotionally satisfying approach (Garcia, Chambers, and Molander, 2005). Modifying diets and liquids is one of the more prevalent strategies used to maintain safe oral intake. In a study of dysphagia practices, speech language pathologists recommended thickened fluids to 59 percent of their patients and modified diets to 93 percent of their patients (Low *et al.*, 2001). Despite this high percentage of use as a compensatory strategy, patients overwhelmingly do not perceive thickened diets as desirable or palatable. Research indicates that less than 36 percent of patients adhere to dysphagia diet recommendations (Leiter and Windsor, 1996). Consequently, effectiveness of thickening protocols remains haphazard. Furthermore, recent literature has questioned a relationship between the strategy of thickening liquids or restricting solids to a puree consistency and the potential for dehydration (Crary *et al.*, 2013). Additionally, dysphagic patients on modified diets are not well transitioned back to more normal diets, significantly affecting a patient's well-being and quality of life. Data suggest that once placed upon a thickened diet, a dysphagic patient may be prescribed that consistency for up to 50 days (Carnaby, Hankey, and Pizzi, 2006). With respect to motor consequences of this prolonged use of modified diets, there may be reduced 'load' on the swallowing mechanism. In this context, 'load' refers to the physiologic demands of foods and liquids on both the effort and timing involved in swallowing (see discussion on bolus accommodation above). If speed demands on swallowing are reduced with slower moving thickened liquids and effort demands are reduced with soft, pureed foods, the swallow mechanism may well accommodate via the processes of disuse weakness and/or learned nonuse. The longer a patient is maintained on these reduced diets, the greater potential for motor 'deterioration' within the swallowing mechanism. Currently, little empirical evidence exists to support or refute this motor deterioration scenario. However, given the prevalence of modified diets as a compensatory strategy, and the duration with which it is applied, future research should evaluate the impact of this strategy on motor aspects of swallowing.

Patient positioning

Changing the patient's body and/or head posture may also be recommended as a compensatory strategy to maintain safe swallowing (see Table 7.2). For example, body posture adjustment may involve 'side-lying'. In a lying posture, gravity is reduced from the swallowing act. Though intended to slow the flow of swallowed materials, this simple technique may also function to strengthen swallowing musculature by requiring more neuromotor activity to propel swallowed materials through the swallowing mechanism without the assistance of gravity. Unfortunately, in the absence of empirical data, this view remains speculative.

Similar to body posture changes, head posture adjustments are frequently recommended as compensatory strategies. For example, a chin tuck posture may be used to facilitate airway protection during swallowing. This posture has the anatomic effect of improving closure of the laryngeal vestibule by narrowing the pharynx. These physiologic changes in swallow performance have been minimally studied but include interference with coordination between swallowing and respiration (Ayuse *et al.*, 2006), and reduction in the strength of pharyngeal muscle contraction (Bulow, Olsson, and Ekberg, 1999). Conversely, turning the head has the functional impact of redirecting a bolus away from a weakened hemipharynx while at the same time increasing physiologic relaxation in the UES. The combined physical and physiologic effects help some patients to swallow greater volumes with less airway compromise or residue.

Available data on the motor impact of modified diets and postural adjustments is limited (and as noted above, nonexistent in some cases). However, these compensatory strategies were not intended to improve swallow motor performance. Rather, the focus of their application is to facilitate safe swallowing. Still, suggestions of negative (e.g., chin tuck posture) or positive (e.g., head turn) influence of some compensatory strategies on swallow motor performance holds both a conceptual value for a better understanding of swallow motor control and a practical value for clinical application.

Rehabilitation strategies

Recently, dysphagia rehabilitation has experienced a changing focus with the development of novel 'exercise-based' rehabilitation therapies. Unlike compensatory strategies, rehabilitation exercises are intended to improve impaired swallow motor function. The underlying rationale of these approaches is based on the recognition of skeletal muscle weakening with aging and/ or disease. Muscles are highly plastic and exercising muscles at a level above their usual load increases muscle strength and results in functional and physiologic improvement in the impaired swallowing mechanism (Crary and Carnaby, 2014). Rehabilitative swallowing exercises use volitional control to augment impaired aspects of pharyngeal swallowing; and their design is grounded in evidence from the fields of sports medicine and exercise physiology. Evidence suggests that activities to volitionally strengthen weakened musculature (weakened from disuse) will serve to improve muscle conditioning and thereby improve control and management of swallowed material through the oropharynx (Seo, Oh, and Han, 2011). These swallowing exercise programs incorporate principles, such as intensity, resistance, load, pacing, and fatigue, in determining the schedule of treatment. Examples of newer exercise programs include the Shaker Head Lift maneuver (Mepani *et al.*, 2009), various lingual pressure resistance training approaches (Juan *et al.*, 2013; Robbins *et al.*, 2005; Steele and Miller, 2010), expiratory muscle strength training (EMST) (Pitts *et al.*, 2009), Pharyngocise (Carnaby-Mann *et al.*, 2012), and the McNeill Dysphagia Therapy Program (Crary *et al.*, 2012).

The Shaker Head Lift technique incorporates repetitive and sustained head raises from a lying position (Mepani *et al.*, 2009). The goal of these exercises is to strengthen the suprahyoid musculature to increase the upward stretch stimulus on the UES, resulting in improved UES relaxation/opening. Positive physiologic (e.g., motoric) changes from this exercise include increased anterior laryngeal excursion and UES opening during swallowing (Shaker *et al.*, 1997). However, the Shaker exercise can be physically demanding to complete, especially in older or weaker patients with dysphagia (Easterling *et al.*, 2005); resulting in reduced adherence and hence, less exercise benefit.

Lingual resistance training was one of the first techniques to utilize progressive resistance in dysphagia therapy (Robbins *et al.*, 2007). Target levels for lingual resistance are increased as a patient increases lingual strength. The overt goal of lingual resistance training is to increase lingual strength, resulting in stronger lingual pressures applied to swallowed materials. In general, lingual resistance programs have been shown to produce increased lingual strength with some indication of improved functional swallowing in patients post-stroke (Robbins *et al.*, 2007) and in patients with progressive neuromotor disease (Malandraki *et al.*, 2012). However, these programs may not benefit all patients with dysphagia, as demonstrated by a randomized control trial by Lazarus *et al.* (2014). In this trial, patients with dysphagia following head and neck cancer did not show improved swallowing from lingual resistance training.

Pharyngocise is a novel approach designed to prophylactically minimize or avoid dysphagia in patients undergoing chemoradiation for head and neck cancer (Carnaby-Mann *et al.*, 2012). This program incorporates performing exercises such as falsetto, tongue press, hard swallow, and jaw stretching, twice daily in cycles. Two randomized control trials demonstrated that Pharyngocise patients show less deterioration in swallow function, salivation, nutritional status, and other dysphagia related morbidities (Carnaby, Crary, and Amdur, 2012; Carnaby-Mann *et al.*, 2012). Furthermore, patients who completed this prophylactic exercise program demonstrated less structural deterioration in the key muscles of swallowing as demonstrated by T2 weighted MRIs. Thus, Pharyngocise as a swallowing exercise 'protects' muscle integrity resulting in maintenance of swallowing functions.

The McNeill Dysphagia Therapy Program (MDTP) is an exercise-based program using 'swallowing as an exercise for swallowing' (Carnaby-Mann and Crary, 2010; Crary *et al.*, 2012). Thus, MDTP addresses the entire upper swallowing mechanism, not just subsystems (as with the head lift or lingual resistance approaches). MDTP is completed daily for three weeks to maintain both frequency and intensity of swallowing exercise. In addition to functional swallowing improvement, motor improvements in swallow performance have been documented in patients completing this program including strength, degree of movement, and speed of swallowing (Crary *et al.*, 2012; Lan *et al.*, 2012).

Each of these exercise-based dysphagia approaches has demonstrated physiologic (motor) improvements in the swallowing mechanism in addition to varying degrees of functional improvement of swallowing. Results indicating change in motor performance during swallowing suggest a degree of neuromotor reorganization following successful swallow rehabilitation. Some evidence indicates that peripheral motor functions are enhanced as reflected by increased strength and range of swallowing movements. However, increased strength could result from central neural control changes resulting in greater motor unit recruitment. Likewise, enhanced timing performance could suggest a degree of central neuromotor reorganization. Little to no data are available on central nervous system changes following successful rehabilitation of neurologically impaired (or other etiologies) swallowing functions. Research addressing the central control of impaired swallow motor functions and the impact of rehabilitation on central control mechanisms is a key focus for the future.

Summary

Human swallowing requires a complex network of neural sensorimotor control from the peripheral neuromuscular system to the cortex. Certain aspects of human swallowing, such as pharyngeal patterns and reciprocity with respiration, are under more automatic brainstem control. Other aspects, such as oral control, initiation, and material-specific swallow patterns appear to be more under a flexible network control of diffuse cortical regions. Aging appears to influence both swallowing performance and neurologic infrastructure supporting human swallowing. A new direction in swallowing rehabilitation is to effect motoric improvement (i.e., strength, range of movement, and speed of movement) in swallowing performance to achieve functional benefit for patients with dysphagia. Methods to achieve this new direction are expanding. However, much remains to be learned, including a broader evaluation of the impact of these strategies on the peripheral neuromotor swallowing system and the 'upstream' impact on central nervous system control of swallowing functions.

References

Ali, G.N., Wallace, K.L., Schwartz, R., Decarle, D.J., Zagami, A.S. and Cook, I.J. (1996), "Mechanisms of oral-pharyngeal dysphagia in patients with Parkinson's disease", *Gastroenterology*, Vol. 110, pp. 383–392.

Ayuse, T., Ayuse, T., Ishitobi, S., Kurata, S., Sakamoto, E., Okayasu, I. and Oi, K. (2006), "Effect of reclining and chin-tuck position on the coordination between respiration and swallowing", *Journal of Oral Rehabilitation*, Vol. 33, pp. 402–408.

Buchholz, D.W., Bosma, J.F. and Donner, M.W. (1985), "Adaptation, compensation, and decompensation of the pharyngeal swallow", *Gastrointestinal Radiology*, Vol. 10, pp. 235–239.

Bulow, M., Olsson, R. and Ekberg, O. (1999), "Videomanometric analysis of supraglottic swallow, effortful swallow, and chin tuck in healthy volunteers", *Dysphagia*, Vol. 14, pp. 67–72.

Carnaby, G., Hankey, G.J. and Pizzi, J. (2006), "Behavioural intervention for dysphagia in acute stroke: A randomised controlled trial", *Lancet Neurology*, Vol. 5, pp. 31–37.

Carnaby, G.D., Crary, M.A. and Amdur, R. (2012), "Dysphagia prevention exercises in head and neck cancer: Pharyngocise dose response study", *Dysphagia Research Society Annual Meeting*. Toronto, Canada.

Carnaby-Mann, G., Crary, M.A., Schmalfuss, I. and Amdur, R. (2012), "'Pharyngocise': Randomized controlled trial of preventative exercises to maintain muscle structure and swallowing function during head-and-neck chemoradiotherapy", *International Journal of Radiation Oncology Biology Physics*, Vol. 83, pp. 210–219.

Carnaby-Mann, G.D. and Crary, M.A. (2010), "McNeill dysphagia therapy program: A case-control study", *Archives of Physical Medicine and Rehabilitation*, Vol. 91, pp. 743–749.

Chen, J. (2009), "Food oral processing – A review", *Food Hydrocolloids*, Vol. 23, pp. 1–25.

Crary, M.A. and Carnaby, G. (2014), "Adoption into clinical practice of two therapies to manage swallowing disorders: Exercise-based swallowing rehabilitation and electrical stimulation", *Current Opinion in Otolaryngology and Head and Neck Surgery*, Vol. 22, pp. 172–180.

Crary, M.A., Carnaby, G.D., Lagorio, L.A. and Carvajal, P.J. (2012), "Functional and physiological outcomes from an exercise-based dysphagia therapy: A pilot investigation of the McNeill Dysphagia Therapy Program", *Archives of Physical Medicine and Rehabilitation*, Vol. 93, pp. 1173–1178.

Crary, M.A., Humphrey, J.L., Carnaby-Mann, G., Sambandam, R., Miller, L. and Silliman, S. (2013), "Dysphagia, nutrition, and hydration in ischemic stroke patients at admission and discharge from acute care", *Dysphagia*, Vol. 28, pp. 69–76.

Dua, K., Surapaneni, S.N., Kuribayashi, S., Hafeezullah, M. and Shaker, R. (2011), "Pharyngeal airway protective reflexes are triggered before the maximum volume of fluid that the hypopharynx can safely hold is exceeded", *American Joural of Physiology: Gastrointestinal and Liver Physiology*, Vol. 301, pp. 197–202.

Easterling, C., Grande, B., Kern, M., Sears, K. and Shaker, R. (2005), "Attaining and maintaining isometric and isokinetic goals of the Shaker exercise", *Dysphagia*, Vol. 20, pp. 133–138.

Garcia, J.M., Chambers, E.T. and Molander, M. (2005), "Thickened liquids: practice patterns of speech-language pathologists", *American Journal of Speech Language Pathology*, Vol. 14, pp. 4–13.

Groher, M.E. and Crary, M.A. (2010), *Dysphagia: Clinical Management in Adults and Children*, Mosby-Elsevier, Maryland Heights, MO, US.

Hamdy, S., Aziz, Q., Rothwell, J.C., Singh, K.D., Barlow, J., Hughes, D.G. *et al.* (1996), "The cortical topography of human swallowing musculature in health and disease", *Nature Medicine*, Vol. 2, pp. 1217–1224.

Hamdy, S., Rothwell, J.C., Aziz, Q. and Thompson, D.G. (2000), "Organization and reorganization of human swallowing motor cortex: implications for recovery after stroke", *Clinical Science (London)*, Vol. 99, pp. 151–157.

Hiiemae, K.M. and Palmer, J.B. (1999), "Food transport and bolus formation during complete feeding sequences on foods of different initial consistency", *Dysphagia*, Vol. 14, pp. 31–42.

Ickenstein, G.W., Kelly, P.J., Furie, K.L., Ambrosi, D., Rallis, N., Goldstein, R. *et al.* (2003), "Predictors of feeding gastrostomy tube removal in stroke patients with dysphagia", *Journal of Stroke and Cerebrovascular Diseases*, Vol. 12, pp. 169–174.

Jean, A. (2001), "Brain stem control of swallowing: neuronal network and cellular mechanisms", *Physiological Reviews,* Vol. 81, pp. 929–969.

Juan, J., Hind, J., Jones, C., Mcculloch, T., Gangnon, R. and Robbins, J. (2013), "Case study: Application of isometric progressive resistance oropharyngeal therapy using the Madison Oral Strengthening Therapeutic device", *Topics in Stroke Rehabilitation,* Vol. 20, pp. 450–470.

Kendall, K.A., Leonard, R.J. and Mckenzie, S.W. (2001), "Accommodation to changes in bolus viscosity in normal deglutition: A videofluoroscopic study", *Annals of Otology, Rhinology and Laryngology,* Vol. 110, pp. 1059–1065.

Kortebein, P., Ferrando, A., Lombeida, J., Wolfe, R. and Evans, W. (2007), "Effect of 10 days of bed rest on skeletal muscle in healthy older adults", *The Journal of the American Medical Association,* Vol. 297, pp. 1769–1774.

Lan, Y., Ohkubo, M., Berretin-Felix, G., Sia, I., Carnaby-Mann, G.D. and Crary, M.A. (2012), "Normalization of temporal aspects of swallowing physiology after the McNeill dysphagia therapy program", *Annals of Otology, Rhinology and Laryngology,* Vol. 121, pp. 525–532.

Lazarus, C.L., Husaini, H., Falciglia, D., Delacure, M., Branski, R.C., Kraus, D., *et al.,* (2014), "Effects of exercise on swallowing and tongue strength in patients with oral and oropharyngeal cancer treated with primary radiotherapy with or without chemotherapy", *International Journal of Oral and Maxillofacial Surgery,* Vol. 43, pp. 523–350.

Leiter, A.E. and Windsor, J. (1996), "Compliance of geriatric patients with safe swallowing instructions", *Journal of Medical Speech-Language Pathology,* Vol. 8, pp. 109–117.

Low, J., Wyles, C., Wilkinson, T. and Sainsbury, R. (2001), "The effect of compliance on clinical outcomes for patients with dysphagia on videofluoroscopy", *Dysphagia,* Vol. 16, pp. 123–127.

Malandraki, G.A., Kaufman, A., Hind, J., Ennis, S., Gangnon, R., Waclawik, A. and Robbins, J. (2012), "The effects of lingual intervention in a patient with inclusion body myositis and Sjogren's syndrome: A longitudinal case study", *Archives of Physical Medicine and Rehabilitation,* Vol. 93, pp. 1469–1475.

Malandraki, G.A., Perlman, A.L., Karampinos, D.C. and Sutton, B.P. (2011), "Reduced somatosensory activations in swallowing with age", *Human Brain Mapping,* Vol. 32, pp. 730–743.

Malandraki, G.A., Sutton, B.P., Perlman, A.L., Karampinos, D.C. and Conway, C. (2009), "Neural activation of swallowing and swallowing-related tasks in healthy young adults: An attempt to separate the components of deglutition", *Human Brain Mapping,* Vol 30, pp. 3209–3226.

Martin, R.E., Macintosh, B.J., Smith, R.C., Barr, A.M., Stevens, T.K., Gati, J.S. and Menon, R.S. (2004), "Cerebral areas processing swallowing and tongue movement are overlapping but distinct: A functional magnetic resonance imaging study", *Journal of Neurophysiology,* Vol. 92, pp. 2428–2443.

Mepani, R., Antonik, S., Massey, B., Kern, M., Logemann, J., Pauloski, B., *et al.,* (2009), "Augmentation of deglutitive thyrohyoid muscle shortening by the Shaker Exercise", *Dysphagia,* Vol. 24, pp. 26–31.

Michou, E. and Hamdy, S. (2009), "Cortical input in control of swallowing", *Current Opinion in Otolaryngology Head Neck Surgery,* Vol. 17, pp. 166–171.

Mihai, P.G., Und Halbach, O.V.B. and Lotze, M. (2013), "Differentiation of cerebral representation of occlusion and swallowing with fMRI", *American Journal of Physiology Gastrointestinal and Liver Physiology,* Vol. 304, pp. 847–854.

Miller, L., Clave, R., Farre, R., Lecea, B., Ruggieri, M.R., Ouyang, A., Regan, J. and McMahon, B.P. (2013), "Physiology of the upper segment, body, and lower segment of the esophagus", *Annals of the New York Academy of Sciences,* Vol. 1300, pp. 261–277.

Pitts, T., Bolser, D., Rosenbek, J., Troche, M., Okun, M.S. and Sapienza, C. (2009), "Impact of expiratory muscle strength training on voluntary cough and swallow function in Parkinson disease", *Chest,* Vol. 135, pp. 1301–1308.

Robbins, J., Gangnon, R.E., Theis, S.M., Kays, S.A., Hewitt, A.L. and Hind, J.A. (2005), "The effects of lingual exercise on swallowing in older adults", *Journal of the American Geriatrics Society,* Vol. 53, pp. 1483–1489.

Robbins, J., Kays, S.A., Gangnon, R.E., Hind, J.A., Hewitt, A.L., Gentry, L.R. and Taylor, A.J. (2007), "The effects of lingual exercise in stroke patients with dysphagia", *Archives of Physical Medicine and Rehabilitation,* Vol. 88, pp. 150–158.

Seo, H.G., Oh, B.M. and Han, T.R. (2011), "Longitudinal changes of the swallowing process in subacute stroke patients with aspiration", *Dysphagia,* Vol. 26, pp. 41–48.

Shaker, R., Kern, M., Bardan, E., Taylor, A., Stewart, E.T., Hoffmann, R.G., *et al.,* (1997), "Augmentation of deglutitive upper esophageal sphincter opening in the elderly by exercise", *American Journal of Physiology,* Vol. 272, pp. 1518–1522.

Shibamoto, I., Tanaka, T., Fujishima, I., Katagiri, N. and Uematsu, H. (2007), "Cortical activation during solid bolus swallowing", *Journal of Medical and Dental Sciences,* Vol. 54, pp. 25–30.

Soros, P., Inamoto, Y. and Martin, R.E. (2009), "Functional brain imaging of swallowing: An activation likelihood estimation meta-analysis", *Human Brain Mapping,* Vol. 30, pp. 2426–2439.

Steele, C. (2010), "Tongue-Pressure resistance training: Workout for dysphagia", *The ASHA Leader.* www.asha.org/Publications/leader/2010/100518/Tongue-Pressure-Resistance-Training.htm.

Steele, C.M. and Miller, A.J. (2010), "Sensory input pathways and mechanisms in swallowing: A review", *Dysphagia,* Vol. 25, pp. 323–333.

Taub, E., Uswatte, G., Mark, V.W. and Morris, D.M. (2006), "The learned nonuse phenomenon: Implications for rehabilitation", *Europa Medicophysica,* Vol. 42, pp. 241–255.

Terre, R. and Mearin, F. (2007), "Prospective evaluation of oro-pharyngeal dysphagia after severe traumatic brain injury", *Brain Injury,* Vol. 21, pp. 1411–1417.

Wijesekera, L.C. and Leigh, P.N. (2009), "Amyotrophic lateral sclerosis", *Orphanet Journal of Rare Diseases,* Vol. 4, No. 1, p. 3, doi: 10.1186/1750-1172-4-3.

8

NEUROPHARMACOLOGIC APPROACHES TO APHASIA REHABILITATION

Marcelo L. Berthier, Guadalupe Dávila
and María José Torres-Prioris

Aphasia is defined as a loss or impairment of the complex process of interpreting and formulating language symbols caused by damage affecting a widely distributed network of cortical and subcortical structures of the language-dominant hemisphere (Berthier *et al.*, 2014a; Hillis, 2007; Varley, 2011). It is a disabling cognitive deficit occurring in about one third of stroke patients (Bersano *et al.*, 2009; Laska *et al.*, 2001; Pedersen *et al.*, 2004) and it causes substantial functional disability and psychological distress (Berthier *et al.*, 2014a; Hilari, 2011). Since spontaneous recovery cannot be expected in a great proportion of post-stroke aphasic patients, they are treated with cognitive-linguistic rehabilitation and, less frequently, with biological treatments (drugs, non-invasive brain stimulation) (Berthier *et al.*, 2011b; Small and Llano, 2009). Nevertheless, the level of evidence of different interventions still remains controversial (Bowen and Patchick, 2014). This chapter reviews the theoretical rationale for using drugs to treat aphasia, and the available evidence on combining rehabilitation with cognitive enhancing drugs to alleviate language and communication deficits in patients with stroke and Alzheimer's disease (AD). Implications will be outlined for future research and clinical practice on the key role of combining rehabilitation with cognitive enhancing drugs.

Cognitive rehabilitation in aphasia: Beyond speech-language therapy

Impact of non-language cognitive deficits on aphasia recovery

Cognitive factors may play a role in the recovery process from aphasia (*see* Lambon Ralph *et al.*, 2010). Several studies have reported an association between aphasic deficits and impairments in non-language cognitive domains (El Hachioui *et al.*, 2014; Kauhanen *et al.*, 2000; van de Sandt-Koenderman *et al.*, 2008). In fact, non-language cognitive impairment seems to be a common feature in chronic aphasia as most patients have at least one cognitive deficit affecting abstract reasoning, visual memory, visual perception and construction, and executive functioning (El Hachioui *et al.*, 2014). Moreover, some studies including large numbers of patients with aphasia found that assessment of non-language cognitive functioning in tasks tapping reasoning, problem-solving, attention and visual recall was a good predictor of therapy outcome (Lambon Ralph *et al.*, 2010; van de Sandt-Koenderman *et al.*, 2008). This is an important piece of information for speech–language pathologists because it advocates testing of non-language cognition in patients with aphasia. Future studies are needed to ascertain whether an integral treatment of aphasic deficits may require supplementing speech-language therapy with rehabilitation of non-language cognitive deficits (Lambon Ralph *et al.*, 2010). It also remains to be determined if complementary strategies (e.g., drugs, non-invasive brain stimulation) currently applied to augment the benefits provided by rehabilitation of language can also impact on non-language cognitive deficits (Allen *et al.*, 2012; Small and Llano, 2009).

The contribution of neuroimaging

Over the last decades, knowledge on cognitive rehabilitation has also been fueled by functional (Price, 2010) and structural (Geva *et al.*, 2011) neuroimaging. One aim of these studies was to examine the neural correlates of language by linking functional models of language with neural systems in healthy subjects (Binder, 1997; Howard *et al.*, 1992; Price *et al.*, 1996) and in patients with aphasia (Rosen *et al.*, 2000; Warburton *et al.*, 1999). A second aim of neuroimaging studies was to analyze the effects of cognitive rehabilitation on neural plasticity in patients with aphasia (Breier *et al.*, 2011; Fridriksson *et al.*, 2012; Richter *et al.*, 2008). These diagnostic and therapeutic advances are greatly contributing to the consolidation of neuroscience-based rehabilitation as a new model of therapeutic intervention for aphasia and other cognitive disorders (e.g., neglect). This consolidation is based on the understanding of how behavioral training and other interventions (drugs, repetitive transcranial magnetic stimulation [rTMS], transcranial direct current stimulation [TDCS]) promote recovery of function through modulation of cellular and circuit plasticity (Barrett *et al.*, 2006; Berthier and Pulvermüller, 2011; Gorgoraptis *et al.*, 2012; Paolucci *et al.*, 2010; Pulvermüller and Berthier, 2008; Small *et al.*, 2013). Non-invasive brain stimulation (rTMS and TDCS) is emerging as a valuable tool to help patients with aphasia regaining 'lost' language functions (Shah *et al.*, 2013). These techniques generate an electrical current which depolarizes or hyperpolarizes neurons on the brain region nearby to the stimulated site. Stimulation may be inhibitory to decrease the activity of abnormally released regions, which presumably interfere with language processing, or may be excitatory to increase the activity of inhibited regions, thus promoting recovery of language function (Shah *et al.*, 2013). (See the chapter by Schwartz, Middleton and Hamilton in this volume for a discussion of neuromodulation).

Current status of drug treatment for aphasia

Drug interventions in clinical practice are increasingly being used in acute care stroke rehabilitation and outpatient settings, accounting for more than 30 percent of cases (Barrett *et al.*, 2007; Engelter *et al.*, 2010, 2012). Results from a recent prospective explorative multicenter study revealed that half of the patients received antidepressant medications to alleviate post-stroke mood and anxiety disorders, whereas in one third of patients drugs were exclusively used with the aim to augment rehabilitation gains (Engelter *et al.*, 2010, 2012). While depression is the most commonly treated psychiatric condition, aphasia, motor deficits, and neglect are the most commonly treated cognitive disorders. Importantly, patients treated with levodopa, cholinesterase inhibitors (e.g., donepezil) and other agents, such as antidepressants and stimulants, achieved greater improvement in a functional independence measure than untreated patients (Engelter *et al.*, 2010, 2012). Although more studies are needed, the prescription of these drugs in clinical practice as "off-label" medications is supported by the results of several well-designed clinical trials. In fact, there is moderate evidence (Level 1b) based on randomized controlled trials ("proof-of-concept" studies) that use of levodopa, donepezil, galantamine, and memantine significantly improve aphasia severity, deficits in speech production (naming), and comprehension in patients with chronic stroke (*see* Berthier *et al.*, 2011b; Salter *et al.*, 2012; Teasell *et al.*, 2012).

Rationale for using cognitive enhancing drugs in aphasia

Focal and diffuse brain lesions interrupt the projections of major neurotransmitter systems (cholinergic, dopaminergic, serotonergic, noradrenergic) from basal forebrain or brainstem to cerebral cortex and subcortical nuclei, causing synaptic depression in both perilesional areas and remote regions in both hemispheres (Berthier and Pulvermüller, 2011; Gotts and Plaut, 2002; Small and Llano, 2009). In addition, stroke lesions induce a pathological activation of N-methyl-D-aspartate receptors (NMDArs) which can result in myelin sheath damage and neuronal cell death (Martin and Wang, 2010; Parsons *et al.*, 2007). The aim of pharmacotherapy is to promote functional and structural neural plasticity by restoring the activity of depleted or pathologically released neurotransmitters in dysfunctional circuits (Berthier *et al.*, 2011b). Drugs may likewise strengthen the activity of systems remote to the structural lesions which did not actively participate in language function in normal conditions (e.g., right hemisphere networks), but which are vicariously recruited to increase recovery further after brain damage (Berthier *et al.*, 2011a; Zipse *et al.*, 2012).

Choosing the right drug

There is evidence that not all aphasic deficits are responsive to a single drug (Galling *et al.*, 2014). Histochemistry studies of the human brain have identified the trajectory of cholinergic pathways (Selden *et al.*, 1998) and mapping approaches have defined the receptor architecture of cholinergic and other major neurotransmitter systems (Amunts and Zilles, 2012; Zilles and Amunts, 2009). In addition, quantitative analysis of the biodistribution of drugs (e.g., donepezil) in the brain using positron emission tomography and [(11)C]-donepezil is now possible in individual patients (Hiraoka *et al.*, 2009; Okamura *et al.*, 2008). Altogether, this valuable information assists in making inferences on how focal and diffuse brain lesions disrupt the neurotransmitter markers in specific anatomical sites (e.g., Broca's area) and also may serve in the selection of specific drugs and appropriate candidates for pharmacological studies of language disorders.

In recent years, the activity of several neurotransmitter systems (dopaminergic, cholinergic, glutamatergic, serotonergic, norepinephrinergic, glutamatergic) has been manipulated in aphasia with variable success using agents (levodopa, bromocriptine, donepezil, galantamine, memantine) originally marketed to alleviate motor and cognitive-behavioral deficits in Parkinson's disease (PD) and AD (*see* Berthier *et al.*, 2011b; Tocco *et al.*, 2014 *for review*). For instance, dopaminergic stimulation may improve aphasic deficits by restoring dopaminergic tone in frontal-basal ganglia circuits (Albert *et al.*, 1988), which modulates motor control, incentive reward, memory, attention, problem-solving, and learning (Berthier *et al.*, 2011b; Gill and Leff, 2014; Seniów *et al.*, 2009). However, initial pharmacological studies on aphasia used dopaminergic agonists in cases with non-fluent speech with mixed results (*for review see* Cahana-Amitay *et al.*, 2014; Gill and Leff, 2014). Although further studies are needed, available evidence indicates that dopaminergic agents, especially when combined with speech–language therapy (Galling *et al.*, 2014; Gill and Leff, 2014), improve speech initiation, pauses in conversation, paraphasias, and naming in patients with reduced drive to generate spontaneous speech (e.g., transcortical motor aphasia and adynamic aphasia) secondary to frontal and/or basal ganglia lesions (Albert *et al.*, 1988; Cahana-Amitay *et al.*, 2014). It should be noted, however, that damage to some structures might deplete the activity of some neurotransmitters while having little impact on others. This would explain why cognitive and language deficits associated with lesions in left posterior perisylvian areas are not responsive to dopaminergic stimulation (Galling *et al.*, 2014). The utility of other drugs targeting catecholaminergic systems (amantadine, dexamphetamine) and other neurotransmitter systems (piracetam, propranolol, cerebrolysin, zolpidem) in the treatment of aphasia requires further assessment (*for recent reviews see* Berthier *et al.*, 2011b; Walker-Batson, 2013).

Expanding the indications for antidementia drugs

During the past decade, cholinergic agents (galantamine, donepezil) and the NMDArs antagonist memantine, drugs used to treat AD, have been added to the pharmacological armamentarium for treating post-stroke aphasia (Berthier and Pulvermüller, 2011; Small and Llano, 2009). Although galantamine was used for the first time to treat aphasic deficits in the late 1960s (Luria *et al.*, 1969), its use in aphasia was abandoned until recently (Hong *et al.*, 2012). A current randomized controlled study of galantamine revealed beneficial effects on aphasia severity and on several language domains in patients with chronic stroke, particularly in those with predominantly left subcortical lesions affecting the trajectory of the lateral cholinergic pathway (Hong *et al.*, 2012). Open-label and controlled studies of donepezil combined with distributed speech–language therapy (two hours per week) also demonstrated significant benefits in aphasia severity, naming, and communication in patients with chronic post-stroke aphasia (*see* Berthier *et al.*, 2011b). The use of memantine in patients with chronic post-stroke aphasia has been associated with significant improvements in aphasia severity and communication deficits and its benefits persisted on long-term follow-up (one year) (Berthier *et al.*, 2009). However, memantine has a different pharmacological profile than cholinergic agents as it tends to downregulate abnormally activated NMDArs to more appropriate levels (Martin and Wang, 2010; Parsons *et al.*, 2007).

Combining neuropharmacologic approaches with cognitive rehabilitation

A growing body of evidence indicates that benefits provided by a pharmacological agent on cognition can be enhanced further when its potential action is combined with cognitive rehabilitation (Berthier *et al.*, 2009; Matsuda, 2007; Rothi *et al.*, 2009). For example, if one considers the case of AD, benefits or stabilization of cognitive deficits are commonly observed in response to cholinesterase inhibitors (Birks, 2006), memantine, or both (McShane *et al.*, 2006; Tocco *et al.*, 2014), even when drug treatment is unpaired with cognitive rehabilitation. In this circumstance, however, treatment effects were not large and their impact on clinical manifestations was considered "modest" (Herrmann, 2002) or "limited" (Schneider, 2013). Fortunately, attempts to strengthen the beneficial effects of drugs with behavioral training are gaining credence. A systematic review on the efficacy of non-pharmacological therapies in AD provided a Grade B recommendation (i.e., benefits of the clinical service outweigh the potential risks) suggesting that rehabilitation (Olazarán *et al.*, 2010) can amplify drug treatment effects in AD (Bottino *et al.*, 2005; Loewenstein *et al.*, 2004; Rozzini *et al.*, 2007). In fact, there is mounting evidence that domain-focused intensive training paired with drugs produces synergistic effects on word relearning in patients with aphasia of various etiologies (Berthier *et al.*, 2009, 2014b; Rothi *et al.*, 2009; Walker-Batson, 2013).

In a recent Phase I study over a three-month interval in six patients with probable AD and anomia, a theory-based cognitive training (errorless learning) (Clare and Jones, 2008) paired with donepezil significantly improved naming in half of the patients (Rothi *et al.*, 2009). The same held true for patients with post-stroke language and communication deficits. Patients with chronic post-stroke aphasia treated with memantine alone showed significant improvement in aphasia severity in comparison to patients treated with placebo alone, but observed benefits in both groups were strengthened further (more in the memantine-treated group) when a short run of intensive aphasia therapy (Constraint-Induced Aphasia Therapy, CIAT) was added (Berthier *et al.*, 2009; Pulvermüller *et al.*, 2001). A recent case-series study found that massed sentence repetition therapy (40 hours; 8 weeks) was associated with better outcomes than distributed speech–language therapy (40 hours; 16 weeks) in chronic post-stroke conduction aphasic patients receiving donepezil (Berthier *et al.*, 2014b). Therefore, combining drugs with intensive neuroscience-based therapies seems to be a highly promising strategy to treat aphasic deficits.

Language is no longer conceptualized as an encapsulated module as it is widely linked to other cognitive functions (e.g., attention, short-term memory, planning) as well as to behavioral dimensions (goal-directed behavior, mood, personality). With this idea in mind, it could be that cholinergic stimulation of non-language brain structures contributes to aphasia recovery by orchestrating the activity of various cognitive processes (attention, learning, cognitive control) (Sarter *et al.*, 2003) linked to language function. In a recent study, treatment with donepezil in combination with CIAT induced structural plasticity in non-damaged areas innervated by the cholinergic system (anterior and posterior cingulate gyrus, peri-insular regions) in both hemispheres (Berthier, 2012). This implies that pharmacological modulation of neurotransmitter systems in aphasia can improve neural efficiency not only in dysfunctional language areas, but also in non-language regions which interact with different language processes through regulation of attention, cognitive control, memory, mood and goal-directed behavior.

Conclusions and directions for future research

The most important lesson to be learnt is that adjunctive drug treatment to rehabilitation can reduce the number of stroke patients with significant disability (Berthier and Pulvermüller, 2011) and also that this strategy can stabilize and even reduce language and communication deficits among patients with degenerative dementias (Rothi *et al.*, 2009; Tocco *et al.*, 2014). Nevertheless, this field is an emergent one and many pending issues remain to be addressed in future research. Studies combining rehabilitation with drugs or other biological treatments (rTMS, TDCS) require a better understanding of intervention interactions. Trials combining drugs (donepezil–memantine) targeting different neurotransmitter systems (cholinergic–glutamatergic), which have already demonstrated benefits in AD (Tocco *et al.*, 2014), may also be useful in the treatment of stroke-related cognitive deficits. Identification of bad and good responders to rehabilitation and biological interventions (drugs, rTMS, TDCS) is important to eradicate "trial and error" prescriptions. This might be accomplished by refining the identification of patient responders/non-responders through the development of responder criteria in multiple outcome cognitive, behavioral and functional measures in individual patients. The ability to identify groups of patients who respond to a specific rehabilitation therapy and/or biological interventions may contribute to more focused assessments and treatments.

The identification of "ideal" candidates for different strategies to remediate aphasic deficits may be integrated with recent advances from structural and functional neuroimaging in the prediction of stroke-deficits evolution (Hope *et al.*, 2013; Menke *et al.*, 2009; Price *et al.*, 2010) and response to treatments (Richter *et al.*, 2008). More understanding of the influence of genetic (Pearson-Fuhrhop *et al.*, 2012) and environmental (McClung *et al.*, 2010) factors on adaptive neural plasticity promoted by different interventions used independently or in combination is necessary.

Victims of post-stroke aphasia may not display only a multiple-domain cognitive impairment as they are also afflicted by motor/sensory deficits and psychiatric comorbidities (depression, apathy, anxiety), which reduce adaptability and quality of life. Preliminary data indicate that motor/sensory deficits can be ameliorated with drugs in conjunction with exercise therapy (Engelter *et al.*, 2012; Nadeau *et al.*, 2004; Walker-Batson, 2013) but further studies are needed to examine the impact of motor rehabilitation on speech, language and communication deficits.

Post-stroke psychiatric conditions negatively impact rehabilitation of physical and cognitive deficits and increase morbidity and mortality. Up to now, efforts have been directed to prevent their occurrence or reduce their severity with drugs and behavioral interventions (Jorge *et al.*, 2010; Mikami *et al.*, 2013) but treatment of psychiatric symptoms in post-stroke aphasia remains to be explored. We hope that gaining further knowledge on the potential role of neuropharmacology to alleviate cognitive, behavioral and functional deficits in aphasia can diminish some of the most negative consequences of stroke.

References

Albert, M.L., Bachman, D.L., Morgan, A. and Helm-Estabrooks, N. (1988), "Pharmacotherapy for aphasia", *Neurology*, Vol. 38, No. 6, pp. 877–879.

Allen, L., Mehta, S., McClure, J.A. and Teasell, R. (2012), "Therapeutic interventions for aphasia initiated more than six months post stroke: a review of the evidence", *Topics in Stroke Rehabilitation*, Vol. 19, No. 6, pp. 523–535.

Amunts, K. and Zilles, K. (2012), "Architecture and organizational principles of Broca's region", *Trends in Cognitive Sciences*, Vol. 16, No. 8, pp. 418–426.

Barrett, A.M., Buxbaum, L.J., Coslett, H.B., Edwards, E., Heilman, K.M., Hillis, A.E. *et al.* (2006), "Cognitive rehabilitation interventions for neglect and related disorders: Moving from bench to bedside in stroke patients", *Journal of Cognitive Neuroscience*, Vol. 18, No. 7, pp. 1223–1236.

Barrett, A.M., Levy, C.E. and Gonzalez Rothi, L.J. (2007), "Pharmaceuticals for poststroke and brain injury rehabilitation", *American Journal of Physical Medicine and Rehabilitation*, Vol. 86, No. 8, pp. 603–604.

Bersano, A, Burgio, F, Gattinoni, M, Candelise, L; PROSIT Study Group. (2009), "Aphasia burden to hospitalised acute stroke patients: Need for an early rehabilitation program", *International Journal of Stroke*, Vol. 4, No. 6, pp. 443–447.

Berthier, M.L. (2012), "Pharmacological interventions boost language and communication treatment effects in chronic post-stroke aphasia", Presented in the symposium Fortschritte in Neurowissenschaft und Neurorehabilitation der Sprache, 85. Kongress der Deutschen Gesellschaft für Neurologie mit Fortbildungsakademie. Hamburg, Germany, Hauptprogramm, p. 23.

Berthier, M.L., Dávila, G., García-Casares, N. and Moreno-Torres, I. (2014a), "Post-stroke aphasia", In: *The Behavioral Consequences of Stroke*. T.A. Schweizer and R.L. Macdonald (Eds.), Springer Science + Business Media. New York, pp. 95–117.

Berthier, M.L., Dávila, G., Green, C., Moreno-Torres, I., Juárez y Ruiz de Mier, R., De Torres, I. and Ruiz-Cruces, R. (2014b), "Massed sentence repetition training can augment and speed up recovery of speech production deficits in patients with chronic conduction aphasia receiving donepezil treatment", *Aphasiology*, Vol. 28, No. 2, pp. 188–218.

Berthier, M.L., García-Casares, N., Walsh, S.F., Nabrozidis, A., Ruíz de Mier, R.J., Green, C., *et al.*, (2011a), "Recovery from post-stroke aphasia: lessons from brain imaging and implications for rehabilitation and biological treatments", *Discovery Medicine*, Vol. 12, No. 65, pp. 275–289.

Berthier, M.L., Green, C., Lara, J.P., Higueras, C., Barbancho, M.A., Dávila, G. and Pulvermüller, F. (2009), "Memantine and constraint-induced aphasia therapy in chronic poststroke aphasia", *Annals of Neurology*, Vol. 65, No. 5, pp. 577–585.

Berthier, M.L. and Pulvermüller, F. (2011), "Neuroscience insights improve neurorehabilitation of poststroke aphasia", *Nature Reviews. Neurology*, Vol. 7, No. 2, pp. 86–97.

Berthier, M.L., Pulvermüller, F., Dávila, G., Casares, N.G. and Gutiérrez, A. (2011b), "Drug therapy of post-stroke aphasia: A review of current evidence", *Neuropsychology Review*, Vol. 21, No. 3, pp. 302–317.

Binder, J.R. (1997), "Neuroanatomy of language processing studied with functional MRI", *Clinical Neuroscience*, Vol. 4, No. 2, pp. 87–94.

Birks, J. (2006), "Cholinesterase inhibitors for Alzheimer's disease", *Cochrane Database of Systematic Reviews*. Jan 25, CD005593.

Bottino, C.M.C., Carvalho, I.A.M., Alvarez, A.M., Avila, R., Zukauskas, P.R., Bustamante, S.E.Z. *et al.*, (2005), "Cognitive rehabilitation combined with drug treatment in Alzheimer's disease patients: A pilot study", *Clinical Rehabilitation*, Vol. 19, No. 8, pp. 861–869.

Bowen, A. and Patchick, E. (2014), "Cognitive rehabilitation and recovery after stroke", In: T.A. Schweizer and R.L. Macdonald (Eds.), *The Behavioral Consequences of Stroke*. Springer Science + Business Media. New York, pp. 315–339.

Breier, J.I., Juranek, J. and Papanicolaou, A.C. (2011), "Changes in maps of language function and the integrity of the arcuate fasciculus after therapy for chronic aphasia", *Neurocase*, Vol. 17, No. 6, pp. 506–517.

Cahana-Amitay, D., Albert, M.L. and Oveis, A. (2014), "Psycholinguistics of aphasia pharmacotherapy: Asking the right questions", *Aphasiology*, Vol. 28, No. 2, pp. 133–154.

Clare, L. and Jones, R.S.P. (2008), "Errorless learning in the rehabilitation of memory impairment: A critical review", *Neuropsychology Review*, Vol. 18, No. 1, pp. 1–23.

El Hachioui, H., Visch-Brink, E.G., Lingsma, H.F., van de Sandt-Koenderman, M.W., Dippel, D.W., Koudstaal, P.J. and Middelkoop, H.A. (2014), "Nonlinguistic cognitive impairment in poststroke aphasia: A prospective study", *Neurorehabilitation and Neural Repair*. Vol. 28, No. 3, pp. 273–281.

Engelter, S.T., Frank, M., Lyrer, P.A. and Conzelmann, M. (2010), "Safety of pharmacological augmentation of stroke rehabilitation", *European Neurology*, Vol. 64, No. 6, pp. 325–330.

Engelter, S.T., Urscheler, N., Baronti, F., Vuadens, P., Koch, J., Frank, M., *et al.*, (2012), "Frequency and determinants of using pharmacological enhancement in the clinical practice of in-hospital stroke rehabilitation", *European Neurology*, Vol. 68, No. 1, pp. 28–33.

Fridriksson, J., Hubbard, H.I., Hudspeth, S.G., Holland, A.L., Bonilha, L., Fromm, D. and Rorden, C. (2012), "Speech entrainment enables patients with Broca's aphasia to produce fluent speech", *Brain*, Vol. 135, No. 12, pp. 3815–3829.

Galling, M.A., Goorah, N., Berthier, M.L. and Sage, K. (2014), "A clinical study of the combined use of bromocriptine and speech and language therapy in the treatment of a person with aphasia", *Aphasiology*, Vol. 28, No. 2, pp. 171–187.

Geva, S., Correia, M. and Warburton, E.A. (2011), "Diffusion tensor imaging in the study of language and aphasia", *Aphasiology*, Vol. 25, No. 5, pp. 543–558.

Gill, S.K. and Leff, A.P. (2014), "Dopaminergic therapy in aphasia", *Aphasiology*, Vol. 28, No. 2, pp. 155–170.

Gorgoraptis, N., Mah, Y.H., Machner, B., Singh-Curry, V., Malhotra, P., Hadji-Michael, M., *et al.*, (2012), "The effects of the dopamine agonist rotigotine on hemispatial neglect following stroke", *Brain*, Vol. 135, No. 8, pp. 2478–2491.

Gotts, S.J. and Plaut, D.C. (2002), "The impact of synaptic depression following brain damage: A connectionist account of 'access/refractory' and 'degraded-store' semantic impairments", *Cognitive, Affective and Behavioral Neuroscience*, Vol. 2, No. 3, pp.187–213.

Herrmann, N. (2002), "Cognitive pharmacotherapy of Alzheimer's disease and other dementias", *Canadian Journal of Psychiatry*, Vol. 47, No. 8, pp. 715–722.

Hilari, K. (2011), "The impact of stroke: Are people with aphasia different to those without?", *Disability and Rehabilitation*, Vol. 33, No. 3, pp. 211–218.

Hillis, A.E. (2007), "Aphasia: progress in the last quarter of a century", *Neurology*, Vol. 69, No. 2, pp. 200–213.

Hiraoka, K., Okamura, N., Funaki, Y., Watanuki, S., Tashiro, M., Kato, M., *et al.*, (2009), "Quantitative analysis of donepezil binding to acetylcholinesterase using positron emission tomography and [5-(11) C-methoxy]donepezil", *Neuroimage*, Vol. 46, No. 3, pp. 616–623.

Hong, J.M., Shin, D.H., Lim, T.S., Lee, J.S. and Huh, K. (2012), "Galantamine administration in chronic post-stroke aphasia", *Journal of Neurology Neurosurgery, and Psychiatry*, Vol. 83, No. 7, pp. 675–680.

Hope, T.M., Seghier, M.L., Leff, A.P. and Price, C.J. (2013), "Predicting outcome and recovery after stroke with lesions extracted from MRI images", *Neuroimage Clinical*, Vol. 2, pp. 424–433.

Howard, D., Patterson, K., Wise, R., Brown, W.D., Friston, K., Weiller, C. and Frackowiak, R. (1992), "The cortical localization of the lexicons. Positron emission tomography evidence", *Brain*, Vol. 115, No. 6, pp. 1769–1782.

Jorge, R.E., Acion, L., Moser, D., Adams, H.P. Jr, and Robinson, R.G. (2010), "Escitalopram and enhancement of cognitive recovery following stroke", *Archives of General Psychiatry*, Vol. 67, No. 2, pp. 187–196.

Kauhanen, M.L., Korpelainen, J.T., Hiltunen, P., Määttä, R., Mononen, H., Brusin, E., *et al.*, (2000), "Aphasia, depression, and non-verbal cognitive impairment in ischaemic stroke", *Cerebrovascular Diseases*, Vol. 10, No. 6, pp. 455–461.

Lambon Ralph, M.A., Snell, C., Fillingham, J.K., Conroy, P. and Sage, K. (2010), "Predicting the outcome of anomia therapy for people with aphasia post CVA: Both language and cognitive status are key predictors", *Neuropsychological Rehabilitation*, Vol. 20, No. 2, pp. 289–305.

Laska, A.C., Hellblom, A., Murray, V., Kahan, T. and Von Arbin, M. (2001), "Aphasia in acute stroke and relation to outcome", *Journal of Internal Medicine*, Vol. 249, No. 5, pp. 413–422.

Loewenstein, D.A., Acevedo, A., Czaja, S.J. and Duara, R. (2004), "Cognitive rehabilitation of mildly impaired Alzheimer disease patients on cholinesterase inhibitors", *The American Journal of Geriatric Psychiatry*, Vol .12, No. 4, pp. 395–402.

Luria, A., Naydyn, V.L., Tsvetkova, L. S. and Vinarskaya, E. N. (1969), "Restoration of higher cortical function following local brain damage", In P.J. Vinken and G.W. Bruyn (Eds.), *Handbook of Clinical Neurology*. North-Holland, Amsterdam, Netherlands. pp. 368–433.

Martin, H.G. and Wang, Y.T. (2010), "Blocking the deadly effects of the NMDA receptor in stroke", *Cell*, Vol. 140, No. 2, pp. 174–176.

Matsuda, O. (2007), "Cognitive stimulation therapy for Alzheimer's disease: The effect of cognitive stimulation therapy on the progression of mild Alzheimer's disease in patients treated with donepezil", *International Psychogeriatrics*, Vol. 19, No. 2, pp. 241–252.

McClung, J.S., Rothi, L.J. and Nadeau, S.E. (2010), "Ambient experience in restitutive treatment of aphasia", *Frontiers in Human Neuroscience*, Nov 2, Vol. 4, p. 183. doi: 10.3389/fnhum.2010.00183.

McShane, R., Areosa Sastre, A. and Minakaran, N. (2006), "Memantine for dementia", *Cochrane Database of Systematic Reviews*. Apr 19; Vol. 2, CD003154.

Menke, R., Meinzer, M., Kugel, H., Deppe, M., Baumgärtner, A., Schiffbauer, H., *et al.*, (2009), "Imaging short- and long-term training success in chronic aphasia", *BMC Neuroscience*, Vol. 10, p. 118.

Mikami, K., Jorge, R.E., Moser, D.J., Arndt, S., Jang, M., Solodkin, A., *et al.*, (2013), "Prevention of poststroke apathy using escitalopram or problem-solving therapy", *The American Journal of Geriatric Psychiatry*. Vol. 21, No. 9, pp. 855–862.

Nadeau, S.E., Behrman, A.L., Davis, S.E., Reid, K., Wu, S.S., Stidham, B.S., *et al.*, (2004), "Donepezil as an adjuvant to constraint-induced therapy for upper-limb dysfunction after stroke: An exploratory randomized clinical trial", *Journal of Rehabilitation Research and Development*, Vol. 41, No. 4, pp. 525–534.

Okamura, N., Funaki, Y., Tashiro, M., Kato, M., Ishikawa, Y., Maruyama, M., *et al.*, (2008), "In vivo visualization of donepezil binding in the brain of patients with Alzheimer's disease", *British Journal of Clinical Pharmacology*, Vol. 65, No. 4, pp. 472–479.

Olazarán, J., Reisberg, B., Clare, L., Cruz, I., Peña-Casanova, J., Del Ser, T., *et al.*, (2010), "Nonpharmacological therapies in Alzheimer's disease: A systematic review of efficacy", *Dementia and Geriatric Cognitive Disorders*, Vol. 30, No. 2, pp. 161–178.

Paolucci, S., Bureca, I., Multari, M., Nocentini, U. and Matano, A. (2010), "An open-label pilot study of the use of rivastigmine to promote functional recovery in patients with unilateral spatial neglect due to first ischemic stroke", *Functional Neurology*, Vol. 25, No. 4, pp. 195–200.

Parsons, C.G., Stöffler, A. and Danysz, W. (2007), "Memantine: a NMDA receptor antagonist that improves memory by restoration of homeostasis in the glutamatergic system—Too little activation is bad, too much is even worse", *Neuropharmacology*, Vol. 53, No. 6, pp. 699–723.

Pearson-Fuhrhop, K.M., Burke, E. and Cramer, S.C. (2012), "The influence of genetic factors on brain plasticity and recovery after neural injury", *Current Opinion in Neurology*, Vol. 25, No. 6, pp. 682–688.

Pedersen, P.M., Vinter, K. and Olsen, T.S. (2004), "Aphasia after stroke: Type, severity and prognosis. The Copenhagen aphasia study", *Cerebrovascular Diseases*, Vol. 17, No. 1, pp.35–43.

Price, C.J. (2010), "The anatomy of language: A review of 100 fMRI studies published in 2009", *Annals of the New York Academy of Sciences*, Vol. 1191, pp. 62–88.

Price, C.J., Seghier, M.L. and Leff, A.P. (2010), "Predicting language outcome and recovery after stroke: The PLORAS system", *Nature Reviews. Neurology*, Vol. 6, No 4, pp. 202–210.

Price, C.J., Wise, R.J., Warburton, E.A., Moore, C.J., Howard, D., Patterson, K., *et al.*, (1996), "Hearing and saying. The functional neuro-anatomy of auditory word processing", *Brain*, Vol. 119, No. 3, pp. 919–931.

Pulvermüller, F. and Berthier, M.L. (2008), "Aphasia therapy on a neuroscience basis", *Aphasiology*, Vol. 22 No. 6, pp. 563–599.

Pulvermüller, F., Neininger, B., Elbert, T., Mohr, B., Rockstroh, B., Koebbel, P. and Taub, E. (2001), "Constraint-induced therapy of chronic aphasia after stroke", *Stroke*, Vol. 32, No. 7, pp. 1621–1626.

Richter, M., Miltner, W.H. and Straube, T. (2008), "Association between therapy outcome and right-hemispheric activation in chronic aphasia", *Brain*, Vol. 131, No. 5, pp. 1391–1401.

Rosen, H.J., Petersen, S.E., Linenweber, M.R., Snyder, A.Z., White, D.A., Chapman, L., *et al.*, (2000), "Neural correlates of recovery from aphasia after damage to left inferior frontal cortex", *Neurology*, Vol. 55, No. 12, pp. 1883–1894.

Rothi, L.J., Fuller, R., Leon, S.A., Kendall, D., Moore, A., Wu, S.S., *et al.* (2009), "Errorless practice as a possible adjuvant to donepezil in Alzheimer's disease", *Journal of the International Neuropsychological Society*, Vol. 15, No. 2, pp. 311–322.

Rozzini, L., Costardi, D., Chilovi, B.V., Franzoni, S., Trabucchi, M. and Padovani, A. (2007), "Efficacy of cognitive rehabilitation in patients with mild cognitive impairment treated with cholinesterase inhibitors", *International Journal of Geriatric Psychiatry*, Vol. 22, No. 4, pp. 356–360.

Salter, K., Teasell, R., Bhogal, S., Zettler, L. and Foley, N. (2012), "The Evidence-Based Review of Stroke Rehabilitation (EBRSR) reviews current practices in stroke rehabilitation", Chapter 14: Aphasia. www.ebrsr.com. Last update November 2012.

Sarter, M., Bruno, J.P. and Givens, B. (2003), "Attentional functions of cortical cholinergic inputs: What does it mean for learning and memory?", *Neurobiology of Learning and Memory*, Vol. 80, No. 3, pp. 245–256.

Schneider, L.S. (2013), "Alzheimer disease pharmacologic treatment and treatment research", *Continuum* (Minneapolis, Minn.), *Vol.* 19 (2 Dementia), pp. 339–357.

Selden, N.R., Gitelman, D.R., Salamon-Murayama, N., Parrish, T.B. and Mesulam, M.M. (1998), "Trajectories of cholinergic pathways within the cerebral hemispheres of the human brain", *Brain*, Vol. 121, No. 12, pp. 2249–2257.

Seniów, J., Litwin, M., Litwin, T., Leśniak, M. and Członkowska, A. (2009), "New approach to the rehabilitation of post-stroke focal cognitive syndrome: Effect of levodopa combined with speech and language therapy on functional recovery from aphasia", *Journal of the Neurological Sciences*, Vol. 283, No. 1–2, pp. 214–218.

Shah, P.P., Szaflarski, J.P., Allendorfer, J. and Hamilton, R.H. (2013), "Induction of neuroplasticity and recovery in post-stroke aphasia by non-invasive brain stimulation", *Frontiers in Human Neuroscience*, Vol. 24, No. 7, p. 888.

Small, S.L., Buccino, G. and Solodkin, A. (2013), "Brain repair after stroke – A novel neurological model", *Nature Reviews. Neurology*, Vol. 9, No. 12, pp. 698–707.

Small, S.L. and Llano, D.A. (2009), "Biological approaches to aphasia treatment", *Current Neurology and Neurosciences Reports*, Vol. 9, No. 6, pp. 443–450.

Teasell, R., Foley, N., Salter, K., Bhogal, S., Jutai, J. and Speechley, M. (2012), "Evidence-based review of stroke rehabilitation. Executive Summary" (15th Edition). Last updated November 2012. www.ebrsr.com.

Tocco, M., Bayles, K., Lopez, O.L., Hofbauer, R.K., Pejović, V., Miller, M.L. and Saxton, J. (2014), "Effects of memantine treatment on language abilities and functional communication: A review of data", *Aphasiology*, Vol. 28, No. 2, pp. 236–257.

van de Sandt-Koenderman, W.M.E., van Harskamp, F., Duivenvoorden, H.J., Remerie, S.C., van der Voort-Klees, Y.A., Wielaert, S.M., *et al.*, (2008), "MAAS (Multi-Axial Aphasia System): Realistic goal setting in aphasia rehabilitation", *International Journal of Rehabilitation Research*, Vol. 31, No. 4, pp. 314–320.

Varley, R. (2011), "Rethinking aphasia therapy: A neuroscience perspective", *International Journal of Speech-Language Pathology*, Vol. 13, No.1, pp. 11–20.

Walker-Batson, D. (2013), "Amphetamine and post-stroke rehabilitation: Indications and controversies", *European Journal of Physical and Rehabilitation Medicine*, Vol. 49, No. 2, pp. 251–260.

Warburton, E., Price, C.J., Swinburn, K. and Wise, R.J. (1999), "Mechanisms of recovery from aphasia: Evidence from positron emission tomography studies", *Journal of Neurology, Neurosurgery and Psychiatry*, Vol. 66, No. 2, pp. 155–161.

Zilles, K. and Amunts, K. (2009), "Receptor mapping: Architecture of the human cerebral cortex", *Current Opinion in Neurology*, Vol. 22, No. 4, pp. 331–339.

Zipse, L., Norton, A., Marchina, S. and Schlaug, G. (2012), "When right is all that is left: Plasticity of right-hemisphere tracts in a young aphasic patient", *Annals of the New York Academy of Sciences*, Vol. 1251, pp. 237–245.

SECTION II

Perceptual-motor systems of communication impairments

9

ORAL SENSORIMOTOR DEVELOPMENT

Research and treatment

Steven M. Barlow and Austin Oder Rosner

Oral sensorimotor development begins before birth. As structures form and nerve fibers make connections *in utero*, the fetus exhibits reflex sensitivity and progressively more complex oromotor activities (Figure 9.1). Oromotor control networks are shaped and refined by network dynamics and competition as a result of sensory experiences and activity-dependent mechanisms (Penn and Shatz, 1999) in the womb and long after birth. As sensory signals proliferate, a cascade of cellular and molecular processes alter neurochemistry, connectivity, and overall brain structure (Als *et al.*, 2012). This chapter will discuss the development of oromotor activities, how the sensory environment plays a role in modulating underlying neural mechanisms that control these activities, and the research and treatment being implemented to improve outcomes in infants with oromotor delays.

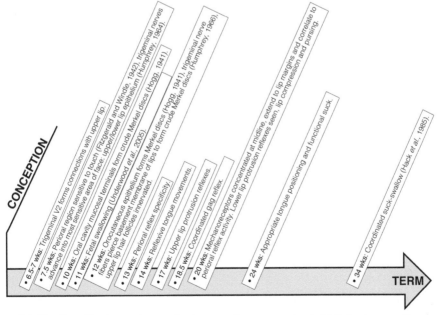

Figure 9.1 Timeline of oral sensorimotor development from conception to birth (post-conceptional age in weeks).

Somatosensory environment of the infant orofacial system

One of the most potent feedback mechanisms for controlling oromotor behaviors is somatosensation. The somatosensory system plays a crucial role during fetal development and beyond, as motor systems rely on touch and proprioceptive information to modulate motor activity. Appropriate somatosensory input during infant maturation is instrumental in promoting proper development of the peripheral and central nervous systems, and can affect all types of oromotor activity (sucking, chewing, deglutition, etc.).

Mechanoreception

Human infants are precocial for trigeminal somatic sensation (Barlow et al., 2001; Humphrey, 1968) which benefits sucking, feeding, airway protection, and state control. The glabrous skin of the lips, perioral hairy skin, oral mucosa, and anterior tongue contain a high density of mechanoreceptors associated with rapidly-conducting Aβ axons, which respond vigorously to subtle mechanical deformation applied to their receptive fields (Trulsson and Essick, 2004). Four types of mechanoreceptors can be distinguished by their adaptation profile, best frequency, and receptive field size (Table 9.1). These orofacial mechanoreceptors have high cortical magnification factors (def^n: ratio between the area of representation in the primary somatosensory cortex to the area of the skin) (Toda and Taoka, 2004). The tongue tip is dominated by fast-adapting (FA) mechanoreceptors with very small receptive fields (~1 mm), whereas the facial skin, lip vermilion, and buccal mucosa are predominantly populated with slow-adapting (SA) mechanoreceptors with small well-defined receptive fields (2–3 mm) which are better suited to encode facial movements (Trulsson and Johansson, 2002).

Building blocks for motor pattern generation

Suck central pattern generator

The mammalian suck is regulated, in part, by a neuronal network in the pontomedullary reticular formation called the suck central pattern generator (sCPG). The sCPG consists of bilateral networks of interneurons that output to lower motoneurons (e.g., trigeminal, facial, hypoglossal nuclei) to activate and sequence rhythmic suck activity (Barlow et al., 2010; Tanaka et al., 1999). The sCPG is highly responsive to sensory inputs, and adapts to changes in task dynamics and local environment (Barlow et al., 2008, 2014b, 2014c; Oder et al., 2013; Zimmerman and Barlow, 2008).

Table 9.1 Classification of cutaneous mechanoreceptors based on their responses to an applied force, the frequency to which each best responds, and the size of their receptive fields.

Mechanoreceptor	Adaptation Profile	Best Frequency (Hz)	Receptive Field diameter (mm)
Meissner corpuscle	Fast-adapting type I (FA I)	< 50	1-2
Pacinian corpuscle	Fast-adapting type II (FA II)	250	8
Merkel cell neurite complex	Slow-adapting type I (SA I)	5-15	2-8
Ruffini ending	Slow-adapting type II (SA II)	0-10	2-3

Non-nutritive sucking and nutritive sucking

Infants demonstrate two distinct types of sucking: non–nutritive sucking (NNS)—a repetitive mouthing action on a pacifier or nipple in the absence of a liquid stimulus (Wolff, 1968), and nutritive sucking (NS)—when a nutrient bolus is obtained from a bottle or breast. NNS begins *in utero* at 15–18 weeks gestational age (GA; Miller *et al.*, 2003) with bursts of 6–12 suck cycles at approximately 2 Hz separated by pause periods to accommodate respiration (Finan and Barlow, 1996). Suck cycles decelerate over the first five cycles (Barlow *et al.*, 2012), with peak compression pressures averaging approximately 25 cmH$_2$0. NNS offers many benefits to the developing infant, including improvements in growth and maturation, behavioral state, stress levels, gastric motility, and oral feeds (Abbasi *et al.*, 2008; Barlow *et al.*, 2008; Field, 1993; Lau and Hurst, 1999; McCain, 1995; Pickler *et al.*, 1996; Woodson *et al.*, 1985).

Failure to successfully transition from NNS to NS can result in long-term feeding difficulties (Barlow, 2009), and is associated with delays in babbling and speech–language acquisition (Adams-Chapman *et al.*, 2013; Mizuno and Ueda, 2005). NS consists of a suction phase followed by an expression phase approximately 100 ms later, in which the tongue tip performs an anterior–posterior stripping motion along the length of the nipple to express milk. The expression of nutrient requires simultaneous coordination of suck, swallow, and respiration (Medoff-Cooper, 2005). NS cycle rate is approximately 1 Hz and is organized as a continuous stream (Gewolb *et al.*, 2001; Lau and Schanler, 1996). Coordination of suck–swallow–breathe is attained when the infant can demonstrate a ratio of 1:1:1 or 2:2:1, respectively. Dyscoordination of the suck–swallow–breathe pattern is associated with aspiration and serious health issues (Lau, 2006). As each action in the suck–swallow–breathe pattern is primarily under the control of its respective pattern generator, dysfunction can occur at any phase of the sequence.

Swallow central pattern generation

The swallow central pattern generator (swCPG) is located in two main groups of interneurons within the medulla oblongata and is modulated by descending cortical inputs. The first is known as the dorsal swallowing group (DSG), which resides in the nucleus tractus solitarii of the dorsomedial medulla, and is involved in initiation and timing of the sequential swallowing pattern. The second is the ventral swallowing group (VSG), localized in the ventrolateral medulla, which is thought to "switch" or modulate activity among lower motor neurons involved in swallowing (Jean and Dallaporta, 2006). Oropharyngeal swallowing involves the precise selection and sequencing of many paired muscle systems, is regulated by the central and peripheral nervous systems, and is continuously modified by sensory mechanisms (Humbert and German, 2013). In preterm infants less than 32 weeks post menstrual age (PMA), this ability is not usually effective enough to sustain full oral feeds. These infants are tube fed (gavage) until they are mature enough to take nutrient directly from the breast/bottle (Pinelli and Symington, 2005). In the neonatal intensive care unit (NICU), NNS is often paired with gavage feeding to satiate and facilitate the transition to independent oral feeds (Barlow *et al.*, 2008), and to develop the timing and coordination of swallow at the correct phase of the respiratory cycle (Reynolds *et al.*, 2010). This ultimately leads to earlier discharge from the NICU.

Masticatory central pattern generation

Mastication requires coordination of over 20 orofacial muscles, in concert with breathing and swallowing (Kolta *et al.*, 2010; Lund, 1991). Infants begin to chew several months after birth, and mastication continues to evolve until the permanent teeth have completely grown in (Barlow *et al.*, 2010). Like sucking, rhythmic mastication is primarily under the control of a CPG in the pons. It is still unclear whether the masticatory central pattern generation (mCPG) is an evolution of the sCPG that undergoes drastic changes in intrinsic properties and network connectivity during development, or if the mCPG emerges as a distinct network during weaning (Barlow *et al.*, 2010; Morquette *et al.*, 2012).

The masticatory sequence has been divided into three functionally different phases: (1) *the preparatory series*, where food in the anterior portion of the mouth is transported back between the molar teeth; (2) *the reduction series*, where food is broken down between the teeth; and (3) *the pre-swallowing series*, where the food is transported posteriorly toward the pharyngeal region to accommodate the swallow (Schwartz *et al.*, 1989).

Suck and mastication share basic features of jaw opening and closing. During mastication, the "power stroke" for breaking or tearing food occurs during *jaw closing*, whereas during NS it occurs during jaw opening to produce a high negative intraoral pressure to facilitate nutrient expression from the teat or bottle nipple (Kolta *et al.*, 2010).

Cortical representation of swallow

Heterarchical organization

A heterarchical control model between cerebral cortex, forebrain, cerebellum and brainstem loci has been proposed to support deglutition (Michou and Hamdy, 2009; Mosier and Bereznaya, 2001). Functional magnetic resonance imaging (fMRI) techniques used during reflexive swallows reveals a cerebral network localized bilaterally to the lateral primary somatosensory (SI) and motor (MI) cortices. In contrast, voluntary swallows produced by neurotypical adults show a more elaborate bilateral activation in the insula, prefrontal cortex, anterior cingulate, parieto-occipital cortex, SI, and MI (Kern *et al.*, 2001). The expanded representation during volitional swallows is presumably related to motor planning and the urge to swallow when presented with a small water bolus. Evidence of a fronto-parietal cortical activation during swallowing has been identified in infants at 45 weeks PMA using near infrared spectroscopy (NIRS) and pharyngoesophageal manometry (Jadcherla *et al.*, in press).

Plasticity

The oropharyngeal system exhibits plasticity in adapting to new tasks and/or sensory experiences in health and disease. The specificity in orofacial gestures and swallowing for targeted neuroplasticity interventions suggests consideration be given for stimulus salience (non-swallowing task training versus swallow-specific task training) to effect beneficial plasticity for safe swallowing (Martin, 2009). Pharyngeal and esophageal motor cortical representations undergo expansion and suppression for extended periods of time, respectively, following brief periods (~10 minutes at 10 Hz) of electrical pharyngeal sensory stimulation in healthy adult participants (Hamdy *et al.*, 1998). Pharyngeal stimulation produces a larger effect on potentiation of the swallowing network compared to voluntary swallowing in adult dysphagic patients, thus peripheral stimulation is favored over volitional exercises (Fraser *et al.*, 2003). Pulse trains or repetitive peripheral stimulation is more effective than single pulse stimulation (Hummel and Cohen, 2005; Luber *et al.*, 2007). Low frequency (<1 Hz) stimulation induces inhibition whereas higher-frequency stimulation (>5 Hz) yields excitatory effects (Pascual-Leone *et al.*, 1994). Clearly, peripheral sensory stimulation is an important tool in swallowing rehabilitation (Martin, 2009).

Promoting suck development in high-risk preterm infants

Critical periods
The perinatal period is especially important for establishing neural networks. Unfortunately, preterm birth can significantly alter developmental processes, as interruption of critical periods can "impair fragile syntheses of central neural representations" of sensory and motor systems (Bosma, 1973 p. 7). In the NICU, many preterm infants' daily oromotor stimulation is centered around medical procedures, such as intubation, continuous positive airway pressure (CPAP), and nasal cannulation (Fucile *et al.*, 2002). These essential care procedures can result in significant forms of sensory deprivation or maladaptive inputs during a critical period of development (Barlow *et al.*, 2008). Even the presence of a nasogastric (NG) gavage tube may negatively impact oral feeding development (Shiao *et al.*, 1995).

Stimulus salience
Controlled orosensory experiences, including oral stroking prior to feeding—with or without simultaneous NNS on a pacifier—facilitate oral feeding performance in preterm infants (Fucile *et al.*, 2002, 2011; Rocha *et al.*, 2007). A pneumatically-charged "pressurized" pacifier can be programmed to provide preterm infants with a pulsatile orocutaneous experience that closely mimics the spatiotemporal pattern of an age-appropriate NNS burst, in an effort to entrain the sCPG (Barlow *et al.*, 2008, 2014b, 2014c; Finan and Barlow, 1996) (Figure 9.2). When applied to preterm infants in the NICU, the result is typically enhanced development of NNS and a timely transition to NS. A recent study involving preterm infants with lung disease and infants of diabetic mothers revealed that a pulsed orocutaneous stimulus regimen with a high-velocity spectral signature was significantly more effective than a low-velocity spectrally-reduced pneumatic stimulus in facilitating the development of NNS (Barlow *et al.*, 2014c). Similar studies now show a link between pulsed orocutaneous stimulation initiated at 32 weeks PMA and modulation of electrocortical activity in the preterm brain in the frequency (Song *et al.*, 2014) and time-amplitude domain (Barlow *et al.*, 2014a). This new form of early

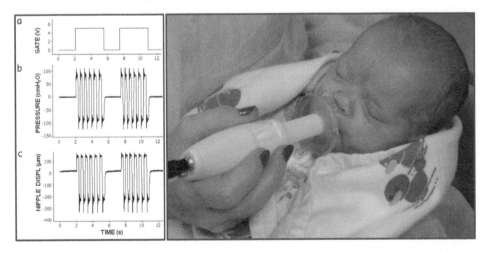

Figure 9.2 Preterm infant receiving pulsed orocutaneous therapy during gavage feeding in the neonatal intensive care unit (nasogastric tube passing through the right nares). Synthesized burst–pause pneumatic stimulus features are shown in the left panel.

Photo courtesy of Innara Health, Inc.

somatosensory experience not only provides behavioral benefits (enhanced sucking and feeding, state control), but also may induce short- and long-term changes in the milieu of cortical activity to enhance brain maturation and offer some degree of neuroprotection.

Pacifiers and their pressurized counterparts play an important role in early oromotor development, as they are often the most readily available form of oral stimulation for infants at the hospital and at home. The mechanical properties of pacifiers, including stiffness (Zimmerman and Barlow, 2008) and texture (Oder *et al.*, 2013), also have significant effects on oromotor behavior during infancy and should be considered when choosing age-appropriate oral stimulation appliances. Because NNS precedes NS, pacifiers can facilitate and strengthen the skills necessary for transitioning to oral feeding.

Transition-to-oral feed

Many infants born preterm or those with neurological disorder do not have the necessary motor skills to safely coordinate the suck–swallow–breathe pattern without aspiration. The transition from tube to independent oral feeding can be tenuous with potential for lifelong detrimental consequences. Success often depends on neurodevelopmental status related to cardiorespiratory and behavioral regulation (i.e., sleep and arousal states), and the ability to produce a safe suck–swallow–breathe pattern (Delaney and Arvedson, 2008). In preterm infants, suck–swallow coordination is attained at the introduction of oral feeding, while swallow–breathe coordination slowly evolves with progression of oral feeds (Lau *et al.*, 2003). Many believe that unsafe oral feeding is due to incoordination of swallow-breathe; however, disruptions in this phase of feeding can be minimized if swallow-related closure of the airway is initiated at times of no airflow (i.e., end of inspiration or expiration) rather than mid-breath. For this to happen, swallowing and breathing must have a stable, constant phase relationship (Bamford *et al.*, 1992).

Links between feeding disorders and speech-language delay

Prematurity can disrupt the development, maturation, and differentiation of key brain structures essential for feeding and later emerging speech–language skills. Preterm infants are highly vulnerable to impairments in speech–language–auditory centers of the brain. A large-scale, longitudinal study conducted by the NICHD Neonatal Research Network has demonstrated that infants born preterm, particularly those with persistent dysfunctional feeding behaviors, have significantly lower cognitive and language scores at 18 months of age as compared to preterm infants with normal feeding behaviors (Adams-Chapman *et al.*, 2013). However, other NICU factors have been shown to predict low language scores at 18–22 months adjusted age, including days of mechanical ventilation, hearing impairment, and Gross Motor Functional Classification System (GMFCS) level ≥2 (Adams-Chapman *et al.*, 2013).

Role of early intervention

Thalamocortical and corticocortical development is diminished in preterm infants (Ball *et al.*, 2013); therefore, sensory stimulation in the correct modality and dose during this critical stage of development is imperative for strengthening neural pathways (Berardi *et al.*, 2000; Hensch, 2004). Agents of neuroprotection during the neonatal period may take the form of brain cooling, pharmacologic intervention (e.g., erythropoietin), or sensory stimulation to spare developing white matter and young neurons engaged in network formation under challenging conditions, such as hypoxic ischemia, intraventricular hemorrhage, or cardiac insufficiency.

Perinatal and adult animal models have demonstrated that neuroprotective strategies, such as mild tactile sensory stimulation of trigeminal afferents within the first two hours after injury, can prevent or mitigate the formation of brain infarcts following middle cerebral artery ligation (Lay *et al.*, 2010, 2011).

The use of supplemental sensory stimulation is gaining support for use among preterm infant populations in an effort to regulate cardiorespiratory and behavioral state, modulate rate and endurance of NNS, and enhance oral feeding skills and weight gain. Of all the sensory modalities, touch and olfaction are regarded as the most salient sensory inputs early in life (Schaal, 2010). One of the most potent and preferential odorants for a newborn is that of his/her own mother's breast milk (Varendi *et al.*, 1994), and exposure to mother's breast milk has a positive effect on sucking behavior and feeding outcomes (Bingham *et al.*, 2003; Raimbault *et al.*, 2007; Yildiz *et al.*, 2011). Auditory stimulation is another form of sensory input, and certain types of auditory stimuli have yielded successful outcomes in preterm infants, including lullabies (Standley *et al.*, 2010), live music (Arnon *et al.*, 2006; Loewy *et al.*, 2013), mother's voice (Chorna *et al.*, 2014; Filippa *et al.*, 2013), and biological maternal sounds (Doheny *et al.*, 2012; Zimmerman *et al.*, 2013). The vestibular system is yet another modality that has been investigated, as it remains largely understimulated during a preterm infant's long stay in the NICU. Vestibular stimulation in the form of rocking (Korner *et al.*, 1975; Tuck *et al.*, 1982) and gliding (Zimmerman and Barlow, 2012) has been shown to effectively modulate respiratory rate, prevent apneic attacks, and decrease the need for respiratory therapies.

A multisensory therapeutic approach known as ATVV (auditory, tactile, visual, vestibular) has shown enhanced physiological stability (heart rate, respiration rate, arousal state) (White-Traut *et al.*, 2004), neuromotor function (Kanagasabai *et al.*, 2013) and decreased length of hospital stay. It also facilitates faster transition to full oral feeds (White-Traut *et al.*, 2002). Another promising multimodal therapy is Kangaroo Care, which utilizes skin-to-skin contact between an infant and their parent, thereby providing an abundance of tactile, kinesthetic, auditory, olfactory, and vestibular stimulation to the infant. Kangaroo Care benefits infants by regulating body temperature, allowing for more periods of quiet sleep, reducing apnea and bradycardia while increasing oxygen saturation levels, reducing length of hospital stay, facilitating breastfeeding (Bauer *et al.*, 1996; Sloan *et al.*, 1994), and accelerating brain maturation (Scher *et al.*, 2009).

Proper oral sensorimotor development is necessary to support life-sustaining functions, such as sucking, chewing, and swallowing, as well as many aspects of communication. Delays in any of these mechanisms can have detrimental effects on an individual's health and quality of life. Clinical research has made great advances in improving patient outcomes and better informing therapeutic strategies, and the body of knowledge in this field is ever-growing.

Acknowledgements

The work was supported in part by the National Institutes of Health R01 DC003311 (Barlow-PI) and the Barkley Trust.

References

Abbasi, S., Sivieri, E., Samuel-Collins, N. and Gerdes, J.S. (2008), "Effect of non-nutritive sucking on gastric motility of preterm infants", Presented at the meeting of the *Pediatric Academic Society*, Honolulu, Hawaii.

Adams-Chapman, I., Bann, C.M., Vaucher, Y.E. and Stoll, B.J. (2013), "Association between feeding difficulties and language delay in preterm infants using Bayley Scales of Infant Development-Third Edition", *The Journal of Pediatrics*, Vol. 163, No. 3, pp. 680–685.

Als, H., Duffy, F.H., McAnulty, G., Butler, S.C., Lightbody, L., Kosta, S., *et al.* (2012), "NIDCAP improves brain function and structure in preterm infants with severe intrauterine growth restriction", *Journal of Perinatology*, Vol. 32, pp. 797–803.

Arnon, S., Shapsa, A., Forman, L., Regev, R., Bauer, S., Litmanovitz, I. and Dolfin, T. (2006), "Live music is beneficial to preterm infants in the neonatal intensive care unit environment", *Birth*, Vol. 33, No. 2, pp. 131–136.

Ball, G., Boardman, J.P., Aljabar, P., Pandit, A., Arichi, T., Merchant, N., *et al.* (2013), "The influence of preterm birth on the developing thalamocortical connectome", *Cortex*, Vol. 49, No. 60, pp. 1711–1721.

Bamford, O., Taciak, V. and Gewolb, I.H. (1992), "The relationship between rhythmic swallowing and breathing during suckle feeding in term neonates", *Pediatric Research,* Vol. 31, No. 6, pp. 619–624.

Barlow, S.M. (2009), "Oral and respiratory control for preterm feeding", *Current Opinion in Otolaryngology: Head and Neck Surgery*, Vol. 17, pp. 179–186.

Barlow, S.M., Dusick, A., Finan, D.S., Coltart, S. and Biswas, A. (2001), "Mechanically evoked perioral reflexes in premature and term human infants", *Brain Research*, Vol. 899, pp. 251–254.

Barlow, S.M., Finan, D.S., Lee, J. and Chu, S.Y. (2008), "Synthetic orocutaneous stimulation entrains preterm infants with feeding difficulties to suck", *Journal of Perinatology*, Vol. 28, pp. 541–548.

Barlow, S.M., Lund, J.P., Estep, M. and Kolta, A. (2010), "Central pattern generators for speech and orofacial activity", in Brudzynski, S.M. (Ed.), *Handbook of Mammalian Vocalization,* Elsevier, Oxford, UK, pp. 351–370.

Barlow, S.M., Burch, M., Venkatesan, L., Harold, M. and Zimmerman, E. (2012), "Frequency modulation and spatiotemporal stability of the sCPG in preterm infants with RDS", *International Journal of Pediatrics*, Article ID 581538, available at: http://dx.doi.org/10.1155/2012/581538.

Barlow, S.M., Jegatheesan, P., Weiss, S., Govindaswami, B., Wang, J., Lee, J., *et al.* (2014a), "Amplitude-integrated EEG and range-EEG modulation associated with pneumatic orocutaneous stimulation in preterm infants", *Journal of Perinatology*, Vol. 32, No. 3, pp. 213–219.

Barlow, S.M., Lee, J., Wang, J., Oder, A., Hall, S., Knox, K., *et al.* (2014b), "Frequency-modulated orocutaneous stimulation promotes non-nutritive suck development in preterm infants with respiratory distress syndrome or chronic lung disease", *Journal of Perinatology*, Vol. 34, No. 2, pp. 136–142.

Barlow, S.M., Lee, J., Wang, J., Oder, A., Oh, H., Hall, S., *et al.* (2014c), "The effects of orocutaneous power spectra on the development of non-nutritive suck in preterm infants with respiratory distress syndrome or chronic lung disease, and preterm infants of diabetic mothers", *Journal of Neonatal Nursing*, Vol. 20, pp. 178–188.

Bauer, J., Sontheimer, D., Fisher, C., Linderkamp, O. (1996), "Metabolic rate and energy balance in very low birthweight infants during kangaroo holding by their mothers and fathers", *Journal of Pediatrics*, Vol. 129, pp. 608–611.

Berardi, N., Pizzorusso, T. and Maffei, L. (2000), "Critical periods during sensory development", *Current Opinion in Neurobiology,* Vol. 10, No. 1, pp. 138–145.

Bingham, P.M., Abassi, S. and Sivieri, E. (2003), "A pilot study of milk odor effect on nonnutritive sucking by premature newborns", *Archives of Pediatrics and Adolescescent Medicine,* Vol. 157, pp. 72–75.

Bosma, J.F. (1973), "Prologue to the symposium", in Bosma, J.F. (Ed.), *Fourth Symposium on Oral Sensation and Perception*, Charles C. Thomas, Bethesda, MD, p. 7.

Chorna, O.D., Slaughter, J.C., Wang, L., Stark, A.R., and Maitre, N.L. (2014), "A pacifier-activated music player with mother's voice improves oral feeding in preterm infants", *Pediatrics*, Vol. 133, No. 3, pp. 462–468.

Delaney, A.L. and Arvedson, J.C. (2008), "Development of swallowing and feeding: Prenatal through first year of life", *Developmental Disabilities Research Reviews*, Vol. 14, No. 2, pp. 105–117.

Doheny, L., Hurwitz, S., Insoft, R., Ringer, S. and Lahav, A. (2012), "Exposure to biological maternal sounds improves cardiorespiratory regulation in extremely preterm infants", *Journal of Maternal-Fetal and Neonatal Medicine*, Vol. 25, No. 9, pp. 1591–1594.

Field, T. (1993), "Sucking for stress reduction, growth and development during infancy", *Pediatric Basics,* Vol. 64, pp. 13–16.

Filippa, M., Devouche, E., Arioni, C., Imberty, M. and Gratier, M. (2013), "Live maternal speech and singing have beneficial effects on hospitalized preterm infants", *Acta Paediatrica*, Vol. 102, pp. 1017–1020.

Finan, D.S. and Barlow, S.M. (1996), "The actifier: A device for neurophysiological studies of orofacial control in human infants", *Journal of Speech and Hearing Research*, Vol. 39, No. 4, pp. 833–838.

Fitzgerald, G.E. and Windle, W.F. (1942), "Some observations on early human fetal movements", *Journal of Comparative Neurology*, Vol. 76, pp. 159–167.

Fraser, C., Rothwell, J., Power, M., Hobson, A., Thompson, D. and Hamdy, S. (2003), "Differential changes in human pharyngoesophageal motor excitability induced by swallowing, pharyngeal stimulation, and anesthesia", *American Journal of Physiology—Gastrointestinal and Liver Physiology*, Vol. 285, pp. G137–G144.

Fucile, S., Gisel, E. and Lau, C. (2002), "Oral stimulation accelerates the transition from tube to oral feeding in preterm infants", *The Journal of Pediatrics*, Vol. 141, No. 2, pp. 230–236.

Fucile, S., Gisel, E., McFarland, D.H. and Lau, C. (2011), "Oral and non-oral sensorimotor interventions enhance oral feeding performance in preterm infants", *Devolpmental Medicine and Child Neurology*, Vol. 53, No. 9, pp. 829–835.

Gewolb, I.H., Vice, F.L., Schwietzer-Kenney, E.L., Taciak, V.L. and Bosma, J.F. (2001), "Developmental patterns of rhythmic suck and swallow in preterm infants", *Developmental Medicine and Child Neurology*, Vol. 43, No. 1, pp. 22–27.

Hack, M., Estabrook, M.M. and Robertson, S.S. (1985), "Development of sucking rhythm in preterm infants", *Early Human Development*, Vol. 11, No. 2, pp. 133–140.

Hamdy, S., Rothwell, J.C., Aziz, Q., Singh, K.D. and Thompson, D.G. (1998), "Long-term reorganization of human motor cortex driven by short-term sensory stimulation", *Nature Neuroscience*, Vol. 1, pp. 64–68.

Hensch, T.K. (2004), "Critical period regulation", *Annual Review of Neuroscience*, Vol. 27, pp. 549–579.

Hogg, I.D. (1941), "Sensory nerves and associated structures in the skin of human fetuses of 8 to 14 weeks of menstrual age correlated with functional capability", *Journal of Comparative Neurology*, Vol. 75, pp. 371–410.

Humbert, I.A. and German, R.Z. (2013), "New directions for understanding neural control in swallowing: The potential and promise of motor learning", *Dysphagia*, Vol. 28, pp. 1–10.

Hummel, F.C. and Cohen, L.G. (2005), "Drivers of brain plasticity", *Current Opinion in Neurology*, Vol. 18, pp. 667–674.

Humphrey, T. (1966), "The development of trigeminal nerve fibers to the oral mucosa, compared with their development to cutaneous surfaces", *Journal of Comparative Neurology*, Vol. 126, pp. 91–108.

Humphrey, T. (1968), "The development of mouth opening and related reflexes involving the oral area of human fetuses", *Alabama Journal of Medicine*, Vol. 5, pp. 126–157.

Jadcherla, S.R., Pakiraih, J.F., Hasenstab, K.A, Dar, I., Gao, X., Bates, D.G., *et al.* (in press), "Esophageal reflexes modulate fronto-parietal response in neonates: Novel application of concurrent NIRS and provocative esophageal manometry", *American Journal of Physiology—Gastrointestinal and Liver Physiology*.

Jean, A. and Dallaporta, M. (2006), "Electrophysiologic characterization of the swallowing pattern generator in the brainstem", *GI Motility online*, available at: www.nature.com/gimo/contents/pt1/full/gimo9.html.

Kanagasabai, P.S., Mohan, K., Lewis, L.E., Kamath, A., Rao, B.K. (2013), "Effect of multisensory stimulation on neuromotor development in preterm infants", *Indian Journal of Pediatrics*, Vol. 80, No. 6, pp. 460–464.

Kern, M.K., Jaradeh, S., Arndorfer, R.C. and Shaker, R. (2001), "Cerebral cortical representation of reflexive and volitional swallowing in humans", *American Journal of Physiology – Gastrointestinal and Liver Physiology*, Vol. 280, pp. G354–G360.

Kolta, A., Morquette, P., Lavoie, R., Arsenault, I. and Verdier, D. (2010), "Modulation of rhythmogenic properties of trigeminal neurons contributing to the masticatory CPG", *Progress in Brain Research*, Vol. 187, pp. 137–147.

Korner, A.F., Kraemer, H.C., Haffner, M.E. and Cosper, L.M. (1975), "Effects of waterbed flotation on premature infants: a pilot study", *Pediatrics*, Vol. 56, pp. 361–367.

Lau, C. (2006), "Oral feeding in the preterm infant", *Neoreviews*, Vol. 7, No. 1, pp. 19–27.

Lau, C. and Schanler, R.J. (1996), "Oral motor function in the neonate", *Clinical Perinatology*, Vol. 23, No. 2, pp. 161–178.

Lau, C. and Hurst, N. (1999), "Oral feeding in infants", *Current Problems in Pediatrics*, Vol. 29, pp. 105–124.

Lau, C., Smith, E.O. and Schanler, R.J. (2003), "Coordination of suck-swallow and swallow respiration in preterm infants", *Acta Paediatrica*, Vol. 92, No. 6, pp. 721–727.

Lay, C.C., Davis, M.F., Chen-Bee, C.H. and Frostig, R.D. (2010), "Mild sensory stimulation completely protects the adult rodent cortex from ischemic stroke", *PLoS One*, Vol. 5, No. 6, p. e11270.

Lay, C.C., Davis, M.F., Chen-Bee, C.H. and Frostig, R.D. (2011), "Mild sensory stimulation reestablishes cortical function during the acute phase of ischemia", *Journal of Neuroscience*, Vol. 31, No. 32, pp. 11495–11504.

Loewy, J., Stewart, K., Dassler, A-M., Telsey, A. and Homel, P. (2013), "The effcts of music therapy on vital signs, feeding, and sleep in premature infants", *Pediatrics*, Vol. 131, No. 5, pp. 902–918.

Luber, B., Peterchev, A.V., Nguyen, T., Sporn, A. and Lisanby, S.H. (2007), "Application of transcranial magnetic stimulation (TMS) in psychophysiology", in Cacioppo, J.T., Tassinary, L.G. and Berntson, G.G. (Eds.), *Handbook of Psychophysiology* (3rd Edition), Cambridge University Press, Cambridge, UK, pp. 120–138.

Lund, J.P. (1991), "Mastication and its control by the brain stem", *Critical Reviews in Oral Biology and Medicine*, Vol. 2, pp. 33–64.

Martin, R. (2009), "Neuroplasticity and swallowing", *Dysphagia*, Vol. 24, pp. 218–229.

McCain, G.C. (1995), "Promotion of preterm infant nipple feeding with nonnutritive sucking", *Journal of Pediatric Nursing*, Vol. 10, pp. 3–8.

Medoff-Cooper, B. (2005), "Nutritive sucking research: From clinical questions to research answers", *Journal of Perinatal and Neonatal Nursing*, Vol. 19, No. 3, pp. 265–272.

Miller, J.L., Sonies, B.C. and Macedonia, C. (2003), "Emergence of oropharyngeal, laryngeal and swallowing activity in the developing fetal upper aerodigestive tract: An ultrasound evaluation", *Early Human Development*, Vol. 71, No. 1, pp. 61–87.

Michou, E. and Hamdy, S. (2009), "Cortical input in control of swallowing", *Current Opinion in Otolaryngology: Head and Neck Surgery*, Vol. 17, No. 3, pp. 166–171.

Mizuno, K. and Ueda, A. (2005), "Neonatal feeding performance as a predictor of neurodevelopmental outcome at 18 months", *Developmental Medicine and Child Neurology*, Vol. 47, No. 5, pp. 299–304.

Morquette, P., Lavoie, R., Fhima, M-D., Lamoureux, X., Verdier, D. and Kolta, A. (2012), "Generation of the masticatory central pattern and its modulation by sensory feedback", *Progress in Neurobiology*, Vol. 96, pp. 340–355.

Mosier, K. and Bereznaya, I. (2001), "Parallel cortical networks for volitional control of swallowing in humans", *Experimental Brain Research*, Vol. 140, No. 3, pp. 280–289.

Oder, A.L., Stalling, D.L. and Barlow, S.M. (2013), "Short-term effects of pacifier texture on NNS in neurotypical infants", *International Journal of Pediatrics*, Article ID 168459, available at: http://dx.doi.org/10.1155/2013/168459

Pascual-Leone, A., Valls-Sole, J., Wassermann, E.M. and Hallett, M. (1994), "Responses to rapid-rate transcranial magnetic stimulation of the human motor cortex", *Brain*, Vol. 117, pp. 847–858.

Penn, A.A. and Shatz, C.J. (1999), "Brain waves and brain wiring: The role of endogenous and sensory-driven neural activity in development", *Pediatric Research*, Vol. 45, pp. 447–458.

Pickler, R.H., Frankel, H.B., Walsh, K.M. and Thompson, N.M. (1996), "Effects of nonnutritive sucking on behavioral organization and feeding performance in preterm infants", *Nursing Research*, Vol. 45, pp. 132–135.

Pinelli, J. and Symington, A. (2005), "Non-nutritive sucking for promoting physiologic stability and nutrition in preterm infants", *Cochrane Database of Systemic Reviews*, Vol. 4, No. CD001071.

Raimbault, C., Saliba, E. and Porter, R.H. (2007), "The effect of the odour of mother's milk on breastfeeding behavior of premature neonates", *Acta Paediatrica*, Vol. 96, pp. 368–371.

Reynolds, E., Grider, D., Caldwell, R., Capilouto, G., Vijaygopal, P., Patwardhan, A., *et al.* (2010), "Swallow-breath interaction and phase of respiration with swallow during nonnutritive suck among low-risk preterm infants", *American Journal of Perinatology*, Vol. 10, pp. 831–840.

Rocha, A.D., Moreira, M.E., Pimenta, H.P., Ramos, J.R. and Lucena, S.L. (2007), "A randomized study of the efficacy of sensory-motor-oral stimulation and non-nutritive sucking in very low birthweight infant", *Early Human Development*, Vol. 83, No. 6, pp. 385–388.

Schaal, B. (2010), "Mammary odor cues and pheromones: Mammalian infant-directed communication about maternal state, mammae, and milk", *Vitamins and Hormones: Pheromones*, Vol. 83, pp. 83–136.

Scher, M.S., Ludington-Hoe, S., Kaffashi, F., Johnson, M.W., Holditch-Davis, D. and Loparo, K.A. (2009), "Neurophysiologic assessment of brain maturation after an 8-week trial of skin-to-skin contact on preterm infants", *Clinical Neurophysiology*, Vol. 120, pp. 1812–1818.

Schwartz, G., Enomoto, S., Valiquette, C. and Lund, J.P. (1989), "Mastication in the rabbit: A description of movement and muscle activity", *Journal of Neurophysiology*, Vol. 62, pp. 273–287.

Shiao, S.Y., Youngblut, J.M., Anderson, G.C., DiFiore, J.M. and Martin, R.J. (1995), "Nasogastric tube placement: Effects on breathing and sucking in very-low-birth-weight infants", *Nursing Research*, Vol. 44, No. 2, pp. 82–88.

Sloan, N., Camacho, L., Rojas, E. and Stern, C. (1994), "Kangaroo mother method: Randomized controlled trial of an alternative method of care for stabilized low birth weight infants", *Lancet*, Vol. 344, pp. 782–785.

Song, D., Jegatheesan, P., Weiss, S., Govindaswami, B., Wang, J., Lee, J., *et al.* (2014), "Modulation of EEG spectral edge frequency during patterned pneumatic oral stimulation in preterm infants", *Pediatric Research*, Vol. 75, No. 1, pp. 85–92.

Standley, J.M., Cassidy, J., Grant, R., Cevasco, A., Szuch, C., Nguyen, J., *et al.* (2010), "The effect of music reinforcement for non-nutritive sucking on nipple feeding of premature infants", *Pediatric Nursing*, Vol. 36, No. 3, pp. 138–145.

Tanaka, S., Kogo, M., Chandler, S.H. and Matsuya, T. (1999), "Localization of oral-motor rhythmogenic circuits in the isolated rat brainstem preparation", *Brain Research*, Vol. 821, pp. 190–199.

Toda, T. and Taoka, M. (2004), "Converging patterns of inputs from oral structures in the postcentral somatosensory cortex of conscious macaque monkeys", *Experimental Brain Research*, Vol. 158, pp. 43–49.

Trulsson, M. and Johansson, R.S. (2002), "Orofacial mechanoreceptors in humans: Encoding characteristics and responses during natural orofacial behaviors", *Behavioral Brain Research*, Vol. 135, pp. 27–33.

Trulsson, M. and Essick, G.K. (2004), "Mechanosensation", in Miles, T.S., Nauntofte, B. and Svensson, P., (Eds.), *Clinical Oral Physiology*, Quintessence Books, Copenhagen, Denmark, pp. 165–197.

Tuck, S.J., Monin, P., Duvivier, C., May, T. and Vert, P. (1982), "Effect of a rocking bed on apnoea of prematurity", *Archives of Disease in Childhood*, Vol. 57, pp. 475–477.

Underwood, M.A., Gilbert, W.M. and Sherman, M.P. (2005), "Amniotic fluid: Not just fetal urine anymore", *Journal of Perinatology*, Vol. 25, pp. 341–348.

Varendi, H., Porter, R.H. and Winberg, J. (1994), "Does the newborn baby find the nipple by smell?", *Lancet*, Vol. 344, pp. 989–990.

White-Traut, R.C., Nelson, M.N., Silvestri, J.M., Vasan, U., Littau, S., Meleedy-Rey, P., *et al.* (2002), "Effect of auditory, tactile, visual, and vestibular intervention on length of stay, alertness, and feeding progression in preterm infants", *Developmental Medicine and Child Neurology*, Vol. 44, No. 2, pp. 91–97.

White-Traut, R.C., Nelson, M.N., Silvestri, J.M., Patel, M., Berbaum, M., Gu, G.G. and Rey, P.M. (2004), "Developmental patterns of physiological response to a multisensory intervention in extremely premature and high-risk infants", *Journal of Obstetric, Gynecological, and Neonatal Nursing*, Vol. 33, No. 2, pp. 266–275.

Wolff, P.H. (1968), "The serial organization of sucking in the young infant", *Pediatrics*, Vol. 42, No. 6, pp. 943–956.

Woodson, R., Drinkwin, J. and Hamilton, C. (1985), "Effects of nonnutritive sucking on state and activity: Term-preterm comparisons", *Infant Behavior and Development*, Vol. 8, pp. 435–441.

Yildiz, A., Arikan, D. Gözüm, S., Taştekin, A. and Budancamanak, I. (2011), "The effect of the odor of breast milk on the time needed for transition from gavage to total oral feeding in preterm infants", *Journal of Nursing Scholarship*, Vol. 43, No. 3, pp. 256–273.

Zimmerman, E. and Barlow, S.M. (2008), "Pacifier stiffness alters the dynamics of the suck central pattern generator", *Journal of Neonatal Nursing*, Vol. 14, pp. 79–86.

Zimmerman, E. and Barlow, S.M. (2012), "The effects of vestibular stimulation rate and magnitude of acceleration on central pattern generation for chest wall kinematics in preterm infants", *Journal of Perinatology*, Vol. 32, pp. 614–620.

Zimmerman, E., Keunen, K., Norton, M. and Lahav, A. (2013), "Weight gain velocity in very low-birth-weight infants: Effects of exposure to biological maternal sounds", *American Journal of Perinatology*, Vol. 30, pp. 863–870.

10

PERCEPTUAL PROCESSING OF SPEECH IN INFANCY

Barbara T. Conboy and Alexis Bosseler

In this chapter we provide a brief overview of pre- and postnatal speech processing abilities; how those skills are shaped by previous experience and learning; and how they permit further learning. We also consider what is available to learners in terms of inputs from multiple modalities (influenced by learners' physical, linguistic, and social environments, including bilingual input), and the "uptake" of those inputs (influenced by basic sensory and cognitive abilities such as attention, memory, computational skills, and processing efficiency).

The prenatal to early postnatal period

Although little is known about the long-term effects of prenatal experience, it is clear that some learning from language input begins prenatally. The cochlea is almost fully mature by 32 weeks gestational age (GA), but only 30 percent of the phonetic information present in speech is heard by fetuses because amniotic fluid attenuates auditory frequencies above approximately 500 Hz (i.e., the acoustic cues that distinguish most vowel and consonant sounds; Granier-Deferre *et al.*, 2011). Thus, the uptake (perception and learning) of many features of speech is limited by the availability of that input in the prenatal environment.

Low-frequency information that reflects speaker identity (e.g., the fundamental frequency and timbre of one's voice) is detected and discriminated by the end of the third trimester (Granier-Deferre *et al.*, 2011; Kisilevsky *et al.*, 2009). Late-term (38 week GA) fetuses detect rapid amplitude modulations in sentences, even when spectral information has been removed (Granier-Deferre *et al.*, 2011). Third-trimester fetuses are also sensitive to the slow modulations in frequency and amplitude, discriminating between languages from different rhythmic classes (Kisilevsky *et al.*, 2009), and between a novel and a familiar passage (DeCasper *et al.*, 1994). Newborn infants show familiarity for a prosodic pattern heard prenatally, such as the maternal vs. an unfamiliar language from a different rhythmic class (Byers-Heinlein *et al.*, 2010; Mehler *et al.*, 1988; Moon *et al.*, 1993), or stimuli they were exposed to experimentally (DeCasper and Spence, 1986; Partanen *et al.*, 2013). They also show familiarity for maternal language vs. unfamiliar speech sounds (i.e., vowels) that are acoustically distinct in lower frequencies, because those sounds can be perceived prenatally (Moon *et al.*, 2013).

By the time of birth, infants possess domain-general computational abilities that allow them to track probabilities between events in their input and to use this information to recognize sequenced patterns, known as *statistical learning* (Kudo et al., 2011; Teinonen et al., 2009) (for elaboration of statistical learning, see the chapter by Bahr, this volume). Newborns can also learn abstract rule-based patterns, such as tone sequences with ascending vs. descending frequencies (Carral et al., 2005), and adjacent repetition patterns (Gervain et al., 2012). Thus, the mechanisms needed to detect regularities in language input are present early in life.

The first year: Tuning in to the phonemes of the native language(s)

The perception of speech gradually becomes aligned with a learner's ambient language(s) during infancy through processes known as "attunement" and "perceptual narrowing." As reviewed in the previous section, sensitivity to features of the native language(s) begins as soon as the human brain is ready to receive and process that input, and increases as the environment provides more input and the brain becomes more efficient at processing that input.

Tuning in

A first step in attunement involves treating speech as a special auditory signal. Newborns prefer listening to speech over nonspeech analogues (Vouloumanos and Werker, 2007), and show greater left- versus right-hemisphere activation when presented with consonant discrimination paradigms (Dehaene-Lambertz and Gliga, 2004; Peña et al., 2003). Other reports suggest that specialized mechanisms for processing speech emerge more gradually (Vouloumanos et al., 2010). Although newborns show left-hemisphere specialization for processing the rapid temporal aspects of speech (e.g., formant frequency transitions in consonant–vowel sequences), left-hemisphere specialization increases throughout development (Minagawa-Kawai et al., 2011).

Research has shown that infants discriminate many vowel and consonant contrasts at birth but do not align their perception with native-language vowel categories until approximatelysix months of age and consonant categories until 10–12 months of age (Kuhl et al., 2008; Maurer and Werker, 2014). Improvements in discrimination of native-language speech sounds have been linked to experience with input that contains those speech sounds throughout the first year and into the second year (Kuhl et al., 2006; Mugitani et al., 2009; Narayan et al., 2010; Sato et al., 2010; Sundara et al., 2006). The size of discriminatory responses to native phoneme contrasts has been linked to the relative amounts of exposure bilingual infants receive to each of their languages (García-Sierra et al., 2011). However, infants with bilingual exposure, as a group, achieve developmental milestones in speech and language perception at the same ages as monolingual infants (Curtin et al., 2011). This is somewhat surprising because bilingual infants receive less exposure to either language than monolingual infants receive to their single language. Bilingual infants learning two lexically close languages (Catalan and Spanish) have been reported to show a slightly different developmental pattern of vowel discrimination compared to monolingual infants, but this pattern may be attributed to exposure to cognates across the two languages that differ in their vowels (Sebastián-Gallés and Bosch, 2009).

Features of exposure other than quantity also may have an effect on phonetic learning. For example, at 9–11 months of age, infants can encode the features of phonemes from a second language after only five hours of exposure to that language in live, naturalistic play-based interactions with adults (Conboy and Kuhl, 2011), but not when the same amount of exposure is delivered via television (Kuhl et al., 2003). Moreover, amounts of phonetic learning from such interactions are linked to the amounts of joint attention episodes that occur between infants and the second language speakers (Conboy *et al.*, in press). Thus, the social contexts in which language experiences occur are important for phonetic learning.

The prosodic modifications of infant-directed speech (IDS) may facilitate phonetic learning by enhancing infants' attention to speech during social interactions (Kuhl, 2007). Other acoustic properties of IDS, which have been observed across several languages (Kuhl *et al.*, 1997; Werker *et al.*, 2007), may also directly facilitate phonetic learning. For example, 10–12-month-old infants whose mothers modified their vowels in IDS, expanding the vowel space between /i/, /a/, and /u/ in terms of the first and second formant (i.e., F1 and F2) values, showed better discrimination of a consonant contrast than infants whose mothers who did not expand their vowel space (Liu *et al.*, 2003). Vowels with exaggerated F1 and F2 values elicit enhanced brain activity (larger ERP responses) than the same vowels produced without that exaggeration, suggesting that the acoustic modifications of IDS may facilitate the neural encoding of vowel properties (Zhang *et al.*, 2011). The distribution of consonants has also been shown to affect infants' discrimination of consonants on experimental tasks. Infants exposed to a bimodal distribution of a continuum of sounds (e.g., variations in /d/ and /t/ presented so that the sounds more acoustically distinct from each other were heard more frequently than those more similar to each other) showed better discrimination of those phonemes than infants exposed to a unimodal distribution of the sounds (Maye *et al.*, 2002; Yoshida *et al.*, 2010).

Visual articulatory cues to speech present in social interactions may also facilitate infants' phonetic learning. Infants match vowels they hear with the corresponding faces articulating those vowels as young as 2–4 months of age (Kuhl and Meltzoff, 1982; Patterson and Werker, 2003) and integrate that auditory and visual information by 3–4 months (Bristow *et al.*, 2009). Infants can discriminate speech when given visual cues alone, and pay attention to visual articulatory cues for a longer period of time in bilingual vs. monolingual learning situations, possibly because visual cues facilitate separation of the statistical properties of each language (Sebastián-Gallés *et al.*, 2012; Weikum *et al.*, 2007).

Individual cognitive abilities may also influence infants' uptake of input in social contexts and affect rates of attunement (Jusczyk, 1997). Increased theta activity (oscillatory brain rhythms occurring between 4 and 8 Hz, believed to index attention and cognitive effort) was observed with native compared to non-native sounds in 12-month-old (but not 6-month-old) infants, possibly reflecting greater attunement to the native language at the later age (Bosseler *et al.*, 2013). Performance on executive function tasks that measure infants' ability to control attention also has been linked to infants' learning of second language phonetic features (Conboy *et al.*, 2008b). In addition, increased attention in bilingual compared to monolingual infants during a speech perception task was noted in an ERP study (Shafer *et al.*, 2011). Bilingual infants, who constantly switch perception and attention between conflicting language features, have enhanced attentional control abilities compared to monolingual infants by as early as seven months of age (Kovács and Mehler, 2009). Such cognitive abilities may allow bilingual infants to keep pace with monolingual infants in learning the features of speech sounds, even when they have less overall exposure to a particular language compared to monolingual learners of that language.

Attunement to the native language's phonology may facilitate subsequent word learning (Werker and Yeung, 2005). Individual differences in infants' rates of attunement to native-language phonetic features – which may stem from extrinsic (input) factors, intrinsic (cognitive, sensory, and/or perceptual) factors, or both – have been linked to current and future vocabulary and grammar skills (Conboy *et al.*, 2008a; García-Sierra *et al.*, 2011; Kuhl *et al.*, 2008; Tsao *et al.*, 2004).

Tuning out: Perceptual narrowing

From early in development, infants can normalize phonetic information within and across speakers, ignoring acoustic information that is not relevant to phoneme category formation, such as fundamental frequency differences, rate, and loudness (Dehaene-Lambertz and Peña, 2001; Jusczyk *et al.*, 1992; Kuhl, 1983). As infants learn the phoneme categories of their ambient language(s), they also increasingly ignore within-category differences and the phonetic features of languages they are not learning. The process of tuning in to relevant information while tuning out irrelevant information (i.e., "perceptual narrowing") is a major achievement in early development that occurs across sensory and cognitive domains (Maurer and Werker, 2014).

In a landmark study, Werker and Tees (1984) found that infants 6–8 months of age discriminated consonants that did not contrast phonemically in their native language (i.e., non-native contrasts) in addition to native-language phonemic contrasts, but infants 10–12 months of age only discriminated native contrasts. Subsequent research has replicated this finding using other speech contrasts (such as vowels and lexical tones) and methods, as these researchers seek to explain factors that are linked to rates of perceptual narrowing (Kuhl *et al.*, 2008; Maurer and Werker, 2014). For example, perceptual narrowing appears to occur for vowels at an earlier age than for consonants (Polka and Werker, 1994), which possibly reflects the relative saliency of the acoustic features of vowels compared to those that differentiate consonants. Perceptual narrowing may be altered by the learning of native-language features, rather than a loss solely due to a lack of exposure to non-native speech sounds. Infants improve on native contrasts at the same time that their discrimination of non-native contrasts declines, and there is a negative correlation between the discrimination accuracy of infants for native and non-native contrasts (Kuhl *et al.*, 2008). Moreover, different patterns of brain activity are observed for non-native compared to native speech sound contrasts at the same ages that perceptual narrowing occurs (Bosseler *et al.*, 2013; Kuhl *et al.*, 2014).

Rates of perceptual narrowing have also been linked to maturation and environmental factors, including health-related factors and bilingualism (Maurer and Werker, 2014). In a study of dual language learning infants, perceptual narrowing was not observed at the same age as in monolingual infants, suggesting that bilingual environments lead infants to maintain a "perceptual wedge," keeping their systems open to multiple phonetic contrasts for a longer period of time than monolingual environments (Petitto *et al.*, 2012). On visual speech discrimination tasks, bilingual infants discriminated a non-native contrast at an age (eight months) when monolingual infants no longer did so (Sebastián-Gallés *et al.*, 2012).

The discriminability of non-native speech sounds may also be affected by features of those sounds. Some perceptually salient non-native contrasts remain discriminable by infants (Burnham, 1986). When non-native sounds cannot be assimilated to a native-language phoneme category, they may remain discriminable (Best *et al.*, 1988). When non-native sounds are similar to native-language sounds that are infrequent, they may remain more discriminable to the learner than ones that are similar to frequent native-language sounds (Anderson *et al.*, 2003).

The narrowing of speech perception to favor native-language contrasts over non-native contrasts varies across infants, and is associated with other aspects of language learning. Whereas infants with stronger native speech discrimination have larger vocabularies than infants with weaker native discrimination, infants with stronger non-native discrimination have slower subsequent language development than infants who have tuned out irrelevant non-native language information (Kuhl *et al.*, 2008). Infants' nonlinguistic cognitive skills are also negatively correlated with the discrimination of non-native (but not native) speech contrasts between 8 and 11 months. Hence, the domain-general cognitive abilities involved in controlling attention to relevant vs. irrelevant stimuli may play a role in the language-specific narrowing of speech perception (Conboy *et al.*, 2008a; Lalonde and Werker, 1995).

In summary, many factors are involved in the formation of a language-specific perceptual system. These include exposure to speech sounds, features of the environment such as bilingualism or monolingualism, relationships between native and non-native phonology, acoustic features of sounds, nonlinguistic cognitive abilities, and brain maturation.

The late first to second and third years: Processing of words

Segmentation/recognition

At the same time that infants are learning the phonetic features of their native language, they are beginning to "crack the code" of their native-language lexicon. In order for infants to begin to comprehend words in their language environment, they must first learn to segment them from continuous speech. This task is difficult as most words infants hear are embedded in ongoing speech without obvious cues to their boundaries, such as silences (van de Weijer, 1998). Segmentation skills are correlated with subsequent vocabulary growth (Kooijman *et al.*, 2013; Newman *et al.*, 2006; Singh *et al.*, 2012). Bottom-up processes (which do not require previous linguistic knowledge) and top-down processes (use of already-learned language) have been shown to facilitate word segmentation at the experimental level.

An example of a bottom-up process that is available for word segmentation by eight months is statistical learning (Saffran, 2003). Infants quickly chunk together sounds that co-occur frequently (i.e., those for which the transitional probability [TP] from one sound to the next is high), and can use that information to determine when within-word sequences (those with higher TPs) and across-word sequences (those with lower TPs) occur. Infants may also use prosody to determine word boundaries. An early sensitivity to the patterns of languages that regularly place stress on the first syllable (e.g., English) would allow infants to adopt a rule about where each word ends and the next one begins. Although not all languages contain reliable prosodic cues to word boundaries, studies have confirmed the use of prosodic cues to word onsets/offsets in English- and French-learning infants by eight months (Goyet *et al.*, 2010; Nazzi *et al.*, 2014; Polka and Sundara, 2012). Infants show sensitivity to native-language allophonic variations and phonotactics, and can use those regularities to segment words from the speech stream by 6–9 months (Friederici and Wessels, 1993; Gonzalez Gomez and Nazzi, 2014; Jusczyk *et al.*, 1999; Mattys and Jusczyk, 2001). However, infants do not initially incorporate all cues (i.e., prosody, statistical regularities, phonotactics) when those cues conflict (Johnson and Jusczyk 2001; Thiessen and Saffran, 2003). In contrast, top-down strategies for word segmentation include the use of highly familiar words as "anchors" for determining the onsets and offsets of surrounding words (Bortfeld *et al.*, 2005; Shi and Lepage, 2008). By 6–8 months, infants recognize many words that may serve as anchors (Bergelson and Swingley, 2011).

Processing efficiency

As infants move into their second and third years, their perception and processing of language improves dramatically. Several studies have suggested that, as infants start learning the meanings of words, they encode only rough approximations of the phonetic information in those words, reflecting cognitive processing limitations (Werker *et al.*, 2009). For example, on structured word-learning tasks, 14-month-old infants treat phonetically similar syllables (e.g., "bih" and "dih"), but not dissimilar syllables (e.g., "neem" and "lif"), as variations of the same "word" for the same referent (Stager and Werker, 1997). Infants this age also show distinct brain activity for phonetically dissimilar words, and like activity for phonetically similar words (Mills *et al.*, 2004). However, younger infants (9-month-olds), as well as older infants (17–20 month-olds), differentiate the similar stimuli, and 14-month-old infants match familiar minimal pairs such as "ball" and "doll" to their referents even when they fail to match "bih" and "dih" to separate referents (Werker *et al.*, 2009). When words on these tasks are pronounced using the phonology of their non-dominant language, bilingual infants fail to encode the phonetic information, even at 17–20 months (Fennell *et al.*, 2007), but when novel words are pronounced in the dominant language phonology) bilingual infants encode this information (Mattock *et al.*, 2010).

Word processing skills in infants have been linked to previous language experience and to subsequent language development. Word processing efficiency (the latency of infants' looks to a visual target that matches a word, or the latency of word recognition ERP responses) is linked to amounts of input and vocabulary size (Hurtado *et al.*, 2008; Mills *et al.*, 2005a). The specialization of brain activity to more focal areas is also thought to reflect processing efficiency, and is associated with better language skills (Mills *et al.*, 2005a). As children gain experience with new words, the brain activity for processing those words becomes specialized to focal brain areas; for words with which a child has less experience, broader, more distributed networks are engaged (Mills *et al.*, 2005b). More focal brain activity and faster processing of words is also noted for the dominant compared to the non-dominant language of bilingual infants (Conboy and Mills, 2006). The ability to associate phonetically similar words with two different objects at 17–20 months predicts language skills up to 30 months later (Bernhardt, Kemp, and Werker, 2007), and the speed of associating a word with a matching picture at 18 months predicts language skills as late as eight years of age (Marchman and Fernald, 2008). Together with the findings reviewed in the previous section, these findings suggest that the processing of speech in infancy provides an important foundation for subsequent language learning.

Conclusion

This chapter has reviewed information about the speech perception and processing skills that allow language learning to take place. We have attempted to highlight the most relevant aspects of the literature for understanding language development. Areas of interest include how infants' perceptual skills are linked to subsequent language learning, how perceptual systems are shaped through experience and previous learning, and how particular features of the input are connected to perceptual learning.

References

Anderson, J.L., Morgan, J.L. and White, K.S. (2003), "A statistical basis for speech sound discrimination", *Language and Speech,* Vol. 46, pp. 155–182.

Bergelson, E. and Swingley, D. (2011), "At 6–9 months, human infants know the meanings of many common nouns", *Proceedings of the National Academy of Sciences of the United States,* Vol. 109, pp. 3253–3258.

Bernhardt, B.M., Kemp, N. and Werker, J.F. (2007), "Early word-object associations and later language development", *First Language,* Vol. 27, pp. 315–328.

Best, C.T., McRoberts, G.W. and Sithole, N.M. (1988), "Examination of perceptual reorganization for non-native speech contrasts: Zulu click discrimination by English-speaking adults and infants", *Journal of Experimental Psychology: Human Perception and Performance,* Vol. 14, pp. 345–360.

Bortfeld, H., Morgan, J.L, Golinkoff, R.M., Rathbun, K. (2005), "Mommy and me: Familiar names help launch babies into speech-stream segmentation", *Psychological Science,* Vol. 16, pp. 298–304.

Bosseler, A.N., Taulu, S., Pihko, E., Mäkelä, J.P., Imada, T., Ahonen, A. and Kuhl, P.K. (2013), "Theta brain rhythms index perceptual narrowing in infant speech perception", *Frontiers in Psychology*, Vol. 4, p. 690.

Bristow, D., Dehaene-Lambertz, G., Mattout, J., Soares, C., Gliga, T., Baillet, S. and Mangin, J.F. (2009), "Hearing faces: How the infant brain matches the face it sees with the speech it hears", *Journal of Cognitive Neuroscience*, Vol. 21, pp. 905–921.

Burnham, D.K. (1986), "Developmental loss of speech perception: Exposure to and experience with a first language", *Applied Psycholinguistics*, Vol. 7, pp. 207–240.

Byers-Heinlein, K., Burns, T.C. and Werker, J.F. (2010), "The roots of bilingualism in newborns", *Psychological Science*, Vol. 21, pp. 343–348.

Carral, V., Huotilainen, M., Ruusuvirta, T., Fellman, V., Näätänen, R. and Escera, C. (2005), "A kind of auditory 'primitive intelligence' already present at birth", *European Journal of Neuroscience*, Vol. 21, pp. 3201–3204.

Conboy, B.T., Brooks, R., Meltzoff, A.N. and Kuhl, P.K. (in press), Social interaction in infants' learning of second-language phonetics: an exploration of brain-behavior relations, *Developmental Neuropsychology*.

Conboy, B.T. and Kuhl, P.K. (2011), "Impact of second-language experience in infancy: brain measures of first- and second-language speech perception", *Developmental Science*, Vol. 14, pp. 242–248.

Conboy, B.T. and Mills, D.L. (2006), "Two languages, one developing brain: Effects of vocabulary size on bilingual toddlers' event-related potentials to auditory words", *Developmental Science*, Vol. 9, pp. F1–11.

Conboy, B.T., Sommerville, J. and Kuhl, P.K. (2008a), "Cognitive control factors in speech perception at 11 months", *Developmental Psychology*, Vol. 44, pp. 1505–1512.

Conboy, B.T., Sommerville, J. and Kuhl, P.K. (2008b), "Cognitive control skills and speech perception after short-term second language experience during infancy", paper presented at the Acoustics '08 Meeting, Paris, FR, 30 June–4 July.

Curtin, S., Byers-Heinlein, K. and Werker, J.F. (2011), "Bilingual beginnings as a lens for theory development: PRIMIR in focus", *Journal of Phonetics*, Vol. 39, pp. 492–504.

DeCasper, A.J., Lecanuet, J.-P., Busnel, M.-C., Granier-Deferre, C. and Maugeais, R. (1994), "Fetal reactions to recurrent maternal speech", *Infant Behavior and Development*, Vol. 17, pp. 159–164.

DeCasper, A.J. and Spence, M.J. (1986), "Prenatal maternal speech influences newborns' perception of speech sounds", *Infant Behavior and Development*, Vol. 9, pp. 133–150.

Dehaene-Lambertz, G. and Gliga, T. (2004), "Common neural basis for phoneme processing in infants and adults", *Journal of Cognitive Neuroscience*, Vol. 16, pp. 1375–1387.

Dehaene-Lambertz, G. and Peña, M. (2001), "Electrophysiological evidence for automatic phonetic processing in neonates", *NeuroReport*, Vol. 12, pp. 3155–3158.

Fennell, C.T., Byers-Heinlein, K. and Werker, J.F. (2007), "Using speech sounds to guide word learning: The case of bilingual infants", *Child Development*, Vol. 78, pp. 1510–1525.

Friederici, A.D. and Wessels, J.M.I. (1993), "Phonotactic knowledge of word boundaries and its use in infant speech perception", *Perception and Psychophysics*, Vol. 54, pp. 287–295.

García-Sierra, A., Rivera-Gaxiola, M., Percaccio, C., Conboy, B.T., Romo, H., Klarman, L., Ortíz, S. and Kuhl, P.K. (2011), "Bilingual language learning: An ERP study relating early brain responses to speech, language input, and later word production", *Journal of Phonetics*, Vol. 39, pp. 546–557.

Gervain, J., Berent, I. and Werker, J. (2012), "Binding at birth: The newborn brain detects identity relations and sequential position in speech", *Journal of Cognitive Neuroscience*, Vol. 24, pp. 564–574.

Gonzalez Gomez, N. and Nazzi, T. (2014), "Effects of prior phonotactic knowledge on infant word segmentation: The case of non-adjacent dependencies", *Journal of Speech, Language, and Hearing Research*, Vol. 56, pp. 840–49.

Goyet, L., de Schonen, S. and Nazzi, T. (2010), "Syllables in word segmentation by French-learning infants: An ERP study", *Brain Research*, Vol. 1332, pp. 75–89.

Granier-Deferre, C., Ribeiro, A., Jacquet, A. Y. and Bassereau, S. (2011), "Near-term fetuses process temporal features of speech", *Developmental Science*, Vol. 14, pp. 336–352.

Hurtado, N., Marchman, V.A. and Fernald, A. (2008), "Does input influence uptake? Links between maternal talk, processing speed and vocabulary size in Spanish-learning children", *Developmental Science*, Vol. 11, pp. F31–39.

Johnson, E.K. and Jusczyk, P.W. (2001), "Word segmentation by 8-month-olds: When speech cues count more than statistics", *Journal of Memory and Language*, Vol. 44, pp. 548–567.

Jusczyk, P.W. (1997), *The Discovery of Spoken Language*, MIT Press, Cambridge, MA, US.

Jusczyk, P.W., Hohne, E.A. and Bauman, A. (1999), "Infants' sensitivity to allophonic cues for word segmentation", *Perception and Psychophysics*, Vol. 62, pp. 1465–1476.

Jusczyk, P.W., Pisoni, D.B. and Mullennix, J. (1992), "Some consequences of stimulus variability on speech processing by 2-month-old infants", *Cognition*, Vol. 43, pp. 253–291.

Kisilevsky, B.S., Hains, S.M.J., Brown, C.A., Lee, C.T., Cowperthwaite, B., Stutzman, S.S., *et al.*, (2009), "Fetal sensitivity to properties of maternal speech and language", *Infant Behavior and Development*, Vol. 32, pp. 59–71.

Kooijman, V., Junge, C., Johnson, E. K., Hagoort, P. and Cutler, A. (2013), "Predictive brain signals of linguistic development", *Frontiers in Psychology*, Vol. 4, p. 25.

Kovács, M.A. and Mehler, J. (2009), "Cognitive gains in 7-month-old bilingual infants", *Proceedings of the National Academy of Sciences*, Vol. 106, pp. 6556–6560.

Kudo, N., Nonaka, Y., Mizuno, N., Mizuno, K. and Okanoya, K. (2011), "On-line statistical segmentation of a non-speech auditory stream in neonates as demonstrated by event-related brain potentials", *Developmental Science*, Vol. 14, pp. 1100–1106.

Kuhl, P.K. (1983), "Perception of auditory equivalence classes for speech in early infancy", *Infant Behavior and Development*, Vol. 6, pp. 263–285.

Kuhl, P.K. (2007), "Is speech learning 'gated' by the social brain?", *Developmental Science*, Vol. 10, pp. 110–120.

Kuhl, P.K., Andruski, J.E., Chistovich, I.A., Chistovich, L.A., Kozhevnikova, E.V., Ryskina, V.L., *et al.*, (1997), "Cross-language analysis of phonetic units in language addressed to infants", *Science*, Vol. 277, pp. 684–686.

Kuhl, P.K., Conboy, B.T., Padden, D., Rivera-Gaxiola, M. and Nelson, T. (2008), "Phonetic learning as a pathway to language: New data and native language magnet theory expanded (NLM-e)", *Philosophical Transactions of the Royal Society B*, Vol. 363, pp. 979–1000.

Kuhl, P.K. and Meltzoff, A.N. (1982), "The bimodal perception of speech in infancy", *Science*, Vol. 218, pp. 1138–1141.

Kuhl, P.K., Ramírez, R.R., Bosseler, A., Lin, J.F.L. and Imada, T. (2014), "Infants' brain responses to speech suggest Analysis by Synthesis", *Proceedings of the National Academy of Sciences*, Vol. 111, pp. 11238–11245.

Kuhl, P.K., Stevens, E., Hayashi, A., Deguchi, T., Kiritani, S. and Iverson, P. (2006), "Infants show a facilitation effect for native language phonetic perception between 6 and 12 months", *Developmental Science*, Vol. 9, pp. F13–21.

Kuhl, P.K., Tsao, F.M. and Liu, H.M. (2003), "Foreign-language experience in infancy: Effects of short-term exposure and social interaction on phonetic learning", *Proceedings of the National Academy of Science*, Vol. 100, pp. 9096–9101.

Lalonde, C. and Werker, J. (1995), "Cognitive influences on cross-language speech perception in infancy", *Infant Behavior and Development*, Vol. 18, pp. 459–475.

Liu, H.-M., Kuhl, P.K. and Tsao, F.-M. (2003), "An association between mothers' speech clarity and infants' speech discrimination skills", *Developmental Science*, Vol. 6, pp. F1–10.

Marchman, V.A. and Fernald, A. (2008), "Speed of word recognition and vocabulary knowledge in infancy predict cognitive and language outcomes in later childhood", *Developmental Science*, Vol. 11, pp. F9–16.

Mattock, K., Polka, L., Rvachew, S. and Krehm, M. (2010), "The first steps in word learning are easier when the shoes fit: Comparing monolingual and bilingual infants", *Developmental Science*, Vol. 13, pp. 229–243.

Mattys, S.L. and Jusczyk, P.W. (2001), "Phonotactic cues for segmentation of fluent speech by infants", *Cognition*, Vol. 78, pp. 91–121.

Maurer, D. and Werker, J.F. (2014), "Perceptual narrowing during infancy: A comparison of language and faces", *Developmental Psychobiology*, Vol. 56, pp. 154–178.

Maye, J., Werker, J.F. and Gerken, L. (2002), "Infant sensitivity to distributional information can affect phonetic discrimination", *Cognition*, Vol. 82, pp. B101–11.

Mehler, J., Jusczyk, P.W., Lambertz, G., Halstead, N., Bertoncini, J. and Amiel-Tison, C. (1988), "A precursor of language acquisition in young infants", *Cognition*, Vol. 29, pp. 143–178.

Mills, D., Prat, C., Stager, C., Zangl, R., Neville, H. and Werker, J. (2004), "Language experience and the organization of brain activity to phonetically similar words: ERP evidence from 14- and 20-month-olds", *Journal of Cognitive Neuroscience*, Vol. 16, pp. 1452–1464.

121

Mills, D.L., Conboy, B.T. and Paton, C. (2005a), "How learning new words shapes the organization of the infant brain", in Namy, L.L. (Ed.), *Symbol Use and Symbolic Representation*, Lawrence Erlbaum Associates, Mahwah, NJ, US, pp. 123–153.

Mills, D., Plunkett, K., Prat, C. and Schafer, G. (2005b), "Watching the infant brain learn words: Effects of language and experience", *Cognitive Development*, Vol. 20, pp. 19–31.

Minagawa-Kawai, Y., Cristià, A. and Dupoux, E. (2011), "Cerebral lateralization and early speech acquisition: A developmental scenario", *Developmental Cognive Neuroscience*, Vol. 2, pp. 194–195.

Moon, C., Cooper, R. and Fifer, W. (1993), "Two-day-olds prefer their native language", *Infant Behavior and Development*, Vol. 16, pp. 495–500.

Moon, C., Lagercrantz, H. and Kuhl, P.K. (2013), "Language experienced *in utero* affects vowel perception after birth: A two-country study", *Acta Pædiatrica*, Vol. 102, pp. 156–160.

Mugitani, R., Pons, F., Fais, L., Dietrich, C., Werker, J.F. and Amano, S. (2009), "Perception of vowel length by Japanese- and English-learning infants", *Developmental Psychology*, Vol. 45, pp. 236–247.

Narayan, C.R., Werker, J.F. and Beddor, P.S. (2010), "The interaction between acoustic salience and language experience in developmental speech perception: Evidence from nasal place discrimination", *Developmental Science*, Vol. 13, pp. 407–420.

Nazzi, T., Mersad, K., Sundara, M., Iakimova, G. and Polka, L. (2014), "Early word segmentation in infants acquiring Parisian French: Task-dependent and dialect-specific aspects", *Journal of Child Language*, Vol. 41, pp. 600–633.

Newman, R., Ratner, N.B., Jusczyk, A.M, Jusczyk, P.W. and Dow, K.A. (2006), "Infants' early ability to segment the conversational speech signal predicts later language development: A retrospective analysis", *Developmental Psychology*, Vol. 42, pp. 643–655.

Partanen, E., Kujala, T., Näätänen, R., Liitola, A., Sambeth, A. and Huotilainen, M. (2013), "Learning-induced neural plasticity of speech processing before birth", *Proceedings of the National Academy of Sciences*, Vol. 110, pp. 15145–15150.

Patterson, M.L. and Werker, J.F. (2003), "Two-month-old infants match phonetic information in lips and voice", *Developmental Science*, Vol. 6, pp. 191–196.

Peña, M., Maki, A., Kovačić, D., Dehaene-Lambertz, G., Koizumi, H., Bouquet, F. and Mehler, J. (2003), "Sounds and silence: An optical topography study of language recognition at birth", *Proceedings of the National Academy of Sciences*, Vol. 100, pp. 11702–11705.

Petitto, L. A., Berens, M.S., Kovelman, I., Dubins, M.H., Williams, L.J. and Shalinsky, M. (2012), "The 'Perceptual Wedge Hypothesis' as the basis for bilingual babies' phonetic processing advantage: New insights from fNIRS brain imaging", *Brain and Language*, Vol. 121, pp. 130–143.

Polka, L. and Sundara, M. (2012), "Word segmentation in monolingual infants acquiring Canadian English and Canadian French: Native language, cross-dialect, and cross language comparisons", *Infancy*, Vol. 17, pp. 198–232.

Polka, L. and Werker, J.F. (1994), "Developmental changes in perception of non-native vowel contrasts", *Journal of Experimental Psychology: Human Perception and Performance*, Vol. 20, pp. 421–435.

Saffran, J.R. (2003), "Statistical language learning mechanisms and constraints", *Current Directions in Psychological Science*, Vol. 12, No. 4, pp. 110–114.

Sato, Y., Sogabe, Y. and Mazuka, R. (2010), "Discrimination of phonemic vowel length by Japanese infants", *Developmental Psychology*, Vol. 46, pp. 106–119.

Sebastián-Gallés, N., Albareda-Castellot, B., Weikum, W.M. and Werker, J.F. (2012), "A bilingual advantage in visual language discrimination in infancy", *Psychological Science*, Vol. 23, pp. 994–999.

Sebastián-Gallés, N. and Bosch, L. (2009), "Developmental shift in the discrimination of vowel contrasts in bilingual infants: is the distributional account all there is to it?", *Developmental Science*, Vol. 12, pp. 874–887.

Shafer, V.L., Yu, Y.H. and Datta, H. (2011), "The development of English vowel perception in monolingual and bilingual infants: Neurophysiological correlates", *Journal of Phonetics*, Vol. 39, pp. 527–545.

Shi, R. and Lepage, M. (2008), "The effect of functional morphemes on word segmentation in preverbal infants", *Developmental Science*, Vol. 11, pp. 407–413.

Singh, L., Reznick, J.S. and Xuehua, L. (2012), "Infant word segmentation and childhood vocabulary development: A longitudinal analysis", *Developmental Science*, Vol. 15, pp. 482–495.

Stager, C.L. and Werker, J.F. (1997), "Infants listen for more phonetic detail in speech perception than in word-learning tasks", *Nature*, Vol. 388, pp. 381–382.

Sundara, M., Polka, L. and Genesee, F. (2006), "Language-experience facilitates discrimination of /d- ð/ in monolingual and bilingual acquisition of English", *Cognition,* Vol. 100, pp. 369–388.

Teinonen, T., Fellman, V., Naatanen, R., Alku, P. and Huotilainen, M. (2009), "Statistical language learning in neonates revealed by event-related brain potentials", *BMC Neuroscience,* Vol. 10, pp. 1–8.

Thiessen, E.D. and Saffran, J.R. (2003), "When cues collide: Use of stress and statistical cues to word boundaries by 7-to 9-month-old infants", *Developmental Psychology*, Vol. 39, pp. 706–716.

Tsao, F.M., Liu, H.M. and Kuhl, P.K. (2004), "Speech perception in infancy predicts language development in the second year of life: A longitudinal study", *Child Development,* Vol. 75, pp. 1067–1084.

van de Weijer, J. (1998), *Language Input for Word Discovery,* Unpublished doctoral dissertation. Radbound University, Nijmegen, The Netherlands.

Vouloumanos, A., Hauser, M.D., Werker, J.F. and Martin, A. (2010), "The tuning of human neonates' preference for speech", *Child Development,* Vol. 81, pp. 517–527.

Vouloumanos, A. and Werker, J.F. (2007), "Listening to language at birth: Evidence for a bias for speech in neonates", *Developmental Science,* Vol. 10, pp. 159–171.

Weikum, W.M., Vouloumanos, A., Navarra, J., Soto-Faraco, S., Sebastián-Gallés, N. and Werker, J.F. (2007), "Visual language discrimination in infancy", *Science,* Vol. 316, p. 1159.

Werker, J.F., Byers-Heinlein, K. and Fennell, C. (2009), "Bilingual beginnings to learning words", *Philosophical Transactions of the Royal Society B: Biological Sciences,* Vol. 364, pp. 3649–3663.

Werker, J.F., Pons, F., Dietrich, C., Kajikawa, S., Fais, L. and Amano, S. (2007), "Infant-directed speech supports phonetic category learning in English and Japanese", *Cognition,* Vol. 103, pp. 147–162.

Werker, J. and Tees, R. (1984), "Cross-language speech perception: Evidence for perceptual reorganization during the first year of life", *Infant Behavior and Development,* Vol. 7, pp. 49–63.

Werker, J.F. and Yeung, H.H. (2005), "Infant speech perception bootstraps word learning", *Trends in Cognitive Sciences,* Vol. 9, pp. 519–527.

Yoshida, K.A., Pons, F., Maye, J. and Werker, J.F. (2010), "Distributional phonetic learning at 10 months of age", *Infancy*, Vol. 15, pp. 420–433.

Zhang, Y., Koerner, T., Miller, S., Grice-Patil, Z., Svec, A., Akbari, D., Tusler, L. and Carney, E. (2011), "Neural coding of formant-exaggerated speech in the infant brain", *Developmental Science,* Vol. 14, pp. 566–581.

11

DEVELOPMENTAL MODELS OF CHILDHOOD APRAXIA OF SPEECH

Ben A.M. Maassen

During the last decade, research suggested that developmental communication disorders have multi-factorial origins at different levels of aggregation. Moreover, the influence of these levels of aggregation on the resulting behavioral output is interactive rather than uni-directional. In this chapter, a developmental, perceptual-motor model of childhood apraxia of speech (CAS) is described that uses this multi-level, multi-factorial concept as its foundation. In the first section, global outlines of the interactive multi-level model are described. This is followed by a discussion of each of the four levels as they relate to CAS, including the interactions between the levels. Since relatively little is known about the genetic and neurological background of CAS, the focus in this chapter is on the perceptual-motor level, including to some extent higher cognitive functions, such as lexical retrieval. In addition, the behavioral level is described, being the most directly observable and accessible level for clinical management. In the final section, implications for clinical practice and future research directions are discussed.

Multi-level models of developmental disorders

A model describing the different levels of causation of developmental disorders is presented in Figure 11.1 (adapted from Bishop and Snowling, 2004). Four levels of aggregation are distinguished, with some of the boxes labeled according to known underlying deficits in CAS. The etiological level describes the genetic constitution of the individual in combination with relevant environmental factors including biological factors, such as ante- and perinatal conditions. The Bishop and Snowling (2004) model also incorporates the influence a child's behavior has on his/ her own environment. An example would be the communicative activity level of an infant. More active infants tend to elicit more communicative response from the care-taker as compared to more passive infants. Hence, during development, the etiological factors unfold into a neurological architecture combined with functionality, i.e., the neurobiological level. The model makes clear that the brain does not develop according to a genetic blueprint, but is continuously adapting to biological and behavioral (environmental) circumstances.

Cognitive functions form the third level of aggregation. The raison d'être of this intermediate level between neurobiology and behavior is that there is no one-to-one relationship between brain functions and behavior. Cognitive functions indeed constitute an intermediate level that operates at a more abstract level than the behaviors that result from it. For example, a deficit in

etiology

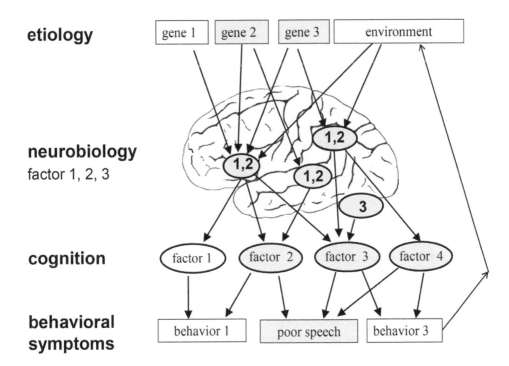

neurobiology

factor 1, 2, 3

cognition

behavioral symptoms

Figure 11.1 Levels of causation for childhood apraxia of speech (CAS) (modified after Bishop and Snowling, 2004, p. 859). Numbered gray cells indicate factors associated with CAS.

Note: Genes 2 and 3 refer to associated genes, such as FOXP2 (Graham and Fisher, 2013). Neurobiology factors 1 and 2 refer to distributed factors in speech areas, such as reduced neurite outgrowth (Graham and Fisher, 2013). Factor 3 depicts cerebellar deficits. Cognition factors 2, 3 and 4 refer to known factors, such as poor sequential motor programming, coordination, and auditory processing.

word and syllable retrieval could have an effect on sentence construction – such as when the speaker experiences difficulty in rapid retrieval of the correct word form for sentence continuation, which could result in speech dysfluencies. In this case, the speaker has difficulty with initiating word articulation. The fourth level is behavioral. It is directly observable and constitutes – in the case of CAS – the speech characteristics and clinical symptoms.

A series of theoretical papers summarizing the main arguments for the notion that developmental disorders are quite unlike acquired disorders in adults has been published. An exhaustive discussion is outside the scope of this chapter, but the key concepts and arguments are briefly presented here. Bishop (1997) argued that dissociation, or even better, double dissociation, which is the ideal neuropsychological evidence in the study of acquired disorders in adults, does not apply to developmental disorders. The reason is that a dysfunction in a developing child (e.g., poor auditory speech perception) will affect the acquisition of other functions and skills that partly depend on this function being intact (e.g., phonological development). Thus, in developmental disorders, it is more likely to find associations between functions than dissociations. From a slightly different perspective, Karmiloff-Smith (2006; Karmiloff-Smith *et al.*, 2003) comes to the same conclusion, arguing that in both normal and disordered development, cognitive modules are the outcome of development rather than its starting point. The progression to the adult system is a gradual and continuous process made up of interactions between emerging modules, resulting in associations among functions.

In an attempt to specify the developmental process for CAS, Maassen (2002) observed that infant speech development starts from random babbling and sensomotoric learning, which forms the basis for more abstract phonological acquisition. Starting from the assumption that the core deficit of CAS is a reduced sensomotoric learning capacity, one can predict not only poor articulation, but also poor auditory and somatosensory representation, and, from there, effects on the psycholinguistic domain because of the impact on phonological and higher-level processes. This contrasts with adults with apraxia of speech (AOS), who already have acquired stable top-down processes. Because the developmental trajectory sketched above is probabilistic and multi-factorial rather than deterministic, Karmiloff-Smith (2006) characterizes the process of childhood disorders as a tortuous route from genes to behavior.

Genetics

The indirect relationship (or tortuous route) between the underlying deficit at the neurological and cognitive level and speech symptoms, seriously complicates the search for heritability and genetic factors involved in CAS. Because the diagnostic speech symptoms of CAS change with age, and are influenced by multiple factors, family members cannot be directly compared at the behavioral level. Even within twins, the commonality of symptoms changes during speech development. The difficulty lies in the changing speech symptoms (Maassen 2002), which seriously complicates the specification of the phenotype. Therefore, Stein *et al.* (2011) have argued that studies comparing siblings, or parent–offspring pairs need to take into account that the expression of a particular underlying, genetically determined trait changes with age and is influenced by environmental factors.

Nevertheless, recent progress in genetic linkage methodology has revealed underlying genetic deficits in speech and language disorders. Since its discovery in 1998 (Fisher *et al.*, 1998), the *FOXP2* gene probably has been the most frequently studied gene in relation to speech and language functions. Its major function has been shown to be regulating the expression of other genes. That is, *FOXP2* encodes a transcription factor that controls the expression of a series of other genes regulating, among other things, language and motor functions. One of these genes regulated by *FOXP2* is *CNTNAP2*, which has been associated with specific language impairment (SLI). Specific parts of *CNTNAP2* also have been associated with phonological short-term memory, and thus with performance on non-word repetition tasks (Newbury *et al.*, 2010).

Whether directly, or in its role as transcription factor, variants of *FOXP2* have been shown to affect the development of the motor cortex, striatum and cerebellum. These structures are involved in neural circuits that facilitate language acquisition, and more specifically sequential speech motor learning. Interestingly, mutations of *FOXP2* lead to difficulties in sequential articulatory movements, like in AOS, and songbird orthologues of *FoxP2* are involved in the vocal learning of the courtship song. Knockdown of FoxP2 expression during song development results in inaccurate and incomplete imitation of tutor songs (Vernes and Fisher, 2009).

Four single cases of individuals with *FOXP2* disruptions have been summarized by Shriberg *et al.* (2012), showing relationships among speech, prosody, voice, cognition, language, and other findings with CAS. Other CAS related genes are *FOXP1, FOXG1, ELP4,* and *RAI1*. These authors note an important difference in CAS as compared to acquired AOS in adults, in that in CAS, cognitive and sensorimotor development may be affected in all brain regions and circuits in which gene expression is disrupted, as compared to more localized impairments in adults.

More detailed discussion is outside the scope of this chapter (the reader is referred to Section I of this volume) but it is important to realize that there are no direct genotype–phenotype links in speech motor disorders. Rather, overlapping and interacting pathways from genes via neurological structure and function to cognition and behavior together result in a disorder with a complex phenotype, such as CAS.

Neurobiology

Direct data on neurobiological determinants of CAS is extremely scarce. No systematic brain imaging studies of young children with CAS are available for obvious ethical reasons, so the scarce studies with MRI, fMRI, or EEG are conducted with children with a medical condition requiring brain imaging. The ASHA Technical Report (American Speech–Language–Hearing Association [ASHA], 2007) notes that CAS can occur in different clinical contexts, the first of which comprises known neurological etiologies, such as intrauterine stroke, infections, and trauma. The second clinical context consists of complex neurobehavioral disorders (e.g., genetic, metabolic). Both contexts are promising sources of information on neural mechanisms underlying CAS. Thus, from a series of heterogeneous studies, it can be determined that associations exist between CAS on the one hand and benign rolandic epilepsy (5 patients), fragile-X syndrome (4 out of 10 patients), galactosemia (14 out of 24 patients), Down syndrome, Rett syndrome, autism, Coffin-Siris syndrome, and increased theta-activity on clinical EEG in parietal-temporal cortical regions (Shriberg, 2010). In these cases, the underlying neurological impairment is known. The contribution of this clinical knowledge to our understanding of underlying mechanisms in CAS is limited, however, because these studies lack detail on the speech and prosody characteristics of the diagnosed children, such that the specific diagnosis CAS cannot be confirmed (ASHA, 2007).

In addition, CAS, which is not associated with any known neurological or complex neurobehavioral disorder, can occur as an *idiopathic neurogenic speech sound disorder* and can be accommodated by Shriberg's (2010) neurodevelopmental framework. This approach, in which core speech and non-speech features are based on diagnostic characteristics as sequelae of a known neurological or neurodevelopmental condition, may have research promise for resolving existing diagnostic controversies for CAS. Speech data from known neurological syndromes (CAS, possibly also AOS) should yield pathognomonic signs and markers, such that the diagnostic circularity – the problem that finding specific diagnostic markers requires clearly diagnosed patients (based on which markers?) – (see further discussion below) – can be breached. Once diagnostic markers are available, further research can be conducted to find the genetic and neural substrates by comparing validated cases of CAS with controls; then idiopathic motor speech disorders can be identified on the basis of established characteristics. A diagnostic category of special interest is dysarthria. There are several subtypes of dysarthria, and also the recently introduced diagnostic category, childhood motor speech disorder – not otherwise specified, which is a cover term for dysarthria and CAS, shows much overlap in symptomatology with CAS.

From a methodological point of view, Weismer and Kim (2010) argued to approach the diagnostic classification of dysarthrias and AOS from a taxonomic perspective, such that not only differential diagnostic, but also commonalities between disorders, are assessed to identify 'core' phenomena of these disorders. An example would be slow speech rate, which is characteristic of almost all speech disorders, and therefore needs to be accounted for rather than discarded because it does not contribute to differential diagnosis.

Cognitive and perceptual-motor processes

More than a decade ago, McNeil and colleagues (2004) made the following comment on the status quo of clinical research in AOS in adults:

> it is not a lack of theory or the inability to select the correct theory from the known alternatives that limits understanding of AOS [..]. It is, likewise, not the lack of neurologic or anatomic instantiation that limits AOS understanding. The most important impediment to theoretical and clinical advancement in AOS is, however, the lack of a comprehensive and clear definition that leads to an agreed-upon set of criteria for subject selection.
>
> *(p. 389)*

This comment still applies to AOS.

The comprehensive ASHA Technical Report (2007) on CAS concludes that: "... there presently is no one validated list of diagnostic features of CAS that differentiates this disorder from other types of childhood speech sound disorders, including those apparently due to phonological level deficits or neuromuscular disorder (dysarthria)" (p. 5). Thus, for both AOS and CAS, there is no consensus with respect to diagnostic criteria. However, as McNeil *et al.* (2004) above and the ASHA Technical Report (2007) conclude, there is consensus with respect to the underlying deficit at the cognitive level, thanks to a series of studies focusing on underlying mechanisms of CAS, by means of measuring kinematic parameters. Thus, as with AOS, in the last decade researchers have agreed on the processes or proximal causes underlying CAS. For CAS, the core impairment lies in planning and/or programming spatiotemporal parameters of movement sequences, resulting in imprecise and inconsistent speech movements (ASHA, 2007, pp. 3–4). Despite this clear definition of the underlying cause of CAS, the major obstacle for clinical management and research is that there is high variability in resulting speech symptoms, particularly if developmental aspects are also taken into account. This variability seriously complicates diagnostic classification.

It is clear that studying only the phonological output (percentage of consonants and vowels correct; number of substitutions – see next paragraph) is insufficient to collect the required data to diagnose the above-mentioned underlying deficits. The study by Bahr (2005) was one of the earliest that focused on the movement of articulators rather than phonemic accuracy. Through comparisons of children with phonological disorder (PD) and CAS, it appeared that both groups evidenced significantly poorer phonemic accuracy than the typically developing children did, but these groups could not be distinguished based on their speech error profile. However, each child group with speech sound disorders (SSD) showed a specific pattern of gesture coordination difficulties. Both groups evidenced difficulty with gestures involving the tongue blade, but children with PD specifically showed poor voicing, and the children with CAS specifically had difficulty with correct coordination of the velum and the lips with the other articulators. An explanation for the coordination difficulty demonstrated by children with CAS might be that the independence of the velum and lips from the tongue is demanding from a gesture coordination point of view, and thus vulnerable to an underlying coordination deficit.

Also, Grigos and Kolenda (2010) studied kinematic parameters in addition to phoneme accuracy. They followed a 3-year-old boy with CAS for eight months during the acquisition of /p/, /b/, and /m/. Transcription analyses showed that consonant and vowel errors decreased across sessions. More importantly, the child's kinematic jaw movement parameters became more similar to controls overall. However, only closing velocity and stability reached a level of accuracy comparable to controls, whereas opening velocities showed a much more erratic pattern over time. Similarly, Terband *et al.* (2011) found higher variability of tongue tip movements trajectories in five children with CAS as compared to controls. Different patterns of coordination between CAS and controls were interpreted as an indication of underlying coordination difficulties.

Such coordination difficulties had been found by Green *et al.* (2002), who measured midsagittal displacements of the lips and jaw in typically developing 1-, 2- and 6-year-olds, as well as adults, while producing utterances 'baba', 'papa', and 'mama'. Their results showed that movement patterns of the jaw matured earlier than those of the lips. Further support for the specific development of lip movement coordination is found in a study by Grigos *et al.* (2005), who studied the development of voicing contrast in /p/ versus /b/. They found that variability of lip and jaw movement of 19-month-old children decreased as they began to acquire the voiceless phoneme /p/ in addition to the earlier acquired voiced /b/.

To summarize, the kinematic studies show that "the precision and consistency of movements underlying speech are impaired" (ASHA, 2007, p. 3) in children with CAS, more so, or perhaps more specifically than in children with SSD. Thus, there seems to be substantial agreement on the basic underlying deficit. Less clear however, is what the sequelae are, both upstream and downstream in the speech production process. Upstream, phonological abilities and lexical storage are involved. Shriberg *et al.* (2012) consider auditory–perceptual encoding processes as proximal causes of CAS. These processes form the input of phonemic and lexical representations, memory processes that store and retrieve these representations, and transcoding processes for the planning and programming of motor gestures. Downstream effects result in speech sound errors that at the perceptual level are classified as substitutions or distortions. For instance, extreme voicing errors could be considered as a substitution. Such distortions and extreme distortions are similar to those found in dysarthria, and therefore contribute to the confusion about differential diagnosis.

Behavior: Speech symptoms

The most accessible, but also the most variable, is the behavioral level, i.e., actual speech production. In the vast majority of cases, clinical intervention starts at this level. A child is referred to a speech–language pathologist (SLP) because parents, other caregivers, or teachers express concern about the observable delays or suspected deviances in speech as compared to their peers. In addition, the diagnostic process takes speech characteristics and symptoms as a starting point. One of the classical issues is whether CAS should be considered as a discrete diagnostic entity that occurs separately from other speech impairments, or if it consists of a symptom complex and should be considered as a syndrome (Guyette and Diedrich, 1981; McCabe *et al.*, 1998).

Approaching differential diagnosis from a multi-level perspective, I personally have never really understood the distinction between a symptom complex and a syndrome. At a purely descriptive level, however, the line of reasoning is that, in order to show that CAS is a discrete diagnostic entity, one searches for a diagnostic marker that is present in all cases with CAS and not with other speech difficulties. Alternatively, CAS as a syndrome presumes a complex of co-occurring underlying deficits that in combination underlie the symptom complex. What is never expressed explicitly, but remains implicit, is the assumption that single and specific causes underlie each single speech symptom, and that no interactions between causes and/or symptoms occur. Although the multi-level model sketched above has – I hope – convincingly shown that the same symptom can refer to different underlying deficits, and the same deficit can result in different symptoms, among other factors due to developmental interactions.

This is why studies relying on clinical judgments alone have shown a wide variety of symptoms and much overlap between different SSDs. For instance, McCabe and colleagues (1998) compiled an inventory of features characteristic of CAS (labeled developmental apraxia of speech [DAS] at the time) from a search of the literature, and came up with 30 different characteristics. To test these characteristics, a retrospective file audit was conducted of 50 pediatric clients, who had been referred to the Communication Disorders Treatment and Research Clinic at The University of Sydney for articulatory or phonological impairment of an unknown origin. Nine children were diagnosed with CAS. It turned out that the order of features was highly similar for the nine children with CAS as compared to the total group of 50 children. The top five characteristics were: decreased performance with increased speech complexity; decreased expressive language level for age; multiple articulation errors; slow development of speech skills; and idiosyncratic sound substitutions. In another study, Forrest (2003) asked 75 SLPs to write down their top three characteristics used to diagnose CAS. This list showed little overlap with that of McCabe et al. The top five characteristics were: inconsistent productions; general–oral motor difficulties; groping; unable to imitate sounds; and increased errors with increased utterance length. These studies indicate that subjective ratings tend to yield variable results; clearer definition and quantification of diagnostic speech characteristics seem to be needed.

A more focused approach is the search for a diagnostic marker. Although this search has not yielded yet "… pathognomonic symptoms or necessary and sufficient conditions…" (Guyette and Diedrich, 1981) to diagnose CAS, it has contributed much to the identification of core symptoms. In a series of papers, Shriberg et al. (1997a, b, c) studied different clinical populations of children with suspected CAS as compared to children with speech delay (SD) and adults with acquired AOS. The aim was to identify speech errors that differentiated CAS from SD, and errors that resembled those produced by adults with AOS. In the first paper, they conclude that children with suspected CAS somehow differed from children with SD and took longer to normalize. The authors further noted that, without a diagnostic marker, there is the problem of circularity. How can one find diagnostic characteristics of CAS if there are no diagnostic criteria available to convincingly identify the subjects of the study? The second and third papers tackled the problem of circularity in the diagnosis of children with suspected CAS as compared to SD. Shriberg et al. concluded that there was no simple pattern of segmental errors that formed a solid basis for diagnosing CAS. However, inappropriate stress, which was characteristic of 52 per cent of the children with suspected CAS as compared to 10 per cent of the children with SD of unknown origin, can be considered a diagnostic marker for CAS. Further elaborations of this characteristic resulted in the lexical stress ratio (Shriberg et al., 2003a) and the coefficient of variation ratio (Hosom et al., 2004; Shriberg et al., 2003b).

Comprehensive studies analyzing segmental error patterns have been conducted by Maassen et al. (1997), Thoonen (1998), and Thoonen et al. (1994). A unique aspect of these studies was the inclusion of the phonotactic context in the analyses. Phonetic transcriptions of consonants produced in word and pseudo-word imitation tasks revealed overall increased substitution and omission rates for the children with CAS in comparison to children with normal speech. However, the overall profile of errors was not distinctive. Because errors were quantified, it was possible to correct for overall error rate, yielding profiles of relative error rates. While children with CAS produced a higher rate of phoneme anticipations, perseverations, and metatheses (i.e., syntagmatic errors) as compared to controls after correction for the overall higher error rate, the relative number of syntagmatic and paradigmatic errors[1] appeared identical for both groups. In general, the error profiles showed very few differences between groups, suggesting that the speech of children with CAS can be characterized by a high rate of 'normal' slips of the tongue. Even so, the children with CAS showed a particularly low percentage of retention of place of articulation in words, and inconsistency with respect to feature realization and feature preference. These two features, high rate of place-of-articulation errors and inconsistency, stood out as possibly diagnostic for CAS (see, however, Forrest and Morrisette, 1999, for counterarguments).

Clinical practice and future research

From the multi-level, multi-factorial model presented above, a series of conclusions can be drawn for clinical practice. One, CAS is not a categorical but a continuous diagnosis, varying from mild to severe. Second, different profiles of CAS should be found, in which the degree of involvement of each of the speech motor functions contributing to fluent speech can vary. Systematic inventories of such profiles could yield subtypes of CAS, for instance, the subtype a) with poor prosody (inappropriate stress), b) with poor co-articulation (syllabic structure errors), and c) with poor place of articulation (many phonemic substitution errors). Recognizing subtypes, as well as the motor aspects involved in each, yields important guidelines for therapy. Third, co-morbidity might be the rule rather than the exception, largely due to the multiple etiologies. For further discussion of this topic, see Nijland *et al.* (in press).

The developmental perspective leads us to approach CAS not as a dissociated, separate condition, but rather as a deficit with possibly far-reaching consequences for speech and language acquisition. As such, impairments of the developing speech motor control system may impact other, related domains, such as phonological and lexical development and auditory–perceptual functions. Thus, the underlying deficit in children with CAS may express itself in different signs and symptoms over the course of development. In the diagnosis of CAS, exclusion criteria should therefore be applied with great caution. Specifically, if speech motor planning difficulties can result in poor phonological development, then a phonological disorder at the behavioral level is not a valid exclusion criterion for CAS. Furthermore, a developmental perspective predicts changing symptomatology across ages.

A dynamic approach is advocated, both for diagnosis and for treatment. From motor theory we know that the acquisition of motor plans and programs requires much practice. The reason is that motor planning and programming are skill-specific: practicing the articulation of English, does not contribute to speaking Chinese, just as practicing playing the piano does not help much in playing the violin. [Note that different learning principles underlie the acquisition of the vocabulary and syntax of languages, as well as the fundamentals of music, as compared to motor learning.] Motor training therefore needs to be adapted to the developmental stage, as expressed in the motor patterns acquired thus far, to other cognitive functions, like memory and attention, and to higher-level language functions. An important aspect is that articulatory movement patterns are not acquired in a vacuum but can be related to meaningful lexical items, so that they can be anchored in lexical memory.

A prerequisite for dynamic diagnosis and treatment is a process-oriented approach. As was discussed above, the speech symptoms at the behavioral level are not transparent regarding the underlying processing deficit. The assumption is that treatment of processes is more effective and yields better generalization than treating symptoms. Recently, we started a process-oriented line of research that applies experimental techniques to directly manipulate speech production processes for dynamic assessment. For instance, the hypothesis that the speech production process of a child with CAS is characterized by overreliance on auditory feedback (Terband, 2011), could be tested in a speech task with auditory masking by presenting the child with noise over headphones. If the speech becomes much poorer, then it can be concluded that, indeed, auditory monitoring plays a role in normal speech production. If the speech barely deteriorates, apparently online feedback is not invoked. Dynamic treatment means that treatment results are continuously assessed and the treatment program is continuously adapted. This requires a dynamic integration of speech motor and phonological treatments.

Note

1 As defined by Thoonen *et al.* (1994), syntagmatic errors are related to context, such as anticipations, perseverations, and transpositions; paradigmatic errors are speech sound errors of place, manner, or voice, not induced by the context.

References

American Speech–Language–Hearing Association (ASHA) (2007), *Childhood Apraxia of Speech [Technical Report]*, Available from www.asha.org/policy

Bahr, R.H. (2005), "Differential diagnosis of severe speech disorders using speech gestures", *Topics in Language Disorders,* Vol. 25, No. 3, pp. 254–265.

Bishop, D.V.M. (1997), "Cognitive neuropsychology and developmental disorders: Uncomfortable bedfellows", *The Quarterly Journal of Experimental Psychology,* Vol. 50A, No. 4, pp. 899–923.

Bishop, D.V.M. and Snowling, M. (2004), "Developmental dyslexia and specific language impairment: Same or different?", *Psychological Bulletin,* Vol. 130, No. 6, pp. 858–886.

Fisher, S.E., Vargha-Khadem, F., Watkins, K.E., Monaco, A.P. and Pembrey, M.E. (1998), "Localisation of a gene implicated in a severe speech and language disorder", *Nature Genetics,* Vol. 18, pp. 168–170.

Forrest, K. (2003), "Diagnostic criteria of developmental apraxia of speech used by clinical speech-language pathologists", *American Journal of Speech-Language Pathology,* Vol. 12, pp. 376–380.

Forrest, K. and Morrisette, M.L. (1999), "Feature analysis of segmental errors in children with phonological disorders", *Journal of Speech, Language, and Hearing Research,* Vol. 42, pp. 187–194.

Graham, S.A. and Fisher, S.E. (2013), "Decoding the genetics of speech and language", *Current Opinion in Neurobiology,* Vol. 23, pp. 43–51.

Green, J.R., Moore, C.A. and Reilly, K.J. (2002), "The sequential development of jaw and lip control for speech", *Journal of Speech, Language, and Hearing Research,* Vol. 45, pp. 66–79.

Grigos, M.I. and Kolenda, N. (2010), "The relationship between articulatory control and improved phonemic accuracy in childhood apraxia of speech: A longitudinal case study", *Clinical Linguistics and Phonetics,* Vol. 24, No. 1, pp. 17–40.

Grigos, M.I., Saxman, J.H. and Gordon, A.M. (2005), "Speech motor development during acquisition of the voicing contrast", *Journal of Speech, Language, and Hearing Research,* Vol. 48, pp. 739–752.

Guyette, T. and Diedrich, W.M. (1981), "A critical review of developmental apraxia of speech" in N. J. Lass, (Ed.), *Speech and Language. Advances in Basic Research and Practice,* Academic Press Inc, New York, pp. 1–49.

Hosom, J.P., Shriberg, L.D. and Green, J.R. (2004), "Diagnostic assessment of childhood apraxia of speech using automatic speech recognition (ASR) methods", *Journal of Medical Speech-Language Pathology,* Vol. 12, pp. 167–171.

Karmiloff-Smith, A. (2006), "The tortuous route from genes to behaviour: A neuroconstructivist approach", *Cognitive, Affective and Behavioural Neuroscience,* Vol. 6, pp. 9–17.

Karmiloff-Smith, A., Scerif, G. and Ansari, D. (2003), "Double dissociations in developmental disorders? Theoretically misconceived, empirically dubious", *Cortex,* Vol. 39, pp. 161–163.

Maassen, B. (2002), "Issues contrasting adult acquired versus developmental apraxia of speech", *Seminars in Speech and Language,* Vol. 23, pp. 257–266.

Maassen, B., Thoonen, G. and Boers, I. (1997), "Quantitative assessment of dysarthria and developmental apraxia of speech", in W. Hulstijn, H.F.M. Peters and P.H.H.M. Van Lieshout, (Eds.), *Speech Production: Motor Control, Brain Research and Fluency Disorders,* Elsevier Science BV, Amsterdam, The Netherlands, pp. 611–619.

McCabe, P., Rosenthal, J.B. and McLeod, S. (1998), "Features of developmental dyspraxia in the general speech-impaired population?", *Clinical Linguistics and Phonetics,* Vol. 12, pp. 105–126.

McNeil, M.R., Pratt, S.R. and Fosset, T.R.D. (2004), "The differential diagnosis of apraxia of speech", in B. Maassen, R.D. Kent, H.F.M. Peters, P.H.H.M. Van Lieshout and W. Hulstijn (Eds.), *Speech Motor Control in Normal and Disordered Speech*, Oxford University Press, Oxford, UK, pp. 389–414.

Newbury, D.F., Fisher, S.E. and Monaco, A.P. (2010), "Recent advances in the genetics of language impairment", *Genome Medicine*, Vol. 2, No. 1 http://genomemedicine.com/content/2/1/6

Nijland, L., Terband, H. and Maassen, B. (in press), "Cognitive functions in childhood apraxia of speech", *Journal of Speech, Language and Hearing Research.*

Shriberg, L.D. (2010), "A neurodevelopmental framework for research in childhood apraxia of speech", in B. Maassen and P.H.H.M. Van Lieshout (Eds.), *Speech Motor Control: New Developments in Basic and Applied Research*, Oxford University Press, Oxford, UK, pp. 259–270.

Shriberg, L.D., Aram, D.M. and Kwiatkowski, J. (1997a), "Developmental apraxia of speech: I. Descriptive and theoretical perspectives", *Journal of Speech and Hearing Research*, Vol. 40, pp. 273–285.

Shriberg, L.D., Aram, D.M. and Kwiatkowski, J. (1997b), "Developmental apraxia of speech: II. Toward a diagnostic marker", *Journal of Speech, Language, and Hearing Research*, Vol. 40, pp. 286–312.

Shriberg, L.D., Aram, D.M. and Kwiatkowski, J. (1997c), "Developmental apraxia of speech: III. A subtype marked by inappropriate stress", *Journal of Speech, Language, and Hearing Research*, Vol. 40, pp. 313–337.

Shriberg, L.D., Campbell, T.F., Karlsson, H., Brown, R.L., McSweeny, J.L. and Nadler, C.J. (2003a), "A diagnostic marker for childhood apraxia of speech: The lexical stress ratio", *Clinical Linguistics and Phonetics*, Vol. 17, pp. 549–574.

Shriberg, L.D., Green, J.R., Campbell, T.F., McSweeny, J.L. and Scheer, A.R. (2003b), "A diagnostic marker for childhood apraxia of speech: The coefficient of variation ratio", *Clinical Linguistics and Phonetics*, Vol. 17, pp. 575–595.

Shriberg, L.D., Lohmeier, H.L., Strand, E.A. and Jakielski, K.J. (2012), "Encoding, memory, and transcoding deficits in childhood apraxia of speech", *Clinical Linguistics and Phonetics*, Vol. 26, pp. 445–482.

Stein, C.M., Lu, Q., Elston, R.C., Freebairn, L.A., Hansen, A.J., Shriberg, L.D., *et al.*, (2011), "Heritability estimation for speech-sound traits with developmental trajectories", *Behavior Genetics*, Vol. 41, pp. 184–191.

Terband, H. (2011), *Speech Motor Function in Relation to Phonology: Neurocomputational Modeling of Disordered Development*, University Medical Centre Groningen, Netherlands. Dissertation. Promotores: Prof. dr. B.A.M. Maassen, Prof.dr. P.H.H.M. van Lieshout (March 2, 2011).

Terband, H., Maassen, B., van Lieshout, P. and Nijland, L. (2011), "Stability and composition of functional synergies for speech movements in children with developmental speech disorders", *Journal of Communication Disorders*, Vol. 44, pp. 59–74.

Thoonen, G. (1998), *Developmental Apraxia of Speech in Children. Quantitative Assessment of Speech Characteristics*, University of Nijmegen, Netherlands. Dissertation. Promotores: Prof.dr. F. Gabreëls, prof.dr. R. Schreuder; copromotor: Dr. B. Maassen.

Thoonen, G., Maassen, B., Gabreëls, F. and Schreuder, R. (1994), "Feature analysis of singleton consonant errors in developmental verbal dyspraxia (DVD)", *Journal of Speech and Hearing Research*, Vol. 37, pp. 1424–1440.

Thoonen, G., Maassen, B., Gabreëls, F., Schreuder, R. and De Swart, B. (1997), "Towards a standardised assessment procedure for developmental apraxia of speech", *European Journal of Disorders of Communication*, Vol. 32, pp. 37–60.

Vernes, S.C. and Fisher, S.E. (2009), "Unravelling neurogenetic networks implicated in developmental language disorders", *Biochemical Society Transactions*, Vol. 37, pp. 1263–1269.

Weismer, G. and Kim, Y. (2010), "Classification and taxonomy of motor speech disorders: What are the issues?", in B. Maassen and P.H.H.M. Van Lieshout, (Eds.), *Speech Motor Control. New Developments in Basic and Applied Research*, Oxford University Press, Oxford, UK, pp. 229–241.

12

SPEECH RECOGNITION SKILLS OF CHILDREN WITH COCHLEAR IMPLANTS

Laurie S. Eisenberg, Dianne Hammes Ganguly, Karen C. Johnson, Amy S. Martinez and Nae-Yuh Wang

Introduction

The cochlear implant (CI) is an auditory sensory device designed for individuals with moderately severe to profound hearing loss who are unable to benefit adequately from conventional amplification. Invented during the second half of the twentieth century, the CI is considered the most significant technological breakthrough to treat both adult and childhood deafness. Children have the most to gain from a CI, particularly those born deaf. For children, the CI fosters the development of listening skills and spoken language, providing the potential for mainstream education.

The CI is composed of internal and external components (Figure 12.1). The externally worn parts consist of a microphone, signal processor, and transmitter. The internal components are surgically implanted. They consist of a receiver and electrode array. The electrode array is threaded through the round window of the scala tympani of the cochlea. Sounds are transduced into electrical signals, digitally processed, and delivered to the different electrodes in a way that approximates the tonotopicity of the cochlea. Today, individuals are implanted with substantial levels of residual hearing, enabling different sensory device configurations, such as a hearing aid in the ear opposite to the CI (bimodal) or a hearing aid and CI in the same ear (electroacoustic or hybrid device).

At the time of this writing, the United States Food and Drug Administration (FDA) has mandated 12 months as the earliest age for surgical implantation. However, many centers implant children younger than 12 months because of noted benefits to the acquisition of spoken language from early access to sound (Dettman *et al.*, 2007; Niparko *et al.*, 2010).

In this chapter we briefly discuss the reasons why a CI might be recommended for a child with hearing loss. We then summarize the speech recognition results from a large-scale, national study on children with CIs, providing insights into the ways in which implanted children progress in their auditory skill development. The processes that underlie spoken word recognition in children with CIs are addressed by summarizing the results from several pediatric studies that test assumptions from the Neighborhood Activation Model (Luce and Pisoni, 1998). Lastly, we conclude with a discussion about clinical considerations.

134

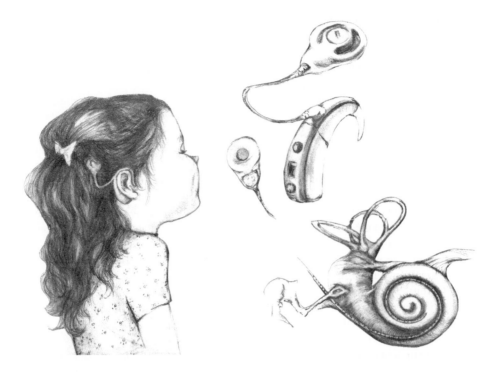

Figure 12.1 Illustration of a cochlear implant. The internal and external components are shown on the right side of the illustration. From "Cochlear Implants in Children: Historical Perspectives and Personal reflections" in *Clinical Management of Children with Cochlear Implants* (p. 2) by Laurie S. Eisenberg. © 2009 Plural Publishing, Inc. All rights reserved. Used with permission.

Why the need for a CI?

For the child born with severe to profound hearing loss, many of the sounds essential for speech recognition are inaudible, even with the use of high-powered hearing aids. For those speech sounds that may be audible, the temporal, intensity, and spectral speech cues are often distorted such that amplification merely increases the level of distortion. Boothroyd (1984) demonstrated that children with losses in the profound range (90 to 115 dB HL) still have access to some speech features, such as vowel height, temporal pattern, talker gender and possibly vowel place and consonant manner when the speech signal is amplified. For children with thresholds of 120 dB HL, only temporal and intensity cues are accessible through detection of the most intensive peaks in the speech signal. Indeed, even children with complete absence of hearing are able to detect low frequency sounds at high presentation levels through the vibrotactile mode (Boothroyd and Cawkwell, 1970). In short, profound hearing loss limits auditory perception to the identification of suprasegmental features and single words presented in a forced-choice or closed-set format (Boothroyd *et al.*, 1991; Erber and Alencewicz, 1976). However, sound detection and rudimentary discrimination represent the lower level skills on the continuum of auditory development. More complex skills encompass speech recognition in open sets (unrestricted choices) and auditory comprehension.

Today, infants and young children with moderately severe to profound hearing loss are referred for CIs when trials with hearing aids determine insufficient access to the acoustic cues essential for recognizing speech. The CI enables the child to detect speech across a broad range of frequencies. For the majority of pediatric CI recipients, this access translates to an ability to discriminate, identify, recognize, and comprehend speech. Such abilities are reliant on articulatory, linguistic, and cognitive development (Blamey *et al.*, 2001; Davidson *et al.*, 2011; Pisoni *et al.*, 2011). The time course over which speech recognition skills emerge varies considerably, as will be illustrated later in the chapter.

Early implantation is an important factor for the development of speech recognition because it promotes maturation of the central auditory nervous system. Sharma and colleagues found that implantation by the age of 3.5 years yields age-appropriate auditory evoked cortical responses by six months following device activation (Sharma *et al.*, 2002). Behavioral studies indicate that infants with CIs can detect differences among various vowel and consonant contrasts by two to three months post-device activation (Uhler *et al.*, 2011). Thus, the behavioral data parallel the cortical data in supporting the time course of maturation.

Another important factor in bolstering auditory development is the processing of sound by both ears. Continued use of a hearing aid is advocated for those children with sufficient residual hearing in the ear opposite to the CI (Ching *et al.*, 2001; Holt *et al.*, 2005), because aided residual hearing provides complementary access to speech cues not made available by the CI. For those children with insufficient hearing for successful use of a hearing aid in the ear opposite to the CI, bilateral CIs have become standard clinical practice. Investigations into the potential benefits of bilateral CIs in school-aged children have shown improved outcomes on measures of speech recognition both in quiet and noise when compared to outcomes with one CI (Galvin *et al.*, 2007; Litovsky *et al.*, 2004, 2006).

To better understand the benefits of bilateral CIs in children, a number of variables have been examined, including: age at initial implantation, duration between CI surgeries, and length of experience after activation of the second implant (Galvin *et al.*, 2008; Peters *et al.*, 2007; Zeitler *et al.*, 2008). Overall, improved speech recognition scores have been found for the second implanted ear post-CI as compared to pre-CI, and under bilateral listening conditions when sequential CIs are implanted within seven years of each other. Children who received both devices before 3.5 to 4 years of age attained greater improvements in background noise than those who received both implants after the age of four years (Dowell *et al.*, 2011).

In short, the CI provides children access to many of the sounds of speech when acoustic amplification has proven to be ineffective. It is important to recognize that the speech recognition abilities of these children do not emerge instantaneously and that wide variability in auditory outcomes characterizes the pediatric CI population. The following section addresses the variability in skill level and rate of improvement based on results from a currently ongoing national study.

Childhood Development after Cochlear Implantation

The Childhood Development after Cochlear Implantation (CDaCI) study is the first longitudinal, multi-center cohort study instituted in the United States for the purpose of tracking young children with CIs (Fink *et al.*, 2007; Niparko *et al.*, 2010). The CDaCI cohort is comprised of 188 children with severe to profound sensorineural hearing loss, recruited through six pediatric CI centers and implanted at a mean age of 2.2 years. In addition, 97 children with typical hearing were enrolled over a similar age range and serve as the hearing controls. The overall objective of the study is to identify factors influencing spoken language development in young children with CIs compared to their typically hearing peers. Additional aims are to understand the downstream impact of language-related outcomes on development in a number of other domains, including: cognition, psychosocial skills, scholastic performance, and quality of life.

One of the early challenges in the CDaCI study was to develop a battery of speech recognition tests that captured and tracked the expanding perceptual capabilities typical of early childhood. Another challenge was to compare performance between the two groups of participants, young children with CIs and their hearing peers. The strategy adopted was to use a hierarchical test battery incorporating a series of developmentally appropriate tests to be administered according to each child's age and functional auditory abilities prior to and following cochlear implantation (Eisenberg *et al.*, 2006).

Table 12.1 lists the measures that comprise the CDaCI speech recognition test battery and includes the type of stimuli, appropriate age for administration, and response format. The early auditory behaviors demonstrated by infants and very young children are probed via a pair of parent-report measures, the Meaningful Auditory Integration Scales (MAIS; Robbins *et al.*, 1991) and the Infant–Toddler version of the MAIS (IT-MAIS: Zimmerman-Phillips *et al.*, 2000). As auditory skills develop and children exhibit the ability to choose among alternates, closed-set identification of words and sentences is assessed via the Early Speech Perception Test (ESP; Moog and Geers, 1990) and Pediatric Speech Intelligibility Test (PSI; Jerger *et al.*, 1980), respectively. Open-set testing is undertaken using a series of word and sentence recognition tests, including: the Lexical Neighborhood Test (LNT) and the multisyllabic version of the LNT. (MLNT; Kirk *et al.*, 1995), Phonetically Balanced Kindergarten Word Lists (PBK; Haskins, 1949), and Hearing in Noise Test for Children (HINT-C; Gelnett *et al.*, 1995). Although all of the measures in the battery are administered in quiet, the two sentence measures are also administered in the presence of varying levels of single-talker competition in the case of the PSI, and speech-shaped noise in the case of the HINT-C.

In working his or her way through the hierarchy, the child is required to achieve minimal performance criteria on one measure before proceeding to the next level of difficulty, thus focusing the child's limited window of attention on speech recognition tasks that are neither too easy nor difficult. Each child moves through the battery at his or her own pace, enabling examination of the rate of individual growth in speech recognition abilities over time. A numerical index, the Speech Recognition Index in Quiet (SRI-Q), has been developed that captures a child's progress through the test battery (Wang *et al.*, 2008). The SRI-Q reflects the highest level achieved within the hierarchy of measures administered in the quiet condition (absence of competing speech or noise) at any given test interval.

Table 12.1 CDaCI Speech Recognition Hierarchical Test Battery. The tests are ordered (top to bottom) from easiest to most difficult, and individual tests are administered on the basis of the child's age and auditory abilities.

Test	Test Age	Stimulus	Response Format
IT-MAIS	1–3 years	10 probes	Parent report
MAIS	≥ 4 years		
ESP: Low-Verbal	≥ 2 years	1- and 2-syllable words	Closed set
ESP: Standard	≥ 3 years		
PSI	≥ 3 years	words and sentences	Closed set
MLNT	≥ 3 years	2- and 3-syllable words	Open set
LNT	≥ 3 years	1-syllable words	
PBK	5 ≥ years	1-syllable words	Open set
HINT-C	5 ≥ years	words and sentences	Open set

Figure 12.2 summarizes the development in speech recognition abilities observed for the CI cohort over the first five years of implant use (Eisenberg, 2013; Johnson, 2013). Shown is the median SRI-Q (i.e., 50th percentile), plotted as a function of follow-up test interval, along with the estimates of the 90th, 75th, 25th, and 10th percentiles of performance. This figure illustrates the variability in speech recognition skills alluded to earlier that is characteristic of the CI population as a whole. The extent of variability is particularly notable at the transition from closed- to open-set speech recognition (denoted by a SRI-Q of 300 and highlighted by a bold line), making this point a significant milestone for CI recipients. In the CDaCI test battery, this occurs when the child has met criterion for the PSI and progresses to the MLNT and LNT measures. Using the length of time taken to transition from closed- to open-set tasks as a benchmark, children in the 90th percentile are advancing to open-set recognition in approximately one year, whereas children at the 50th percentile are taking between 2 and 2.5 years to achieve this same milestone. Children at the 25th percentile move into open-set recognition around 3.5 years. However, 10 percent of the sample have not made their way out of the most basic of closed-set identification tasks by 5 years post-implant, with some children demonstrating little beyond consistent sound detection, if that. Taken together, it can be seen that the top 75 percent of children in the CI cohort reached open-set speech recognition by 5 years post-implant, which, despite the delays shown by some, still speaks to the effectiveness of this form of sensory intervention for deaf children.

To better understand why some children in the CDaCI study did not progress beyond closed-set speech recognition, an analysis was performed to identify potential characteristics that

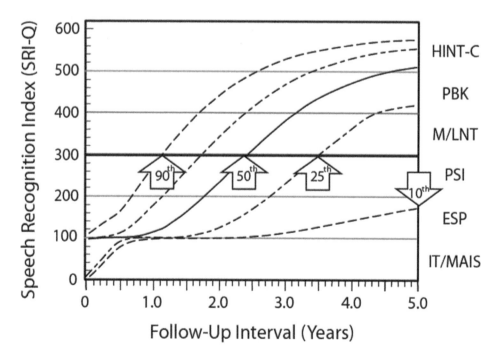

Figure 12.2 Speech Recognition Index in Quiet (SRI-Q) growth curves from baseline to five years post-CI from the CDaCI study. The curves represent the 90th, 75th, 50th, 25th, and 10th percentiles of the CI sample. Highlighted is the point of transition from closed- to open-set speech recognition (score of 300).

differentiated the children with SRI-Q scores below and above 300 at the five-year test interval (Barnard *et al.*, in press). The analysis identified the following factors associated with SRI-Q scores below 300: less access to sound with hearing aids prior to CI surgery, older ages when hearing aids were fitted, lower scores on a measure of maternal sensitivity, minority status, and complicated perinatal history (i.e., premature birth and/or admission to the NICU). From a communication standpoint, the inability of a child with a CI to advance in auditory skill development would also be expected to have an adverse effect on the development of spoken language. An additional analysis conducted on the data set confirmed this assumption. All but one of the 18 children in < 300 group (94 percent) relied on some level of sign support to communicate.

The transition point from closed- to open-set speech recognition occurs when children advance to the MLNT and LNT word measures (SRI-Q = 300–399). Of all the tests that comprise the CDaCI speech recognition hierarchy, the MLNT and LNT are the only ones that are theoretically motivated. That is, these two tests were designed to explore the underlying processes that support the development of spoken word recognition in children with CIs. They also were derived directly from the Neighborhood Activation Model (Luce and Pisoni, 1998). In the next section, we briefly describe this model and cite some of the relevant research specific to the pediatric CI population.

The Neighborhood Activation Model

The Neighborhood Activation Model (Luce and Pisoni, 1998) has been the one conceptual model proposed to explore spoken word recognition in pediatric CI users. This model addresses the underlying processes of word recognition through an activation/lexical selection paradigm. The model posits that an incoming word activates similar acoustic–phonetic representations stored in long-term memory with stimulation levels proportional to the similarity of the target word. The lexical properties implemented in the model are word frequency, neighborhood density, and neighborhood frequency. Word frequency represents how often a word occurs in the language. Neighborhood density denotes the number of similar sounding words to the target word, determined by substituting, deleting, or adding one phoneme to generate other words. Neighborhood frequency refers to the average number of words in the similarity neighborhood.

The open-set MLNT and LNT measures were based on the Neighborhood Activation Model to explore the ways in which pediatric CI users organize, store, and access words from memory (Kirk *et al.*, 1995). Both tests are composed of lexically easy words (high word frequency in low-density neighborhoods; e.g., *food*) and lexically hard words (low word frequency in high-density neighborhoods; e.g. *cap*). Results from Kirk and colleagues showed that children with CIs recognized the lexically easy words more accurately than the lexically hard words, suggesting that pediatric CI users are sensitive to the lexical properties of speech and that words are organized in ways similar to listeners with normal hearing.

Subsequent to the development of the MLNT and LNT, two sets of lexically controlled sentences were created by Eisenberg *et al.* (2002) to test specific hypotheses about how children with CIs access words in memory when those words are presented in isolation and in sentences. The sentences were constructed to be syntactically correct but semantically neutral in order to examine the effects of syntactic context in the lexical selection task. Lexically easy and hard sentences were generated with each sentence containing three key words. The subjects were instructed to repeat the sentence or word presented. For the group of children with CIs, results confirmed that the lexically easy words were recognized with greater accuracy than the lexically hard words, and that sentence context was advantageous. Of particular interest was the finding that children who presented with poor receptive vocabulary skills (as measured by the Peabody Picture Vocabulary Test—Third Edition; Dunn and Dunn, 1997), also recognized words in sentences with less accuracy than words in isolation, a result later replicated by other investigators (Conway *et al.*, in press; Kirk *et al.*, 2007). This pattern suggested an inability to retain a sequence of words in memory. The findings from this study further underscored the importance of linguistic knowledge on the acoustic–phonetic processing of words. The following section addresses the practical implications of speech recognition in the broader context of speech and language.

Clinical considerations

Speech perception is a major underpinning for speech production, spoken language, and literacy development. Good speech perception supports better lexical knowledge and clearer speech, which in turn support better speech perception (Davidson *et al.*, 2011). The more impoverished the child's perceptual capabilities or the more degraded the auditory signal, the more difficult it will be for that child to develop speech, spoken language, and print communication. Thus, it is vital that clinicians understand the variables that may compromise the reception of speech and the repercussions that hearing loss can have relative to communication development.

Optimizing speech reception

Maintaining optimal speech audibility is essential for children with CIs who are learning spoken language. Speech reception can be optimized by ensuring on a daily basis that the child's hearing devices are functioning optimally and by attending to talker variables and classroom acoustics.

Talker variables

Talker variables include characteristics such as talker volume, speaking rate, and clarity of speech. In quiet environments, whereas children with normal hearing can generally attain near perfect scores on speech recognition measures at soft conversational levels (e.g., 50 dB SPL), children with CIs typically require conversationally loud (e.g., 70 dB SPL) levels to score their best (Davidson *et al.*, 2011). Even simple strategies, such as a talker's use of "clear speech" (either automatically or through conscious effort when the talker believes the listener to be having difficulty), provides a distinct listening advantage for children with CIs (Liu *et al.*, 2004).

Although CIs can improve many aspects of speech perception, some aspects remain difficult. In particular, these children tend to have trouble with indexical components of spoken language, such as identifying emotional content or distinguishing talkers. In one study, Geers and colleagues (Geers *et al.*, 2013), found that only 30 percent of the children with CIs were able to identify the talker's actual emotion. Moreover, while 65 percent of the children with CIs could distinguish a male from a female voice, only 8 percent could discriminate one female talker from another female talker. In a classroom setting, children with CIs may not recognize who is talking based on vocal cues. Miscommunication may also occur if children misread the emotion behind classroom conversations or discussions.

Acoustic variables

Key acoustic variables impacting speech recognition include: the presence of background noise, the signal-to-noise ratio (SNR) (i.e., the level of the talker's voice relative to the level of background noise), the distance of the talker from the listener, and reverberation time (Crandell and Smaldino, 2000). In general, the louder the talker in relation to noise, the more advantageous the situation is for the listener. Children with hearing loss or other distinctive learning needs (e.g., language delays, limited English proficiency, neurological immaturity) require a SNR of at least 15 dB in the classroom to support learning (American National Standards Institute [ANSI], 2002).

To improve the SNR and thereby more effectively facilitate communication, assistive listening devices, such as frequency-modulated (FM) systems, are often recommended for children with hearing loss. In addition, preferential seating close to the teacher and away from hallway, street, or heating and cooling system noises is also instrumental for mitigating background noise at school.

Repercussions of hearing loss for communication development

Speech production

The ability to perceive and produce the acoustic cues of speech is predictive of a child's speech intelligibility (Osberger and McGarr, 1982). Prior to the availability of CIs, even with the use of hearing aids, mean intelligibility scores tended to fall below 20 percent for children with profound hearing loss (Smith, 1975). CIs have improved prospects greatly. In a recent study, children implanted between 35 to 40 months of age attained a mean intelligibility score of 80 percent and children implanted between 8 and 24 months obtained a mean score of 93 percent (Habib *et al.*, 2010). Impressively, there are some children with CIs that attain speech intelligibility scores comparable to hearing peers. Yet, even among early implanted children, variability in performance remains wide.

Before treating articulation and intelligibility, clinicians should first ensure that the child with a CI is able to detect and discriminate speech contrasts or features using audition alone. Without this ability, remediation will need to begin at this level. If auditory-only detection and discrimination are not possible, the use of other compensatory strategies should be explored (e.g., visual phonics). Developing speech production in the absence of auditory perception is laborious, requiring much effort, and often has unsatisfactory outcomes (Smith, 1975).

Spoken language development

Children learn spoken language through direct and indirect interactions with others. The greater the degree of hearing loss or the poorer the speech recognition abilities, the more restricted the child's ability to learn through hearing. CIs can improve capacity for auditory learning, but outcomes vary greatly and CIs never provide normal hearing.

As mentioned earlier, age at implantation, length of auditory deprivation, and amount of residual hearing loss prior to CI are factors that impact outcomes following implantation. Up to 40 percent of children with hearing loss have one or more additional developmental disabilities (Gallaudet Research Institute, 2011). Depending on the circumstances and child's rate of progress, very different intervention strategies or supportive services will be necessary for this group of children. In general, early implanted children without additional disabilities often progress well using a combination of direct, structured practice paired with naturalistic, language-enriched learning opportunities (Ganek *et al.*, 2012). In contrast, children who are late-implanted or who have secondary learning disabilities often need a more structured and directed intervention plan. Due to language delays or gaps that often exist for these children, classroom accommodations, such as gaining a child's attention before speaking, asking frequent comprehension questions, allowing ample processing time and pre-/post-teaching of vocabulary, may be necessary.

Literacy development

Deficits in oral language or phonological abilities (common for children with hearing loss, regardless of CI use), contribute to deficits in reading and writing in children with severe or profound hearing loss (Mayberry *et al.*, 2011). Describing the findings from their analysis of empirical studies about the effects of cochlear implantation on children's reading and academic achievement, Marschark and colleagues (2007) noted that even when children with CIs demonstrated literacy skills similar to hearing peers in early grade school, divergence of skills from the hearing norm was common by the teenage years. These investigators concluded that it is unsafe to assume that strong skill development in the early years will lead to strong skills at later points. Explicit instruction in reading and writing may need to continue into the upper grade levels for children with CIs.

In summary, the CI is considered the most significant technological breakthrough to treat deafness. Although most children reach open-set speech understanding within five years of implantation, a significant portion of children never reach open-set understanding. Some children retain delays or subtle gaps in speech reception, production, language, or literacy. Daily listening checks, optimizing talker variables and managing classroom acoustics combine to facilitate auditory learning in children with CIs.

Acknowledgment

The CDaCI study is supported by grant R01DC004797 (P.I. John Niparko).

References

American National Standards Institute (ANSI) (2002), *Acoustical Performance Criteria, Design Requirements, and Guidelines for Schools*. ANSI/ASA S12.60. New York: American National Standards Institute.

Barnard, J.M., Fisher, L.M., Johnson, K.C., Eisenberg, L.S., Wang, N-Y., Quittner, A.L., Carson, C.M., Niparko, J.K. and the CDaCI Investigative Team. (in press), "A prospective, longitudinal study of US children unable to achieve open-set speech recognition five years after cochlear implantation", *Otology and Neurotology*.

Blamey, P.J., Sarant, J.Z., Paatsch, L.E., Barry, J.G., Bow, C.P., Wales, R.J., *et al.*, (2001), "Relationships among speech perception, production, language, hearing loss, and age in children with impaired hearing", *Journal of Speech, Language, and Hearing Research*, Vol. 44, pp. 264–285.

Boothroyd, A. (1984), "Auditory perception of speech contrasts by subjects with sensorineural hearing loss", *Journal of Speech and Hearing Research*, Vol. 27, pp. 134–144.

Boothroyd, A. and Cawkwell, S. (1970), "Vibrotactile thresholds in pure-tone audiometry", *Acta Otolaryngologica*, Vol. 69, pp. 384–387.

Boothroyd, A., Geers, A.E. and Moog, J.S. (1991), "Practical implications of cochlear implants in children", *Ear and Hearing*, 12(Suppl.), pp. 81S–89S.

Ching, T.Y.C., Psarros, C., Hill, M., Dillon, H. and Incerti, P. (2001), "Should children who use cochlear implants wear hearing aids in the opposite ear?", *Ear and Hearing*, Vol. 22, pp. 365–380.

Conway, C.M., Deocampo, J.A., Walk, A.M., Anaya, E.M. and Pisoni, D.B. (2014), "Deaf children with cochlear implants do not appear to use sentence context to help recognize spoken words", *Journal of Speech, Language, and Hearing Research*, Vol. 57, No. 6, pp. 2174–2190.

Crandell, C. and Smaldino, J. (2000), "Classroom acoustics for children with normal hearing and with hearing impairment", *Language, Speech, and Hearing Services in Schools*, Vol. 31, pp. 362–370.

Davidson, L.S., Geers, A.E., Blamey, P.J., Tobey, E.A. and Brenner, C. (2011), "Factors contributing to speech perception scores in long-term pediatric cochlear implant users", *Ear and Hearing*, Vol. 32 (1 Suppl.), pp. 19S–26S.

Dettman, S.J., Pinder, D., Briggs, R.J., Dowell, R.C. and Leigh, J.R. (2007), "Communication development in children who receive the cochlear implant younger than 12 months", *Ear and Hearing,* Vol. 28 (Suppl.), pp. 11S–18S.

Dowell, R.C., Galvin, K.L, Dettman, S.J., Leigh, J.R., Hughes, K.C. and van Hoesel, R. (2011), "Bilateral cochlear implants in children", *Seminars in Hearing,* Vol. 32, pp. 53–72.

Dunn, L.M. and Dunn, L.M. (1997), *Peabody Picture Vocabulary Test—Third Edition.* Circle Pines, MN, US: American Guidance Service.

Eisenberg, L.S. (2013), "The consequences of being born deaf in the 21st century", *The 2013 Libby Harricks Memorial Oration.* Australia: Deafness Forum Limited.

Eisenberg, L.S., Johnson, K.J., Martinez, A.S., Cokely, C.G., Tobey, E.A., Quittner, A.L., Fink, N.E., Wang, N-Y., Niparko, J.K, and the CDaCI Investigative Team (2006), "Speech recognition at 1-year follow-up in the Childhood Development after Cochlear Implantation Study: Methods and preliminary findings", *Audiology and Neurotology,* Vol. 11, pp. 259–268.

Eisenberg, L.S., Martinez, A.S., Holowecky, S.R. and Pogorelsky, S. (2002), "Recognition of lexically controlled words and sentences in children with normal hearing and children with cochlear implants", *Ear and Hearing,* Vol. 23, pp. 450–462.

Erber, N. and Alencewicz, C. (1976), "Audiologic evaluation of the deaf children", *Journal of Speech and Hearing Disorders,* Vol. 41, pp. 256–267.

Fink, N.E., Wang, N-Y., Vusaya, J., Niparko, J.K., Quittner, A., Eisenberg, L.S., Tobey, E.A. and the CDaCI Investigative Team (2007), "Childhood Development after Cochlear Implantation (CDaCI) study: Design and baseline characteristics", *Cochlear Implants International,* Vol. 8, pp. 92–116.

Gallaudet Research Institute (2011), *Regional and National Summary Report of Data from the 2009–10 Annual Survey of Deaf and Hard of Hearing Children and Youth,* Washington, DC, US: GRI, Gallaudet University.

Galvin, K.L., Mok, M. and Dowell, R.C. (2007), "Perceptual benefit and functional outcomes for children using sequential bilateral cochlear implants", *Ear and Hearing,* Vol. 28, pp. 470–482.

Galvin, K.L., Mok, M., Dowell, R.C. and Briggs, R.J. (2008), "Speech detection and localization results and clinical outcomes for children receiving sequential bilateral cochlear implants before four years of age", *International Journal of Audiology,* Vol. 47, pp. 636–646.

Ganek, H., McConkey Robbins, A. and Niparko, J.K. (2012), "Language outcomes after cochlear implantation", *Otolaryngologic Clinics of North America,* Vol. 45, pp. 173–185.

Geers, A.E., Davidson, L.S., Uchanski, R.M. and Nicholas, J.G. (2013), "Interdependence of linguistic and indexical speech perception skills in school-age children with early cochlear implantation", *Ear and Hearing,* Vol. 34, pp. 562–574.

Gelnett, D., Sumida, A., Nilsson, M. and Soli, S.D. (1995), "Development of the Hearing in Noise Test for Children (HINT-C)", Presented at the Annual Meeting of the American Academy of Audiology, Dallas, TX, US.

Habib, M.G., Waltzman, S.B., Tajudeen, B. and Svirsky, M.A. (2010), "Speech production intelligibility of early implanted pediatric cochlear implant users", *International Journal of Pediatric Otorhinolaryngology,* Vol. 74, pp. 855–859.

Haskins, H. (1949), *A Phonetically Balanced Test of Speech Discrimination for Children,* Master's thesis. Northwestern University, Evanston, IL, US.

Holt, R.F., Kirk, K.I., Eisenberg, L.S., Martinez, A.S. and Campbell, W. (2005), "Spoken word recognition development in children with residual hearing using cochlear implants and hearing aids in opposite ears", *Ear and Hearing,* Vol. 26 (4 Suppl.), pp. 82S–91S.

Jerger, S., Lewis, S., Hawkins, J. and Jerger, J. (1980), "Pediatric speech intelligibility test: 1. Generation of test materials", *International Journal of Pediatric Otolaryngology,* Vol. 2, pp. 217–230.

Johnson, K.C. (2013), "The childhood development after cochlear implant (CDaCI) study", American Academy of Audiology Annual Meeting. Anaheim, California, US.

Kirk, K.I., Hay-McCutcheon, M.J., Holt, R.F., Gao, S., Rong, Q. and Gehrlein, B.L. (2007), "Audiovisual spoken word recognition by children with cochlear implants", *Audiological Medicine,* Vol. 5, pp. 251–260.

Kirk, K.I., Pisoni, D.B. and Osberger, M.J. (1995), "Lexical effects of spoken word recognition by pediatric cochlear implant users", *Ear and Hearing,* Vol. 16, pp. 470–481.

Litovsky, R.Y., Johnstone, P.M. and Godar, S.P. (2006), "Benefits of bilateral cochlear implants and/or hearing aids in children", *International Journal of Audiology,* Vol. 45 (Suppl 1), pp. S78–91.

Litovsky, R.Y., Parkinson, A., Arcaroli, J., Peters, R., Lake, J., Johnstone, P., *et al.* (2004), "Bilateral cochlear implants in adults and children", *Archives of Otolaryngology–Head and Neck Surgery,* Vol. 130, pp. 648–655.

Liu, S., Del Rio, E., Bradlow, A. and Zeng, F-G. (2004), "Clear speech perception in acoustic and electric hearing", *Journal of the Acoustical Society of America,* Vol. 116, pp. 2374–2383.

Luce, P.A. and Pisoni, D.B. (1998), "Recognizing spoken words: The Neighborhood Activation Model", *Ear and Hearing,* Vol. 19, pp. 1–36.

Marschark, M., Rhoten, C. and Fabich, M. (2007), "Effects of cochlear implants on children's reading and academic achievement", *Journal of Deaf Studies and Deaf Education,* Vol. 12, No. 3, pp. 269–282.

Mayberry, R.I., del Giudice, A.A. and Lieberman, A.M. (2011), "Reading achievement in relation to phonological coding and awareness in deaf readers: A meta-analysis", *Journal of Deaf Studies and Deaf Education*, Vol. 16, pp. 164–188.

Moog, J.S. and Geers, A.E. (1990), "Early Speech Perception Test for profoundly hearing-impaired children", St. Louis, US: Central Institute for the Deaf.

Niparko, J.K, Tobey, E.A., Thal, D.J., Eisenberg, L.S., Wang, N-Y., Quittner, A.L. and Fink, N.E., for the CDaCI Investigative Team (2010), "Spoken language development in children following cochlear implantation", *Journal of the American Medical Association*, Vol. 303, pp. 1498–1506.

Osberger, M.J. and McGarr, N.S. (1982), "Speech production characteristics of the hearing impaired", In N. Lass (Ed.), *Speech and Language: Advances in Basic Research and Practice,* Vol. 8, New York, NY: Academic Press, pp. 227–288.

Peters, B.R., Litovsky, R.Y., Parkinson, A. and Lake, J. (2007), "Importance of age and postimplantation experience on speech perception measures in children with sequential bilateral cochlear implants", *Otology and Neurotology,* Vol. 28, pp. 649–657.

Pisoni, D.B., Kronenberger, W.G., Roman, A.S. and Geers, A.E. (2011), "Measures of digit span and verbal rehearsal speed in deaf children after more than 10 years of cochlear implantation", *Ear and Hearing,* Vol. 32 (1 Suppl.), pp. 60S–74S.

Robbins, A.M., Renshaw, J.J. and Berry, S.W. (1991), "Evaluating meaningful auditory integration in profoundly hearing-impaired children", *American Journal of Otology,* Vol. 12 (Suppl.), pp. 144–150.

Sharma, A., Dorman, M.F. and Spahr, A.J. (2002), "A sensitive period for the development of the central auditory system in children with cochlear implants: Implications for age of implantation", *Ear and Hearing,* Vol. 23, pp. 532–539.

Smith, C.R. (1975), "Residual hearing and speech production in deaf children", *Journal of Speech and Hearing Research,* Vol. 18, pp. 795–811.

Uhler, K., Yoshinaga-Itano, C., Gabbard, S.A., Rothpletz, A.M. and Jenkins, H. (2011), "Longitudinal infant speech perception in young cochlear implant users", *Journal of the American Academy of Audiology,* Vol. 22, pp. 129–142.

Wang, N-Y., Eisenberg, L.S., Johnson, K.C., Fink, N.E., Tobey, E.A., Quittner, A.L., Niparko, J.K. and the CDaCI Investigative Team (2008), "Tracking development of speech recognition: Longitudinal data from hierarchical assessments in the Childhood Development After Cochlear Implantation Study", *Otology and Neurotology,* Vol. 29, pp. 240–245.

Zeitler, D.M., Kessler, M.A., Terushkin, V., Roland, T.J. Jr., Svirsky, M.A., Lalwani, A.K. and Waltzman, S.B. (2008), "Speech perception benefits of sequential bilateral cochlear implantation in children and adults: A retrospective analysis", *Otology and Neurotology,* Vol. 29, pp. 314–325.

Zimmerman-Phillips, S., Robbins, A.M. and Osberger, M.J. (2000), "Assessing cochlear implant benefit in very young children", *Annals of Otology, Rhinology, and Laryngology,* Vol. 109 (Suppl. 185), pp. 42–43.

13

INSTRUMENTAL ANALYSIS OF ATYPICAL SPEECH

Sara Howard and Barry Heselwood

Introduction

Researchers have made attempts to measure aspects of vocal organ behaviour for centuries but it has only been with refinements in computer processing that instrumental speech analysis techniques have expanded and are more accessible for clinical use. Different techniques provide objective information on the individual subsystems of speech production (articulation, phonation, resonance, airflow) and on how these subsystems coordinate to produce speech. Often in clinical assessment, the auditory impression of speech is captured by phonetic transcription alone (Heselwood and Howard, 2008). However, comparing and combining perceptual analyses of atypical speech production with instrumental data provides a powerful basis for assessment (Howard and Heselwood, 2013). In addition, instrumental techniques often provide visual representations and feedback, which can be effectively used in therapy. In this chapter, we present an overview of instrumental techniques covering acoustic, articulatory and aerodynamic analysis, with particular emphasis on their clinical application to acquired and developmental speech disorders.

Measuring speech production acoustically

Acoustic analysis can reveal much about speech production processes if we know what to look for and how to make the appropriate measurements. Here, we will consider Voice Onset Time, vowel formant centre-frequencies, vowel formant transitions, and C-centre analysis.

Voice Onset Time

Voice Onset Time (VOT) measurements give insight into the coordination of phonation and articulation in plosive-plus-vowel sequences. The time interval between the release of the plosive occlusion and the moment when voicing begins is measured (see Figure 13.1). VOT is negative if voicing begins before the release, positive if it begins after, and zero if it begins simultaneously with the release. Interpretation of VOT requires norms that are specific to language varieties. In most English dialects, we expect VOT values for /p, t, k/ to be in excess of +25ms, and those for /b, d, g/ to be less than that. Values will be higher when place of articulation is more posterior, and when the following vowel is close (high) rather than open (low).

VOT differences that reflect voicing are part of the phonology, while those due to place of articulation and vowel height are mostly determined by non-linguistic aerodynamic factors. The latter, however, may be significantly affected by structural atypicalities, such as cleft palate. Children typically have low positive VOT values for all plosives early in phonological acquisition, gradually introducing longer VOTs for voiceless plosives in languages such as English, and negative VOTs for voiced plosives in languages such as French (Vihman, 1996). Some children with developmental phonological problems have been reported to use VOT idiosyncratically, e.g., to signal place of articulation instead of voice distinctions (see Kent and Kim, 2008).

Formant centre-frequencies

Vowels have an acoustic structure characterized by bands of resonance called formants. It is largely these frequencies, particularly the lowest two (F1 and F2), which give vowels their distinctive qualities. Open vowels have a higher F1 than close vowels, and front vowels have a higher F2 than back vowels. Rounding affects vowels differently depending on openness and frontness, but in general it lowers F2 in all vowels and F1 in open vowels (Stevens, 1998). Formants are measured in Hertz at the midpoint of the vowel's duration by locating their centre-frequencies, displayed as peaks on spectra (see Figure 13.2). When typical vowel formant values are known for a language variety, vowels in atypical speech can be compared to them, providing the formant values are normalized for age and gender differences.

Some caution, however, has to be exercised when relating vowel formant values to tongue and lip positions. Ladefoged *et al.* (1978) demonstrated that different vocal tract shapes can generate the same formant structure, and Maurer *et al.* (1993) present articulographic evidence to confirm this. Howard and Heselwood (2013), however, suggest that these results, obtained

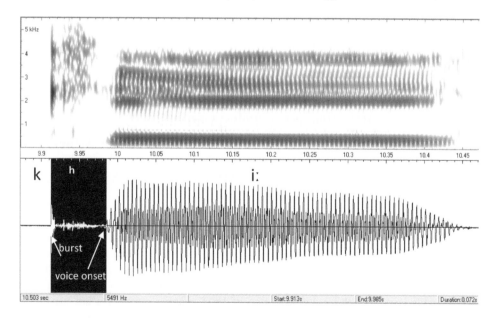

Figure 13.1 Spectrogram (upper pane) and waveform (lower panel) of the word 'key' with the VOT highlighted and the measuring points identified. In this example, VOT = 72ms.

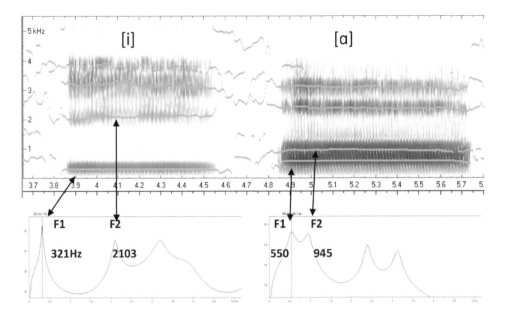

Figure 13.2 Spectrogram with formant tracks (upper panel) and spectra (lower panels) of the vowels [i] (front, close) and [ɑ] (back, open).

in experimental conditions with sustained vowels, may not be representative of conversational speech. If this is the case, then a client's acoustic vowel formant data could be used as a basis for articulatory intervention (see Ciocca and Whitehill [2013] for a review of formant frequencies in atypical speech). For example, if F1 is too high and F2 is too low for a typical /i/ vowel, then the client can be encouraged to raise the tongue and push it further forward.

Formant transitions

Formant transitions reflect articulator movement during the onset and offset phases of articulatory gestures. In Figure 13.3, vowel formants "bend" their edges in different patterns depending on the place of articulation of the adjacent consonants. Of particular interest are the F2 transitions, which are important in speech perception, and the approximation of F2 and F3 adjacent to the velar stop. Transitions are termed "positive" if the extremity of the formant is

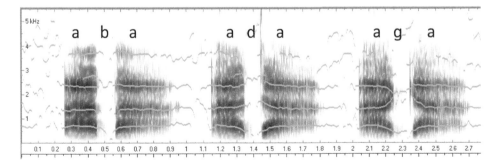

Figure 13.3 Formant transitions for different places of articulation.

higher in frequency than the midpoint, and "negative" if it is lower. Lack of clear transition patterns can have an adverse effect on perception and speech intelligibility (Smits *et al.*, 1996). In addition, patterns have been reported to be more variable in speakers with motor speech difficulties (Ryalls, 1986); that is, their transitions are likely to be longer and shallower because the active articulator is not moving as fast or as far (e.g., Weismer *et al.* 1992).

C-centre analysis

C-centre analysis investigates the extent of coarticulation in onset–vowel sequences and compares it with vowel-coda sequences. It is hypothesized that, in typical English syllable productions, the onset and the vowel are "in phase", meaning that their underlying articulatory gestures begin synchronously (Honorof and Browman, 1995). A durational measurement is taken from the centre of the syllable onset (the C-centre) to the end of the vowel (the anchor point). This duration should remain constant across singleton and cluster onsets. For example, the /l/ gesture in *clap* will overlap with the vowel to make room for the /k/, thus shortening vowel duration. However in *claps*, the /s/ simply appends to /p/ with no effect on /p/. The distance from the centre of the coda to the start of the vowel thus increases as more consonants are added to the coda. Figure 13.4 presents schematic representations of these relationships.

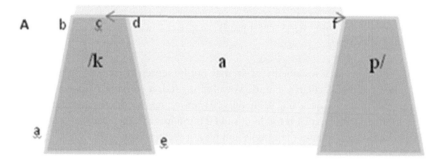

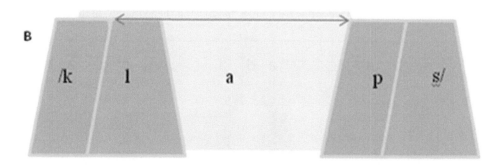

Figure 13.4 A: Gesture for /k/ begins in phase with gesture for /a/. B: To maintain stability of C-centre to anchor duration, gesture for /k/ begins slightly earlier, gesture for /l/ extends into the vowel gesture. a = gesture onset, b = target, c = C-centre, d = gesture release, e = gesture offset, f = anchor point.

Instrumental investigations of articulation

The instrumental techniques described here directly capture information about the movements of the articulators. For clinical purposes, being able to visualize the speed, direction, and range of articulator movement is advantageous both for the clinician and the client. For the clinician, it allows for identification of the atypical behaviours underlying the perception of atypical speech. For the client, it provides visual feedback on the needed adjustments to articulatory patterns, which would yield more perceptually acceptable speech.

Electropalatography

Electropalatography (EPG) provides spatial and temporal information about tongue contact with the upper surface of the oral cavity from the margins of the upper teeth and alveolar ridge at the front to the margins of the hard and soft palate/velum at the rear. An EPG recording is usually combined with a simultaneous acoustic recording. The speaker wears a thin acrylic dental plate studded with electrodes. The concentration of electrodes is relatively greater in the alveolar region of this dental plate, reflecting the importance of this place of articulation in consonant production. Contact between the tongue and an electrode is registered by the EPG system, which converts this signal into visual feedback on a computer.

EPG has proved to be a popular technique for investigating typical and atypical speech production and for providing therapy for many types of speech impairment. EPG patterns in typical speakers show a range of variation in speech sound production; however, different sounds demonstrate recognizable patterns of contact. By viewing the EPG data of a sound's production as it emerges and decays over time, typical and atypical spatial and temporal patterns can be identified. Figure 13.5 shows the linguapalatal contact patterns for a typical speaker's

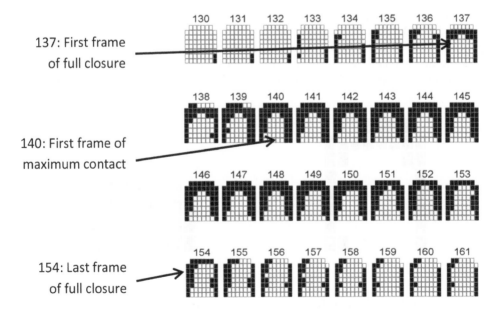

Figure 13.5 Lingual palatal contact patterns for [t], showing key reference points in the production of that sound.

production of the voiceless alveolar plosive /t/. The sides of the tongue are raised to make lateral contact with the palate before the tongue tip gradually forms complete closure in the alveolar region, creating a characteristic horseshoe-shaped pattern of contact. While identifying when complete closure is first achieved (frame 137) and the point at which it is released (frame 154), a phase of maximum lingual palatal contact is also identified, starting at frame 140.

Figure 13.6 compares the frame of maximum contact for a typical speaker's production of /t/ with the midpoint for /t/ produced by a child with a cleft palate, which is perceived as the voiceless palatal plosive [c]. Hence, the EPG data confirms the perception of [c], by revealing complete asymmetrical closure in the region of the hard palate, with no alveolar ridge contact. EPG investigations have proved particularly valuable in illuminating covert contrasts, where a speaker is making a consistent articulatory contrast, which is not auditorily perceptible (Gibbon, 1990), and in identifying aspects of tongue behaviour in connected speech versus single sounds or words (Howard, 2007).

EPG has been used for both assessment and intervention across a number of speech impairments, including: a) developmental phonological and motor speech disorders (Gibbon, 1999; Nordberg *et al.*, 2011); b) speech production with cleft palate (Howard, 2013, Gibbon 2004); c) speech production with hearing impairment (Bacsfalvi and Bernhardt, 2011); d) acquired motor speech disorders (McAuliffe and Ward, 2007); e) speech production associated with Down syndrome (Cleland *et al.*, 2009); f) dysfluency (Wood, 1995); and g) glossectomy (Fletcher, 1988). The easily interpretable visual feedback provided by EPG appears to be particularly useful for speakers who have difficulty changing their speech behaviours using traditional therapy approaches. Small, portable EPG systems (Wrench *et al.*, 2002) can be used for therapy outside the traditional clinic.

Ultrasound

Ultrasound is a technique for providing visual information on internal anatomical structures (Stone, 2005). Ultrasound uses very high frequency sound waves which, when directed at physical structures, such as those in the oral cavity, either pass through them or are deflected back, creating an echo. The greater the density of the target structure, the more difficulty sound waves have travelling through the structure, making it more likely they will bounce back.

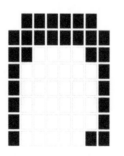

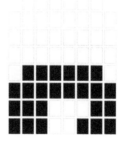

(a) /t/ realised as [t]   (b) /t/ realised as [c]

Figure 13.6 Midpoints of lingual palatal contact for realisations of /t/ as (a) a typical alveolar [t], and (b) a palatal [c].

To monitor speech production, a transducer is placed under the speaker's chin, directing sound waves upwards through the tongue musculature. When the sound waves hit the tissue-to-air boundary created by the upper surface of the tongue, the resulting echo creates a clear image which reflects the shape of the tongue surface. Ultrasound can thus capture both still and moving images of the tongue during speech production and swallowing. A mid-sagittal view of the tongue surface is usually provided, but a coronal view is also possible, which captures aspects of midline lingual activity, such as tongue grooving. Figure 13.7 shows the ultrasound images of a typical adult British speaker during the production of the voiceless alveolar fricative /s/ in /asa/. The mid-sagittal view illustrates the elevation of the tongue tip and blade in the anterior of the vocal cavity; the coronal view reveals the characteristic grooving of the tongue for this sound.

One drawback of ultrasound is that both bony structures and pockets of air can impede the imaging of the tongue. Although ultrasound provides clear images of the surface of the main body of the tongue, both the tip and root may be obscured by the jaw and hyoid bone. Furthermore, because the palate is not visible, the precise location of the tongue can only be inferred.

Nevertheless, ultrasound is a valuable technique for speech analysis, particularly for depicting vowel production and investigating tongue shape and movement for alveolar and postalveolar fricatives, affricates and approximants, as well as alveolar and velar plosives. In the clinical context, ultrasound has been used to explore tongue behaviour in a range of developmental and acquired disorders of speech, including glossectomy (Bressman *et al.*, 2010), hearing impairment (Bernhardt *et al.*, 2003), cleft palate (Gibbon and Wolters, 2005), and residual developmental misarticulations (Lipetz and Bernhardt, 2013).

Bernhardt, Bacsfalvi and colleagues have demonstrated effective therapy for individuals with a range of developmental speech difficulties and described how ultrasound therapy can be provided to clients living in remote rural locations (Bernhardt *et al.*, 2008). Cleland *et al.* (2013) report that typical adult speakers are able to "read" ultrasound and EPG displays, which makes it useful for biofeedback purposes in speech therapy. Although current ultrasound systems for speech analysis require the speaker to wear a headset, ongoing technical developments suggest production of a more user-friendly version in future (Articulate Instruments: www.articulateinstruments.com).

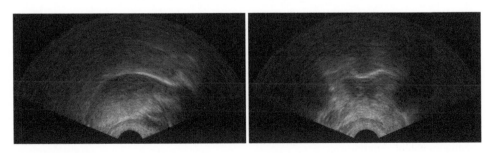

Mid-sagittal view   Coronal view

Figure 13.7 Mid-sagittal (left-to-right = posterior-to-anterior) and coronal views of the tongue producing /s/: the tongue's surface appears as a white line.

Electromagnetic articulography

Electromagnetic articulography (EMA) provides information on the tongue, as well as the movement and position of other oral articulators, including the jaw, lips and velum, in a mid-sagittal view. Electromagnetic transducers, situated in a headset worn by the speaker, induce an alternating current in a series of sensors fixed to chosen sites in and around the vocal organs. Depending on the speech behaviours of interest, these locations may include the chin, velum, upper and lower lips, upper and lower gums and various points along the tongue surface, and the bridge of the nose, which acts as a fixed reference point. These sensors track the position and movement of individual articulators over time and capture how different articulators coordinate movement with each other.

EMA is relatively expensive. Its use requires considerable technical knowledge and support and (as with ultrasound) it requires the speaker to wear a fairly substantial headset. Therefore, it has rarely been used for assessment or intervention in clinical contexts (but see Katz *et al.*, 2010, for a report of successful EMA-based therapy for an adult with acquired apraxia of speech).

However, EMA does provide a rich source of information about speech articulation, and can be combined with other instrumental techniques, such as EPG, to enhance our understanding of the coordination of the articulators during speech development production of typical and atypical speech. The number of publications using EMA to investigate articulatory behaviours in a wide range of speech disorders has been steadily increasing. These include developmental phonological disorders (Terband *et al.*, 2011), speech associated with cleft palate (van Lieshout *et al.*, 2002), acquired and developmental motor speech disorders (Nijland *et al.*, 2004, Rong *et al.*, 2012) and dysfluency (*Namasivayam and van Lieshout, 2008*). A common feature of many of these studies has been their identification of reduced coordination of different articulators and greater speech variability, in comparison with typical speakers. EMA studies often take the form of single case studies or small case series, and vary from those examining a single articulator to those investigating coordination of several articulators. Many studies using EMA to examine speech production combine it with other instrumental methods, such as EPG and acoustic analysis.

Measuring nasal resonance and airflow

Difficulties directing airflow appropriately through the nasal and oral cavities are characteristic of a number of different types of speech impairment, including developmental and acquired motor speech disorders, speech associated with hearing impairment, and speech associated with cleft palate and craniofacial anomalies. In each case, the causes of the problems will differ and may have their origins in neuromuscular, perceptual or structural difficulties. However, they may all have negative implications for listener perceptions, and all may be investigated instrumentally. In terms of the speech behaviours to be investigated, we need to distinguish between resonance (sound vibration in the oral and nasal cavities) and airflow, as the investigative techniques will be different.

Measuring nasal resonance

There are currently three main systems which provide objective measurements of nasal resonance (and the ratio of oral resonance to nasal resonance) in speech production: the Nasometer (KayPENTAX, Lincoln Park, NJ), NasalView (Tiger DRS Inc., Seattle, WA) and the Nasality Visualization System (Glottal Enterprises Inc., Syracuse, NY), which also measures nasal emission. Of the three systems, the Nasometer is currently the most widely employed for clinical evaluation. These systems employ similar techniques to separate out oral and nasal signals and to compute measures of their relative acoustic energy. For example, the Nasometer requires the speaker to wear a helmet which contains two microphones, separated by a baffle. One microphone picks up acoustic energy from the oral cavity; the other from the nasal cavity. The system automatically computes a "nasalance" score, which reflects the ratio of nasal to nasal-and-oral acoustic energy. In addition, detailed quantitative data is generated and a visual representation of nasalance across time is provided which is particularly useful for client feedback. Figure 13.8 shows a screen display for the syllable string /apa/, /ama/, /apa/, /ama/, revealing clear differences in nasalance between the oral and nasal targets.

Nasometry is used to identify or characterize suspected hypernasality (excessive nasal resonance) in a patient's speech. This process entails using carefully devised test materials, comprised of sentences or short passages, which have been designed to be free from nasal consonants, so that nasal resonance would not be expected in typical speech production. In investigating suspected hyponasality, sentences which are heavily loaded with nasal consonants will most easily identify a reduction in expected nasal resonance in a speaker's productions. However, it is very apparent from many instrumental studies of nasal resonance that a great deal of intra- and inter-speaker variability exists. Individual speakers may vary from one recording session to the next (van Doorn and Purcell, 1998), which alerts us to take great care in the comparison and interpretation of results obtained over time in successive clinical sessions.

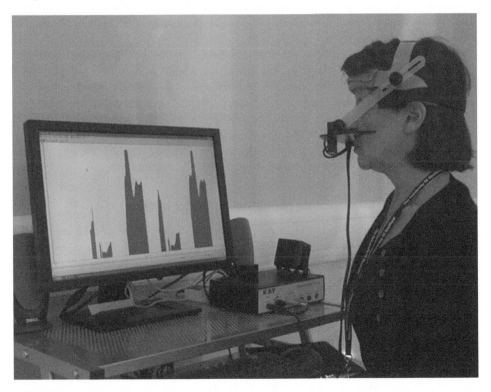

Figure 13.8 A speaker wearing the helmet for the Nasometer demonstrates contrasting visual feedback for nasalance values in productions of /apa/, /ama/, /apa/, /ama/.

Inter-speaker variability includes numerous factors, such as age, gender, language, accent, speech rate, the speech material used and even, in women, stage of menstrual cycle. In terms of clinical evaluation, then, we clearly need to be sensitive to a range of biological, social and linguistic factors in estimating the appropriateness of a nasalance score for an individual speaker. Particular care is also necessary when using Nasometry with young children. Van der Heijden *et al.* (2011) observed that older children (age 6 years) coped well with the demands imposed by wearing the headset. The youngest children (age 4 years) found the situation challenging and were not able to cooperate well during data collection. Overall, the consensus is that Nasometry is a useful and informative technique for clinical observation, and that it should always be used in combination with perceptual analysis (Karnell, 2011) since satisfactory levels of agreement between nasalance measurements and perceptual ratings of resonance have been observed (Sweeney and Sell, 2008).

Measuring air pressure and airflow

Another useful clinical measurement for velopharyngeal function is oral–nasal air pressure and flow. It has most commonly been measured using the Perci-SARS technique (Speech-Aeromechanics Research System: MicroTronics Inc.), originally developed by Warren and Dubois (1964) (for other techniques see Bunton *et al.*, 2011). Perci-SARS uses oral and nasal catheters to measure oral and nasal air pressure and nasal airflow, providing clear visual representations for comparative purposes. However, caution is advised. As Ladefoged (2003) comments, "[t]he same pressure can result in very different flows depending on the resistance to the flow". Atypical resistance may relate to atypical velopharyngeal structure or function, or a nasal cavity obstruction.

A key principle in the use of pressure-flow measurement is that the degree of nasal airflow at a given moment is directly related to, and therefore predicts, the size of the velopharyngeal port. This relationship has been reported in both typical and atypical speech production, particularly with cleft palate (Searl and Knollhoff, 2013), although reservations have been expressed about its validity for larger velopharyngeal port openings (Warren, 2004). A strong correlation between nasal airflow and nasal resonance has been suggested by Dalston *et al.* (1991) in a study comparing data from the Nasometer and Perci-SARS and both measures have been reported to correlate with perceptual ratings (Sweeney and Sell, 2008).

Measuring phonation and voice quality

In addition to the production of the voiced–voiceless distinction, the vocal folds are used for the habitual laryngeal settings which contribute to overall voice quality. While all speakers of English need to make appropriate distinctions between /p/ and /b/ and other phonological pairs, some may produce these phonemes using voice which is more breathy or less tense.

Electrolaryngography

Electrolaryngography (ELG) captures data about a speaker's vocal fold activity while wearing a collar with two electrodes attached. These electrodes are positioned on either side of the thyroid protuberance to measure a very weak flow of electrical current from one electrode to the other across the glottis. When the glottis is closed, the flow is high because there is continuous conduction through the tissue. When the glottis is open, the flow is reduced by the impedance of the gap. One advantage of using ELG is that physiological information about vocal fold activity is measured directly instead of being inferred from acoustic data. For example, ELG measures the rate of vocal fold vibration—the physiological correlate of pitch—and is not subject to the errors, such as pitch-doubling and pitch-halving, which commonly occur when making acoustic estimates of F0 (Hillenbrand and Houde, 1996).

Additional advantages of ELG are that the dynamics of individual vocal fold vibrations can be seen on larynx (Lx) waveforms and quantified. Figure 13.9 compares a waveform from a healthy 21-year-old female with that of an 86-year-old female. In the former, the steeper closing and opening slopes reflect faster movements of the vocal folds, which are indicative of greater elasticity and better muscle tone. The more sluggish vocal fold movement in older speakers often results in slower vibrations (i.e., a lower pitch), as is the case here.

Lx waveforms also show different types of phonation more clearly than an acoustic waveform or spectrogram. Figure 13.10 presents Lx waveforms of breathy voice and creak in which the long open phases characteristic of breathy voice are readily apparent, as are the short open phases and the "double-pulse" vibration pattern often observed in creak.

A useful measure for quantifying properties of larynx waveforms is the closed quotient (or its inverse, the open quotient). The closed quotient (CQ) is the proportion of a full vocal fold cycle of voicing during which the vocal folds are in contact (Abberton *et al.*, 1989), expressed as a percentage. The measure is normally taken at a point on the waveform 70 per cent below the peak, and is calculated by the equation

CQ = ((closed phase duration/cycle duration)*100)%

A CQ value of approximately 40 per cent or less is indicative of breathiness which can be a habitual phonation type in some speakers, a symptom of a voice disorder in others, a coarticulatory effect on vowels adjacent to voiceless consonants, or a phonologically distinctive phonatory feature. Gujarati (an Indian language), for example, contrasts non-breathy voice and breathy voice in minimal pairs, such as /mɛl/ "dirt" and /mɛ̤l/ "palace" (Ladefoged and Johnson 2011). However, the acoustic and physiological correlates of breathy voice are far from agreed upon in the literature (Gerratt and Kreiman, 2001).

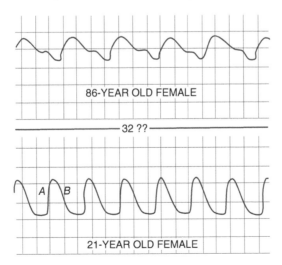

Figure 13.9 Lx waveforms showing lack of elasticity in the vocal folds with ageing. A = closing slope, B = opening slope.

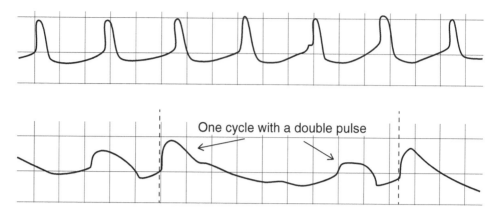

Figure 13.10 Lx waveforms of breathy voice (upper) and creak (lower).

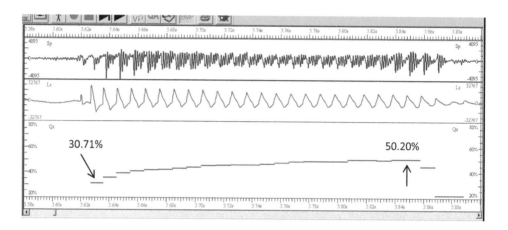

Figure 13.11 Lx waveform (middle panel) and CQ trace (lower panel) showing coarticulatory effects on voicing of the vowel from initial aspirated [kʰ] and final glottalised [ʔp] in "carp".

The CQ trace in Figure 13.11 shows the coarticulatory effects on vowel phonation of the initial and final stops in English *carp*. We can see the low CQ value at voice onset after the open-glottis aspirated [kʰ], and the high value at voice offset immediately before the closed-glottis [ʔp].

Excessive instability of phonatory action can be quantified using jitter and shimmer measures. Jitter refers to variation in the time-periods of successive glottal cycles that are not due to the pitch dynamics of prosody. Shimmer refers to variation in their amplitudes. Typical values for jitter and shimmer are problematic to establish and are sensitive to the method of calculation, but for a sustained vowel at a level pitch, any value over about 1.0 per cent for jitter or 4.0 per cent for shimmer (Kay Elemetrics 2008) is considered outside the normal range.

Conclusion

We have presented a range of instrumental techniques that explore aspects of articulation, phonation, resonance, and airflow, both separately and in combination. They have all provided researchers with insights into vocal organ activity underpinning atypical speech production.

Many of them are also available for use in clinical intervention, where their ability to provide visual feedback to a speaker can be particularly effective in facilitating change in speech behaviours. Our aim has been to show how such techniques are valuable in both assessment and intervention, not as a replacement for the perceptual analysis of the listener's impression of atypical speech production, but as a complementary approach with exciting possibilities. As observed elsewhere, "instrumental and perceptual analyses are … not competing to represent 'the truth' about an utterance. Rather, each is offering a perspective which is inaccessible to the other" (Howard and Heselwood, 2013, p. 948).

Acknowledgments

The authors would like to thank Joanne Cleland and Alan Wrench, Queen Margaret University Edinburgh/Articulate Instruments, for assistance with the ultrasound figure.

References

Abberton, E., Howard, D.M. and Fourcin, A.J. (1989), "Laryngographic assessment of normal voice: A tutorial", *Clinical Linguistics and Phonetics*, Vol. 3, pp. 281–296.

Bacsfalvi, P. and Bernhardt, B. (2011), "Long-term outcomes of speech therapy for seven adolescents with visual feedback technologies: Ultrasound and electropalatography", *Clinical Linguistics and Phonetics,* Vol. 25, pp. 1034–1043.

Bernhardt, B., Gick, B., Bacsfalvi, P. and Ashdown, J. (2003), "Speech habilitation of hard of hearing adolescents using ultrasound as evaluated by trained listeners", *Clinical Linguistics and Phonetics*, Vol. 17, pp. 199–216.

Bernhardt, B., Bacsfalvi, P., Adler-Bock, M., Shimizu, R., Chenay, A., Giesbrecht, N., *et al.*, (2008), "Ultrasound as visual feedback in speech habilitation: Exploring consultative use in rural British Columbia, Canada", *Clinical Linguistics and Phonetics*, Vol. 22, pp. 149–162

Bressman, T., Flowers, H., Wong, W. and Irish, J. (2010), "Coronal view ultrasound imaging of movement in different segments of the tongue during paced recital: Findings from four normal speakers and a speaker with partial glossectomy", *Clinical Linguistics and Phonetics,* Vol. 24, pp. 589–601.

Bunton, K., Hoit, J. and Gallagher, K. (2011), "A simple technique for determining velopharyngeal status during speech production", *Seminars in Speech and Language,* Vol. 32, pp. 69–80.

Ciocca, V. and Whitehill, T.L. (2013), "The acoustic measurement of vowels", in Ball, M.J. and Gibbon, F.E. (Eds.), *Handbook of Vowels and Vowel Disorders*, Psychology Press, New York, pp. 113–137.

Cleland, J., Timmins, C., Wood, S., Hardcastle, W. and Wishart, J. (2009), "Electropalatographic therapy for children and young people with Down's syndrome". *Clinical Linguistics and Phonetics*, Vol. 23, pp. 926–939.

Cleland, J., McCron, C. and Scobbie, J. (2013), "Tongue reading: Comparing the interpretation of visual information from the inside of the mouth, from electropalatographic and ultrasound displays of speech sounds", *Clinical Linguistics and Phonetics*, Vol. 27, pp. 299–311.

Dalston, R., Warren, D. and Dalston, E. (1991), "Use of nasometry as a diagnostic tool for identifying patients with velopharyngeal impairment", *Cleft Palate-Craniofacial Journal*, Vol. 28, pp. 184–189.

Fletcher, S. (1988), "Speech production following partial glossectomy", *Journal of Speech and Hearing Disorders,* Vol. 53, pp. 232–238.

Gerratt, B. and Kreiman, J. (2001), "Toward a taxonomy of nonmodal phonation", *Journal of Phonetics*, Vol. 29, pp. 365–381.

Gibbon, F. (1990), "Lingual activity in two speech-disordered children's attempts to produce velar and alveolar stop consonants: Evidence from electropalatographic (EPG) data", *British Journal of Disorders of Communication*, Vol. 25, pp. 329–340.

Gibbon, F. (1999), "Undifferentiated lingual gestures in children with articulation/phonological disorders", *Journal of Speech, Language, and Hearing Research,* Vol. 42, pp. 382–397.

Gibbon, F. (2004), "Abnormal patterns of tongue-palate contact in the speech of individuals with cleft palate", *Clinical Linguistics and Phonetics*, Vol. 18, pp. 285–311.

Gibbon, F. and Wolters, M. (2005), "A new application of ultrasound to image tongue behaviour in cleft palate speech", Presentation at the Craniofacial Society of Great Britain and Ireland Annual Conference, Swansea, UK, 13–15 April 2005.

Heselwood, B. and Howard, S. (2008), "Clinical phonetic transcription", in M. Ball, M. Perkins, N. Müller and S. Howard (Eds.), *The Handbook of Clinical Linguistics*, Blackwell, Oxford, UK, pp. 381–399.

Hillenbrand, J. and Houde, R.A. (1996), "Acoustic correlates of breathy vocal quality: Dysphonic voices and continuous speech", *Journal of Speech and Hearing Research*, Vol. 39, pp. 311–321.

Honorof, D. and Browman, C.P. (1995), "The center or the edge: How are consonant clusters organized with respect to the vowel?", in Elenius, K. and Branderud, P. (Eds.), *Proceedings of the XIIIth International Congress of Phonetic Sciences*, University of Stockholm, Stockholm, pp. 552–555.

Howard, S. (2007), "The interplay between articulation and prosody in children with impaired speech: Observations from electropalatographic and perceptual analysis", *International Journal of Speech-Language Pathology*, Vol. 9, pp. 20–35.

Howard, S. (2013), "A phonetic investigation of single word versus connected speech production in children with persisting speech difficulties relating to cleft palate", *Cleft Palate-Craniofacial Journal*, Vol. 20, pp. 207–223.

Howard, S. and Heselwood, B. (2013), "The contribution of phonetics to the study of vowel development and disorders", in M. Ball and F. Gibbon (Eds.), *Handbook of Vowels and Vowel Disorders*, Psychology Press, New York, NY, pp. 61–112.

Karnell, M. (2011), "Instrumental assessment of velopharyngeal closure for speech", *Seminars in Speech and Language*, Vol. 32, pp. 168–178.

Katz, W., McNeil, M. and Garst, D. (2010), "Treating apraxia of speech (AOS) with EMA-supplied visual augmented feedback", *Aphasiology*, Vol. 24, pp. 826–837.

Kay Elemetrics (2008), *Multi-Dimensional Voice Program, Model 5105*, Kay Elemetrics Corporation, Lincoln Park, NJ, US.

Kent, R.D. and Kim, Y. (2008), "Acoustic analysis of speech", in Ball, M.J., Perkins, M.R., Müller, N. and Howard, S.J. (Eds.), *The Handbook of Clinical Linguistics*, Blackwell, Malden, MA, US, pp. 360–380.

Ladefoged, P. (2003), *Phonetic Data Analysis*, Blackwell, Malden, MA, US.

Ladefoged, P. and Johnson, K. (2011), *A Course in Phonetics*, (6th Edition), Wadsworth, Belmont, CA, US.

Ladefoged, P., Harshman, R., Goldstein, L. and Rice, L. (1978), "Generating vocal tract shapes from formant frequencies", *Journal of the Acoustical Society of America*, Vol. 64, pp. 1027–1035.

Lipetz, H. and Bernhardt, B. (2013), "A multi-modal approach to intervention for one adult's frontal lisp", *Clinical Linguistics and Phonetics*, Vol. 27, pp. 1–17.

McAuliffe, M. and Ward, E. (2007), "The use of electropalatography in the assessment and treatment of acquired motor speech disorders in adults: Current knowledge and future directions", *Neurorehabilitation*, Vol. 21, pp. 189–203.

Maurer, D., Gröne, B., Landis, T., Hoch, G. and Schönle, P. (1993), "Re-examination of the relation between the vocal tract and the vowel sound with electromagnetic articulography (EMA) in vocalizations", *Clinical Linguistics and Phonetics*, Vol. 7, pp. 129–143.

Namasivayam, A. and van Lieshout, P. (2008), "Investigating speech motor practice and learning in people who stutter", *Journal of Fluency Disorders*, Vol. 33, pp. 32–51.

Nijland, L., Maassen, B., Hulstijn, W. and Peters, H. (2004), "Speech motor coordination in Dutch-speaking children with DAS studied with EMA", *Journal of Multilingual Communication Disorders*, Vol. 2, pp. 50–60.

Nordberg, A., Carlsson, C. and Lohmander, A. (2011), "Electropalatography in the description and treatment of speech disorders in five children with cerebral palsy", *Clinical Linguistics and Phonetics*, Vol. 25, pp. 831–852.

Rong, P., Loucks, T., Kim, H. and Hasegawa-Johnson, M. (2012), "Relationship between kinematics, F2 slope and speech intelligibility in dysarthria due to cerebral palsy", *Clinical Linguistics and Phonetics*, Vol. 26, pp. 806–822.

Ryalls, J. (1986), "An acoustic study of vowel production in aphasia", *Brain and Language*, Vol. 29, pp. 48–67.

Searl, J. and Knollhoff, S. (2013), "Oral pressure and nasal flow on /m/ and /p/ in 3- to 5-year-old children without cleft palate", *Cleft Palate-Craniofacial Journal*, Vol. 50, pp. 40–50.

Smits, R., Bosch, L.T. and Collier, R. (1996), "Evaluation of various sets of acoustic cues for the perception of prevocalic stop consonants", *Journal of the Acoustical Society of America*, Vol. 100, pp. 3852–3864.

Stevens, K.N. (1998), "Vowels: Acoustic events with a relatively open vocal tract", Stevens K.N., *Acoustic Phonetics*, MIT Press, Cambridge, MA, pp. 257–322.

Stone, M. (2005), "A guide to analysing tongue motion from ultrasound images", *Clinical Linguistics and Phonetics*, Vol. 19, pp. 455–501.

Sweeney, T. and Sell, D. (2008), "Relationship between perceptual ratings of nasality and Nasometry in children/adolescents with cleft palate and/or velopharyngeal dysfunction", *International Journal of Language and Communication,* Vol. 43, pp. 265–282.

Terband, H., Maassen, B., van Lieshout, P. and Nijland, L. (2011), "Stability and composition of functional synergies for speech movements in children with developmental speech disorders", *Journal of Communication Disorders,* Vol. 44, pp. 59–74.

Van der Heijden, P., Hobbel, H.H., van der Laan, B.F.A.M., Korsten-Meijer, A.G.W. and Gorrhuis-Brouwer, S.M. (2011), "Nasometry cooperation in children 4-6 years of age", *International Journal of Pediatric Otorhinolaryngography,* Vol. 75, pp. 627–630.

Van Doorn, J. and Purcell, A. (1998), "Nasalance levels in the speech of normal Australian children", *The Cleft Palate Craniofacial Journal,* Vol. 35, pp. 287–292.

Van Lieshout, P., Rutjens, C. and Spauwen, P. (2002), "The dynamics of interlip coupling in speakers with a repaired unilateral cleft-lip history", *Journal of Speech, Language and Hearing Research,* Vol. 45, pp. 5–19.

Vihman, M. (1996), *Phonological Development: The Origins of Language in the Child,* Blackwell, Oxford, UK.

Warren, D. (2004), "Aerodynamic assessments and procedures to determine extent of velopharyngeal inadequacy", in Bzoch, K. (Ed.), *Communicative Disorders Related to Cleft Lip and Palate,* (5th Edition), Pro-Ed, Austin, TX, US, pp. 595–628.

Warren, D. and Dubois, A. (1964), "A pressure-flow technique for measuring velopharyngeal orifice area during continuous speech", *Cleft Palate Journal,* Vol. 1, pp. 52–71.

Weismer, G., Martin, R., Kent, R.D. and Kent, J.F. (1992), "Formant trajectory characteristics of males with amyotrophic lateral sclerosis", *Journal of the Acoustical Society of America,* Vol. 91, pp. 1085–1098.

Wood, S. (1995), "An electropalatographic analysis of stutterers' speech", *European Journal of Disorders of Communication,* Vol. 30, pp. 226–236.

Wrench, A., Gibbon, F., McNeill, A. and Wood, S. (2002), "An EPG therapy protocol for remediation and assessment of articulation disorders", in Hansen, J.H.L. and Pellom, B. (Eds.) *Proceedings of the ICSLP-2002,* www.isca-speech.org/archive/icslp02, pp. 965-968.

14

CONTEMPORARY ISSUES IN DYSARTHRIA

Kris Tjaden, Jennifer Lam and Lynda Feenaughty

Introduction

The seminal studies of Darley, Aronson, and Brown (1969a, b) laid the foundation for the systematic study of adult dysarthria more than 45 years ago. Despite a fair amount of research, however, a comprehensive theory of dysarthria that accounts for the complex mapping between different forms of nervous system disease, the impact on underlying movements of the speech mechanism, and the resulting auditory–acoustic speech signal recovered by the listener is still lacking. The purpose of this chapter is to consider several themes emerging from contemporary studies of dysarthria that ultimately will bear on development of such a theory, including; 1) classification; 2) measurement of intelligibility and related perceptual constructs; 3) severity; and 4) cognitive–linguistic factors and their relationship to dysarthria.

Classification

There is no doubt that a valid dysarthria classification system would facilitate patient communication within and across clinics, as well as comparisons across studies. The perceptually-based system of Darley *et al.* (1969a, b) also referred to as the Mayo Clinic System, remains the "gold standard". The most recent version of the system summarized in Duffy (2013) includes seven dysarthria subtypes (i.e., flaccid, spastic, ataxic, hypokinetic, hyperkinetic, unilateral upper motor neuron, and mixed) as well as the designation of undetermined dysarthria. Each subtype reflects a distinct form of nervous system disease and accompanying speech mechanism pathophysiology which in turn is associated with a unique perceptual profile reflecting voice, resonance, articulation, prosody and rate characteristics. While the Mayo Clinic System has been the dominant classification scheme since its inception, it is not without problems as suggested by Duffy's acknowledgment that "no classification system is perfect" (Duffy, 2007, p. 30). Assertions concerning pathophysiology in the speech mechanism (i.e., incoordination, spasticity) have not been strongly supported by research nor has the relationship between pathophysiology and auditory–perceptual characteristics been established. Many studies also have reported poor inter-judge reliability and limited accuracy in identifying dysarthria subtypes (e.g., Bunton *et al.*, 2007; Fonville *et al.*, 2008). For these and other reasons, it has been suggested that progress might be hindered by continued use of the Mayo Clinic System (Weismer and

Kim, 2010). Research therefore has begun to explore alternate approaches to dysarthria classification.

Recent studies employing acoustic measures to classify individuals with dysarthria according to their Mayo Clinic subtype has revealed classification accuracy as high as 80 percent (Kim *et al.*, 2011; Liss *et al.* 2010). The 80 percent classification accuracy reported by Liss *et al.* (2010) may be related to the fact that only speakers with cardinal perceptual characteristics of the Mayo dysarthria subtypes were included. Medical etiology and dysarthria subtype also overlapped, thus precluding conclusions as to whether acoustic metrics were predicting medical etiology (i.e., Parkinson's disease) or Mayo Clinic dysarthria subtype (i.e., hypokinetic). Interestingly, Kim *et al.*, (2011) found that acoustic measures were more successful in classifying speakers on the basis of medical etiology (i.e., 68 percent accuracy) or sentence intelligibility (i.e., 55 percent accuracy) versus Mayo Clinic dysarthria subtype (i.e., 32 percent accuracy). Similarly, Lansford and Liss (2014) found that acoustic metrics were unreliable classifiers of Mayo Clinic System dysarthria subtypes, but did distinguish healthy speakers from those with dysarthria with classification accuracy as high as 84 percent. These results were interpreted as support for the taxonomical approach to dysarthria classification (Weismer and Kim, 2010).

Unlike the Mayo Clinic System which focuses on identifying differences among speakers, a taxonomical approach seeks to identify a core set of deficits shared by all speakers, regardless of medical diagnosis or etiology. For example, Lansford, Liss and Norton (2014) employed an auditory, free-classification approach to dysarthria classification in which listeners were asked to group stimuli by how similar they sound. Acoustic and perceptual metrics of rate, intelligibility and vocal quality were important for identifying six clusters of perceptually-similar speakers. Of note, speakers representing multiple Mayo Clinic dysarthria subtypes were members of the same cluster.

A potential criticism of using acoustic measures in a dysarthria classification scheme is the level of expertise and training involved in performing the measures, and a similar criticism has been leveled with respect to the perceptual skills needed to implement the Mayo Clinic System. Importantly, there is evidence that an automated acoustic metric termed the Envelope Modulation Spectra (EMS) can successfully differentiate neurotypical speakers from speakers with dysarthria (Liss *et al.*, 2010). Although interpretation of the measure with respect to underlying speech subsystem impairment is not straightforward, the Liss *et al.* (2010) study demonstrates the feasibility of employing an automated acoustic measure to distinguish speakers with and without dysarthria. Ongoing research will move the field closer towards the goal of "parametric assessment of speech function" (Kent and Kim, 2003, p. 441).

The role of a dysarthria classification system in management remains to be seen. At present, the same therapeutic techniques (i.e., rate manipulation, increased vocal intensity, increasing prosodic variation) are recommended for individuals representing a range of Mayo Clinic dysarthria diagnoses and medical etiologies (Duffy, 2013; Yorkston *et al.*, 2007a). Whether different dysarthria clusters or groups identified in studies exploring acoustic-based classification schemes benefit from different forms of therapy is an important matter for future research.

Measurement of intelligibility and related perceptual constructs

Numerous factors can impact the extent to which a speaker's intended message is recovered by the listener. In recent years, a fair amount of attention has been devoted to the role of the listener in determining the intelligibility deficit of dysarthria. The focus here, however, is on work that bears more generally on measurement of intelligibility or the closely related perceptual construct of Speech Severity, as operationally defined in Sussman and Tjaden (2012).

Types of intelligibility metrics

Intelligibility measures can be broadly categorized as objective or subjective metrics. Orthographic transcription in which the listener writes or types the speaker's message word-for-word is a common objective metric. An overall percent-correct score can then be used as an indication of the magnitude of speech impairment or severity of dysarthria. Transcription is widely used to quantify intelligibility in dysarthria, as suggested by its long standing use in research as well as published intelligibility tests (Yorkston and Beukelman, 1984; Yorkston et al., 1996).

Scaling tasks are considered to be subjective metrics and do not require a computation. There is no standard definition of intelligibility used in dysarthria studies employing scaling tasks. In our recent work, listeners have been instructed to judge the "understandability" of speech (Tjaden et al., 2013a; Tjaden et al., 2013b). Other studies have defined intelligibility as the "ease with which speech is understood," which may tap into the cognitive effort used by the listener. Whether different definitions of intelligibility impact outcomes in studies employing scaling tasks is an important topic for future research and has implications for using scaling tasks in clinical practice to quantify intelligibility.

A variety of subjective scaling tasks are available. Equal-appearing interval (EAI) scaling requires listeners to designate a number, most often on a five to nine-point scale, representing their overall judgment of intelligibility. Although EAI scaling continues to be employed in dysarthria tests (Enderby and Palmer, 2008) and research (e.g., Neel, 2009), interval scaling is not as well-suited to quantifying intelligibility as other scaling techniques involve proportional or ratio-level judgments (Schiavetti, 1992).

Direct magnitude estimation (DME) is another technique in which listeners assign a numerical value to speech samples representing proportional differences in intelligibility (Hustad and Weismer, 2007). In some instances, speech samples are judged relative to a modulus or standard (i.e., another speech sample). The choice of a standard influences intelligibility outcomes, precluding comparison of studies employing different standards (Weismer and Laures, 2002). In modulus-free DME, speech samples are judged relative to one another rather than a standard, and scale values from different listeners are then converted to a common scale. However, listeners may find the task unusual, and this may account for the modest listener reliability in some studies (Tjaden and Wilding, 2004, 2011). Relatedly, for statistical reasons, listener reliability for modulus-free DME is likely to be more robust when speakers span a wide range of overall dysarthria severity (Kim et al., 2011; Kim and Kuo, 2012).

Our recent work has employed visual analog scaling (VAS) to quantify intelligibility for speakers with Parkinson's disease (PD) or Multiple Sclerosis (MS), as well as neurotypical speakers (Feenaughty et al., 2013; Kuo et al., 2014; Sussman and Tjaden, 2012; Tjaden et al., 2013a, b; Tjaden et al., 2014). VAS is superior to interval scaling because the data are ratio-level and are more amenable to parametric statistical analysis. Moreover, because the data are continuous, the probability of chance agreement is reduced compared to interval scales using a small number of categories. Although VAS may be completed using a printed scale which is then converted to a numerical value using a ruler (McHenry, 2011), computerized scales are available. Similar to transcription, speech samples for a given talker are pooled and scale values may be averaged to provide an indication of the overall magnitude of speech impairment relative to neurotypical speech.

Strengths and weaknesses of objective and subjective metrics

Transcription is undoubtedly the most common method for quantifying intelligibility both in research and clinical practice. Because error patterns may be examined, transcription not only can provide an indication of the overall severity of speech impairment, but also affords evaluation of listener-related factors that might explain a reduction or change in intelligibility (Liss, 2007). In theory, error patterns might also be used to direct management. For example, in the case of the target word "dip" being transcribed as "tip," treatment might focus on the word-initial voicing distinction to improve intelligibility (see Kent et al., 1989).

On the other hand, transcription is time-consuming for the listener writing down what is being said as well as for the person scoring the transcript. Even computerized scoring requires that responses be manually reviewed for typos and homonyms (Yorkston et al., 1996). Individual listeners also vary in the ability to accurately transcribe speech produced by individuals with dysarthria, as well as speech of neurotypical speakers presented in an adverse perceptual environment (e.g., Choe et al., 2012; Lam and Tjaden, 2013; McHenry, 2011; Tjaden and Wilding, 2011). Interestingly, both inter-listener and intra-listener variation for transcription is almost never reported, and listeners are expected to vary in the ability to use their perceptual strategies to recover the intended message (see Liss, 2007; McHenry, 2011). Transcription has also been criticized for not being wholly representative of perceptual processes used to understand connected speech (Hustad, 2008; Weismer, 2008).

Percent-correct scores for words and sentences also may not be sensitive to speech impairment for individuals with mild dysarthria. Sussman and Tjaden (2012) therefore proposed an operationally-defined construct termed "Speech Severity" (SS) to capture the perceptual consequences of mild dysarthria. Listeners were directed not to judge intelligibility, but to pay attention to overall speech naturalness and prosody when judging SS for a paragraph reading task using a computerized VAS (Sussman and Tjaden, 2012). Single word intelligibility and sentence intelligibility were obtained using percent-correct scores from word identification and orthographic transcription tasks, respectively. Only scaled judgments of SS distinguished disordered groups from neurotypical speakers. SS was further examined in a study that obtained computerized VAS judgments of SS and intelligibility for the same speech materials (Tjaden et al., 2013a). Judgments of SS correlated with sentence intelligibility judgments for all groups. The correlation was less robust for non-habitual conditions (i.e., Clear, Loud, Slow) compared to habitual speech style. Most importantly, the pattern of results for intelligibility versus SS differed for disordered and neurotypical speakers. Hence, the construct of SS may be sensitive to aspects of speech impairment not captured by traditional percent-correct word and sentence intelligibility scores and might prove useful for documenting treatment-related changes in speech production.

These studies, as well as others, suggest that scaling tasks have advantages and disadvantages. A global or overall judgment of intelligibility (or SS) does not require any computation, making it efficient and cost-effective. Scaling techniques also may be readily applied to extended speech samples, such as paragraphs or spontaneous speech. However, listener misperceptions cannot be examined, providing little insight into the listener's role in evaluating intelligibility. Since only an overall indication of overall speech impairment is supplied, scaling tasks may be used to document treatment progress or disease progression, but provide little direction for treatment to enhance intelligibility.

Perhaps the greatest concern with using subjective metrics, however, is reliability (Miller, 2013). For this reason, studies employing scaling tasks routinely include statistics of intra-judge and inter-judge reliability. However, standards for what constitutes adequate listener reliability for scaled intelligibility are lacking and metrics for quantifying reliability vary across studies (e.g., Kim and Kuo, 2012; Neel, 2009; Tjaden *et al.*, 2013a; Weismer *et al.*, 2001). The requirement that listener reliability be reported for scaled intelligibility stands in stark contrast to dysarthria studies employing transcription (e.g., Hustad, 2008; Hustad and Lee, 2008; Liss *et al.*, 1998; Liss *et al.*, 2000; McHenry, 2011). The different standards appear to stem from the expectation that reliability is often poorer for subjective metrics, as well as the lack of research directly comparing subjective and objective intelligibility metrics in dysarthria (Weismer *et al.*, 2008). Tjaden *et al.* (2014) sought to address this issue. Results indicated two key findings. First, VAS may provide a more conservative estimate of intelligibility change in dysarthria compared to transcription. Second, listener reliability (i.e., intra-judge and inter-judge) was virtually identical for both methods. Thus, regardless of whether an objective or subjective metric is employed, listeners vary within themselves, as well as among one another, in their judgments of intelligibility for mild dysarthria. Additional studies directly comparing subjective and objective intelligibility metrics in dysarthria are clearly needed. However, the Tjaden *et al.*, (2014) study is an important step in strengthening the scientific evidence base for using VAS in research as well as clinical practice to index overall intelligibility.

Perceptual environment and intelligibility

With few exceptions, listeners judge speech in a quiet room, the audio signal is presented at a comfortable loudness level, and there is no competing signal (i.e., white noise, multi-talker babble). Communication does not always occur in ideal contexts, however, and the importance of investigating speech intelligibility measurement in dysarthria in adverse listening conditions has been noted (Yorkston *et al.*, 2007a).

Multi-talker babble is an ecologically-valid adverse listening condition that has long been used to eliminate ceiling effects when studying intelligibility for neurotypical speakers (e.g., Lam and Tjaden, 2013; Smiljanić and Bradlow, 2009). Babble is only beginning to be used to study how intelligibility in dysarthria is impacted by an adverse perceptual environment, however. Unpublished data suggest that background noise impacts intelligibility in dysarthria in a slightly different way than for neurotypical talkers and may even differ depending on the perceptual characteristics of the dysarthria (McAuliffe *et al.*, 2008; McAuliffe *et al.*, 2009). Published studies are needed to substantiate these preliminary findings. We recently investigated intelligibility for speakers with mild dysarthria as well as neurotypical speakers in which sentence stimuli were mixed with 20-talker babble (Feenaughty *et al.*, 2013; Kuo *et al.*, 2014; Tjaden *et al.*, 2013 a, b; Tjaden *et al.*, 2014). The multi-talker babble not only eliminated expected ceiling effects, but is an adverse listening condition with high ecological validity. It should be noted that these studies did not compare intelligibility in quiet to intelligibility in background noise.

Knowledge of how adverse listening conditions impact intelligibility in dysarthria has important implications for developing an acoustically-based model of intelligibility. A first step is to establish whether acoustic variables explanatory for intelligibility in dysarthria in quiet also are explanatory for intelligibility in adverse listening conditions. The challenge of identifying acoustic variables truly explanatory for intelligibility is not trivial. Studies employing speech resynthesis to parametrically manipulate the acoustic signal of dysarthria are one approach to this complex problem (Neel, 2009; Weismer, 2008). Indeed, we recently demonstrated the feasibility of using the innovative speech resynthesis technique of "hybridization" to identify segmental, as well as suprasegmental variables explaining the improved intelligibility of clearly produced sentences for talkers with mild dysarthria secondary to PD (Tjaden *et al.*, 2014). If separate acoustically-based models of intelligibility in dysarthria are necessary for optimal (i.e., quiet) and adverse (i.e., multi-talker babble) listening conditions, this also would have implications for management. It seems plausible that a behavioral therapy technique could elicit changes in production that benefit intelligibility in an optimal listening condition, but the same technique may not elicit production changes that benefit intelligibility in adverse listening conditions.

Severity

The overall level of speech impairment or involvement in dysarthria is commonly described with labels like "mild," "moderate" or "severe" (Yorkston *et al.*, 2010). While the construct of severity is useful for describing speakers in both research and clinical practice, several inter-related factors are deserving of careful consideration moving forward, including the appropriate metric(s) for characterizing overall impairment, as well as procedures for classifying degree of speech impairment.

The construct of dysarthria severity has been approached in a variety of ways. Some studies simply refer to "mild, moderate or severe" dysarthria with no explanation as to how these labels were obtained (Fager *et al.*, 2010; Van Nuffelen *et al.*, 2010). In other studies, descriptors of severity reflect the impressionistic judgments of clinicians or researchers (Huber and Darling, 2011; Tjaden and Wilding, 2004). In other studies, severity descriptors have been derived from intelligibility metrics (Lansford and Liss, 2014; McHenry, 2003; Sussman and Tjaden, 2012). For example, Hustad (2008) designated speakers as mild, moderate, severe or profound on the basis of Sentence Intelligibility Test (SIT) scores (Yorkston *et al.*, 1996). Using intelligibility metrics as the basis for designating dysarthria severity is the most objective approach currently available, but is not without problems. First, intelligibility metrics vary across studies. One study may use transcriptions scores from a published intelligibility metric while another study uses transcription scores for experimental speech stimuli unique to that study. Still other studies use DMEs of intelligibility to designate severity. Scores for assigning severity also vary across study. For example, in Liss *et al.* (1998), speakers with "at least a moderate impairment" could score 96 percent on the SIT – a score that has carried the designation of mild dysarthria in other studies (Hustad, 2008; Sussman and Tjaden, 2012). A standard metric of dysarthria severity would help to facilitate direct comparison of speakers across studies and clinics. An existing, transcription-based published metric, such as the SIT (Yorkston *et al.*, 1996), is one solution. Alternatively, a set of speech stimuli explicitly for use in indexing severity could be developed along with standardized procedures for administration and scoring.

Finally, several issues pertaining to the study and management of speakers with "mild" dysarthria deserve comment. The designation of "mild" dysarthria here refers to individuals for whom intelligibility on the SIT (Yorkston *et al.*, 1996) approximates 90 percent. When transcription-based, sentence intelligibility is well preserved, the perceptual construct of SS, as operationally defined in Sussman and Tjaden (2012) and obtained for an extended sample of connected speech using a VAS, may prove a useful supplement for documenting the presence of dysarthria. Second, therapeutic techniques that aim to maximize intelligibility are appropriate for mild dysarthria. That is, unlike persons with moderate and severe involvement who require supplemental support to enhance or replace speech (i.e., iconic gestures, topic cues, augmentative communication), persons with mild involvement use natural speech for all of their communication needs, but have difficulty being understood in certain situations (Hustad and Weismer, 2007). Thus, persons with mild dysarthria can benefit from treatments that facilitate the ability to participate in life situations, such as being understood in a noisy restaurant (Yorkston *et al.*, 2010).

Cognitive–linguistic factors and dysarthria

Cognitive processes refer to mental processes that serve to facilitate attention, memory, and executive functions (i.e., reasoning, planning, and organizing behavior). There is growing appreciation that cognitive deficits can accompany acquired neurologic disorders associated with dysarthria, including progressive neurologic conditions traditionally thought to be sensorimotor in nature (i.e., PD, Amyotrophic Lateral Sclerosis). In many cases, even subtle changes in memory and attention, as well as slowing of the executive functions of reasoning, can have a large effect on daily activities important for life quality (Baylor *et al.*, 2010; Yorkston *et al.*, 2007b). It further seems likely that the co-occurrence of dysarthria and cognitive impairment may exacerbate the perceived deviancy of spoken communication and also may obscure the primary source of the communication deficit.

A great deal has been learned from previous research separately investigating dysarthria and cognitive deficits that may accompany neurologic diseases or conditions, such as MS. However, the role of cognitive variables in the speech production deficit of dysarthria is only beginning to be understood. The available empirical evidence for adults with acquired neurologic conditions includes studies investigating global speech timing characteristics (e.g., Feenaughty *et al.*, 2013; Huber and Darling, 2011; Lowit *et al.*, 2006; Rodgers *et al.*, 2013), linguistic characteristics (Feenaughty *et al.*, 2013) or perceptual characteristics (Wang *et al.*, 2005). Results of these studies suggest that speech rate, prosody, silent pause frequency, duration and grammatical appropriateness of pauses are most sensitive to cognitive deficits. Poorer judgments of sentence intelligibility have also been linked to cognitive deficits (Mackenzie and Green, 2009). In addition, cognitive deficits appear to manifest differently depending on the speech task (Feenaughty *et al.*, 2013). It is difficult to determine the underlying mechanism explaining findings in many of these studies because of the co-occurring effects of dysarthria and cognitive deficits. One way to address this problem is to pursue studies investigating the relative contributions of cognitive deficits versus dysarthria on spoken language characteristics as well as perceived speech adequacy using carefully selected clinical groups (e.g., speakers with dysarthria, speakers with and without cognitive deficits). Speech tasks thought to be sensitive to even subtle changes in cognition (e.g., oral reading, narrative) also may be helpful in evaluating the separate effects of dysarthria versus cognitive impairment on spoken language production. There are several clinical implications of this line of inquiry. Results will not only guide development of tools to detect the contribution of cognitive versus speech motor variables to spoken language deficits, but also may help to identify the most favorable window of opportunity to simultaneously address cognitive and speech motor variables in treatment. This work also will contribute to a comprehensive theory of spoken language and thus provide a foundation upon which to advance understanding of how cognitive function and motor speech behaviors interact for adults with acquired neurologic conditions.

Summary and conclusions

Several issues in contemporary research have emerged that have implications for development of a comprehensive theory of dysarthria. First, an acoustically-based classification system for distinguishing speakers with and without dysarthria appears to be feasible, although the implications of such a system for clinical practice remain to be determined. Intelligibility continues to be an important construct in the study and management of dysarthria, including individuals with mild speech impairment. For mild dysarthria, as suggested by transcription-based intelligibility metrics approaching 90 percent, the operationally-defined perceptual construct of SS (Sussman and Tjaden, 2012) may prove a useful supplement for indexing a reduction in prosodic adequacy and speech naturalness. Relatedly, VAS is an efficient way to globally index intelligibility (or the closely related construct of SS), with levels of intra-judge and inter-judge reliability comparable to transcription. The impact of ecologically-valid adverse listening conditions on intelligibility in dysarthria is an important topic for future research as is development of standards for designating levels of dysarthria severity. Finally, there is growing appreciation that cognitive impairment and dysarthria may co-occur in progressive neurologic diseases affecting seniors (i.e., PD), as well as progressive (i.e., MS) and acquired neurologic conditions (i.e., blast-related brain injury) affecting younger adults. Effective clinical management of the spoken language deficit in these individuals requires better understanding of how cognitive and motor speech variables interact.

Acknowledgment

Writing of this chapter supported in part by R01 DC004689.

References

Baylor, C., Yorkston, K., Bamer, A., Britton, D. and Amtmann, D. (2010), "Variables associated with communicative participation in people with multiple sclerosis: A regression analysis", *American Journal of Speech-Language Pathology*, Vol. 19, pp. 143–153.

Bunton, K., Kent, R.D., Duffy, J.R., Rosenbek, J.C. and Kent, J.F. (2007), "Listener agreement for auditory perceptual ratings of dysarthria", *Journal of Speech, Language and Hearing Research*, Vol. 50, pp. 1481–1495.

Choe, Y.-K., Liss, J.M., Azuma, T. and Mathy, P. (2012), "Evidence of cue use and performance differences in deciphering dysarthric speech", *The Journal of the Acoustical Society of America,* Vol. 131, No. 2, pp. EL112–EL118.

Darley, F.L., Aronson, A.E. and Brown, J.R. (1969a), "Differential diagnostic patterns of dysarthria", *Journal of Speech and Hearing Research*, Vol. 12, pp. 246–269.

Darley, F.L., Aronson, A.E. and Brown, J.R. (1969b), "Clusters of deviant speech dimensions in the dysarthrias", *Journal of Speech, Language, and Hearing Research*, Vol. 12, pp. 462–496.

Duffy, J. (2007), "Motor speech disorders: History, current practice, future trends and goals", in Weismer, G., (Ed.) *Motor Speech Disorders: Essays for Ray Kent*, Plural Publishing, San Diego, CA, US, pp. 7–56.

Duffy, J. (2013), *Motor Speech Disorders: Substrates, Differential Diagnosis, and Management*, 3rd Edition, Elsevier, St. Louis, MO, US.

Enderby, P.M. and Palmer, R. (2008), *Frenchay Dysarthria Assessment*, 2nd Edition, Pro-Ed, Austin, TX, US.

Fager, S.K., Beukelman, D.R., Jakobs, T. and Hosom, J.P. (2010), "Evaluation of a speech recognition prototype for speakers with moderate and severe dysarthria: A preliminary report", *Augmentative and Alternative Communication*, Vol. 26, pp. 267–277.

Feenaughty, L., Tjaden, K., Benedict, R.H. and Weinstock-Guttman, B. (2013), "Speech and pause characteristics in multiple sclerosis: A preliminary study of speakers with high and low neuropsychological test performance", *Clinical Linguistics and Phonetics*, Vol. 27, pp. 134–151.

Feenaughty, L., Tjaden, K. and Sussman, J. (2014), "Relationship between acoustic measures and judgments of intelligibility in Parkinson's disease: A within-speaker approach", *Clinical Linguistics and Phonetics*, Vol. 28, pp. 1–22.

Fonville, S., van der Worp, H.B., Maat, P., Aldenhoven, M., Algra, A. and van Gijn, J. (2008), "Accuracy and inter-observer variation in the classification of dysarthria from speech recordings", *Journal of Neurology*, Vol. 255, pp. 1545–1548.

Huber, J.E. and Darling, M. (2011), "Effect of Parkinson's disease on the production of structured and unstructured speaking tasks: Respiratory physiologic and linguistic considerations", *Journal of Speech, Language, and Hearing Research*, Vol. 54, pp. 33–46.

Hustad, K.C. (2008), "The relationship between listener comprehension and intelligibility scores for speakers with dysarthria", *Journal of Speech, Language, and Hearing Research*, Vol. 51, pp. 562–573.

Hustad, K.C. and Weismer, G. (2007), "Interventions to improve intelligibility and communicative success for speakers with dysarthria", in Weismer, G. (Ed.), *Motor Speech Disorders,* Plural Publishing, San Diego, CA, US, pp. 261–303.

Hustad, K.C. and Lee, J. (2008), "Changes in speech production associated with alphabet supplementation", *Journal of Speech, Language, and Hearing Research,* Vol. 51, pp.1438–1450.

Kent, R.D. and Kim, Y.J. (2003), "Toward an acoustic typology of motor speech disorders", *Clinical Linguistics and Phonetics,* Vol. 17, pp. 427–445.

Kent, R.D., Weismer, G. and Rosenbek, J.C. (1989), "Toward phonetic intelligibility testing in dysarthria", *Journal of Speech and Hearing Disorders,* Vol. 54, pp. 482–499.

Kim, Y. and Kuo, C. (2012), "Effect level of presentation to listeners on scaled speech intelligibility of speakers with dysarthria", *Folia Phoniatrica et Logopaedica,* Vol. 64, pp. 26–33.

Kim, Y., Kent, R.D. and Weismer, G. (2011), "An acoustic study of the relationships among neurologic disease, dysarthria type, and severity of dysarthria", *Journal of Speech, Language, and Hearing Research,* Vol. 54, pp. 417–429.

Kuo, C., Tjaden, K. and Sussman, J. (2014), "Acoustic and perceptual correlates of faster-than-habitual speech produced by speakers with Parkinson's disease and multiple sclerosis", *Journal of Communication Disorders,* Vol. 52, pp. 156–169.

Lam, J. and Tjaden, K. (2013), "Intelligibility of clear speech: Effect of instruction", *Journal of Speech, Language and Hearing Research,* Vol. 56, pp. 1429–1440.

Lansford, K.L. and Liss, J.M. (2014), "Vowel acoustics in dysarthria: Speech disorder diagnosis and classification", *Journal of Speech, Language, and Hearing Research,* Vol. 57, pp. 57–67.

Lansford, K.L., Liss, J.M. and Norton, R.E. (2014), "Free-classification of perceptually-similar speakers with dysarthria", *Journal of Speech, Language, and Hearing Research,* Vol. 57, pp. 2051–2064.

Liss, J.M. (2007), "The role of speech perception in motor speech disorders", in Weismer, G. (Ed.), *Motor Speech Disorders,* Plural, San Diego, CA, US, pp. 187–220.

Liss, J.M., Spitzer, S., Caviness, J.N., Adler, C. and Edwards, B. (1998), "Syllabic strength and lexical boundary decisions in the perception of hypokinetic dysarthric speech", *The Journal of the Acoustical Society of America,* Vol. 104, pp. 2457–2466.

Liss, J.M., Spitzer, S.M., Caviness, J.N., Adler, C. and Edwards, B.W. (2000), "Lexical boundary error analysis in hypokinetic and ataxic dysarthria", *Journal of the Acoustical Society of America,* Vol. 107, No. 6, pp. 3415–3424.

Liss, J.M., LeGendre, S. and Lotto, A.J. (2010), "Discriminating dysarthria type from envelope modulation spectra", *Journal of Speech, Language, and Hearing Research,* Vol. 53, pp. 1246–1255.

Lowit, A., Brendal, B., Dobinson, C. and Howell, P. (2006), "An investigation into the influence of age, pathology and cognition on speech production", *Journal of Medical Speech-Language Pathology,* Vol. 12, pp. 253–262.

Mackenzie, C. and Green, J. (2009), "Cognitive-linguistic deficit and speech intelligibility in chronic progressive multiple sclerosis", *International Journal of Language and Communication Disorders,* Vol. 44, pp. 401–420.

McAuliffe, M.J., Good, P.V., O'Beirne, G.A. and LaPointe, L.L. (2008), "Influence of auditory distraction upon intelligibility ratings in dysarthria", Poster presented at the Fourteenth Biennial Conference on Motor Speech - Motor Speech Disorders & Speech Motor Control, Monterey, CA, US, 6-9 Mar 2008. http://hdl.handle.net/10092/3398.

McAuliffe, M.J., Schaefer, M., O'Beirne, G.A. and LaPointe, L.L. (2009), "Effect of noise upon the perception of speech intelligibility in dysarthria", Poster presented at the American Speech-Language and Hearing Association Convention, New Orleans, LA, US, pp. 18-21 Nov, 2009. http://hdl.handle.net/10092/3410.

McHenry, M. (2003), "The effect of pacing strategies on the variability of speech movement sequences in dysarthria", *Journal of Speech, Language, and Hearing Research,* Vol. 46, pp. 702–710.

McHenry, M. (2011), "An exploration of listener variability in intelligibility judgments", *American Journal of Speech-Language Pathology,* Vol. 20, pp. 119–123.

Miller, N. (2013), "Measuring up to speech intelligibility", *International Journal of Language and Communication Disorders,* Vol. 48, pp. 601–612.

Neel, A. (2009), "Effects of loud and amplified speech on sentence and word intelligibility in Parkinson disease", *Journal of Speech, Language, and Hearing Research,* Vol. 52, pp. 1021–1033.

Rodgers, J.D., Tjaden, K., Feenaughty, L., Weinstock-Guttman, B. and Benedict, R.H.B. (2013), "Influence of cognitive function on speech and articulation rate in multiple sclerosis", *Journal of the International Neuropsychological Society*, Vol. 19, pp. 173–180.

Schiavetti, N. (1992), "Scaling procedures for the measurement of speech intelligibility", in Kent, R.D. (Ed.), *Intelligibility in Speech Disorders: Theory, Measurement and Management*, John Benjamins Publishing, Philadelphia, PA, US, pp. 11–34.

Smiljanić, R. and Bradlow, A.R. (2009), "Speaking and hearing clearly: Talker and listener factors in speaking style changes", *Language and Linguistics Compass*, Vol. 3, pp. 236–264.

Sussman, J.E. and Tjaden, K. (2012), "Perceptual measures of speech from individuals with Parkinson's disease and multiple sclerosis: Intelligibility and beyond", *Journal of Speech, Language, and Hearing Research*, Vol. 55, pp. 1208–1219.

Tjaden, K. and Wilding, G.E. (2004), "Rate and loudness manipulations in dysarthria: Acoustic and perceptual findings", *Journal of Speech, Language, and Hearing Research*, Vol. 47, pp. 766–783.

Tjaden, K. and Wilding, G. (2011), "Effects of speaking task on intelligibility in Parkinson's disease", *Clinical Linguistics and Phonetics*, Vol. 25, pp. 155–168.

Tjaden, K., Richards, E., Kuo, C., Wilding, G. and Sussman, J. (2013a), "Acoustic and perceptual consequences of clear and loud speech", *Folia Phoniatrica et Logopaedica*, Vol. 65, pp. 214–220.

Tjaden, K., Sussman, J.E. and Wilding, G.E. (2013b), "Impact of clear, loud and slow speech on scaled intelligibility and speech severity in Parkinson's disease and multiple sclerosis", *Journal of Speech, Language, and Hearing Research*, Vol. 57, pp. 779–792.

Tjaden, K., Kain, A. and Lam, J. (2014), "Hybridizing conversational and clear speech to investigate the source of increased intelligibility in Parkinson's disease", *Journal of Speech, Language and Hearing Research*, Vol. 57, No. 4, pp. 1191–1205.

Van Nuffelen, G., De Bodt, M., Vanderwegen, J., Van de Heyning, P. and Wuyts, F. (2010), "Effect of rate control on speech production and intelligibility in dysarthria", *Folia Phoniatrica et Logopaedica*, Vol. 62, pp. 110–119.

Wang, Y.T., Kent, R.D., Duffy, J.R. and Thomas, J.E. (2005), "Dysarthria associated with traumatic brain injury: Speaking rate and emphatic stress", *Journal of Communication Disorders*, Vol. 38, pp. 231–260.

Weismer, G. (2008), "Speech intelligibility", in Ball, M.J., Perkins, M.R., Muller, N. and Howard, S. (Eds.), *The Handbook of Clinical Linguistics*, Blackwell, Oxford, UK, pp. 568–582.

Weismer, G. and Laures, J.S. (2002), "Direct magnitude estimates of speech intelligibility in dysarthria: Effects of a chosen standard", *Journal of Speech Language, and Hearing Research*, Vol. 45, No. 3, pp. 421–433.

Weismer, G. and Kim, Y.J. (2010), "Classification and taxonomy of motor speech disorders: What are the issues", in Maassen, B. and Van Lieshout, P. (Eds.), *Speech Motor Control: New Developments in Basic and Applied Research*, Oxford University Press, New York, NY, pp. 229–241.

Weismer, G., Jeng, J-Y., Laures, J., Kent, R.D. and Kent, J.F. (2001), "Acoustic and intelligibility characteristics of sentence production in neurogenic speech disorders", *Folia Phoniatrica et Logopaedics*, Vol. 53, pp. 1–18.

Weismer, G., Barlow, S., Smith, A. and Caviness, J. (2008), "Special panel session: Driving critical initiatives in motor speech", *Journal of Medical Speech-Language Pathology*, Vol. 16, p. 283.

Yorkston, K.M. and Beukelman, D.R. (1984), *Assessment of Intelligibility of Dysarthric Speech*, Pro-Ed, Austin, TX, US.

Yorkston, K.M., Beukelman, D.R. and Hakel, M. (1996), *Speech Intelligibility Test for Windows Intelligibility Test*, Pro-Ed, Austin, TX, US.

Yorkston, K.M., Hakel, M., Beukelman, D.R. and Fager, S. (2007a), "Evidence for effectiveness of treatment of loudness, rate, or prosody in dysarthria: A systematic review", *Journal of Medical Speech–Language Pathology*, Vol. 15, pp. XI–XXXVI.

Yorkston, K.M., Baylor, C.R., Klasner, E.R., Deitz, J., Dudgeon, B.J., Eadie, T., *et al.*, (2007b), "Satisfaction with communicative participation as defined by adults with multiple sclerosis: A qualitative study", *Journal of Communication Disorders*, Vol. 40, pp. 433–451.

Yorkston, K., Beukelman, D., Strand, E. and Hakel, M. (2010), *Management of Motor Speech Disorders in Children and Adults*, Pro-Ed, Austin, TX, US.

SECTION III

Cognitive and linguistic-discourse systems of communication impairments

15

WHAT BILINGUALISM TELLS US ABOUT PHONOLOGICAL ACQUISITION

Elena Babatsouli and David Ingram

The study of bilingual language acquisition is a daunting area of research. First, there is the extensive number of possible language combinations. For example, suppose we restrict our initial investigations into the one hundred most linguistically diverse languages in the world. The permutation of those languages leads to 4,950 bilingual contexts. Next, each of these bilingual contexts needs to be examined for a wide range of research variables. There is the issue of when the child becomes bilingual, i.e. whether acquisition of the languages is simultaneous or dual, where simultaneous means both languages are present from birth, and dual means that the second language begins acquisition later, say from age three on. If the latter, there is the variable of which language is acquired earlier. Then we need to consider the contexts of the input in these bilingual contexts. Does the child hear one and/or both languages from a single speaker or multiple speakers? There are design issues concerning the number of necessary participants, and whether to conduct case studies or cross-sectional studies. We also have the various components of language (e.g. phonology, morphology, syntax, semantics) and the range of research questions, some of which are discussed below, to consider. When the math is done, the number of possible bilingual studies approaches one million. From this perspective, every study on bilingual language acquisition is one in a million!

This chapter reviews one piece of this daunting task, that being phonological acquisition in bilingual children. We begin with a brief discussion of the role of the lexicon in phonological acquisition, an integral role that is sometimes overlooked when the focus is restricted to just speech sounds. This is followed by an examination of when bilingual children identify and separate the input languages into two phonological systems. This is a central issue in determining the influence of bilingualism on phonological acquisition and its understanding is necessary for determining the extent to which bilingual acquisition informs our understanding of phonological acquisition. With the emergence of separation, the question arises regarding the extent and nature of interaction during the separation process. Does the language of bilingual children come to look the same as that of monolingual children and if not, to what extent are they different? We then briefly review bilingualism in relation to speech sound disorders, and the implications for typical and atypical bilingual phonological development. Lastly, we describe three examples of bilingual acquisition informing phonological acquisition in a way that studies restricted to monolingual acquisition could not.

The bilingual lexicon and phonological acquisition

The understanding of phonological acquisition in both monolingual and bilingual children involves the study of lexical development. A basic question is whether bilingual children begin with single or separate lexicons. The idea of a single vocabulary would fit if children acquired a single word for a particular concept, and avoided using words from both of the languages being acquired. The early research by Volterra and Taeschner (1978) proposed that this was the case. Later, Yavaş (1995) found that there were phonological properties of the words being acquired in the two languages that were influencing the words being used. In his study of a young Portuguese and Turkish bilingual girl, Yavaş found that the words selected by the girl were phonologically simple and she avoided words that contained more difficult sounds. Though the identification of lexical separation is no simple matter (e.g. Kehoe, 2011; Pearson *et al.*, 1993; Stoel-Gammon, 2011; Vihman, 1985, 2014), the results lean more toward relatively early vocabulary separation, and support the view that phonological characteristics influence the acquisition of the bilingual child's vocabulary.

Besides the question of vocabulary separation, there is the issue of how the phonological properties of the target languages influence the bilingual child's speech acquisition. Languages differ from one another in a variety of ways, such as in their rhythm patterns, phonological inventories, and syllabic structures. For phonological studies, these differences also have to be considered in relation to the vocabulary that children acquire. For example, English has a large number of polysyllabic words, that is, words that contain three or more syllables. Their acquisition will be a challenge to English learners (James, 2006). That challenge, however, does not take place during the acquisition of the early vocabulary which tends to be a majority of simple monosyllabic words. Individual speech sounds also show variation in this regard. English children show later acquisition of 'ch' (e.g. 'cheese') and 'l' (e.g. 'letter'), and this, in part, is likely influenced by their relatively low occurrence in early vocabulary. This is not the case, however, for children acquiring K'iche', a Mayan language spoken in Guatemala. These sounds are common in early words acquired in K'iche', and they are pronounced accurately from the onset of vocabulary acquisition (Pye, Ingram and List, 1987).

The influence of a language's rhythm pattern and syllabic structures in relation to age of acquisition also need to be considered. English, for example, has a stress-based system where stress may occur on the first, middle or last syllable depending on the word considered. Stress acquisition in English, therefore, will eventually be a problem when the child needs to determine the rules for placing stress in these more complex words. It is not a problem, however, for early vocabulary because most early words are monosyllabic or disyllabic with stress on the first syllable ('bottle', 'mommy' etc.). On the other hand, stress acquisition will be a problem for Russian-learning children since Russian stress placement is lexically based and needs to be learned for the individual words.

There is a trade off in complexity between English and Spanish when it comes to timing of syllables when compared to stress. Spanish timing is relatively even from syllable to syllable since Spanish does not shorten unstressed syllables while English reduces the vowel in that syllable to a schwa vowel (e.g. Spanish 'mañana' vs. English 'banana', both stressed on the second syllable). Determining how monolingual children acquire these early word patterns is a challenging enough task. Imagine the task for the bilingual child who needs to figure them out for each language along with determining in the early stages which words belong to which language (cf. Bunta and Ingram, 2007).

In summary, the study of bilingual phonological acquisition needs to begin with a careful assessment of the phonological properties of the early target vocabulary. These characteristics will influence the rate of acquisition of individual sounds, rhythm patterns, and syllable structures. This assessment will be crucial in identifying when language separation takes place. It is also important in determining possible influences between the two languages that will help identify in turn differences in bilingual versus monolingual phonological acquisition.

One vs. two phonological systems

When does phonological separation take place? The attempts to answer this question have led to a long-standing 'one versus two phonological systems' controversy, mirroring similar arguments for the lexicon and syntax (Swain, 1972; Swain and Wesche, 1975). The earliest position on this matter was that there is an integrated phonological system initially, a proposal based on the lack of adequate phonetic evidence for 100 percent, clear-cut separation (Burling, 1959/1978; Leopold, 1949; Schnitzer and Krasinski, 1994; Vogel, 1975). Children were believed eventually to 'split' the languages (Leopold, 1953/1954, p. 141) sometime in their development. Subsequent interpretations of these studies (e.g. Krasinski, 1989) have led to a position known as the 'unitary language systems hypothesis' (Genesee, 1989).

There were already indications in the early studies, however, that the unitary hypothesis might not accurately capture the phonological organization of young bilingual children. When Leopold (1953/1954, p. 24) writes "infants … weld *the double presentation* [our italics] into one unified speech system," he may well be talking about two languages immaturely communicated by the child as if they were one. Burling (1959/1978) discussed the possibility that bilingual children may favor a mechanism for separating the vowels in each language, but not the consonants. Even Vogel (1975, p. 51) who is often cited as supporting the unitary hypothesis, discussed "analogous phonological/phonotactic processes" with differences reflecting the "phonological distribution of the two languages." All of these comments are suggestive of subtle language interaction rather than one linguistic system.

The shift to a 'differentiated language systems hypothesis' (Genesee, 1989), whereby children acquire separate phonologies from the onset of word acquisition begins with Ingram (1981). In a case study of an Italian–English bilingual child, the study found differences in the child's syllables and distribution of consonants in each language that suggested early emergent differences, even though the phonetic inventories were highly similar. This led to new studies that took a closer look for more subtle phonological differences. Separation of phonological systems has been subsequently supported with evidence on phonemes (e.g. Schnitzer and Krasinski, 1996), the voicing contrast and VOT (Deuchar and Clark, 1996; Kehoe *et al.*, 2004), prosodic patterns (e.g. Gut, 2000; Johnson and Lancaster, 1998; Keshavarz and Ingram, 2002; Paradis, 1996), and other processes (Brulard and Carr, 2003).

Interestingly, the issue of when bilingual children separate the two phonological systems may be independent from other aspects of bilingual acquisition, such as the time of exposure and the nature of the input, though the issue is far from resolved. Holm and Dodd (1999) reported separation of systems in dual language acquisition. A study on simultaneous Greek/English acquisition of phonology (Babatsouli, 2013) documented separated phonologies, based on consonant inventories and phonotactic rules. These differences occurred despite the fact that the child, raised in Greece and was only exposed to the mother's second-language English from age 1;0 on. The ability to determine when separation takes place, however, does become more difficult to determine when there is 'interlanguage ambiguity' (Paradis, 2000) that is, when there are overlapping characteristics of the two languages. One such example is when similar languages have a number of cognates, i.e. etymologically related words (Bosch and Ramon-Casas, 2011; see also Bunta *et al.*, 2006).

As the focus of research shifted from the unitary approach to one of emerging separation, so did the effort to identify more explicit patterns of possible development. Keshavarz and Ingram (2002) discussed possible variations of phonological acquisition in bilingual children based on ideas expressed in Paradis and Genesee (1996). One possibility is that of *autonomy*, whereby bilingual children acquire the phonologies separately, so that each language is acquired in a fashion comparable to that of monolingual children (Schnitzer and Krasinski, 1996). A variation of autonomy would be *delay*, whereby the patterns of acquisition are autonomous, but the rate of acquisition is slowed down due to acquiring two languages simultaneously. An alternative possibility is that each language to some extent influences the acquisition of the other, such that there is *interdependence* (Johnson and Lancaster, 1998). Another option is that the direction of influence may only be in one direction, that is, that there is *transfer* from a dominant language to the other less dominant language. Still another way that one language might influence another is a situation of *acceleration* whereby the existence of a phonological characteristic in one language might accelerate the acquisition of the same characteristic in the other.

It is a complex challenge to research all the aspects of bilingual phonological acquisition so that we can see if one or even all of these possibilities take place. It requires the detailed study of all the different ways that languages phonologically differ from each other. Further, it requires accurate identification of the ages at which monolingual and bilingual children acquire these different phonological characteristics. Only then can we say with any confidence that one thing is acquired before something else.

The focus in recent years has shifted toward identifying the general characteristics of interdependence, transfer, and acceleration (Fabiano-Smith and Barlow, 2010; Lleó and Kehoe, 2002; Paradis, 1996). For example, Fabiano-Smith and Bunta (2012) provide some evidence that bilingual children have VOT characteristics that are different from those of monolinguals (e.g. shorter values). Barlow *et al.* (2013) compared monolinguals vs. bilinguals' acoustic correlates of [l] and found evidence of merged phonetic categories specific to the bilinguals only. Given the complexity of the issue, it is likely that determining the exact nature and degree of interaction will remain elusive for some time.

Monolingual vs. bilingual acquisition

There is a range of evidence that suggests bilingual and monolingual phonological acquisition are simultaneous in the sense that both are guided by the same underlying principles (e.g. Bunta *et al.*, 2009; Ingram, 1981; Lleó and Kehoe, 2002; Paradis, 1996, 2001). Examples of milestones found in both monolingual and bilingual acquisition include meaningful holophrases beginning in the second year (e.g. Brulard and Carr, 2003; Ingram, 1989; Ronjat, 1913); an early silence period (e.g. Paradis, 2011); individual variation (e.g. Leonard *et al.*, 1980; Paradis, 2011); the same phonological processes, e.g. #sC cluster reduction patterns in English monolinguals and Spanish–English, Haitian Creole–English bilinguals (Yavaş, 2011), etc. Comparable similarities are found for bilinguals with speech sound disorders and language impairment (Bunta and Douglas, 2013; Ingram, 2012).

Despite an overall similarity in monolingual and bilingual acquisition, researchers have identified subtle differences in the individual languages of bilingual children. For example, Lleó *et al.* (2003) reported greater use of coda consonants in Spanish for bilingual English–Spanish children than for monolingual Spanish children. Keshavarz and Ingram (2002) found examples of mutual influence in their study of an English–Farsi bilingual child. Ball *et al.* (2001) found that Welsh–English bilingual children acquired trills earlier in Welsh than in English. The dominance of one language over another did not lead to differences for bilingual Cantonese–

Putonghau children, however, where Cantonese was acquired earlier regardless of which language was dominant (Law and So, 2010). These and other examples are reviewed in Goldstein and McLeod (2012), where they concluded that the overall rate of such phenomena was relatively low (7 percent of potential instances).

Speech sound disorders and assessment

There is no consensus regarding speech sound disorders in monolingual children, much less in bilingual children. In monolingual children, the distinction is often one of a *delay* versus a *disorder*. It seems reasonable that the same distinction may be made for bilingual children (Goldstein and Gildersleeve-Neumann, 2012). The question of what is a disorder in monolingual children needs to be resolved before much progress regarding bilingualism can be made.

Research on multilingual speech disorders is selectively reviewed in Ingram (2012) who reports that cross-linguistic differences in typical development are also mirrored in children with speech sound disorders, based on the few available studies. For example, [v] is a late acquisition for English, but an earlier one in Swedish and Italian. Data reported for children with speech sound disorders in Swedish (Nettelbladt, 1983) and in Italian (Ingram *et al.*, 1993) revealed early usage of [v] as well (see also Topbaş, 2007 for similar results on other sounds in Turkish). A difference between monolingual vs. bilingual children in speech development, however, is reported for Canadian French–English bilinguals with specific language impairment (SLI) when compared to monolingual Canadian French children with SLI (MacLeod and McCauley, 2003). Measures of word complexity revealed lower rates of consonant correctness in the bilingual group, related to their tendency to attempt more complex words. The result, however, may be more the consequence of language impairment than of a speech sound disorder.

One important strategy in better understanding bilingual acquisition is to explore the extent to which current approaches in assessing monolingual children are appropriate for the assessment of bilingual acquisition (Paradis *et al.*, 2013). For example, it is currently recommended that assessment and/or intervention on disordered and impaired speech should be: *phonological*, accounting for phonetic complexity/frequency and functional load; and *multidimensional*, evaluating phonetic inventories, articulation, word complexity/correctness and shape (Ingram and Dubasik 2011); while tackling treatment on both the *auditory and production* front (c.f. Ingram, 2012 and references therein). Some current assessment guidelines in bilingual speech disorders are described by Fabiano-Smith and Goldstein (2010), McLeod (2012), and Topbaş and Yavaş (2010) for a comprehensive list of tests employed in child speech pathology cross-linguistically (also check: www.csu.edu.au/research/multilingual-speech/speech-assessments).

Bilingualism informing phonological acquisition

The study of bilingual phonological acquisition is an important component for understanding phonological acquisition in general. The study of cross-linguistic acquisition provides a broader understanding than can be obtained by the study of a single language, such as English. So far the review has identified the primary areas of bilingual phonological acquisition and some of the main findings to date. The assumption is that identifying both similarities and differences between monolingual and bilingual acquisition would provide the foundation for determining specific insights into the understanding of phonological acquisition. We conclude the review with three examples of bilingual acquisition informing phonological acquisition in a way distinct from the study of monolingual development.

The first example deals with the question of what determines the order in which children acquire the phonological characteristics of their language. The prominent view for many years is what Bunta, Davidovich and Ingram (2006) referred to as the *Constraint-driven* model. Simply stated, this view is that the order of acquisition of phonology is determined by phonetic/ phonological complexity such that simple sounds are acquired early, while complex sounds are acquired later. Such a viewpoint, however, does not capture the findings discussed earlier whereby K'iche' children acquired 'ch' and 'l' much earlier than English children. Pye, Ingram and List (1987) proposed that it was due to the *functional load* of these sounds, that is, that their lexical frequency in K'iche' was greater than in English. Bunta *et al.* (2006) expand this latter account to a *Target-driven* model, which proposes that the complexity of the target language plays an important role in phonological acquisition in addition to speech complexity. They tested the two models in the analysis of a bilingual girl's acquisition of English and Hungarian. The Constraint-driven model predicts that the speech/phonology of the child would be similar for both languages, since complexity constraints should apply uniformly across the languages. They found, however, that her speech production in the two languages in terms of word length and consonant correctness was significantly different, with the English productions being less complex. There was no significant difference, however, in the proximity of her productions to the target words in both languages (approximately 68 percent in both cases). This is consistent with the Target-driven model, which states that the child's primary attention is to make sure that her speech forms are relatively close to the target language so that intelligibility is maintained.

The second example concerns the study of the influence of environment on phonological development. Babatsouli (2013) reported a case study of a bilingual English–Greek child who acquired English primarily from the mother, and Greek from a much wider range of speakers. The difference in input did not have a negative impact on the acquisition of either language. An even more striking example of 'environmental plasticity' is found in Tse and Ingram (1987). They report the phonological development of a Cantonese girl, Wai, who was acquiring two dialects of Cantonese, one dialect that distinguished /l/ and /n/ (the mother's dialect), and one that merged /l/ and /n/ into a single phoneme /l/ (the father's dialect). The child was primarily exposed to the mother's /l/ dialect, while she occasionally heard the /l, n/ dialect from the father and the father's parents. The child did not use the strategy of acquiring the dialect of one parent or the other, but treated the input of /l/ and /n/ words as a single linguistic input. Thus, she treated them as allophones of a single phoneme and used [l] and [n] in free variation, both for words she heard with just /l/ and the other words she would hear with both (the /n/ words in the mother's dialect that would be produced with /l/ in the father's dialect). The child took over a year before she finally sorted out the difference. As with the previous example, the effect of the input can be determined most clearly in a bilingual (or in this case bi-dialectal) context.

The third example concerns the speech disorder in which a child shows disfluency, a situation traditionally referred to as stuttering. One central question concerns whether there are cases in which the disfluency is not just a motor problem, but rather also one resulting from linguistic factors. A preliminary study by Carias and Ingram (2006) explored this issue in four English–Spanish bilingual children identified by a speech–language pathologist as having a fluency problem. If the disfluencies were the result of a motor speech problem, then the patterns of disfluency should be similar in both languages. They categorized the disfluencies of each child by language, examining repetitions, insertions, prolongations, and revisions. They found that the patterns of disfluency were linguistically different for each child, and that the specific differences varied with each child. Two of the children showed greater disfluencies for English, while two others did so for Spanish. Interestingly, there was a pattern whereby the language with the greatest number of disfluencies also tended to be the one with larger mean length of utterances (MLUs). That is, disfluencies correlated with linguistic complexity. Though just a preliminary study, it demonstrates the value of exploring this issue with bilingual participants.

Summary

A bilingual child is one who is acquiring two languages from an early age either simultaneously or successively where the onset of acquiring the second occurs before the first one is completed. Given the wide diversity of phonological characteristics in the languages of the world, the child will most likely be exposed to a wide range of phonological patterns that will need to be sorted out. This child will likely show an early awareness of some of these characteristics, and will do remarkably well at keeping them separated. Some differences from monolingual development of either language, however, will occur, and the exact pattern of those will require careful study. Given ample input in both languages, we predict that he or she will show environmental plasticity, and will make a subconscious effort to be equally intelligible in both languages. These general findings provide a good start for sorting out all the details in future studies. One down and only 995,000 or so studies to go!

References

Babatsouli, E. (2013), *Phonological Development of a Child's L2 English in Bilingualism*, Unpublished Doctoral Dissertation, University of Crete.

Ball, M., Mueller, N. and Munro, S. (2001), "The acquisition of rhotic consonants by Welsh-English bilingual children", *International Journal of Bilingualism*, Vol. 5, pp. 71–86.

Barlow, J.A., Branson, P.E. and Nip, I.S.B. (2013), "Phonetic equivalence in the acquisition of /l/ by Spanish-English bilingual children", *Bilingualism: Language and Cognition*, Vol. 16, pp. 68–85.

Bosch, L. and Ramon-Casas, M. (2011), "Variability in vowel production by bilingual speakers: Can input properties hinder the early stabilization of contrastive categories?", *Journal of Phonetics*, Vol. 39, pp. 514–526.

Brulard, I. and Carr, P. (2003), "French-English bilingual acquisition of phonology: One production system or two?", *International Journal of Bilingualism*, Vol. 7, pp. 177–202.

Bunta, F. and Ingram, D. (2007), "The acquisition of speech rhythm by bilingual Spanish and English-speaking 4- and 6-year-old children", *Journal of Speech, Language, and Hearing Research*, Vol. 50, pp. 999–1014.

Bunta, F. and Douglas, M. (2013), "The effects of dual language support on the English skills of bilingual children with cochlear implants and hearing aids as compared to monolingual peers", *Language, Speech and Hearing Services in the Schools*, Vol. 44, pp. 281–290.

Bunta, F., Davidovich, I. and Ingram, D. (2006), "The relationship between the phonological complexity of a bilingual child's words and those of the target languages", *International Journal of Bilingualism*, Vol. 10, pp. 71–88.

Bunta, F., Fabiano-Smith, L., Goldstein, B.A. and Ingram, D. (2009), "Phonological whole-word measures in three-year-old bilingual children and their age-matched monolingual peers", *Clinical Linguistics and Phonetics*, Vol. 23, pp. 156–175.

Burling, R. (1959/1978), "Language development of a Garo and English child", *Word*, Vol. 15, pp. 45–68. Reprinted in E.M. Hatch (Ed.) (1978), *Second Language Acquisition*, Newbury House, Rowley, MA, US, pp. 54–75.

Carias, S. and Ingram, D. (2006), "Language and disfluency: Four case studies on Spanish-English bilingual children", *Journal of Multilingual Communication Disorders*, Vol. 4, pp. 149–157.

Deuchar, M. and Clark, A. (1996), "Early bilingual acquisition of the voicing contrast in English and Spanish", *Journal of Phonetics*, Vol. 24, pp. 351–365.

Fabiano-Smith, L. and Barlow, J. (2010), "Interaction in bilingual phonological acquisition: Evidence from phonetic inventories", *The International Journal of Bilingual Education and Bilingualism*, Vol. 13, pp. 81–97.

Fabiano-Smith, L. and Goldstein, B. (2010), "Assessment and intervention in bilingual children", in S. Levey (Ed.) *Language Development, Disorders, and Differences*, Sage Publishing, Inc., Thousand Oaks, CA, US.

Fabiano-Smith, L. and Bunta, F. (2012), "Voice onset time of voiceless bilabial and velar stops in 3-year-old bilingual children and their age-matched monolingual peers", *Clinical Linguistics and Phonetics*, Vol. 26, pp. 148–163.

Genesee, F. (1989), "Early bilingual development: One language or two?", *Journal of Child Language*, Vol. 6, pp. 161–179.

Goldstein, B. and Gildersleeve-Neumann, C. (2012), "Phonological development and disorders", in B. Goldstein (Ed.) *Bilingual Language Development and Disorders*, 2nd Edn., Paul Brookes, Baltimore, MD, US, pp. 285–307.

Goldstein, B. and McLeod, S. (2012), "Typical and atypical multilingual speech acquisition", In S. McLeod and B. Goldstein (Eds.), *Multilingual Aspects of Speech Sound Disorders in Children*, Multilingual Matters, Bristol, UK, pp. 84–95.

Grosjean, F. (2013), "Bilingualism: A short introduction", in F. Grosjean, F. and P. Li, *The Psycholinguistics of Bilingualism*, Wiley Blackwell, Malden, MA, US and Oxford, UK, pp. 5–26.

Gut, U. (2000), *Bilingual Acquisition of Intonation: A Study of Children Speaking German and English*, Niemeyer, Tübingen, Germany.

Holm, A. and Dodd, B. (1999), "A longitudinal study of the phonological development of two Cantonese-English bilingual children", *Applied Psycholinguistics*, Vol. 20, pp. 349–376.

Ingram, D. (1981), "The emerging phonological system of an Italian-English bilingual child", *Journal of Italian Linguistics*, Vol. 2, pp. 95–113.

Ingram, D. (1989), *First Language Acquisition: Method, Description and Explanation*. Cambridge University Press, Cambridge, UK.

Ingram, D. (2012), "Prologue: Cross-linguistic and multilingual aspects of speech sound disorders in children", in S. McLeod and B. Goldstein (Eds.), *Multilingual Aspects of Speech Sound Disorders in Children*, Multilingual Matters, Bristol, UK, pp. 3–12.

Ingram, D. and Dubasik, V.L. (2011), "Multidimensional assessment of phonological similarity within and between children", *Clinical Linguistics and Phonetics*, Vol. 25, pp. 962–967.

Ingram, D. and Dubasik, V.L. (2014), "Sibling rivalry: Comparing phonological similarity between twin and non-twin siblings", in A.W. Farris-Trimble and J.A. Barlow (Eds.), *Perspectives on Phonological Theory and Development*, John Benjamins Publishing Co., Philadelphia, PA, US, pp. 53–70.

Ingram, D., Bortolini, U. and Dykstra, K. (1993), "The acquisition of the feature [voice] in normal and phonologially delayed children", Paper presented to the Symposium on Research in Child Language Disorders, U. Wisconsin, US.

Ingram, D., Dubasik, V.L., Liceras, J. and Fernandez-Fuertes, R. (2011), "Early phonological acquisition in a set of English-Spanish bilingual twins", in C. Sanz and R. Leow (Eds.), *Implicit and Explicit Language Learning*, Georgetown University Press, Washington, DC, US, pp. 195–205.

James, D.G.H. (2006), *Hippopotamus Is So Hard to Say: Children's Acquisition of Polysyllabic Words*, Unpublished Doctoral Dissertation, University of Sydney, Australia.

Johnson, C.E. and Lancaster, P. (1998), "The development of more than one phonology: A case study of a Norwegian-English bilingual child", *International Journal of Bilingualism*, Vol. 2, pp. 265–300.

Kehoe, M. (2011), "Relationships between lexical and phonological development: A look at bilingual children – A commentary on Stoel-Gammon's 'Relationships between lexical and phonological development in young children'", *Journal of Child Language*, Vol. 38, pp. 75–81.

Kehoe, M., Lleó, C. and Rakow, M, (2004), "Voice onset time in bilingual German-Spanish children", *Bilingualism: Language and Cognition*, Vol. 7, No. 1, pp. 71–88.

Keshavarz, M.H. and Ingram, D. (2002), "The early phonological development of a Farsi-English bilingual child", *International Journal of Bilingualism*, Vol. 6, No. 3, pp. 255–269.

Krasinski, E. (1989), *Simultaneous Acquisition and the Bioprogram: A Case Study*, Unpublished doctoral dissertation, University of the West Indies, Kingston, Jamaica.

Law, N.C.W. and So, L.K.H. (2010), "The relationship of phonological development and language dominance in bilingual Cantonese-Putonghua children", *International Journal of Bilingualism*, Vol. 10, No. 4, pp. 405–427.

Leonard, L.B., Newhoff, M. and Mesalam, L. (1980), "Individual differences in early child phonology", *Applied Psycholinguistics*, Vol. 1, pp. 7–30.

Leopold, W.F. (1949), *Speech Development of a Bilingual Child: A Linguist's Record*, Northwestern University Press, Evanston, IL, US.

Leopold, W.F. (1953/54), "Patterning in children's language learning", *Language Learning*, Vol. 5, pp. 1–14.

Lleó, C. and Kehoe, M. (2002), "On the interaction of phonological systems in child bilingual acquisition", *International Journal of Bilingualism*, Vol. 6, pp. 233–237.

Lleó, C., Kuchenbrandt, I., Kehoe, M. and Trujillo, C. (2003), "Syllable final consonants in Spanish and German monolingual and bilingual acquisition", in N. Miller (Ed.), *(In)vulnerable Domains in Multilingualism*, John Benjamins, Amsterdam, pp. 191–220.

MacLeod, A.A. and McCauley (2003), "The phonological abilities of bilingual children with specific language impairment: A descriptive study", *Journal of Speech-Language Pathology and Audiology*, Vol. 27, pp. 29–44.

McLeod, S. (2012), "Multilingual speech assessment", in S. McLeod and B.A. Goldstein (Eds.), *Multilingual Aspects of Speech Sound Disorders in Children*, Multilingual Matters, Bristol, UK, pp. 113–143.

Nettelbladt, E. (1983), *Developmental Studies of Dysphonology in Children*, Travaux de L'Institut de Linguistique de Lund, CWK Gleerup, Lund, Sweden.

Paradis, J. (1996), "Prosodic development and differentiation in bilingual first language acquisition", in A. Stringfellow, A.D. Cahana-Amitay, E. Hughes and A. Zukowski (Eds.), *Proceedings of the 20th Annual Boston University Conference on Language Development*, Cascadilla Press, Somerville, MA, US, pp. 528–539.

Paradis, J. (2000), "Beyond 'one system or two': Degrees of separation between languages of French English bilingual children", in S. Döpke (Ed.), *Cross-linguistic Structures in Simultaneous Bilingualism*, John Benjamins, Amsterdam/Philadelphia, US, pp. 175–200.

Paradis, J. (2001), "Do bilingual two-year-olds have separate phonological systems?", *International Journal of Bilingualism*, Vol. 5, pp. 19–38.

Paradis, J. (2011), "Individual differences in child English second language acquisition: Comparing child-internal and child-external factors", *Linguistic Approaches to Bilingualism*, Vol. 1, No. 3, pp. 213–237.

Paradis, J. and Genesee, F. (1996), "Syntactic acquisition in bilingual children: Autonomous or interdependent?", *Studies in Second Language Acquisition*, Vol. 18, pp. 1–25.

Paradis, J., Schneider, P. and Sorenson Duncan, T. (2013), "Discriminating children with language impairment among English language learners from diverse first language backgrounds", *Journal of Speech, Language and Hearing Research*, Vol. 56, pp. 971–981.

Pearson, B., Fernandez, S. and Oller, D.K. (1993), "Lexical development in bilingual infants and toddlers: Comparison to monolingual norms", *Language Learning*, Vol. 43, pp. 93–120.

Pye, C., Ingram, D. and List, H. (1987), "A comparison of initial consonant acquisition in English and Quiché", in K.E. Nelson and A. van Kleeck (Eds.), *Children's Language*, Vol. 6. Lawrence Erlbaum, Hillsdale, NJ, US, pp. 175–190.

Ronjat, J. (1913), *Le développement du langage observé chez un enfant bilingue*, Champion, Paris.

Schnitzer, M.L. and Krasinski, E. (1994), "The development of segmental phonological production in a bilingual child", *Journal of Child Language*, Vol. 21, pp. 585–622.

Schnitzer, M.L. and Krasinski, E. (1996), "The development of segmental phonological production in a bilingual child: A contrasting second case", *Journal of Child Language*, Vol. 23, pp. 547–571.

Stoel-Gammon, C. (2011), "Relationships between lexical and phonological development in young children", *Journal of Child Language*, Vol. 38, pp. 1–34.

Swain, M. (1972), *Bilingualism as a First Language*, Unpublished doctoral dissertation, University of California, Irvine, US.

Swain, M. and Wesche, M. (1975), "Linguistic interaction: Case study of a bilingual child", *Language Sciences*, Vol. 37, pp. 17–22.

Topbaş, S. (2007), "Turkish speech acquisition", in S. McLeod (Ed.), *The International Guide to Speech Acquisition*, Thomson Delmar Learning, Clifton Park, NY, US, pp. 566–579.

Topbaş S. and Yavaş, M, (2010), *Communication Disorders in Turkish*, Multilingual Matters, Bristol, UK.

Tse, S-M. and Ingram, D. (1987), "The influence of dialect variation on phonological acquisition: A case study on the acquisition of Cantonese", *Journal of Child Language*, Vol. 14, pp. 281–294.

Vihman, M.M. (1985), "Language differentiation by the bilingual infant", *Journal of Child Language*, Vol. 12, pp. 297–324.

Vihman, M.M. (2014), *Phonological Development: The First Two Years*, John Wiley and Sons, West Sussex, UK.

Vogel, I. (1975), "One system or two: An analysis of a two-year-old Romanian-English bilingual's phonology", *Papers and Reports on Child Language Development*, Vol. 9, pp. 43–62.

Volterra, V. and Taeschner, T. (1978), "The acquisition and development of language by bilingual children", *Journal of Child Language*, Vol. 5, pp. 311–326.

Yavaş, M. (1995), "Phonological selectivity in the first fifty words of a bilingual child", *Language and Speech*, Vol. 38, pp. 189–202.

Yavaş, M. (2011), "Patterns of cluster reduction in the acquisition of #sC onsets: Are bilinguals different from monolinguals?", *Clinical Linguistics and Phonetics*, Vol. 25, pp. 981–988.

16

INFORMATION PROCESSING IN CHILDREN WITH SPECIFIC LANGUAGE IMPAIRMENT

James W. Montgomery, Ronald B. Gillam and Julia L. Evans

Children with specific language impairment (SLI) are those who demonstrate normal-range hearing and nonverbal intelligence and an absence of developmental disability (e.g., Autism, Fragile X syndrome) yet show marked receptive and/or expressive language difficulties for their age. Despite demonstrating normal-range nonverbal intelligence, however, these children evidence limitations in a wide range of cognitive or information processing abilities. Information processing refers to the mechanisms within human cognition that allow humans, for example, to perceive, attend, remember, interpret, learn, and problem solve. In this chapter, we provide a brief overview of children with SLI and focus on the following: 1) information processing abilities (i.e., memory, attention); 2) the association between information processing and language; and 3) clinical assessment and intervention implications. We focus on school-age children between the ages of 6 and 12 years.

Information processing in children with SLI

Memory

Memory is a broad mental construct for explaining the storage, retrieval, and use of information. Numerous theories and models have been proposed to characterize its architecture and function. Within the SLI literature, memory has been examined mainly from the perspective of working memory. For this reason, we will review this literature. Working memory concerns the concurrent short-term storage and manipulation of information.

Working memory

Because working memory (WM) is strongly related to a variety of higher-order cognitive abilities (Cowan *et al.*, 2005; Engle *et al.*, 1999), it has been the subject of much research focus. There exist a number of different models of WM varying in architectural and functional detail. Irrespective of theory-dependent differences, there is general agreement among researchers that WM is a multi-mechanism construct involving the ability to store information while concurrently performing some kind of mental activity (Baddeley, 1998; Barrouillet *et al.*, 2009).

WM performance is conventionally measured using complex span tasks that require both information storage and processing. Within the verbal domain, a conventional listening span task requires children to listen to sets of sentences. Each sentence has a corresponding separate item (word or digit) that needs to be recalled later. Children are asked to: 1) judge the truth value of each sentence (processing component) and; 2) immediately after each sentence set, recall as many of the items as they can in serial order (storage component). Item recall is typically the score of interest and reflects children's storage capacity while performing a concurrent processing activity. Such tasks are complex because in order to perform at age-appropriate levels children must engage various attentional control (or executive function) mechanisms (see the subsequent section titled "Attentional control") as they coordinate the processing and storage requirements of the task.

In addition to some kind of limited-capacity storage components (verbal, nonverbal/visuo-spatial), all WM models assume a resource-limited attention mechanism comprising various control mechanisms that play a crucial role in WM performance (Barrouillet et al., 2009; Unsworth and Engle, 2007). During a WM task, an individual switches his/her attentional focus (mental focus) between the processing and storage components such that he/she: 1) allocates attentional focus to the processing activity immediately followed by; 2) a momentary switch of attentional focus away from processing to storage in order to refresh the to-be-recalled items (Barrouillet et al., 2009). These control mechanisms are domain general in that they participate in the performance of both verbal and nonverbal cognitive tasks.

Relative to age peers, many children with SLI show marked deficits in WM-related storage capacity (Hoffman and Gillam, 2004; Archibald and Gathercole, 2007). Storage capacity can be indexed as either simple storage, referred to as short-term memory (STM), or complex storage (WM). Simple storage reflects the ability to remember and recall as many items (digits, words) in the same order they were presented in the absence of performing any other (concurrent) task. Relative to age peers, children with SLI tend to exhibit reduced simple storage capacity for verbal material (Archibald and Gathercole, 2007; Ellis Weismer et al., 1999; Gillam et al., 1995). By contrast, preliminary findings suggest that children with SLI and age peers may have similar nonverbal storage capacity (Archibald and Gathercole, 2007) although considerably more work is required in this area.

Unlike simple storage tasks that require information storage only, complex memory tasks invite children to store information in the face of performing some kind of cognitive processing task. Much evidence suggests that, relative to age mates, children with SLI, have significant limitations in complex verbal and nonverbal memory (Archibald and Gathercole, 2007; Hoffman and Gillam, 2004; Montgomery, 2000; Windsor et al., 2008). Ellis Weismer et al. (1999), for instance, compared the complex storage capacity of children with SLI and age peers using a conventional listening span task. Children were presented sets of simple sentences, such as "*Pumpkins are purple*," and asked to comprehend the truth value of each sentence and then recall as many of the sentence-final words as possible after each set. The SLI and control groups yielded similar comprehension. But the group with SLI showed significantly poorer word recall. Similar results have been reported by others (Archibald and Gathercole, 2007; Mainela-Arnold and Evans, 2005). All of these studies show that children with SLI have the ability to manage both processing and storage, but they are more vulnerable to storage loss than age peers when the number of to-be-stored/recalled items increases. Archibald and Gathercole (2007), Windsor et al. (2008), and Henry et al. (2012) have extended these findings to the nonlinguistic domain. Collectively, such findings imply that children with SLI have domain-general (not verbal-specific) WM limitations compared with age peers. (For an individual profile perspective on memory abilities, see Wingert et al. in this volume.)

Two final comments about the nature of WM in SLI are in order. First, some researchers (Archibald and Joanisse, 2009) argue that the SLI population is heterogeneous regarding memory problems. For Archibald and colleagues, the SLI population is marked by individual differences in memory ability, with such differences possibly leading to variations in language performance patterns across children with SLI. Second, linguistic factors may also play a role. Mainela-Arnold and Evans (2005) showed that, relative to age peers, word recall on complex verbal span tasks by children with SLI is significantly affected by the frequency of the to-be-recalled words. Children with SLI recalled low-frequency words with less accuracy than high-frequency words. The authors argued that WM capacity and linguistic knowledge were not separable mental constructs. Instead memory capacity reflected the activation and reactivation/recall of specific word representations in long-term memory (Cowan *et al.*, 2005; MacDonald and Christiansen, 2002). In this view, limited memory capacity (WM and even short-term) in SLI could be a reflection of weak linguistic representations (Kidd, 2013; Mainela-Arnold, Evans, and Coady, 2008), with strength, access, and retrieval of representation dependent on input frequencies (MacDonald and Christiansen, 2002). Low-frequency words reflect a case of weak representation driving poor storage and retrieval because such words are experienced less often and hence subject to slower/less accurate processing and retrieval than high-frequency words (Juhasz, 2005). It is critical to reiterate however, that despite the role linguistic knowledge can play in the WM performance of children with SLI, it is clear that the WM deficits in SLI span both verbal and nonverbal modalities. Such findings indicate that these children's WM limitations are domain-general in nature, not specific to verbal WM.

Attention

There are a number of theoretical views regarding the structure and function of attention. In this chapter, we review what is known about attention in SLI from a more neuropsychological perspective. The primary focus is on attentional capacity and attentional control mechanisms.

Attentional capacity

Attentional capacity refers to the limited mental energy (activation) available to an individual to perform a given mental and/or physical activity. Any given task requires some degree of attentional/mental effort and energy. Well-learned, highly-familiar activities require minimal attentional capacity to perform. By contrast, complex activities (e.g., comprehending complex sentences, making inferences) invite greater use of attentional effort and capacity. Relative to age peers, children with SLI show reduced attentional capacity, irrespective of whether the task is verbal or nonverbal (Archibald and Gathercole, 2007; Ellis Weismer *et al.*, 1999; Mainela-Arnold and Evans, 2005; Montgomery, 2000). Reduced attentional capacity has been used to help explain, for example, the difficulty children with SLI have learning and using grammatical morphology (Leonard *et al.*, 1997). Leonard and associates propose that morpheme learning/use involves attentional capacity as children must simultaneously perceive an inflected word, compare it with its bare stem counterpart, hypothesize the grammatical function of the marker, and place it in a morphological paradigm. Children with SLI presumably have insufficient attentional resources to complete all of these operations in a timely manner.

Attentional control

As a group, children with SLI tend to show poorer attentional control than age mates (Henry *et al.*, 2012; Hoffman and Gillam, 2004; Im-Bolter *et al.*, 2006). A variety of broad, domain-general control mechanisms have been assessed in children with SLI, including, for example, sustaining, shifting, updating, and inhibition. Sustained attention relates to the ability to maintain focus of attention over time. Shifting refers to the ability to devote attention (mental focus) between two different tasks (Im-bolter *et al.*, 2006). Updating refers to maintaining focus at a given level of a task and adding new content to the focus of attention, e.g., adding to a list of to-be-remembered items in memory in a WM task. Inhibition refers to preventing irrelevant stimuli from entering the focus of attention. Emerging evidence suggests that, relative to age mates, children with SLI may have: 1) comparable attention shifting skills; 2) poorer sustained attention; 3) poorer memory updating; and 4) poorer inhibitory control. Such findings advance the SLI literature by showing that children with SLI have domain-general deficits across a range of attentional control mechanisms.

In summary, relative to age peers, children with SLI demonstrate a range of memory and attention problems. The memory and attentional control deficits of children with SLI are not specific to the verbal domain but rather represent domain-general deficits. Such weaknesses place these children at greater risk for language problems.

Association between information processing and language in SLI

The majority of research examining the association between information processing and language abilities in SLI has focused on sentence comprehension. Relatively little research has explored the association between information processing and lexical learning and even less has focused on sentence production. We therefore focus on sentence comprehension.

Memory and sentence comprehension

Relative to age peers, children with SLI exhibit poorer comprehension of non-canonical sentences that violate typical subject–verb–object (SVO) word order. These include passives (*The girl was kissed on the head by the lady*) and object relatives (*The dog that the cat bit was running away*), and also complex relative clauses that express SVO word order (*The boy who is standing is hugging the girl who is sitting*).

Non-canonical sentences, however, are especially difficult for children with SLI (Friedman and Novogrodsky, 2004; van der Lely, 2005) because a noun phrase (NP) occupies a syntactic position that is different from the position that determines its semantic role. For example, in the passive and object relative sentences above, NP1 appears in a subject position but functions as a patient. To recover the SVO order of such sentences, children must move NP1 to behind the verb or syntactic gap. Researchers proposing a syntax-specific view of sentence comprehension problems in SLI argue that children's problems are due to a faulty "syntactic movement" operation. Children with SLI appear to treat the obligatory movement of NP1 as optional, resulting in inconsistent comprehension (van der Lely, 2005). By contrast, there are researchers who ascribe to a more domain-general processing limitation perspective to explain the wider range of comprehension problems in SLI; these investigators propose that SLI comprehension deficits are associated with general cognitive processing limitations, most notably WM (Bishop, 1997; Leonard *et al.*, 2013; Montgomery *et al.*, 2010; Robertson and Joanisse, 2010).

The role played by memory storage, either simple (STM) or complex (WM), in SLI sentence comprehension is mixed. The inconsistency owes much to the fact that research in this area has not been systematic and there have been vast methodological differences across studies. Nonetheless, with respect to the relation of simple (STM) storage and offline (picture pointing) comprehension, children with SLI, relative to age peers, show greater difficulty comprehending: 1) SVO-like structures containing extra verbiage and/or dependent clausal material (Leonard *et al.*, 2013; Montgomery, 1995; Robertson and Joanisse, 2010); 2) subject relatives involving extra verbiage (e.g., *This is the boy in the dark blue pants that taps the girl with the nice blond hair*)

(Robertson and Joanisse, 2010); and 3) *wh*-questions including extra verbiage (Deevy and Leonard, 2004). Such findings suggest that it is not only more complex grammatical structures that require significant STM from children with SLI but also simple SVO structures. This latter finding suggests that, because children with SLI are slower to process spoken input in the moment than age peers (Montgomery, 2005, 2006), they need to retain the lexical material of even simple SVO-like structures in STM longer to interpret it. Emerging direct and indirect evidence also suggests that the complex (WM) storage deficits in children with SLI place them at greater risk than age peers for difficulty comprehending both early-acquired non-canonical passive sentences (Montgomery and Evans, 2009) and later-acquired object relative constructions (Robertson and Joanisse, 2010).

Controlled attention and sentence comprehension

Only two studies have directly examined the relation of controlled attention and sentence comprehension in SLI, with one focusing on the relation of auditory sustained attention on real-time sentence comprehension (Montgomery, 2008) and the other on offline comprehension (Montgomery *et al.*, 2009). The children, in each study, completed a sustained attention task in which they responded to a target word (*dog*) while listening to a continuous stream of words containing both target and non-target words. The real-time study used a word recognition task in which the children listened for a highly-familiar target word within a pair of simple sentences (e.g., *The man went to the park. There he walked his dog around the pond*) and made a timed response thereby indexing the speed of linguistic processing. In the offline comprehension task, children listened to simple sentences varying in length depending on the inclusion of extra verbiage (e.g., *The little brown cat is walking under the old broken fence*) or one or two dependent clauses (e.g., *The little boy who is standing is hugging the girl who is sitting*) and pointed to a picture best matching the input from an array of four pictures. In each study, we predicted a relation between sustained attention and sentence processing/comprehension. Our assumption was that for both groups accurate sentence processing/comprehension should require sustaining attention over the course of the sentence. Relative to age peers, the SLI group in each study showed: 1) significantly poorer sustained attention; 2) significantly poorer sentence processing (slower word recognition) and sentence comprehension; and 3) a correlation between attention and comprehension (but no correlation in the control group). We interpreted such results to mean that the processing/ comprehension of simple grammar entails significant mental effort by children with SLI but not age peers, implying that simple grammar is not yet processed automatically by children with SLI.

In summary, accumulating evidence suggests that the sentence comprehension problems of children with SLI may be related to limitations in basic cognitive functions, including at least auditory memory storage and sustained attention. This said, however, considerable need exists for further research in the area of SLI sentence comprehension. For example, these efforts might take a more systematic approach to the study of the intersection of cognition and sentence comprehension by examining the influence of a range of mechanisms such as memory storage, memory retrieval, and attentional control on the comprehension of a wider range of syntactic structures. Future studies might also include both verbal and nonverbal memory and attention tasks thereby addressing the modality issue, i.e., whether WM and attention as domain-general constructs are associated with sentence comprehension. Results of such efforts would advance our understanding of the nature of the intersection of cognition and sentence comprehension.

Bridging research to practice: Intervention implications and future research

The language intervention literature for children with SLI is seriously underdeveloped, as little systematic and sustained research effort has been conducted. The lack of activity has resulted in several shortcomings in the field of speech–language pathology (SLP). First, there exists no literature focusing on interventions designed to improve the language abilities of children with SLI in the middle grades and beyond (Cirrin and Gillam, 2008). Second, there are no published evidence based practice (EBP) guidelines for providing language intervention to school-age children with SLI (Gillam and Gillam, 2006). Third, children with SLI appear to show inconsistent response to language-specific treatments designed to remediate their sentence-level syntactic limitations (Ebbels, 2007). (See Brinton and Fujiki, this volume; Wingert *et al.*, this volume, for factors that may account for individual differences in responsiveness to intervention). The lack of intervention research on comprehension has major implications because children with such impairments are at higher risk for academic failure than those with just expressive deficits (Botting and Conti-Ramsden, 2000; Conti-Ramsden *et al.*, 2009).

The final section of the chapter touches on two intervention issues: 1) a memory intervention approach from psychology that might be useful to the SLP field; and 2) a contextualized language intervention that has been shown to improve narrative comprehension and production. This latter issue is important because it has been suggested by some SLI researchers (Bishop *et al.*, 2006) that failure to consider the cognitive limitations of SLI during language intervention will likely lead to poor outcomes.

WM training: Some potential intervention implications and caveats

New developments have taken place in the past few years in the experimental psychology literature regarding the potential impact of explicit WM training. Emerging developmental data show that training WM may lead to increases in WM capacity and perhaps also to increases in higher-order cognitive abilities, both in typically developing children and children with various learning difficulties. For instance, WM capacity training has been shown to lead to improved reading comprehension accuracy and reading speed in young elementary school-age children (Loosli *et al.*, 2012). Training also has been shown to transfer to improvements in sustained attention in typically developing preschool-age children (Thorell *et al.*, 2009). WM training has also been shown to lead to increases in WM capacity, nonverbal reasoning, and attention functioning in children diagnosed with Attention Deficit Hyperactivity Disorder (Klingberg *et al.*, 2002, 2005). The purpose of training is to help children enhance their WM capacity, thereby allowing them to better manage the dual demands of information processing and storage during the performance of various cognitive tasks. In fact, several computerized WM training programs have been developed and are now commercially available, including Lumosity (2011), Jungle Memory (2011), and Cogmed (2011).

Despite the apparent promise of such findings and applicability of the findings and programs to children with SLI, the evidence for WM training efficacy to enhance WM capacity and improve cognitive functioning must be taken with caution. Many of the studies had inadequate designs to allow such claims to be made. There is also accumulating direct counterevidence suggesting that such training does not improve WM capacity and/or cognitive functioning (see Gillam and Gillam, 2012; Melby-Lervag and Hulme, 2013; and Shipstead *et al.*, 2012 for reviews). Finally, WM is a complex construct and it is therefore difficult to tease out in many of these studies just which sub-mechanism(s) of WM had been affected by training and were thus potentially responsible for any improvement of cognitive functioning.

Speech–language pathologists (SLPs) often use hybrid approaches to language intervention in which they model and elicit target language structures during functional activities, such as reading and discussing children's literature. A variety of linguistic, social and cognitive skills may be learned simultaneously under these conditions. In a recent study, Gillam, Gillam and Reese (2012) compared the narrative comprehension and production outcomes of contextualized and decontextualized intervention. In the contextualized intervention, clinicians read simple stories and engaged children in a variety of activities that required them to talk about the story content, use vocabulary and grammatical structures from the stories, answer comprehension questions, and retell the stories. In the decontextualized intervention, children played a commercially packaged grammar game and completed situational drill cards designed to improve vocabulary, sentence complexity, and social language. Both interventions were effective for improving children's sentence-level language production skills, but the effect sizes for the children in the contextualized language intervention group were 81 percent larger than the effect sizes for the children in the decontextualized language intervention group. With respect to language comprehension, only the children who received contextualized intervention performed differently than the controls on measures of story comprehension and production. The results of this early-stage efficacy study suggest that interventions that incorporate contextualized activities could have larger effects on children's sentential and narrative language abilities than interventions that incorporate decontextualized activities.

Future SLI intervention research must proceed with the ultimate aim of developing EBP interventions designed to improve a range of language abilities in children with SLI. Research designed to examine the potential benefits of WM training on language learning/performance should be developed with an eye toward training specific WM sub-mechanisms (Shipstead *et al.*, 2012) that are likely to influence language-related mechanisms. There is some suggestive evidence in the adult language processing literature that adults receiving training of various executive memory functions leads to improved sentence processing (Hussey and Novick, 2012; Novick *et al.*, 2013). Future intervention research may also explicitly include procedural learning principles in interventions to determine whether grammatical processing can be improved. Meantime, clinicians who employ contextual language intervention procedures similar to those used by Gillam *et al.* (2012) are likely to influence children's general comprehension skills. Whether these kinds of intervention procedures will improve the comprehension of complex sentences is yet to be determined.

Chapter summary

School-age children with SLI demonstrate a range of information processing limitations, including memory and attention. These limitations are not restricted to the verbal domain but rather are domain-general in nature. Accumulating experimental evidence suggests that these general processing limitations are associated with a wide range of SLI sentence comprehension deficits involving not just difficulty understanding complex sentences but also SVO-like structures that contain extra verbiage and dependent clausal material. Future SLI research might explore from a more theoretically systematic perspective the relation of cognition and sentence comprehension, as well as other language abilities, to better understand the intersection of cognition and language.

Finally, the SLI language intervention literature is sparse with respect to EBP intervention approaches designed to improve the cognitive and sentence comprehension abilities of children with SLI. It is essential that future SLI research theoretically and systematically expands its intervention scope to include a range of cognitive- and language-based therapy approaches to determine whether they can improve the cognitive and language functioning of children with SLI.

References

Archibald, L. and Gathercole, S. (2007), "The complexities of complex memory span: Storage and processing deficits in specific language impairment", *Journal of Memory and Language*, Vol. 57, pp. 177–194.

Archibald, L. and Joanisse, M. (2009), "On the sensitivity and specificity of nonword repetition and sentence recall to language and memory impairments in children", *Journal of Speech, Language, and Hearing Research*, Vol. 52, pp. 899–914.

Baddeley, A. (1998), *Human memory: Theory and practice*, Hove, UK: Psychology Press.

Barrouillet, P., Gavens, N., Vergauwe, E., Gaillard, V. and Camos, V. (2009), "Working memory span development: A time-based resource-sharing model account", *Developmental Psychology*, Vol. 45, pp. 277–290.

Bishop, D. (1997), "Cognitive neuropsychology and developmental disorders: Uncomfortable bedfellows", *The Quarterly Journal of Experimental Psychology*, Vol. 50, pp. 899–923.

Bishop, D., Adams, C. and Rosen, S. (2006), "Resistance of grammatical impairment to computerized comprehension training in children with specific and non-specific language impairments", *International Journal of Language and Communication Disorders*, Vol. 41, pp. 19–40.

Botting, N. and Conti-Ramsden, G. (2000), "Social and behavioral difficulties in children with language impairment", *Child Language Teaching and Therapy*, Vol. 16, pp. 105–120.

Cirrin, F. and Gillam, R. (2008), "Language intervention practices for school-age children with spoken language disorders: A systematic review", *Language, Speech, and Hearing Services in Schools*, Vol. 39, pp. 110–137.

Cogmed. (2011), "Frequently asked questions: What is Cogmed all about?", Available at www.cogmed.com/faq

Conti-Ramsden, G., Durkin, K., Simkin, Z. and Knox, E. (2009), "Specific language impairment and school outcomes. I: Identifying and explaining variability at the end of compulsory education", *International Journal of Language and Communication Disorders*, Vol. 44, pp. 15–35.

Cowan, N., Elliott, M., Saults, S., Morey, C., Mattox, S., Hismjatullina, A. and Conway, A. (2005), "On the capacity of attention: Its estimation and its role in working memory and cognitive aptitudes", *Cognitive Psychology*, Vol. 51, pp. 42–100.

Deevy, P. and Leonard, L. (2004), "The comprehension of *wh*-questions with specific language impairment", *Journal of Speech, Language, and Hearing Research*, Vol. 47, pp. 802–815.

Ebbels, S. (2007), "Teaching grammar to school-aged children with specific language impairment using shape coding", *Child Language Teaching and Therapy*, Vol. 23, pp. 67–93.

Ellis Weismer, S., Evans, J. and Hesketh, L. (1999), "An examination of verbal working memory capacity in children with specific language impairment", *Journal of Speech, Language, and Hearing Research*, Vol. 42, pp. 1249–1260.

Engle, R.W., Tuholski, S.W., Laughlin, J.E. and Conway, A. (1999), "Working memory, short-term memory, and general fluid intelligence: A latent variable approach", *Journal of Experimental Psychology: General*, Vol. 128, pp. 309–331.

Friedman, N. and Novogrodsky, R. (2004), "The acquisition of relative clause comprehension in Hebrew: A study of SLI and normal development", *Journal of Child Language*, Vol. 31, pp. 661–681.

Gillam, R., Cowan, N. and Day, L. (1995), "Sequential memory in children with and without language impairment", *Journal of Speech and Hearing Research*, Vol. 38, pp. 393–402.

Gillam, R. and Gillam, S. (2012), "N-back and CogMed working memory training: Proceed with caution", *Perspectives on Language, Learning, and Education*, Vol. 19, pp. 108–116.

Gillam, R., Gillam, S., and Reese, K. (2012), "Language outcomes of contextualized and decontextualized language intervention: Results of an early efficacy study", *Language Speech and Hearing Services in Schools*, Vol. 43, pp. 276–291.

Gillam, S. and Gillam, R. (2006), "Making evidence-based decisions about child language intervention in schools", *Language, Speech, and Hearing Services in Schools*, Vol. 37, pp. 304–315.

Henry, L., Messer, D. and Nash, G. (2012), "Executive functioning in children with specific language impairment", *The Journal of Child Psychology and Psychiatry*, Vol. 53, pp. 37–45.

Hoffman, L.M., and Gillam, R.B. (2004), "Verbal and spatial information processing constraints in children with specific language impairment", *Journal of Speech, Language, and Hearing Research*, Vol. 47, pp. 114–125.

Hussey, E. and Novick, J. (2012), "The benefits of executive control training and the implications for language processing", *Frontiers in Psychology,* Vol. 3, pp. 1–14.

Im-Bolter, N., Johnson, J. and Pascual-Leone, J. (2006), "Processing limitations in children with specific language impairment: The role of executive function", *Child Development,* Vol. 77, pp. 1822–1841.

Juhasz, B. (2005), "Age-of-acquisition effects in word and picture identification", *Psychological Bulletin,* Vol. 131, pp. 684–712.

Jungle Memory. (2011), "How it works", available at: www.junglememory

Kidd, E. (2013), "The role of verbal working memory in children's sentence comprehension: A critical review", *Topics in Language Disorders,* Vol. 33, pp. 208–233.

Klingberg, T., Forssberg, H., and Westerberg, H. (2002), "Training of working memory in children with ADHD", *Journal of Clinical and Experimental Neuropsychology,* Vol. 24, pp. 781–791.

Klingberg, T., Fernell, E., Olesen, P., Johnson, M., Gustafsson, P., Dahlstrom, K., *et al.,* (2005), "Computerized training of working memory in children with ADHD: A randomized, controlled trial", *Journal of American Academy of Child and Adolescent Psychiatry,* Vol. 44, pp. 177–186.

Leonard, L., Eyer, J., Bedore, L. and Grela, B. (1997), "Three accounts of the grammatical morpheme difficulties of English speaking children with specific language impairment", *Journal of Speech, Language, and Hearing Research,* Vol. 40, pp. 741–753.

Leonard, L., Deevy, P., Fey, M. and Bredin-Oja, S. (2013), "Sentence comprehension in specific language impairment: A task designed to distinguish between cognitive capacity and syntactic complexity", *Journal of Speech, Language and Hearing Research,* Vol. 56, pp. 577–589.

Loosli, S., Buschkuehl, M., Perrig, J. and Jaeggi, M. (2012), "Working memory training improves reading processes in typically developing children", *Child Neuropsychology,* Vol. 15, pp. 1–17.

Lumosity. (2011), "Enhance creativity", available at: www.lumosity.com/how-we-help/enhance-creativity

MacDonald, M. and Christiansen, M. (2002), "Reassessing working memory: Comment on Just and Carpenter (1992) and Waters and Caplan (1996)", *Psychological Review,* Vol. 109, pp. 35–54.

Mainela-Arnold, E. and Evans, J. (2005), "Beyond capacity limitations: Determinants of word-recall performance on verbal working memory span tasks in children with SLI", *Journal of Speech, Language, and Hearing Research,* Vol. 48, pp. 897–909.

Mainela-Arnold, E., Evans, J. and Coady, J. (2008), "Lexical representations in children with SLI: Evidence from a frequency manipulated gating task", *Journal of Speech, Language, and Hearing Research,* Vol. 51, pp. 381–393.

Melby-Lervag, M. and Hulme, C. (2013), "Is working training effective? A meta-analytic review", *Developmental Psychology,* Vol. 49, pp. 270–291.

Montgomery, J. (1995), "Sentence comprehension in children with specific language impairment: The role of phonological working memory", *Journal of Speech and Hearing Research,* Vol. 38, pp. 187–199.

Montgomery, J. (2000), "Verbal working memory and sentence comprehension in children with specific language impairment", *Journal of Speech, Language, and Hearing Research,* Vol. 43, pp. 293–308.

Montgomery, J. (2005), "Effects of input rate and age on the real-time lexical processing of children with specific language impairment", *International Journal of Language and Communication Disorders,* Vol. 40, pp. 171–188.

Montgomery, J. (2006), "Real-time language processing in school age children with specific language impairment", *International Journal of Language and Communication Disorders,* Vol. 41, pp. 275–291.

Montgomery, J. (2008), "Role of auditory attention in the real-time sentence processing of children with specific language impairment: A preliminary investigation", *International Journal of Language and Communication Disorders,* Vol. 43, pp. 499–527.

Montgomery, J. and Evans, J. (2009), "Complex sentence comprehension and working memory in children with specific language impairment", *Journal of Speech, Language, and Hearing Research,* Vol. 52, pp. 269–288.

Montgomery, J., Evans, J. and Gillam, R. (2009), "Relation of auditory attention and complex sentence comprehension in children with specific language impairment: A preliminary study", *Applied Psycholinguistics,* Vol. 30, pp. 123–151.

Montgomery, J., Magimairaj, B., and Finney, M. (2010), "Working memory and specific language impairment: An update on the relation and perspectives on assessment and treatment", *American Journal of Speech-Language Pathology,* Vol. 19, pp. 78–94.

Novick, J., Hussey, E., Teubner-Rhodes, S., Harbison, J. and Bunting, M. (2013), "Clearing the garden-path: Improving sentence processing through cognitive control training", *Language and Cognitive Processes,* Vol. 29, pp. 186–217.

Robertson, E. and Joanisse, M. (2010), "Spoken sentence comprehension in children with dyslexia and language impairment: The roles of syntax and working memory", *Applied Psycholinguistics,* Vol. 31, pp. 141–165.

Shipstead, Z., Hicks, K. and Engle, R. (2012), "Cogmed working memory training: Does the evidence support the claims?", *Journal of Applied Research in Memory and Cognition,* Vol. 1, pp. 185–193.

Thorell, L., Lindqvist, S., Nutley, S., Bohlin, G. and Klingberg, T. (2009), "Training and transfer effects of executive functions in preschool children", *Developmental Science,* Vol. 12, pp. 106–113.

Unsworth, N. and Engle, R. (2007), "On the division of short-term and working memory: An examination of simple and complex span and their relation to higher order abilities", *Psychological Bulletin,* Vol. 133, pp. 1038–1066.

van der Lely, H. (2005), "Domain-specific cognitive systems: Insight from Grammatical-SLI", *Trends in Cognitive Sciences,* Vol. 9, pp. 53–59.

Windsor, J., Kohnert, K., Loxtercamp, A. and Kan, P. (2008), "Performance on nonlinguistic visual tasks by children with language impairment", *Applied Psycholinguistics,* Vol. 29, pp. 237–268.

17

SPELLING STRATEGIES AND WORD FORMATION PROCESSES

Evidence from developmental and spelling ability data

Ruth Huntley Bahr

Spelling is more than rote memory. It represents the integration of phonology, orthography and morphology to represent word meaning (Bahr *et al.*, 2009, 2012; Silliman *et al.*, in press). Misspellings then provide a window into what students understand about word formation as the following spelling test of a young girl in kindergarten (5 years, 8 months) illustrates (reproduced verbatim):

Jup for *jump*	*Jut* for *jumped*	*Juping* for *jumping*
play for *play*	*plaed* for *played*	*plaing* for *playing*

Analysis of the misspellings indicates that this child relies on spelling–sound correspondences to represent words. She is struggling with sonorant clusters (-*mp*; as noted in Treiman *et al.*, 1995), the spelling of long vowel digraphs (-*ay*) but has a partial understanding of the different ways that the past tense in English can be represented (Deacon and Bryant, 2006). All of these errors are typical of young spellers; however, they also illustrate how young children combine their knowledge of phonology, orthography, and basic morphology to create words.

This chapter illustrates how children use phonology, orthography, and morphology to form words. The first section describes spelling as a linguistic process that draws on multiple sources of linguistic knowledge and processing resources. The second section explores factors that underlie the differences between good and poor spellers, including students with dyslexia. Next, examples of spelling errors are discussed in terms of the linguistic properties described by Newman (2010): granularity, stability, and accessibility. The chapter concludes with suggestions for teaching spelling.

Spelling as a linguistic process

Spelling is more than the graphic representation of sounds with letters. It is a complex linguistic process, which integrates the phonological, orthographic, and morphological processing of words with aspects of visual processing, visual memory, and strategic thinking (Westwood, 2014). This process is accomplished, in part, by the abstraction of linguistic patterns from language input to identify regularities and structure within a language. This process, known as statistical learning (Saffran, 2003), has been embraced by researchers in spelling development (among others, Bourassa and Treiman, 2014; Pacton *et al.*, 2001). These studies show that early spelling patterns are characterized by: 1) relative preservation of the phonological structure of words (e.g., Treiman, 1991; Treiman *et al.*, 1995); 2) adherance to orthographic patterns that characterize the native language (Cassar and Treiman, 1997; Conrad *et al.*, 2013); and 3) a basic understanding of inflectional and derivational morphology (Bourassa and Treiman, 2008; Deacon and Dhooge, 2010). These studies stress the importance of determining the rules that underlie the phonological structure of a language (phonotactics), the regularity of letter patterns (orthotactics), and the rules governing the addition of prefixes and suffixes to root words (morphotactics). These terms are further defined with examples below.

Phonotactics

Segmentation of words into syllables and individual phonemes is critical in early spelling acquisition and this develops through the identification of phonological patterns (phonotactics) within children's oral language. For instance, early misspellings demonstrate the child's ability to represent each sound with a letter, as in *dag* for *dog* or *fit* for *fight* (Bourassa and Treiman, 2014). At times, the child's perception of a sound in a particular word position is affected, as noted for sonorant consonants within consonant clusters (Treiman, 1991; Treiman *et al.*, 1995). Sonorant consonants are more difficult to perceive in clusters because of their vowel-like quality, which results in their frequent omission, as in *had* for *hand* and *sow* for *snow*. Bourassa and Treiman (2014) suggest these misspellings are related to a young child's tendency to treat initial clusters as a unit. As new phonological rules are learned, these types of errors decline.

Orthotactics

Orthotactics involves knowledge of the phoneme–grapheme correspondences and orthographic rules within a language (Conrad *et al.*, 2013; Holmes *et al.*, 2008; Rothe *et al.*, 2014). Early on, children operate with a one phoneme–one grapheme strategy, which generally results in accurate spelling for many of the more transparent monosyllabic words in English. However, misspellings arise when a particular sound is represented by more than one grapheme. For instance, the *g* can be a /g/ or a /dʒ/ sound, as in *give* and *gypsy* and a long vowel can be represented by multiple spellings, as in *seem, team, grieve,* and *eve.* In addition, there are positional constraints that determine how a phoneme is spelled, such as in letter doubling or when to use *-ck* or *k* in the word-final position, as in *duck* or *cake* (Bourassa and Treiman, 2014). Such knowledge is generally strengthened through experiences with reading and writing.

Morphotactics

Like phonology and orthography, morphology also provides statistically predictable patterns, concerning the graphemes that compose individual morphemes and the rules by which morphemes are affixed to words (Deacon *et al.*, 2008). Morphotactics limits the range of possible spelling options and is noted in spelling as early as grades 1–2 (Bourassa and Treiman, 2014; Deacon *et al.*, 2008). Development of morphotactics improves spelling accuracy because the speller becomes aware of how affixation (through prefixes and suffixes) alters the root word meaning, as opposed to a phonological extension of a novel word, as in *freely* and *freeze.* Therefore, the roles of phonotactics, orthotactics, and morphotactics are essential in the word formation process underlying spelling. Their interrelationships are described in triple word form theory.

Triple word form theory

Triple word form theory (Bahr *et al.*, 2009; Richards *et al.*, 2006) considers the essential roles of phonology, orthography and morphology in learning to spell new word forms. This theory proposes that spelling acquisition does not rely completely on the alphabetic principle for encoding written forms from spoken words. Rather, children acquire considerable knowledge of spelling through implicit abstraction of phonological patterns (Bourassa and Treiman, 2014), orthographic regularities (e.g., Pacton *et al.*, 2001) and morphological adaptations (e.g., Apel *et al.*, 2012; Pacton *et al.*, 2005).

Simply stated, learning to spell reflects dynamic tensions among phonology, orthography, and morphology. Children discern how spellings bridge spoken and written language by abstracting, progressively applying, and interconnecting phonotactic, orthotactic, and morphotactic knowledge (Apel *et al.*, 2006; Deacon *et al.*, 2008; Treiman and Cassar, 1996). Breakdowns in any of these processes can lead to spelling errors, which might be indicative of a developmental delay or language impairment. Examination of misspelling patterns also provides insight into why some people are better spellers than others.

The role of spelling ability: Good vs. poor spellers

Several studies have shown that poor spellers are generally delayed in their spelling development (Cassar *et al.*, 2005; Schwartz, 1983; Schwartz and Doehring, 1977); while others indicate that good and poor spellers differ qualitatively in the nature of the spelling errors they make (Arndt and Foorman, 2010; Holmes *et al.*, 2008; Lennox and Siegel, 1996; Waters *et al.*, 1985). These differences are explored from three perspectives: phonological and orthographic processing, the relationship between reading and spelling, and consideration of word-general and word-specific knowledge.

Phonological and orthographic processing perspective

At first, it was proposed that poor spellers had difficulty with phonological processing (Bourassa and Treiman, 2014). In other words, they struggled with identifying the phonological structure of a word, having to rely more on the visual aspects of spelling. If this were so, Kamhi and Hinton (2000) proposed that poor spellers should produce more nonphonetic misspellings, spell common words correctly while struggling with novel and nonsense words, and experience difficulty using morphology when spelling. However, their review of the literature revealed more similarities than differences between good and poor spellers when matched for age and/ or ability. They found that good and poor spellers made the same basic types of errors, but differed in the number of errors made, even when the speller's age was taken into account (Friend and Olson, 2008). Poor spellers demonstrated errors that were phonological in nature, such as omitting graphemes in words that incorporated consonant clusters, as in *sop* for *stop* and *bet* for *belt* (Bourassa and Treiman, 2014; Friend and Olson, 2008; Treiman, 1991; Treiman *et al.*, 1995) and often struggled with rhotic vowels (Silliman *et al.*, 2006; Bourassa and Treiman, 2014). Phonologically implausible spellings, like *gej* for *book*, were rarely noted in either group and little evidence was found for their reliance on the visual aspects of a word (Fischer *et al.*, 1985).

As researchers determined that phonological processing alone did not account for the types of spelling errors made by good and poor spellers, interest increased in orthographic processing (Bourassa and Treiman, 2014). Studies in this area have confirmed the idea that poor spellers demonstrate adequate knowledge of the orthographic patterns in their language, but struggle with the word-specific applications of this knowledge (Arndt and Foorman, 2010; Cassar et al., 2005). Fischer et al. (1985) demonstrated differences in good and poor adult spellers as a function of word transparency and task. Specifically, good spellers were better than poor spellers at recognizing and utilizing orthographic and morphophonemic structure in their spelling attempts. Berninger and Chanquoy (2012) also noted that the regularity of stress patterns within a language affects the speller's ability to segment words. If word segmentation is easier, then orthographic processing predominates. In conclusion, good spellers apply their knowledge of orthographic conventions and allowable phoneme sequences better as they spell novel words (Bourassa and Treiman, 2014).

The equality of reading and spelling perspective

Many researchers have considered the role of reading skill as it relates to spelling ability (Bruck, 1988; Bruck and Waters, 1988; Cassar et al., 2005; Fayol et al, 2009; Savage et al., 2005). Since both reading and spelling draw on many of the same linguistic skills, the premise was that spelling and reading should be affected in similar manners. In fact, when the top 25 percent of readers were compared to the lowest 25 percent, based on standardized reading test performance, or to students with dyslexia, investigators were able to verify this claim (Bruck, 1988; Bruck and Treiman, 1990; Cassar et al., 2005).

However, poor spellers are not always poor readers because of the linguistic differences in spelling and reading tasks (Waters et al., 1985; Fayol et al., 2009). While reading, individuals can draw on context to decipher a written word, suggesting there is no need to sound out every unfamiliar word in order to be able to read it. However, spelling depends upon identification of the phonological structure of a word and accurate phoneme-to-grapheme correspondences that take into account orthographic regularities within the language, such as *tote, coat, toe, snow* when spelling a long -o vowel. Increasing task difficulty is the fact that the same spelling can be pronounced differently in words, like *mow* and *cow* or *proof* and *foot*. Context may help with the reading of such words, but word-specific knowledge is necessary to assist the student in accurately spelling these words (Fischer et al., 1985; Holmes and Ng, 1993; Silliman et al., in press). Such discrepancies in spelling can influence the strength of a word's lexical representation and affect both reading speed and spelling accuracy. Words with strong lexical representations are read and spelled accurately; however, misspelled words tend to have weaker lexical representations as represented by a slower word reading rate (Martin-Chang et al., 2014). Hence, lexical quality, as opposed to participant or word characteristics, seems to be the stronger determinant of spelling accuracy.

Word-specific and word-general knowledge perspective

Other investigators have considered the roles of word-general and word-specific knowledge in evaluating the orthographic abilities of good and poor adult spellers (Conrad et al., 2013; Holmes and Ng, 1993; Holmes et al., 2008). *Word-general knowledge* about the alphabetic system can include knowing about letter-sound correspondences in words, like smaller grapheme–phoneme correspondences and larger rime–rhyme correspondences, as well as morphemic knowledge about root words and affixes (Davis and Drouin, 2010). On the other hand, knowledge about the spellings of individual words that become stored in memory because of experiences with reading or writing those particular words is commonly referred to as *word-specific knowledge* (Davis and Drouin, 2010).

Research in this area of orthographic processing also has focused on the differences between reading and spelling skill. For instance, Holmes and Ng (1993) found that poor spellers were no different than good spellers in reading/spelling high frequency words, regardless of word length or regularity. However, poor spellers struggled with less familiar and longer words. Holmes and Ng demonstrated that poor spellers did not completely analyze the target word and made decisions based on partial word analysis, especially involving the interiors of longer words. These investigators concluded that poor spellers have not developed enough knowledge of orthographic regularities to speed up word processing. In other words, it took too much time to analyze the middles of words. In another experiment, Holmes *et al.* (2008) demonstrated that difficulties in orthographic processing for poor spellers were not related to visual sequential memory, but instead to slower orthographic processing.

Whereas the studies described above focus on adults, Conrad *et al.* (2013) targeted the use of orthographic knowledge in young children (ages 7–9 years) as they developed spelling skill. These investigators reported that word-specific knowledge is used to read familiar words and words that can be read by analogy. Such knowledge is developed through the child's ability to abstract word-general knowledge about orthographic regularities and patterns in a language.

While experiences with print are important in this process, some orthographic knowledge is apparent before written word recognition in children (Cassar and Treiman, 1997; Pacton *et al.*, 2001). Recent research by Silliman and colleagues (in press) suggests that vocabulary knowledge is critical in the development of word-specific knowledge. They have shown that children initially rely on word-general knowledge as they learn to spell and when they are confronted with novel words. As word representations become lexically richer, the individual child hones in on the correct spelling.

Spelling impairment associated with dyslexia

As our understanding of spelling development increased, researchers wondered if the quality of the misspelling would differ in children with a presumed phonological processing deficit, such as dyslexia. Research in this area has shown that children with dyslexia perform as well as or better than spelling-matched controls on tasks involving orthographic processing (Bourassa and Treiman, 2003; Cassar *et al.*, 2005; Friend and Olson, 2008); however, results on phonological processing tasks have been mixed (Bruck, 1988; Friend and Olson, 2008). With more careful control of the stimuli and stronger methods for misspelling analysis, other research (Bourassa and Treiman, 2003; Cassar *et al.*, 2005) indicates that children with dyslexia perform similarly to spelling-matched controls in spelling initial consonant clusters, letter name sequences, and schwa vowels. In addition, they indicated that orthographic knowledge was similar between groups. In other words, children with dyslexia produced misspelling patterns that were similar to younger spellers. When morphological knowledge is considered, research has focused on children's recognition of the root word when constructing derived forms (i.e., root constancy), with no significant differences noted (see Bourassa and Treiman, 2014 for details).

In summary, research in the area of spelling ability has focused in three areas: phonological/orthographic processing, the relationship of reading ability to spelling skill, and the development of word-general and word-specific knowledge. Results indicated that spelling errors did not differ as much by error type as they did by developmental ability. Older poor spellers made errors that were similar to younger spelling age-matched peers, a pattern also noted for children with dyslexia and language impairment (Bourassa and Treiman, 2014; Kamhi and Hinton, 2000; Silliman *et al.*, 2006). While the nature of the errors was similar across spelling ability groups, some researchers have noted persisting difficulties with some of the more difficult phoneme–grapheme correspondences, like rhotic and schwa vowels, and orthographic patterns, like letter doubling and silent -e (Bourassa and Treiman, 2003; Silliman *et al.*, 2006). More recent investigations suggest that differences between good and poor spellers lie in the quality of their lexical representations (Fayol *et al.*, 2009; Martin-Chang *et al.*, 2014) and the development of word-specific knowledge (Fischer *et al.*, 1985; Holmes and Ng, 1993; Silliman *et al.*, in press). Differences in word knowledge will be explored further in the next section, which describes error patterns produced by superior, average, and poor spellers.

Linguistic feature patterns from dictated and spontaneous spellings

Children draw on all three sources of linguistic knowledge as they learn to spell. However, reliance on these sources of linguistic knowledge alone provides a restricted view of how spelling develops over time. One must also consider the nature of the orthography to be learned, whether it is deep (e.g., English, French, Hebrew) or shallow (e.g., Italian, Spanish, Finnish). Newman (2010) provides a framework for contrasting deep and shallow orthographies in alphabetic and alphasyllabary languages in terms of interactions among three linguistic dimensions: a) *granularity* (the linguistic grain-size level at which phonology is mapped to the orthography, e.g., phoneme, onset-rime, syllable); b) *stability* (regularity) of the mapping across phonology–orthography relationships; and c) *accessibility* of the mapping level in the structure of the spoken language, e.g., the extent to which phonological features are sufficiently salient for transcription into word forms. Analysis of misspellings within this framework assists in describing the development of spelling patterns over time and within the complexity of a specific language.

Bahr and colleagues analyzed spelling errors within triple word form theory with the Phonological, Orthographic, Morphological Assessment of Spelling (POMAS). The POMAS allowed the analysis of linguistic feature errors within the written compositions of typically developing children in grades 1–9 (Bahr *et al.*, 2012) and the dictated spelling test performances of typically developing children identified by spelling ability level (superior, good and poor) over time (cohorts in overlapping time frames, grades 1–5 and 3–7) (Silliman *et al.*, in press). What became apparent was that children incorporated both word-general (i.e., information about syllable composition and structure) and word-specific knowledge (e.g., the suffix spelling in *attention* vs. *confusion*) to spell words; hence, an analysis of linguistic feature use over time can illustrate the transition from word-general to word-specific spellings. Examples of misspellings of children on a dictated spelling test (St. John *et al.*, 2014) and from writing samples (Bahr *et al.*, 2012) are provided next to illustrate how children deal with granularity, stability and accessibility (Newman, 2010) in applying both word-general and word-specific knowledge in learning to spell.

Granularity

At the level of fine-grained analysis, students are faced with two ongoing judgments: a) decisions about phoneme-to-grapheme correspondences and the application of general word knowledge in terms of possible phonotactic, orthotactic, and morphotactic patterns; and b) decisions about how to interconnect these various linguistic cues. In our database of dictated spellings from grades 1–7, knowledge of the alphabetic principle in English was generally not a problem for superior, average, or poor spellers. For instance, in the 81 spellings of the word *careless* in grades

1–7, only five participants (6 percent) used a grapheme other than *c* to represent the first letter in the word. In four cases, the *k* represented *c* and in the last instance, a *ch* was used. Likewise, in all 28 of the attempts at spelling the word *conscientious* in grades 1–4, the letter *c* was used to represent the initial sound in the word (as obtained from superior and average spellers only; poor spellers did not attempt this word).

However, issues with granularity surfaced with two-letter sequences (or bigrams). Specifically, children utilized the wrong spelling of a phoneme pattern for a particular sound. This problem was noted in the grade 5 spellings of *conscientious* as *contiantiose and concientious*. In this case, *ti*, *si*, and *ci* can represent the /ʃ/ sound, as in *physician*; however, some children may be unfamiliar with the spelling of this word and select the wrong bigram. It is proposed that these students applied their general word knowledge of bigram possibilities when attempting to spell this word.

A final example of granularity was evidenced when children demonstrated knowledge of acceptable orthographic patterns, but used them in the wrong word position. Although the dictated spellings of the superior, good and poor spellers evidenced procedural knowledge of letter doubling (St. John *et al.*, 2014), many students struggled with knowing when to double a grapheme. Two good examples were noted in the misspelling of *careless*. Several children wrote *carlees*, which illustrates difficulty segmenting the word and further suggests that no morphemic analysis occurred. A few others wrote *carelless,* indicating that the morphemic structure was parsed, but in integrating the two units, the child reverted to a non-lexicalized strategy for doubling. Given that errors involving granularity occur at the level of phoneme–grapheme correspondences, explicit instruction on spelling rules and their exceptions should be beneficial.

Stability

Stability refers to the consistency of a spelling and can be noted when a word is spelled numerous times in a writing sample. For example, one adolescent misspelled *score* as *socor* in the second paragraph of a narrative and then spelled it as *scoor* when it followed the word *floor* in the third paragraph. Such occurrences were often noted in our analysis of writing samples.

Another frequently encountered strategy influencing stability was recursion or the returning to earlier stages of spelling development when spelling more complex words. This was illustrated in the spellings of *careless* for two children followed longitudinally from grades 1–5: Child 1 (a poor speller) – *carls, cerles, carlees, careles, carless* and Child 2 (an average speller) – *carlisse, karles, carlis, carless, careless*. Child 1 did not provide direct evidence of parsing the compound word into two units until grade 2. Recursion is noted in grade 3, when this child represented the root more accurately (*carlees*) but struggled with the doubling sequence in *-less*. By grade 4, the root *care* was solidified with another approximation for *-less*; this time without doubling. At grade 5, another recursion involved difficulty with combining the two word forms (*carless*). Child 2 demonstrated a different recursive pattern. His initial spelling (*carlisse*) was an attempt at representing both word parts. In grades 2 and 3, there was reversion, which involved phoneme-to-grapheme matches (*karles, carlis*). While in grade 4 the word was more accurately represented as two word parts (carless), but problems with word combination still remained. The correct spelling in this case was mastered by grade 5.

In contrast to the poor and average spellers, a superior speller appeared to display a more linear, developmental trajectory for the word *absence* from grades 1–4: *absent, absents, absense, absence*. The root word was spelled correctly from the beginning, consistent with the predictions of prior research (see Bourassa and Treiman, 2014 for a discussion of root constancy). By grade 2, the child was experimenting with possible morphological spellings of the suffix by using his phonotactic and orthotactic knowledge, and possibly semantic knowledge, to produce a plausible spelling (*absents*). By grade 4, he produced the correct spelling, showing he had probably succeeded in changing the root word (an adjective) into a noun.

The morphological complexity of particular derivations can influence the stability of word-specific knowledge (Bourassa and Treiman, 2014). However, the orchestration of orthographic knowledge for certain spellings can produce regressions even for higher frequency, more transparent derivations, as in an average speller from grades 1–5 who spelled *excitement* as *excitmint, excitement* (which was correct), *ecxitement,* and, finally, *excitement* (for both grades 4 and 5). These examples of instability in morphemic analysis suggest that word-specific knowledge takes time to develop.

Accessibility

At least two factors influence the accessibility of specific word forms from the mental lexicon. One finding in our spontaneous writing data (Bahr *et al.*, 2012) involved the syllable reductions (i.e., syncope) which are often associated with speaking. For example, grade 5 students spelled *dangerous* as *dangrous* and *favorite* as *favrot*, while a grade 7 student produced *usly* for *usually* and a grade 8 student wrote *diffrent* for *different*. Another error involved the writer's attempt to phonologically reproduce the target word, as in *jewlery* for *jewelry* (grade 5) and *probilly* for *probably* (grade 8). While these spellings reflect the colloquial pronunciations of the target words, failure to focus on morphological decomposition is prominent. In these examples, granularity restricted accessibility in that students reverted to a syllable parsing strategy.

A second access issue involved the semantic context. Misspellings of this type were frequent in both dictated spellings (St. John *et al.*, 2014) and spontaneous writing samples (Bahr *et al.*, 2012) as students accessed the wrong homophone for the desired word, as in *addition* for *edition* and *patience* for *patients*. This type of error results from the weak integration of form, meaning, and context (Bahr *et al.*, 2012). A form that matches the desired phonological representation is retrieved, but the outcome is not the desired word meaning. A variation of this error is the inclusion of a real word as an orthographic image that represents the target phonology, as in *exsightment* for *excitement* or *farmersuitical* for *pharmaceutical* (noted in young superior spellers from the dictated spelling data). In the latter case, children are associating a possibly more familiar orthographic sequence with the phonology of a less familiar word. Inadequate lexical representations influence accessibility, resulting in the student's reliance on the access of smaller units of meaning to spell.

These fine-grained analyses of misspellings revealed that the poor spellers never caught up to the average spellers. In addition, poor spellers continued to make spelling errors that were more typical of younger students, even though their overall spelling test scores improved. So, if these poor spellers are to improve, it would appear that they need continued instruction in middle and high school, especially since these students are encountering more and more complex academic vocabulary that they will need to spell (see Silliman and Wilkinson, this volume).

Conclusion

Phonological, orthographic, and morphemic awareness all contribute to successful spelling. Information about the development and integration of the three linguistic skills at a given point in time can be gathered, because, depending on the strength of a given source of linguistic knowledge, students will employ different strategies to spell, resulting in different misspellings (Bahr *et al.*, 2012). By analyzing misspellings over time, researchers can provide empirical insights into variations in the process of word formation, differentiating when students resort to a previous spelling strategy (i.e., recursion) versus a linear strategy.

Thinking of spelling as a word formation process encourages teachers to focus on the identification of rules and alternations (i.e., exceptions to the silent -e rule: *lone, home, come,* and *some*). Pattern abstraction encourages the child to analyze words as units, which can be modified by affixation, as well as assisting in the identification of spelling alternatives (e.g., knowing different ways to spell long vowels). Use of naturalistic writing can expose other factors that influence spelling accuracy, like syntactic complexity. Finally, instruction should continue through the upper grades, as students will encounter new vocabulary to spell. In order to generate quality lexical representations, students require repeated experiences with the foundational processes for word formation.

References

Apel, K., Wilson-Fowler, E.B., Brimo, D. and Perrin, N.A. (2012), "Metalinguistic contributions to reading and spelling in second and third grade students", *Reading and Writing*, Vol. 25, pp. 1283–1305.

Apel, K., Wolter, J.A. and Masterson, J.J. (2006), "Effects of phonotactic and orthotactic probabilities during fast mapping on 5-year-olds' learning to spell", *Developmental Neuropsychology*, Vol. 29, pp. 21–42.

Arndt, E.J. and Foorman, B.R. (2010), "Second graders as spellers: What types of errors are they making?", *Assessment for Effective Intervention*, Vol. 36, pp. 57–67.

Bahr, R.H., Silliman, E.R. and Berninger, V.W. (2009), "What spelling errors have to tell", In Woods, C. and Connolly, V. (Eds.), *Contemporary Perspectives on Reading and Writing*. Routledge, New York, NY, US, pp. 109–129.

Bahr, R.H., Silliman, E.R., Berninger, V.W. and Dow, M. (2012), "Linguistic pattern analysis of misspellings of typically developing writers in grades 1–9", *Journal of Speech, Language and Hearing Research*, Vol. 55, pp. 1587–1599.

Berninger, V.W. and Chanquoy, L. (2012), "What writing is and how it changes across early and middle childhood development", In Grigorenko, E.L., Mambrio, E. and Preiss, D.D. (Eds.), *Writing: A Mosaic of New Perspectives*. Psychology Press, New York, US, pp. 65–84.

Bourassa, D. and Treiman, R. (2003), "Spelling in children with dyslexia: Analyses from the Treiman-Bourassa Early Spelling Test", *Scientific Studies of Reading*, Vol. 7, pp. 309–333.

Bourassa, D. and Treiman, R. (2008), "Morphological constancy in spelling: A comparison of children with dyslexia and typically developing children", *Dyslexia*, Vol. 14, pp. 155–169.

Bourassa, D.C. and Treiman, R. (2014), "Spelling development and disability in English", In Stone, C.A., Silliman, E.R., Ehren, B.J. and Wallach, G.P. (Eds.), *Handbook of Language and Literacy Second Edition*. The Guilford Press: New York, NY, US, pp. 569–601.

Bruck, M. (1988), "The word recognition and spelling of dyslexic children", *Reading Research Quarterly*, Vol. 23, pp. 51–69.

Bruck, M. and Treiman, R. (1990), "Phonological awareness and spelling in normal children and dyslexics: The case of initial consonant clusters", *Journal of Experimental Child Psychology*, Vol. 50, pp. 156–178.

Bruck, M. and Waters, G. (1988), "An analysis of the spelling errors of children who differ in their reading and spelling skills", *Applied Psycholinguistics*, Vol. 9, pp. 77–92.

Cassar, M. and Treiman, R. (1997), "The beginnings of orthographic knowledge: Children's knowledge of double letters in words", *Journal of Educational Psychology*, Vol. 89, pp. 631–644.

Cassar, M., Treiman, R., Moats, L., Pollo, T.C. and Kessler, B. (2005), "How do the spellings of children with dyslexia compare with those of nondyslexic children?", *Reading and Writing*, Vol. 18, pp. 27–49.

Conrad, N.J., Harris, N. and Williams, J. (2013), "Individual differences in children's literacy development: The contribution of orthographic knowledge", *Reading and Writing*, Vol. 26, pp. 1223–1239.

Davis, C. and Drouin, M. (2010), "Relations between specific and general word learning", *Reading Psychology*, Vol. 31, pp. 327–346.

Deacon, S.H. and Bryant, P. (2006), "Getting to the root: Young writers' sensitivity to the role of root morphemes in the spelling of inflected and derived words", *Journal of Child Language*, Vol. 33, pp. 401–417.

Deacon, S.H., Conrad, N. and Pacton, S. (2008), "A statistical learning perspective on children's learning about graphotactic and morphological regularities in spelling", *Canadian Psychology on Literacy Development*, Vol. 49, pp. 118–124.

Deacon, S.H. and Dhooge, S. (2010), "Developmental stability and changes in the impact of root constancy on children's spellings", *Reading and Writing: An Interdisciplinary Journal*, Vol. 23, pp. 1005–1069.

Fayol, M., Zorman, M. and Lété, B. (2009), "Associations and dissociations in reading and spelling French: Unexpectedly poor and good spellers", *British Journal of Educational Psychology Monograph Series*, Vol. 2, No. 6, pp. 63–75.

Fischer, F.W., Shankweiler, D. and Liberman, I.Y. (1985), "Spelling proficiency and sensitivity to word structure", *Journal of Memory and Language*, Vol. 24, pp. 423–441.

Friend, A. and Olson, R.K. (2008), "Phonological spelling and reading deficits in children with spelling disabilities", *Scientific Studies of Reading*, Vol. 12, pp. 90–105.

Holmes, V.M. and Ng, E. (1993), "Word-specific knowledge, word-recognition strategies, and spelling ability", *Journal of Memory and Language*, Vol. 32, pp. 230–257.

Holmes, V.M., Malone, A.M. and Redenbach, H. (2008), "Orthographic processing and visual sequential memory in unexpectedly poor spellers", *Journal of Research in Reading*, Vol. 31, pp. 136–156.

Kamhi, A.G. and Hinton, L.N. (2000), "Explaining individual differences in spelling ability", *Topics in Language Disorders*, Vol. 20, No. 3, pp. 37–49.

Lennox, C. and Siegel, L.S. (1996), "The development of phonological rules and visual strategies in average and poor spellers", *Journal of Child Psychology*, Vol. 62, pp. 60–83.

Martin-Chang, S., Ouellette, G. and Madden, M. (2014), "Does poor spelling equate to slow reading? The relationship between reading, spelling, and orthographic quality", *Reading and Writing*, Vol. 27, pp. 1485–1505.

Newman, E.H. (2010), "The role of phonology in orthographically different languages", In M. Shatz, and L.C. Wilkinson (Eds.), *The Education of English Language Learners: Research to Practice*. Guilford Press, New York, US, pp. 108–132.

Pacton, S., Fayol, M. and Perruchet, P. (2005), "Children's implicit learning of graphotactic and morphological regularities", *Child Development*, Vol. 76, pp. 324–339.

Pacton, S., Perruchet, P., Fayol, M. and Cleeremans, A. (2001), "Implicit learning out of the lab: The case of orthographic regularities", *Journal of Experimental Psychology: General*, Vol. 130, pp. 401–426.

Richards, T.L., Aylward, E.H., Field, K.M., Grimme, A.C., Raskind, W., Richards, A.L., *et al.*, (2006), "Converging evidence for triple word form theory in children with dyslexia", *Developmental Neuropsychology*, 30, pp. 547–589.

Rothe, J., Schulte-Körne, G. and Ise, E. (2014), "Does sensitivity to orthographic regularities influence reading and spelling acquisition? A 1-year prospective study", *Reading and Writing*, Vol. 27, pp. 1141–1161.

Saffran, J.R. (2003), "Statistical language learning: Mechanisms and constraints", *Current Directions in Psychological Science*, Vol. 12, No. 4, pp. 110–114.

Savage, R.S., Frederickson, N., Goodwin, R., Patni, U., Smith, N. and Tuersley, L. (2005), "Relationships among rapid digit naming, phonological processing, motor automaticity, and speech perception in poor, average, and good readers and spellers", *Journal of Learning Disabilities*, Vol. 38, pp. 12–28.

Schwartz, S. (1983), "Spelling disability: A developmental linguistic analysis of pattern abstraction", *Applied Psycholinguistics*, Vol. 4, pp. 303–316.

Schwartz, S. and Doehring, D.G. (1977), "A developmental study of children's ability to acquire knowledge of spelling patterns", *Developmental Psychology*, Vol. 13, pp. 419–420.

Silliman, E.R., Bahr, R.H. and Peters, M. (2006), "Spelling patterns in preadolescents with atypical language skills: Phonological, morphological, and orthographic factors", *Developmental Neuropsychology*, Vol. 29, pp. 93–123.

Silliman, E.R., Bahr, R.H., Nagy, W. and Berninger, V.W. (in press), "Language basis of spelling in writing during early and middle childhood: Grounding applications to struggling writers in typical writing development", In B. Miller, P. McCardle and V. Connelly (Eds.), *Development of writing skills in individuals with learning difficulties*. Leiden, The Netherlands: Brill.

St. John, E., Bahr, R.H., Silliman, E.R. and Barker, R.M. (2014), "Misspellings are developmentally complex I: Longitudinal analysis of spelling errors", Poster presented at the annual convention of the American Speech-Language-Hearing Association,

Treiman, R. (1991), "Children's spelling errors on syllable-initial consonant clusters", *Journal of Educational Psychology*, Vol. 83, pp. 346–360.

Treiman, R. and Cassar, M. (1996), "Effects of morphology on children's spelling of final consonant clusters", *Journal of Experimental Child Psychology*, Vol. 63, pp. 141–170.

Treiman, R., Zukowski, A. and Richmond-Welty, E.D. (1995), "What happened to the 'n' of sink? Children's spellings of final consonant clusters", *Cognition*, Vol. 55, pp. 1–38.

Waters, G.S., Bruck, M. and Seidenberg, M. (1985), "Do children use similar processes to read and spell words?", *Journal of Experimental Child Psychology*, Vol. 39, pp. 511–530.

Westwood, P. (2014), "Spelling: Do the eyes have it?", *Australian Journal of Learning Difficulties*, ahead of print, pp. 1–11.

18

LITERACY DEVELOPMENT

The interdependent roles of oral language and reading comprehension

Kate Cain

Reading comprehension is a core aspect of literacy and our success in understanding what we read impacts on many aspects of our lives, including our education, employment, and recreation. This chapter concerns reading comprehension development and its relation to oral language skills. A clear understanding of the skills that support the development of reading comprehension will inform early curricula so that they provide the appropriate foundations for beginner readers and also targeted interventions for children who struggle to understand what they read. In the first section, I discuss what it means to comprehend a text, highlighting key features of the product and the process of comprehension. In the second, I review what we know about the development of reading comprehension and its relation with word reading and oral language. The third section focuses on the reading and language profiles of children with poor reading comprehension to identify why some children struggle specifically with text comprehension. In the fourth and final section, I consider how this research base can inform educational and clinical practice.

Reading and listening comprehension: The product and the process

The product of reading a text and listening to someone else read a text aloud is the same: a memory-based representation of the text's meaning called a mental model (Johnson-Laird, 1980; Kintsch, 1998). With the exception of written word recognition, the knowledge, skills and processes involved in extracting meaning from written or spoken text and constructing that mental model are the same. Therefore, a good starting point for discussing the development of text comprehension and the skills that support it is an examination of the product of skilled comprehension and how this is achieved.

The product of skilled comprehension

A mental model of a text is a representation of the state of affairs described by the text, not a verbatim record. This was illustrated in a seminal study in which adult participants were presented with sentences such as, *Three turtles rested on a floating log, and some fish swam beneath them*. In a subsequent recognition test, they could not reliably distinguish between the original sentence and one that described the same scene. With a word change, as in, *Three turtles rested on a floating log, and some fish swam beneath it*, the adult participants could discriminate the original sentence from one that described a different scene such as, *Three turtles rested beside a floating log....* (Bransford *et al.*, 1972).

The same is true for syntax. When asked to judge if they have heard a sentence before, adults are guided by the meaning of the sentence, not its wording. As a result, adult listeners will "falsely recognise" a sentence that shares its meaning with one heard previously but which has a different word order and/or voice (e.g., active for passive) (Sachs, 1967). Together these (and other) studies clearly demonstrate that good comprehenders do not remember a verbatim record of a text; they encode its meaning.

The process of skilled comprehension

To construct this representation of a text's meaning, readers and listeners draw on a range of language skills and knowledge. Consider the following text:

> Bridget was getting ready for her big night out. She always got nervous before a date. After phoning her sister, she felt much better.

This text did not probably cause you any significant comprehension difficulties, but you engaged in several complex processes to extract its sense and construct a mental model of its meaning. To understand text, words are decoded and their meanings retrieved and put together to form meaningful sentences. Good comprehenders go beyond individual words and sentences: they make links between different elements in a text to integrate their meanings and they draw on their background knowledge to make sense of details that are not fully specified (Garnham, 2010). Cohesive devices, such as pronouns, are resolved as part of the integration process: above, the pronoun *she* refers back to Bridget, which enables us to link the meanings of those sentences. Other cohesive devices, such as connectives, signal the relation between elements in a text: here *after* indicates the temporal order of events.

In addition to information integration within the text, comprehenders often draw on background knowledge when generating inferences to make sense of unspecified or missing details (Graesser *et al.*, 1994). Some inferences are guided by knowledge of text structure. For example, knowledge about narrative leads comprehenders to generate causal inferences to understand a character's actions (Van den Broek, 1997), such as why Bridget phoned her sister. Good comprehenders reflect on their understanding as the text unfolds, a process referred to as comprehension monitoring. This can alert them to the need to engage in the inference making that is necessary to construct an accurate and coherent mental model. Thus, the construction of a mental model involves the higher-level skills of integration and inference, application of knowledge about text structure, and monitoring for meaning (Paris and Paris, 2003). Finally, it is important to note that comprehension is a dynamic process. The mental model constructed so far provides the context for interpreting specific words or phrases. As a result, *date* in the above is taken to refer to a romantic date rather than a fruit.

This analysis of a text demonstrates how "comprehension is greater than the sum of its perceptual and conceptual parts" (Caccamise and Snyder, 2005 p. 10). The construction of a mental model helps readers to learn from texts, both narrative and expository, and to apply that knowledge in other situations, because the information has been integrated with existing knowledge structures (Graesser *et al.*, 2003).

Reading comprehension development and its relation to oral language skills

Reading comprehension is a construct determined by many different aspects of language. As noted by Scarborough (2003), learning to read begins before the start of formal reading instruction because reading comprehension builds on a foundation of oral language skills and experience. I next review research on reading comprehension development during middle childhood and the precursors of reading comprehension.

Reading comprehension development and word reading

Word reading and language comprehension skills are both necessary for reading comprehension, a viewpoint encapsulated in the simple view of reading (Gough and Tunmer, 1986). The relative importance of each for the prediction of reading comprehension changes during development. In the early years, word reading is more strongly predictive of reading comprehension than is listening comprehension of text (Catts *et al.*, 2005). Word reading is supported by a range of phonological skills, such as phonological awareness, short-term memory and rapid naming, as well as letter-sound knowledge and word-specific orthographic knowledge (Ehri, 2014). As these skills and knowledge develop, word reading becomes more accurate and less effortful. However, in the early stages of reading development, key words in a text may be inaccurately decoded and cognitive resources will be focused on word identification rather than meaning construction, such that word reading can limit reading comprehension (Perfetti, 1985).

As word reading becomes more fluent, listening comprehension becomes the stronger predictor of reading comprehension (Catts *et al.*, 2005). The correlations between reading and listening comprehension are very high in adulthood (Gernsbacher *et al.*, 1990), when individual differences in word reading ability are small.

Which oral language skills support reading and listening comprehension development?

In the same way that various phonological processing skills and print knowledge are important to word reading development (Wagner and Torgesen, 1987), different meaning-related oral language skills underpin text-level reading and listening comprehension. In relation to text, vocabulary and grammar have been referred to as lower-level (Hogan *et al.*, 2012) or foundational skills (Lepola *et al.*, 2012) because words form sentences and sentences describe events, which form the critical building blocks of connected prose. Research to date indicates a stronger role for vocabulary than for syntactic knowledge in predicting reading comprehension concurrently (Oakhill *et al.*, 2003; Vellutino *et al.*, 2007) and longitudinally (Muter *et al.*, 2004; Oakhill and Cain, 2012) in young beginner readers.

It would be premature to conclude that grammar is not important for reading comprehension. Components of grammar such as pronouns and connectives help to integrate the meanings of clauses and sentences, and knowledge of these features is related to text comprehension (Cain and Nash, 2011; Garcia *et al.*, in press; Williams *et al.*, 2009). Particular grammatical structures common to written text but not conversation, such as embedded relative clauses, can be difficult to understand because of the distance between dependent elements (Scott, 2009). Thus, the strength of the relationship between syntax and comprehension of extended text may depend on the degree to which grammar signals integration of meaning and the complexity of the syntax in that text.

The language skills of inference and integration, knowledge and use of text structure, and comprehension monitoring have been referred to as higher-level skills because of the specific role they play in the construction of mental models of text (Oakhill and Cain, 2007). As with vocabulary and grammar, these skills develop before reading instruction. For example, knowledge about narrative structure and sensitivity to the causal structure and critical events in a narrative are evident in preschoolers (Lynch *et al.*, 2008; Paris and Paris, 2003), probably because children have experience with narrative from an early age through picture books, the retelling of autobiographical memories, and play. Vocabulary, grammar, inference and integration, knowledge of text structure, and monitoring will also all contribute to comprehension of expository text. Pre-readers are familiar with expository text as well and demonstrate an awareness of the differences in language between narrative and expository text (Pappas, 1993).

During their first couple of years of reading instruction, children engage in comprehension monitoring (Kinnunen *et al.*, 1998) and inference making (Barnes *et al.*, 1996) to make sense of text, and use knowledge of story structure to remember and recall narratives (Mandler and Johnson, 1977). Sensitivity to narrative structure is separable from vocabulary knowledge and both are related to concurrent standardised measures of reading comprehension in beginner readers (Lynch *et al.*, 2008; Paris and Paris, 2003), as well as in children with several years' reading instruction (Cain *et al.*, 2004; Oakhill and Cain, 2012). Similarly, inference and integration explain performance in broader measures of listening comprehension in addition to vocabulary knowledge in 4- to 6-year-olds (Florit *et al.*, 2011; Kendeou *et al.*, 2008; Tompkins *et al.*, 2013) and 7- to 11-year-olds (Cain *et al.*, 2004). The same is true for high-school students: vocabulary and background knowledge, inference and knowledge of cohesive devices all contribute to expository text comprehension (Cromley and Azevedo, 2007; Eason *et al.*, 2012; Garcia *et al.*, in press).

Longitudinal studies have also demonstrated a unique role for inference and knowledge of story structure between 4 to 6 years in the prediction of narrative reading and listening comprehension (Kendeou *et al.*, 2009; Lepola *et al.*, 2012)[1]. Inference, knowledge of story structure, and comprehension monitoring, also predict reading comprehension development between 7 to 14 years beyond the contribution of general cognitive ability, word reading, and vocabulary (Cain and Oakhill, 2009; Oakhill and Cain, 2012).

Thus, from the outset of reading development, vocabulary, grammar, and higher-level language skills all contribute to reading and listening comprehension outcomes. This conclusion accords with the meta-analysis conducted by the National Early Literacy Panel (2008), which found the strongest prediction of reading comprehension from studies that used composite measures of oral language that went beyond single word vocabulary to include sentence and text-level measures (see Hogan *et al.*, 2012, for a review). Clearly, all levels of oral language are important to the construction of a mental model of a text's meaning.

The interdependence of comprehension skills

A range of oral language skills support reading comprehension and its development. In turn, reading comprehension further promotes the development of oral language skills. Both reading and listening comprehension share reciprocal relations in the early grades, and furthermore, reading and listening comprehension and vocabulary are predictive of each other across Grades 1 to 6 (Verhoeven and Van Leeuwe, 2008).

There are two reasons for this interdependence. First, good reading and listening comprehension both involve the construction of a mental model of the text's meaning. Second, reading may support vocabulary and grammatical development (as well as vice versa) because good reading comprehension is associated with greater out-of-school reading experience, such that better readers have greater opportunities, as well as the skills, to acquire knowledge of our language system when reading (Cain and Oakhill, 2011). These reciprocal relations may become particularly important for later literacy and learning from content areas. For these, texts include a greater density of morphologically complex and content-specific words and complex grammatical constructions. Knowledge of morphosyntax and inference from context will help readers to derive meaning.

Reading and listening comprehension difficulties

Although the vast majority of children develop good comprehension skills, some fail to understand adequately what they read. A recent large-scale study indicates that around 16 per cent of children in Grades 2 through 10 fit the criteria of poor reader and have difficulties with word reading, text comprehension, or both (Catts *et al.*, 2012). We need to consider how best to identify poor readers who have comprehension rather than word reading difficulties and the nature and range of the language difficulties that they experience.

Unexpected reading comprehension difficulties

Some children will experience poor reading comprehension as a consequence of weak word recognition skills. Other children experience reading comprehension difficulties that cannot be attributed to weak word reading. For these children, comprehension problems are evident when text is read aloud to them (Cain *et al.*, 2001; Megherbi and Ehrlich, 2005), indicating difficulty with language comprehension in both modalities. To be clear, we are not talking about difficulties with conversational language here; rather with text that is read aloud and contains vocabulary, grammatical, and discourse structures common to written text. Unexpected comprehension difficulties are not simply a product of an opaque orthography such as English or a particular education system: children with a similar profile have been identified across Europe and North America (Cornoldi *et al.*, 1996; Megherbi and Ehrlich, 2005; Nation and Snowling, 1998; Paris *et al.*, 2005; Swanson and Berninger, 1995).

There is no single procedure for the identification of children with unexpectedly poor comprehension: they have been selected using percentile cut offs for achievement in word reading and reading comprehension (Adlof *et al.*, 2010) and also regression techniques to identify poor reading comprehension relative to word reading and other variables (Tong *et al.*, 2011). Poor reading comprehenders have been matched to peers for both word reading and vocabulary (Cain, 2006) or for nonword reading and nonverbal reasoning (Nation *et al.*, 1999). These differences may explain, in part, why the range and magnitude of language and cognitive processing difficulties differs across studies. These differences do not mean that the category of "poor reading comprehender" is not valid: different measures and thresholds are used to identify children with dyslexia (Catts *et al.*, 2012; Snowling *et al.*, 2007), for which different core deficits have been proposed (Ramus *et al.*, 2003). To note, a child who performs significantly below the population average is clearly a struggling reader.

Correlates and causes of poor text-level comprehension

Cross-sectional studies that compare poor comprehenders with same-age good comprehenders reveal difficulties on a wide range of language tasks. These include semantic processing (Nation and Snowling, 1998), grammatical contrasts (Stothard and Hulme, 1992), and the higher-level skills critical to the construction of the mental model (Cain and Oakhill, 2006). Poor comprehenders often have poor working memory as well (Cain 2006; Cornoldi *et al.*, 1996), which may in part explain their higher-level language weaknesses. It is not the case that all language skills are weak. Rather, weaknesses, where found, are in the aspects of oral language specific to meaning. To reiterate, poor comprehenders have intact phonological processing skills in line with their relative strength in word reading (Cain *et al.*, 2000).

There are a handful of retrospective longitudinal studies that have identified poor comprehenders and examined their earlier oral language. These demonstrate a strong relation between weak oral language and subsequent reading comprehension difficulties. Seven-year-olds with poor reading comprehension but age-appropriate word reading, demonstrate poor language production and comprehension (Justice *et al.*, 2013), vocabulary, grammar, and narrative comprehension in preschool (Catts *et al.*, 2006) or in the first year of schooling (Nation *et al.*, 2010).

There is unlikely to be a single cause of poor reading comprehension or a single factor implicated in success. Indeed, when researchers have examined the language skills in groups of poor comprehenders, they find heterogeneity: some poor comprehenders have weak semantic skills but intact morphosyntax (Nation *et al.*, 2004), and others have intact semantic skills but weak inference and monitoring skills (Cain and Oakhill, 2006). In addition, some children may have a late-emerging reading difficulty. Their performance on early measures of language and literacy does not indicate a cause for concern but later on, around Grades 2 and 4, difficulties are apparent (Catts *et al.*, 2012). One reason for such transitions from good to poor reader may be the changing nature of text: those used in reading assessments for beginner readers likely use fewer complex multisyllabic words and also simpler event sequences, which require less complex mental models.

The interdependence of reading and oral language comprehension: The implications for practice

Two core conclusions arise from our review of the research base on the relationship between written and spoken language. First, text-level reading comprehension and listening comprehension both draw on the same range of oral language skills that are specific to meaning. Second, children with poor reading comprehension often have weaknesses with language comprehension and production in the preschool years, before reading instruction begins. In this section, we focus on the implications for assessment to identify poor comprehenders and also on how this information can inform effective interventions for poor comprehenders and curricula for all children to foster good reading comprehension.

Assessment: What should we assess and when should we do so?

Some children have poor reading comprehension as a result of poor word reading skills. However, as noted above, children with specific reading comprehension difficulties will also do poorly on measures of listening comprehension. Thus, one recommendation is to compare comprehension in these two presentation modalities. If comprehension is weak only for text that the individual has to read, then weak word reading skills are the most likely source of reading comprehension problems; if comprehension is weak in both modalities, the child most probably has a general comprehension deficit (Keenan *et al.*, 2006). However, understanding text read aloud can pose its own challenges. Spoken language is temporary and the pace of delivery is determined by the speaker, not the comprehender, which may cause problems for those with memory or attention difficulties (Cain and Bignell, 2014).

Identification of children at risk of poor reading comprehension before reading instruction begins provides the opportunity to intervene early and minimise the risk of reading failure. That does not mean that we can necessarily identify *all* prospective poor comprehenders because some children have late-emerging reading difficulties (Catts *et al.*, 2012). Thus, it is important to assess a range of language skills at different grades, in order to identify both children at risk of reading comprehension failure and those with late-emerging reading difficulties.

Intervention and curricula

Whilst some have argued that vocabulary and grammar are the key language skills that underpin comprehension failure (and presumably comprehension success) (Hulme and Snowling, 2011), the evidence reviewed here suggests that higher-level skills are also critical to good reading comprehension and the construction of a mental model. Indeed, a range of successful interventions with poor comprehenders have included higher-level skill instruction (Center *et al.*, 1999; Clarke *et al.*, 2010; Gersten *et al.*, 2001; Johnson-Glenberg, 2005; McKeown *et al.*, 2009; Williams *et al.*, 2009; Yuill and Oakhill, 1991). Although different skills were included in these interventions, at their core each encourages a deeper engagement with the constructive processing necessary to build an accurate and coherent mental model.

The critical skills for reading comprehension can be fostered through oral language activities. For example, joint book reading allows questioning to assess comprehension and also scaffolding to develop vocabulary and the construction of meaning in preschoolers (Silva *et al.*, 2014; Zevenbergen *et al.*, 2003). Interventions in the oral modality that target vocabulary, comprehension monitoring and narrative have proven successful (Clarke *et al.*, 2010). The use of expository texts for read-alouds with young children provides exposure to the range of text structures in this genre (Williams *et al.*, 2009) and facilitates discussion that enriches vocabulary knowledge and inferential processing (Pentimonti *et al.*, 2010). A clear recommendation is that the foundations of comprehension can and should be fostered in the early years, that is even before children can decode words. Through the use of oral language activities, we can also enable children with weak word reading skills to engage with age-appropriate written materials to develop their text-processing skills and language base.

In sum, reading comprehension is a complex construct that draws on a range of oral language skills. Because reading comprehension is multi-faceted, there are many reasons for why comprehension might break down and many skills that need to be fostered to develop skilled readers. As noted by Dickinson *et al.*(2012), a focus on a single dimension of language runs the risk of overlooking the contributions made by other aspects of language and will not result in effective curricula and robust interventions for struggling readers.

Note

1   There are no published studies that include comprehension monitoring in this age range to date, nor studies of the longitudinal prediction of expository text comprehension in young children.

References

Adlof, S.M., Catts, H.W. and Lee, J. (2010), "Kindergarten predictors of second versus eighth grade reading comprehension impairments", *Journal of Learning Disabilities*, Vol. 43, pp. 332–345.

Barnes, M.A., Dennis, M. and Haefele-Kalvaitis, J. (1996), "The effects of knowledge availability and knowledge accessibility on coherence and elaborative inferencing in children from six to fifteen years of age", *Journal of Experimental Child Psychology*, Vol. 61, pp. 216–241.

Bransford, J.D., Barclay, J.R. and Franks, J.J. (1972), "Sentence memory; A constructive versus interpretive approach", *Cognitive Psychology*, Vol. 3, pp. 193–209.

Caccamise, D. and Snyder, L.S. (2005), "Theory and pedagogical practices of text comprehension", *Topics in Language Disorders*, Vol. 25, pp. 5–20.

Cain, K. (2006), "Individual differences in children's memory and reading comprehension: An investigation of semantic and inhibitory deficits", *Memory*, Vol. 14, pp. 553–569.

Cain, K. and Bignell, S. (2014), "Reading and listening comprehension and their relation to inattention and hyperactivity", *British Journal of Educational Psychology*, Vol. 84, pp. 108–124.

Cain, K. and Nash, H. (2011), "The influence of connectives on young readers' processing and comprehension of text", *Journal of Educational Psychology*, Vol. 103, pp. 429–441.

Cain, K. and Oakhill, J. (2006), "Profiles of children with specific reading comprehension difficulties", *British Journal of Educational Psychology*, Vol. 76, pp. 683–696.

Cain, K. and Oakhill, J. (2009), "Reading comprehension development from 8 to 14 years: The contribution of component skills and processes", in R.K. Wagner, C. Schatschneider and C. Phythian-Sence, (Eds.), *Beyond Decoding: The Behavioural and Biological Foundations of Reading Comprehension*. New York: Guilford Press, pp. 143–175.

Cain, K. and Oakhill, J.V. (2011), "Matthew Effects in young readers: Reading comprehension and reading experience aid vocabulary development", *Journal of Learning Disabilities*, Vol. 44, pp. 431–443.

Cain, K., Oakhill, J.V., Barnes, M.A. and Bryant, P.E. (2001), "Comprehension skill, inference making ability and their relation to knowledge", *Memory and Cognition*, Vol. 29, pp. 850–859.

Cain, K., Oakhill, J.V. and Bryant, P.E. (2000), "Phonological skills and comprehension failure: A test of the phonological processing deficit hypothesis", *Reading and Writing*, Vol. 13, pp. 31–56.

Cain, K., Oakhill, J.V. and Bryant, P.E. (2004), "Children's reading comprehension ability: Concurrent prediction by working memory, verbal ability, and component skills", *Journal of Educational Psychology*, Vol. 96, pp. 671–681.

Catts, H.W., Adlof, S.M. and Weismer, S.E. (2006), "Language deficits in poor comprehenders: A case for the simple view of reading", *Journal of Speech, Language, and Hearing Research*, Vol. 49, pp. 278–293.

Catts, H.W., Compton, D.L., Tomblin, J.B. and Bridges, M.S. (2012), "Prevalence and nature of late-emerging poor readers", *Journal of Educational Psychology*, Vol. 104, pp. 166–181.

Catts, H.W., Hogan, T.P. and Adlof, S.M. (2005), "Developmental changes in reading and reading disabilities", in H.W. Catts and A.G. Kamhi, (Eds.), *The Connections between Language and Reading Disabilities*. Mahwah, NJ, US: Lawrence Erlbaum Associates, pp. 25–40.

Center, Y., Freeman, L., Robertson, G. and Outhred, L. (1999), "The effect of visual imagery training on the reading and listening comprehension of low listening comprehenders in Year 2", *Journal of Research in Reading*, Vol. 22, pp. 241–256.

Clarke, P.J., Snowling, M.J., Truelove, E. and Hulme, C. (2010), "Ameliorating children's reading-comprehension difficulties: A randomised controlled trial", *Psychological Science*, Vol. 21, pp. 1106–1116.

Cornoldi, C., De Beni, R. and Pazzaglia, F. (1996), "Profiles of reading comprehension difficulties: An analysis of single cases", in C. Cornoldi and J. Oakhill, (Eds.), *Reading Comprehension Difficulties: Processes and Intervention*. Mahwah, NJ, US: Lawrence Erlbaum Associates, pp. 113–136.

Cromley, J.G. and Azevedo, R. (2007), "Testing and refining the direct and inferential mediation model of reading comprehension", *Journal of Educational Psychology*, Vol. 99, pp. 311–325.

Dickinson, D.K., Griffith, J.A., Golinkoff, R.M. and Hirsh-Pasek, K. (2012), "How reading books fosters language development around the world", *Child Development Research*. http://www.hindawi.com/journals/cdr/contents/, pp. 1–15.

Eason, S.H., Goldberg, L.F., Young, K.M., Geist, M.C. and Cutting, L.E. (2012), "Reader–text interactions: How differential text and question types influence cognitive skills needed for reading comprehension", *Journal of Educational Psychology*, Vol. 104, pp. 515–528.

Ehri, L.C. (2014), "Orthographic mapping in the acquisition of sight word reading, spelling memory, and vocabulary learning", *Scientific Studies of Reading*, Vol. 18, pp. 5–21.

Florit, E., Roch, M. and Levorato, M.C. (2011), "Listening text comprehension of explicit and implicit information in preschoolers: The role of verbal and inferential skills", *Discourse Processes*, Vol. 48, pp. 119–138.

Garcia, J.R., Sanchez, E. and Bustos, A. (in press), "The contribution of knowledge about anaphors, organisational signals and refutations to reading comprehension", *Journal of Research in Reading*.

Garnham, A. (2010), "Models of processing: Discourse", *Wiley Interdisciplinary Reviews: Cognitive Science*, Vol. 1, pp. 845–853.

Gernsbacher, M.A., Varner, K.R. and Faust, M. (1990), "Investigating differences in general comprehension skill", *Journal of Experimental Psychology: Learning, Memory and Cognition*, Vol. 16, pp. 430–445.

Gersten, R., Fuchs, L.S., Williams, J.P. and Baker, S.K. (2001), "Teaching reading comprehension strategies to students with learning disabilities: A review of research", *Review of Educational Research*, Vol. 71, pp. 279–320.

Gough, P.B. and Tunmer, W.E. (1986), "Decoding, reading and reading disability", *Remedial and Special Education*, Vol. 7, pp. 6–10.

Graesser, A.C., Mcnamara, D.S. and Louwerse, M.M. (2003), "What do readers need to learn in order to process coherence relations in narrative and expository text?", in A.P. Sweet and C.E. Snow, (Eds.), *Rethinking Reading Comprehension*. New York, NY: Guilford, pp. 82–98.

Graesser, A.C., Singer, M. and Trabasso, T. (1994), "Constructing inferences during narrative text comprehension", *Psychological Review*, Vol. 101, pp. 371–395.

Hogan, T.P., Cain, K. and Bridges, M.S. (2012), "Young children's oral language abilities and later reading comprehension", in T. Shanahan and C.J. Lonigan, (Eds.), *Early Childhood Literacy: The National Early Literacy Panel and Beyond*. Baltimore, US: Brookes Publishing Co, pp. 217–232.

Hulme, C. and Snowling, M.J. (2011), "Children's reading comprehension difficulties: Nature, causes, and treatments", *Curent Directions in Psychological Science*, Vol. 20, pp. 139–142.

Johnson-Glenberg, M.C. (2005), "Web-based training of metacognitive strategies for text comprehension: Focus on poor comprehenders", *Reading and Writing*, Vol. 18, pp. 755–786.

Johnson-Laird, P.N. (1980), "Mental models in cognitive science", *Cognitive Science*, Vol. 4, pp. 71–115.

Justice, L.M., Mashburn, A. and Petscher, Y. (2013), "Very early language skills of fifth-grade poor comprehenders", *Journal of Research in Reading*, Vol. 36, pp. 172–185.

Keenan, J.M., Betjemann, R.S., Wadsworth, S.J., Defries, J.C. and Olson, R.K. (2006), "Genetic and environmental influences on reading and listening comprehension", *Journal of Research in Reading*, Vol. 29, pp. 75–91.

Kendeou, P., Bohn-Gettler, C., White, M. and Van Den Broek, P. (2008), "Children's inference generation across different media", *Journal of Research in Reading*, Vol. 31, pp. 259–272.

Kendeou, P., Van Den Broek, P., White, M. and Lynch, J.S. (2009), "Predicting reading comprehension in early elementary school: The independent contributions of oral language and decoding skills", *Journal of Educational Psychology*, Vol. 101, pp. 765–778.

Kinnunen, R., Vauras, M. and Niemi, P. (1998), "Comprehension monitoring in beginning readers", *Scientific Studies of Reading*, Vol. 2, pp. 353–375.

Kintsch, W. (1998), *Comprehension: A Paradigm for Cognition*, New York, NY: Cambridge University Press.

Lepola, J., Lynch, J.S., Laakkonen, E., Silven, M. and Niemi, P. (2012), "The role of inference making and other language skills in the development of narrative listening comprehension in 4–6-year-old children", *Reading Research Quarterly*, Vol. 47, pp. 259–282.

Lynch, J.S., Van Den Broek, P., Kremer, K., Kendeou, P., White, M.J. and Lorch, E.P. (2008), "The development of narrative comprehension and its relation to other early reading skills", *Reading Psychology*, Vol. 29, pp. 327–365.

Mandler, J.M. and Johnson, N.S. (1977), "Remembrance of things parsed: story structure and recall", *Cognitive Psychology*, Vol. 9, pp. 111–151.

McKeown, M.G., Beck, I.L. and Blake, R.K. (2009), "Rethinking reading comprehension instruction: A comparison of instruction for strategies and content approaches", *Reading Research Quarterly*, Vol. 44, pp. 218–253.

Megherbi, H. and Ehrlich, M.F. (2005), "Language impairment in less skilled comprehenders: The on-line processing of anaphoric pronouns in a listening situation", *Reading and Writing*, Vol. 18, pp. 715–753.

Muter, V., Hulme, C., Snowling, M. and Stevenson, J. (2004), "Phonemes, rimes, vocabulary and grammatical skills as foundations of early reading development: Evidence from a longitudinal study", *Developmental Psychology*, Vol. 40, pp. 665–681.

Nation, K., Adams, J.W., Bowyer-Crane, C.A. and Snowling, M.J. (1999), "Working memory deficits in poor comprehenders reflect underlying language impairments", *Journal of Experimental Child Psychology*, Vol. 73, pp. 139–158.

Nation, K., Clarke, P., Marshall, C.M. and Durand, M. (2004), "Hidden language impairments in children: Parallels between poor reading comprehension and specific language impairment?", *Journal of Speech, Language, and Hearing Research*, Vol. 47, pp. 199–211.

Nation, K., Cocksey, J., Taylor, J.S.H. and Bishop, D.V.M. (2010), "A longitudinal investigation of early reading and language skills in children with poor reading comprehension", *Journal of Child Psychology and Psychiatry*, Vol. 51, pp.1031–1039.

Nation, K. and Snowling, M.J. (1998), "Semantic processing and the development of word-recognition skills: Evidence from children with reading comprehension difficulties", *Journal of Memory and Language*, Vol. 39, pp. 85–101.

National Early Literacy Panel (2008), "Developing early literacy: Report of the National Early Literacy Panel", Washington, DC: National Institute for Literacy.

Oakhill, J. and Cain, K. (2007), "Introduction to comprehension development", in K. Cain and J. Oakhill, (Eds.), *Children's Comprehension Problems in Oral and Written Text: A Cognitive Perspective*. New York: Guilford Press, pp. 3–40.

Oakhill, J. and Cain, K. (2012), "The precursors of reading comprehension and word reading in young readers: Evidence from a four-year longitudinal study", *Scientific Studies of Reading*, Vol. 16, pp. 91–121.

Oakhill, J., Cain, K. and Bryant, P.E. (2003), "The dissociation of word reading and text comprehension: Evidence from component skills", *Language and Cognitive Processes*, Vol. 18, pp. 443–468.

Pappas, C.C. (1993), "Is narrative 'primary'? Some insights from kindergarteners' pretend readings of stories and information books", *Journal of Reading Behavior*, Vol. 25, pp. 97–129.

Paris, A.H. and Paris, S.G. (2003), "Assessing narrative comprehension in young children", *Reading Research Quarterly*, Vol. 38, pp. 36–76.

Paris, S.G., Carpenter, R.D., Paris, A.H. and Hamilton, E.E. (2005), "Spurious and genuine correlates of children's reading comprehension", in S.G. Paris and S.A. Stahl, (Eds.), *Children's Reading Comprehension and Assessment*. Mahwah, NJ, US: Erlbaum, pp. 131–160.

Pentimonti, J.M., Zucker, T.A., Justice, L.M. and Kaderavek, J.N. (2010), "Informational text use in preschool classroom read-alouds", *The Reading Teacher*, Vol. 63, pp. 656–665.

Perfetti, C.A. (1985), *Reading Ability*, New York: Oxford University Press.

Ramus, F., Rosen, S., Dakin, S., Day, B.L., Castellote, J.M., White, S. and Frith, U. (2003), "Theories of developmental dyslexia: Insights from a multiple case study of dyslexic adults", *Brain*, Vol. 126, pp. 1–25.

Sachs, J.S. (1967), "Recognition of semantic, syntactic, and lexical changes in sentences", *Psychonomic Bulletin*, Vol. 1, pp. 17–18.

Scarborough, H.S. (2003), "Connecting early language and literacy to later reading (dis)abilities: Evidence, theory, and practice", in S.B. Neuman and D.K. Dickinson, (Eds.), *Handbook of Early Literacy Research*. Guilford Press, New York, pp. 97–110.

Scott, C.M. (2009), "A case for the sentence in reading comprehension", *Language, Speech, and Hearing Services in Schools*, Vol. 40, pp. 184–191.

Silva, M., Straesser, K. and Cain, K. (2014), "Early narrative skills in Chilean preschool: Questions scaffold the production of coherent narratives", *Early Childhood Research Quarterly*, Vol. 29, pp. 205–213.

Snowling, M.J., Muter, V. and Carroll, J. (2007), "Children at family risk of dyslexia: A follow-up in early adolescence", *Journal of Child Psychology and Psychiatry*, Vol. 48, pp. 609–618.

Stothard, S.E. and Hulme, C. (1992), "Reading comprehension difficulties in children: The role of language comprehension and working memory skills", *Reading and Writing*, Vol. 4, pp. 245–256.

Swanson, H.L. and Berninger, V. (1995), "The role of working memory in skilled and less skilled readers' comprehension", *Intelligence*, Vol. 21, pp. 83–108.

Tompkins, V., Guo, Y. and Justice, L.M. (2013), "Inference generation, story comprehension, and language skills in the preschool years", *Reading and Writing*, Vol. 26, pp. 403–429.

Tong, X., Deacon, S.H., Kirby, J., Cain, K. and Parrila, R. (2011), "Morphological awareness: A key to understanding poor reading comprehension in English", *Journal of Educational Psychology*, Vol. 103, pp. 523–534.

Van Den Broek, P.W. (1997), "Discovering the cement of the universe: The development of event comprehension from childhood to adulthood", in P.W. v. d. Broek, P.J. Bauer, and T. Bourg, (Eds.), *Developmental Spans in Event Comprehension and Representation*. Mahwah, NJ, US: Lawrence Erlbaum Associates, pp. 321–342.

Vellutino, F.R., Tunmer, W.E., Jaccard, J.J. and Chen, R. (2007), "Components of reading ability: Multivariate evidence for a convergent skill model of reading development", *Scientific Studies of Reading*, Vol. 11, pp. 3–32.

Verhoeven, L. and Van Leeuwe, J. (2008), "Prediction of the development of reading comprehension: A longitudinal study", *Applied Cognitive Psychology*, Vol. 22, pp. 407–423.

Wagner, R.K. and Torgesen, J.K. (1987), "The nature of phonological processing and its causal role in the acquisition of reading skills", *Psychological Bulletin*, Vol. 101, pp. 192–212.

Williams, J.P., Stafford, K.B., Lauer, K.D., Hall, K.M. and Pollini, S. (2009), "Embedding reading comprehension training in content-area instruction", *Journal of Educational Psychology*, Vol. 101, pp. 1–20.

Yuill, N.M. and Oakhill, J.V. (1991), *Children's Problems in Text Comprehension: An Experimental Investigation*, Cambridge, UK: Cambridge University Press.

Zevenbergen, A.A., Whitehurst, G.J. and Zevenbergen, J.A. (2003), "Effects of a shared-reading intervention on the inclusion of evaluative devices in narratives of children from low-income families", *Journal of Applied Developmental Psychology*, Vol. 24, pp. 1–15.

19

CHILD WORD FINDING

Differential diagnosis guides comprehensive intervention

Diane J. German

Word Finding (WF) refers to the ability to retrieve words in single word or discourse contexts. Prevalence rates for learners with word finding difficulties (WFD) are high; 25 percent of learners with specific language impairment (SLI) and 49 percent of students classified as learning disabled (LD) have been reported with WFD (Dockrell, *et al.*, 1998; German, 1998). These learners' WF complications interfere with their communication. They manifest difficulties when answering questions (single word contexts) and when relating events (discourse contexts). Further, problems in WF compromise learners' ability to succeed in school, especially when faced with tasks that require lexical access of words, facts, etc. (Borodkin and Faust, 2012). Learners with WFD manifest problems in oral reading (German and Newman, 2007) and reading fluency (Wolf and Bowers, 2000; Faust *et al.*, 2003). Together these prevalence rates and research reports make this oral language challenge worthy of further study. Therefore, to provide professionals with information that will aid them in their work with learners with WFD, this chapter considers: (1) the sources of oral WFD; (2) theoretical underpinnings of WFD; (3) differential diagnosis of WFD; (4) comprehensive intervention; and (5) a summary and future directions.

Sources of oral WFD

WFD have been viewed as either a difficulty in the storage or retrieval of a word's semantic (concepts/meanings) attributes and/or phonological/lexical forms. In part, these views are based on a memory model that indicates that items in memory have both storage and retrieval strength (Bjork and Bjork, 1992). Storage strength refers to the permanence and completeness of an entry (i.e., its accuracy of representation). Retrieval strength refers to how reliably, consistently, and efficiently the entry can be accessed from memory on a given occasion.

Research supports both explanations. This may be because of methodology differences or because children with WFD represent a heterogeneous group (Best, 2005; Lahey and Edwards, 1999; Messer and Dockrell, 2006; Thomas, 2003). Perhaps researchers are studying different children with different lexical profiles and, thus, learners who have different kinds of vocabulary difficulties. For example, some learners, like those with SLI, may have difficulties using words due to weak conceptual understandings and incomplete semantic representations of words or imprecise phonological information (the storage deficit hypothesis) (Alt and Plante, 2006; Gray,

2005; McGregor and Appel, 2002). In contrast, students with LD, dyslexia, or traumatic brain injury, may manifest WFD due to disruptions in underlying retrieval processes or lexical access (Borodkin and Faust, 2012; Faust *et al.*, 2003; German and Newman, 2004; Messer and Dockrell, 2006; Ramus and Szenkovits, 2008; Wolf and Bowers, 2000). These learners are thought to have lexical access difficulties underlying their WFD. They demonstrate problems accessing the semantic and/or phonological attributes of known words (the retrieval deficit hypothesis) for oral and/or written language.

In summary, some learners with WFD may demonstrate vocabulary problems due to difficulties learning word meanings and underlying concepts (storage deficit hypothesis) while others may experience vocabulary difficulties due to problems accessing known words for spontaneous usage (retrieval deficit hypothesis). Although this chapter is focused on the latter, learners with lexical access difficulties, professionals are encouraged to consider both of these explanations when programming since intervention varies depending on the underlying source of learners' vocabulary difficulties.

Theoretical underpinnings of WF disruptions

WFD represent a class of lexical access disruptions that occur at different points in the lexical process and are uniquely manifested in single word and discourse contexts. A helpful way to view the origins of these WFD is to map them onto psycholinguistic and connectionist models of lexical access. This process furthers one's understanding of the WF error patterns that represent retrieval based WFD.

Model of lexical access

The Test of Word Finding, Third Edition (TWF-3, German, 2015) presents a model for the differential diagnosis of WFD. Adapted from Levelt's (1989) and other adult speech production models (Goldrick and Rapp, 2002; Roelofs, 2000), the TWF-3 adapted lexical model illustrates the architectural structure underlying lexical access for single words (see Figure 19.1). This adapted model postulates three levels of representation—the conceptual repository of the word, the abstract lexical representation of the word, and the speech motor program. These levels are involved in the four stages of lexical access.

- Stage 1. The stimulus (a teacher's question, a picture, or a thought) elicits the conceptual structure (e.g., a shallow drum-like instrument) associated with a word (tambourine).
- Stage 2. The conceptual structure for the word (tambourine) activates the word's lemma (its semantic features [a link back to the concept] and syntax specification [a noun]), as well as priming neighboring entries (drum, guitar, and instrument).
- Stage 3. The lemma, via cascading connections, accesses the entries' corresponding form features (lexeme) to create the word's phonological schema. After lemma selection, a corresponding morphological frame (stem + affix) is created in which retrieved morphological codes are inserted in Stage 3 (Levelt, 2001) (tambourine + singular). Similarly, in the case of progressive (e.g., pouring) and past tense verbs (e.g., poured) corresponding tense rules generate target frames representing two units also, the verb + suffix. In all, a word's form includes lexical and post-lexical phonological representations (Goldrick and Rapp, 2007). Lexical phonological representations include the word's morphological properties, while post-lexical form representations include a word's segmental sound units (t-æ-m-b-ə-r-i-n) and syllabic structure (tæm bə rin).

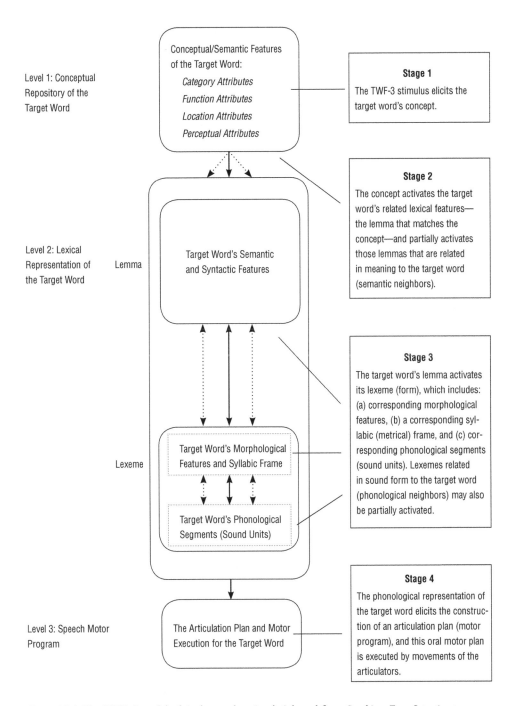

Level 1: Conceptual
Repository of the
Target Word

Conceptual/Semantic Features
of the Target Word:
   Category Attributes
   Function Attributes
   Location Attributes
   Perceptual Attributes

Stage 1
The TWF-3 stimulus elicits the
target word's concept.

Level 2: Lexical
Representation of
the Target Word

Lemma

Target Word's Semantic
and Syntactic Features

Stage 2
The concept activates the target
word's related lexical features—
the lemma that matches the
concept—and partially activates
those lemmas that are related
in meaning to the target word
(semantic neighbors).

Lexeme

Target Word's Morphological
Features and Syllabic Frame

Target Word's Phonological
Segments (Sound Units)

Stage 3
The target word's lemma activates
its lexeme (form), which includes:
(a) corresponding morphological
features, (b) a corresponding syllabic (metrical) frame, and (c) corresponding phonological segments
(sound units). Lexemes related
in sound form to the target word
(phonological neighbors) may also
be partially activated.

Level 3: Speech Motor
Program

The Articulation Plan and Motor
Execution for the Target Word

Stage 4
The phonological representation of
the target word elicits the construction of an articulation plan (motor
program), and this oral motor plan
is executed by movements of the
articulators.

Figure 19.1 The TWF-3 model of single-word retrieval. Adapted from *Speaking: From Intention to Articulation*, by W. M. J. Levelt, 1989, Cambridge, MA, US: MIT Press, and from *Lexical Access in Speech Production*, by W. M. J. Levelt, 1991, Cambridge, MA, US: Blackwell. Adapted with permission.

- Stage 4. The phonological schema elicits an articulation plan. The speaker creates a motor program, and then executes the program by controlling the movements of the articulators. The word (tambourine) is then said.

During lexical access, semantic and phonological processes influence each other (Goldrick and Blumstein, 2006; Morsella and Miozzo, 2002) through a series of cascading (feed forward) and feedback (backward) activation systems. The cascading activation allows semantic processing to influence form selection while the feedback systems enable the phonological system to impact semantic selection (Blanken *et al.*, 2002). Cascading and feedback systems are represented by multi-directional arrows on the TWF-3 model (see Figure 19.1).

Differential diagnosis of WF errors

Most important to our understanding of the differential diagnosis of learners' WF errors is the assumption that the semantic and phonological aspects of words are accessed from two systems. This assumption suggests two potential causes of WF errors: either the semantic aspects of words are inaccessible to a learner, making the phonological features unavailable also, or the semantic features are accessible while subsequent retrieval of the word's phonological features is blocked. If this assumption has reality for children with WFD, one could hypothesize WF disruptions at one of three points in the lexical process depicted in our theoretical model: (1) a disruption in accessing the semantic features of the word; (2) a disruption in accessing the phonological features of the word; or (3) a disruption at the juncture point between the semantic and phonological lexicons. In contrast to these three WF disruptions, it is assumed that disruptions at the conceptual level would lead to storage difficulties, while disruptions at the speech motor program area would lead to articulation difficulties.

The extent to which this model or corresponding error patterns are descriptive of children's lexical retrieval awaits further investigation. However, there is evidence from the fields of psycholinguistics (Newman and German, 2002), child language (German, 2014; German and Newman, 2004, 2007; German *et al.*, 2012; Lahey and Edwards, 1999; McGregor and Appel, 2002), and reading (Faust *et al.*, 2003) to suggest that, in children's language, a word's semantic and phonological information is stored in two different components of the lexicon and that the three corresponding error patterns, described next, do have reality.

Error Pattern 1: Lemma related semantic error

In this error type, the eliciting concept cannot find or select the corresponding lemma (semantic and syntactic features). Causes of Error Pattern 1 are believed to be the result of competition between word neighbors primed along with the word during lemma selection (Goldinger *et al.*, 1992; Ovchinnikova, 2007). For example, in naming *Monday*, *Wednesday* is also primed and competes with *Monday* for selection. Error Pattern 1 occurs when a competing semantic neighbor is chosen instead of the word, e.g., *Wednesday, no I mean Monday* (known as a slip of the tongue).

In single word naming contexts, Error Pattern 1 disruptions are observed as fast/inaccurate responses that may or may not be self-corrected. The speaker retrieves a semantic substitution, a semantic neighbor of the target embedded in its taxonomy. In discourse, two word reformulations (*I was, we were going fast*) as well as one word noun phrase substitutions (*Bob, no Bill is going*) are often produced. Anecdotal evidence and research verifies the presence of these underlying lexical access difficulties in children. Seiger-Gardner and Schwartz (2008) used a picture word interference paradigm and instructed learners to ignore phonologically or semantically related competing words while naming pictures. Learners with SLI had slower naming times than Typical Learners (TL) when semantically similar competitors were presented. Inadequate suppression of semantic alternatives that were also primed was said to cause this effect. Such findings are consistent with the weakness thought to underlie Error Pattern 1, which reflects an inability to inhibit competing lemmas (semantic neighbors) primed during the WF process.

Error Pattern 2: Word form related blocked error

Error Pattern 2 represents difficulties in accessing the phonological features of the word. The lemma cannot find the lexeme or corresponding phonological information as the morphological and segmental features of the word are evasive (e.g., *Today is … um … um*, known as a tip of the tongue [TOT] error). This error pattern is observed most often as slow and inaccurate responses, delays, and no responses, along with extra verbalizations or insertions (*I can't think of it* or *I know it*). Speakers may also produce time fillers (*um, uh*), empty words (*you know*), repetitions (*The name is… the name is…*) and gestures (finger snapping) as they search for the elusive word.

The presence of Error Pattern 2 has been verified in numerous studies and is the typical WF error pattern studied in child language research (Borodkin and Faust, 2012; Faust *et al.*, 2003; Stackhouse and Wells, 1997). Error Pattern 2 has been identified in learners with SLI (Messer and Dockrell, 2006), LD (Conca, 1989; German and Newman, 2004), and dyslexia. For example, Borodkin and Faust (2012) studied Error 2 Patterns in learners with dyslexia and SLI, using a TOT-based paradigm—picture naming, cueing and multiple choice. They concluded that these learners had difficulty accessing the phonological features of the word and not the semantic word features as evidenced by a higher frequency of TOT states, phonological substitutions, less ability to provide partial phonological information or to resolve TOT states from phonological cueing. Similarly, Ramus and Szenkovits (2008) indicated that their learners with dyslexia manifested difficulties with phonological lexical access.

Linguistic causes of Error Pattern 2 are believed to be the result of either blocking or transmission deficits (Borodkin and Faust, 2012). The former is due to phonological neighbors blocking access to the word's form (Jones, 1989) whereas the latter represents weakened connections between the various levels in the lexical process, making linguistic transmission inefficient (Burke *et al.*, 1991). Reasons for retrieval based weakened pathways may include fragile retrieval algorithms, low frequency of usage, or non-recent use (German and Newman, 2004), although reduced word elaboration or maturation may contribute to transmission deficits also (Stamatakis *et al.*, 2011).

Error Pattern 3: Word form and segment related phonologic errors

Error Pattern 3 describes difficulties in accessing the complete phonological schema for the word. Here the lemma partially accesses the syllabic frame and/or segmental sound content associated with the target word lemmas evidenced by phonological substitutions, e.g., *Today is Wesday* (known as a twist of the tongue). Or, in other situations, a real word phonological neighbor may be retrieved, like, *Today is Wendy* (known as a malapropism). In discourse, learners who produce Error Pattern 3, manifest difficulties with multisyllabic words by producing phonological approximations of targets. These learners may also use time fillers or produce empty words (*you know*) in place of long or phonologically complex words whose phonological schema is evasive. Lahey and Edwards (1999) noted Error Pattern 3 responses among learners with expressive language difficulties, reporting both phonological approximations of words (*pumplin* for *pumpkin*, *brana* for *banana*) and real word substitutions (*hat* for *cat*) in their language. Similarly, phonological substitutions have been observed in the language of learners with dyslexia (Borodkin and Faust, 2012). These form based substitutions indicate WF disruptions in the phonological lexicon, suggesting that learners with dyslexia may also manifest Error Pattern 3 in their expressive language, an area meriting further investigation.

To further explore these WF error patterns in learners' language, German and Newman (2004, 2007) switched the focus from WF characteristics to word characteristics. They studied the properties of words that elicit the WF error patterns in both oral language (OL) and oral reading (OR). In OL they considered whether a word's lexical factors—length, frequency of occurrence, familiarity, and neighborhood density—might predict WF error patterns. Their findings indicated that: (a) neighborhood density predicted Error Pattern 2—children produce more form related blocked errors on words from sparse neighborhoods; and (b) word frequency and neighborhood frequency predicted Error Pattern 3—more form segment related phonologic errors occurred on rare words and words whose neighbors were lower frequency. The presence of these lexical factor effects on learners' WF error patterns supports their presence in these learners' OL.

In a second study, lexical factor effects emerged for these three WF error patterns in both learners with and without WFD (German *et al.*, 2013). Error Pattern 1 disruptions were manifested on shorter, high frequency, more familiar words, residing in dense neighborhoods, while more Error Pattern 2 and 3 disruptions occurred on longer words, of lower frequency. For learners with WFD, word frequency and neighborhood frequency predicted the likelihood of Error Patterns 2 and 3, respectively, while word frequency and length predicted the likelihood of TL learners producing Error Patterns 2 and 3.

Adding to this data base, these researchers also reported lexical factor effects on learners' WF error patterns during OR: Error Pattern 1, semantic and syntactic miscues, occurred when orally reading words that were highly familiar; Error Pattern 2, form related blocked errors, occurred when orally reading words lower in frequency with lower phonotactic probability (rare phonologic patterns); and Error Patten 3, phonologic miscues, occurred when reading low frequency words which had higher phonotactic probability, such that partial phonotactic information was available (e.g., *cyote* for *coyote*). In summary, lexical factors elicited the three WF error patterns implying their presence in OR and the OL of both learners with and without WFD.

Procedures for the differential diagnosis of WF error patterns

Differential diagnosis of WF error patterns is the goal of WF assessment. The TWF-3 (German, 2015) is a standardized measure designed to complete a differential diagnosis of WF in single word naming contexts. The TWF-3 provides normative data for ages 4 years, 6 months to 12 years, 11 months. TWF-3 target word selection considered word properties other than meaning to draw out each of the error patterns, e.g., form based lexical factors such as word frequency, neighborhood density, phonotactics, and length. Six informal diagnostic procedures are provided to determine learners' individual WF error patterns. These procedures and corresponding error patterns include:

- contrasts between word knowledge (comprehension) and word production (lexical access) on the same words to identify performance discrepancies (needed to diagnose WFD);
- phonemic cueing procedures to assess blocked pathways between semantic and phonological representations (identifies Error Pattern 2);

- imitation procedure to rule out articulation difficulties (identifies Error Pattern 3);
- response analysis to observe if access to semantic and/or form features are derailed or blocked during the WF process (semantic substitutions can identify Error Pattern 1, no responses identify Error Pattern 2 and phonemic substitutions identify Error Pattern 3);
- response time analysis to observe WF efficiency (fast/inaccurate profile identifies Error Pattern 1, slow/inaccurate profile identifies Error Pattern 2 or 3 and slow/accurate profile identifies Error Pattern 2);
- secondary characteristics tally (gestures or extra verbalizations during the WF disruption) to determine the learner's metacognitive knowledge of the WF process, (*I know it, but can't think of it*) and metalinguistic awareness (*It starts with the P sound*) of the evasive target word (identifies Error Pattern 2).

In summary, an in-depth WF assessment is needed to carry out a differential diagnosis in WF so as to maximize the efficacy of intervention. Such an evaluation requires knowledge of learners' naming accuracy (selection) and response time (efficiency), responsiveness to phonemic cueing, nature of target word substitutions, and the manifestation of secondary characteristics (gestures and extra verbalizations) in the WF process. Further, to identify the performance discrepancy between receptive and expressive language, the hallmark of a WF disruption, language comparisons need to be made on the same words. Together, data from all these assessments enables examiners to predict the nature of learners, WF disruptions. The use of vocabulary tests that simply assess picture-naming accuracy is not comprehensive enough to identify the three WF error patterns.

WF intervention based on differential diagnosis

WF intervention must be comprehensive with respect to its focus and application (German, 2005). Based on learners' differential diagnosis, at least two programming areas need to be considered: retrieval strategy training and differentiated instruction.

Retrieval strategy training based on learners' differential diagnosis

WF intervention is applied to words whose (a) meanings learners comprehend (conceptual structure and lemma are stored), (b) phonological schema (form or lexeme) they recognize, and (c) motor plan and capacity to articulate they possess. For these words, instruction is focused on elaboration of words' retrieval strength, thereby increasing the ease with which these known words can be accessed. Described next are retrieval strategies for each of the WF error patterns.

Error Pattern 1: Lemma related semantic errors (known as the slip of the tongue)
Metacognitive strategies are employed to reduce semantic-based WF disruptions. These include Strategic Pausing, Self-Monitoring (Hanson, 1996), and Self-Correction (Paul, 2001) designed to reduce fast inaccurate responses that may be due to competition in the semantic lexicon. Strategic Pausing helps the learner slow down the speaking process by inserting a pause before the noun in the noun phrase and/or before the verb or adverb in the verb phrase. When strategically placed, the pause provides the speaker time to inhibit competing names or words and select the target. Self-Monitoring and Self-Correcting are taught with Strategic Pausing and are designed to reduce misspeaking and aid self-corrections. Both are important in maintaining accurate communication for learners who manifest Error Pattern 1.

Retrieval strategies for Error Pattern 2, word form related blocked errors, and Error Pattern 3, word form segment related phonologic errors

A three-pronged strategic approach is recommended to stabilize retrieval of words whose form learners cannot access consistently (Error Pattern 2) or retrieve partially (Error Pattern 3). It differs from the cueing hierarchy protocols (Nickels, 2002), which utilize phonemic, semantic, gestural, and/or graphemic cues to trigger lost or blocked word forms for on-demand usage (Best, 2005; Conca, 1989; McGregor, 1994). Although cueing hierarchy approaches aid learners' retrieval for the moment, the learner is dependent on a listener to provide the phonemic or semantic cue to achieve retrieval success. Thus, its benefits can be limited to the cueing context making carry over hard to achieve. In contrast, the three-pronged strategic approach, described next, strives to make evasive words salient in the learner's lexicon, anchoring retrieval of these words for future usage.

Treatment of evasive words begins with the first strategy, the metalinguistic reinforcement of target vocabulary, e.g., segmentation to reinforce awareness of the word's syllabic structure, such as *daffodil* (dæ fə dıl). Researchers (German *et al.*, 2012; Montgomery, 2007) have reported that focusing students on the metalinguistic properties of words can *reinforce* their awareness of words' phonological structure. This metalinguistic strategy is used in tandem with the second strategy, the phonological mnemonic strategy.

Mnemonic retrieval strategies target lexical access between semantic and form based processes, between Stages 2 and 3 in the lexical model discussed earlier. Learners associate phonological mnemonics to their evasive targets to anchor their retrieval for future usage. This involves linking words similar in sound form to the target word or word parts (e.g., dæfy for *daffodil*). These linking words (dæfy), or phonological mnemonics, are believed to be phonological neighbors of the target word (Luce and Pisoni, 1998; Vitevitch and Sommers, 2003). Use of these cues makes the implicit linguistic process of priming explicit by requiring the learner to consciously think of a word's phonological form and neighbors to remember the target.

Child studies (German, 2002; German *et al.*, 2012) have reported improved WF skills on words and syllables treated, in part, with form base mnemonic cues. Adult studies too have reported that primes similar in sound form to words, like phonological mnemonics, (*coat* for *goat*), facilitate activation and retrieval of word forms during WF disruptions (Demke *et al.*, 2002; Fisher *et al.*, 2009; James and Burke, 2000). More TOT states were resolved after adults read phonologically related words than unrelated words.

The third strategy is rehearsal. Learners are taught to think of their phonological mnemonic cue (dæfy), while rehearing aloud their target alone (*daffodil, daffodil*) and in a sentence (*The daffodils grow every year*) until they are automatic in its usage.

In conclusion, the phonological mnemonic protocol makes the word's form more salient in the phonological lexicon by providing: (a) metalinguistic reinforcement of the word's syllabic structure; (b) a phonological neighbor prompt as a mnemonic link to the word form; and (c) rehearsal. It differs from other intervention protocols as its focus is on anchoring word forms to facilitate future retrieval rather than on demand.

Differentiated classroom instruction for learners with WFD

Currently in US schools, Common Core State Standards (CCSS) are being used to guide school curricula. Unfortunately, many aspects of the CCSS are not aligned with best practice for learners with WFD because they mandate modes of expression that are barriers to students demonstrating their learning. One example is the first grade CCSS for reading which requires students to read grade level text orally with accuracy, appropriate rate, and expression on successive readings. First grade learners with WFD find OR challenging since it requires good oral WF. Even though they are decoding silently at grade level, they are frequently not able to meet this CCSS because of its focus on oral fluency. A significant performance discrepancy exists between their oral and silent reading skills.

German and Newman (2007) studied this performance discrepancy and reported that learners with WFD manifested a significant discrepancy between their OR and silent reading (SR) of the same words (sight and multisyllabic) greater than that of younger learners who had not yet been taught the reading competencies embedded in the text. Thus, these researchers concluded that the OR performance of learners with WFD may not represent their decoding abilities, but rather some aspect of their oral word production such as their lexical access skills. Based on these findings, they recommend that differentiated reading assessment and instruction for learners with WFD utilize SR measures (not OR). Similarly, the first grade CCSS for reading comprehension focuses on learners' OL. These CCSS require students with WFD to answer oral questions about text details, retell stories, and describe characters, settings, and major events even though assessing their reading comprehension with recognition response formats (multiple choice, find the answer, or select the answer) would better determine their understanding of read text.

In conclusion, for learners with WFD, differentiated instruction requires reducing the expressive language demands inherent in learners' curriculum so that their achievement is not underestimated due to their weak expressive language skills (WFD). Red flag response-types (e.g., read orally, retell, list, describe, summarize, or write the answer) required in academic work are barriers to learners expressing their knowledge. Rather, best practice for learners with WFD incorporates alternate assessments like SR to determine reading instructional level, mnemonic supports, and resources to aid retrieval of factual information, and recognition response formats (e.g., multiple choice frames, *select, circle, or highlight the answer*) in place of *tell me* or *write the answer* assessments (Newman, 2010).

Summary and future directions

High prevalence rates of learners with WFD warrant this language difficulty an important area of study. Theoretical underpinnings of lexical access can aid in the differential diagnosis of their WF error patterns and deep assessment in WF is available to carry out this differential diagnosis. These learners are in need of comprehensive intervention if they are going to succeed in school. Broad base programming for learners with WFD should include retrieval strategy instruction in the speech and language room and differentiated instruction in the classroom. Continued research is needed to isolate those factors that will contribute to improving learners' WF skills and facilitate their academic success.

References

Alt, M. and Plante, E. (2006), "Factors that influence lexical and semantic fast-mapping of young children with specific language impairment", *Journal of Speech, Language, and Hearing Research*, Vol. 49, pp. 941–954.

Best, W. (2005), "Investigation of a new intervention for children with word-finding problems", *International Journal of Language and Communication Disorders*, Vol. 4, No. 3, pp. 279–318.

Bjork, R. and Bjork, L. (1992), "A new theory of disuse and an old theory of stimulus fluctuation", In Healy, A.F., Kosslyn, S.M. and Shiffrin, R.M. (Eds.), *From Learning Process to Cognitive Processes: Essays in Honor of William K. Estes*, Erlbaum, Hillsdale, NJ, US, pp. 35–67.

Blanken, G., Dittman, J. and Wallesch, C.W. (2002), "Parallel or serial activation of word forms in speech production? Neurolinguistic evidence from an aphasic patient", *Neuroscience Letters, Vol.* 325, pp. 72–74.

Borodkin, K. and Faust, M. (2012), "Word retrieval in developmental language impairments: Application of the tip of the tongue paradigm", *Handbook in the Neuropsychology of Language.* Volumes 1 and 2, Wiley-Blackwell, Oxford, UK, pp. 963–982.

Burke, D.M., MacKay, D.G., Worthley, J.S. and Wade, E. (1991), "On the tip of the tongue: What causes word finding failures in young and older adults"?, *Journal of Memory and Language*, Vol. 30, No 5, pp. 542–579.

Conca, L. (1989), "Strategy choice by LD children with good and poor naming ability in a naturalistic memory situation", *Learning Disabilities Quarterly*, Vol. 12, pp. 92–106.

Demke, T.L., Graham, S.A. and Siakaluk, P.D. (2002), "The influence of exposure to phonological neighbours on preschoolers' novel word production", *Journal of Child Language*, Vol. 29, pp. 379–392.

Dockrell, J.E., Messer, D., George, R. and Wilson, G. (1998), "Children with word-finding difficulties – Prevalence, presentation and naming problems", *International Journal of Language and Communication Disorders,* Vol. 33, No. 4, pp. 445–454.

Faust, M., Dimitrovsky, L. and Schacht, T. (2003), "Naming difficulties in children with dyslexia: Application of the tip of the tongue paradigm", *Journal of Learning Disabilities*, No. 36, pp. 203–216.

Fisher, C., Wilshire, C. and Ponsford, J. (2009), "Word discrimination therapy: A new technique for the treatment of a phonologically based word-finding impairment", *Aphasiology*, Vol. 23, No. 6, pp. 676–693.

German, D.J. (1998, February), "Prevalence estimates for word finding difficulties in students with learning disabilities: Implications for assessment/instructional accommodation", Poster session presented at the annual meeting of the Learning Disability Association of America, Washington, DC.

German, D.J. (2002), "A phonologically based strategy to improve word-finding abilities in children", *Communication Disorders Quarterly*, Vol. 23, pp. 179–192.

German, D.J. (2005), *Word Finding Intervention Program, Second Edition (WFIP-2).* PRO.ED. Austin, TX, US.

German, D. (2014), *Test of Word Finding, Third Edition (TWF-3).* PRO.ED, Austin, TX, US.

German, D.J. and Newman, R.S. (2004), "The impact of lexical factors on children's word finding errors", *Journal of Speech, Language, and Hearing Research*, Vol. 47, pp. 624–636.

German, D.J. and Newman, R.S. (2007), "Oral reading skills of children with oral language (word finding) difficulties", *Reading Psychology*, Vol. 28, No. 5, pp. 397–442.

German, D.J., Newman, R.S. and Jagielko, J. (2013, November), "The impact of lexical factors on error patterns of children with and without word-finding difficulties", Poster session presented at the annual meeting of the American Speech and Hearing Association (ASHA), Chicago, IL, US.

German, D.J., Schwanke, J. and Ravid, R. (2012), "Word finding difficulties: Differentiated vocabulary instruction in the speech and language room", *Communication Disorders Quarterly*, Vol. 28, No. 5, pp. 397–442.

Goldinger, S., Luce, P., Pisoni, D. and Marcario, J. (1992), "Form-based priming in spoken word recognition: The roles of competition and bias", *Journal of Experimental Psychology: Learning, Memory, and Cognition*, Vol. 18, pp. 1211–1238.

Goldrick, M. and Blumstein, S.E. (2006), "Cascading activation from phonological planning to articulatory processes: Evidence from tongue twisters", *Language and Cognitive Processes*, Vol. 21, pp. 649–683.

Goldrick, M. and Rapp, B. (2002), "A restricted interaction account (RIA) of spoken word production: The best of both worlds", *Aphasiology*, Vol. 16, pp. 20–55.

Goldrick, M. and Rapp, B. (2007), "Lexical and post lexical phonological representations in spoken production", *Cognition,* Vol. 102, pp. 219–260.

Gray, S. (2005), "Word learning by preschoolers with specific language impairment: Effect of phonological or semantic cues", *Journal of Speech, Language, and Hearing Research,* Vol. 48, No. 6, pp. 1452–1467.

Hanson, M. (1996), "Self-management through self-monitoring", In Jones, K. and Charlton, T. (Eds.), *Overcoming Learning and Behaviour Difficulties: Partnership with Pupils,* Routledge, London, pp. 173–191.

James, L.E. and Burke, D.M. (2000), "Phonological priming effects on word retrieval and tip-of-the-tongue experiences in young and older adults", *Journal of Experimental Psychology: Learning, Memory, and Cognition,* Vol. 26, pp. 1378–1391.

Jones, G.V. (1989), "Back to Woodworth: Role of interlopers in the tip-of-the-tongue phenomenon", *Memory and Cognition*, Vol. 17, No. 1, pp. 69–76.

Lahey, M. and Edwards, J. (1999), "Naming errors of children with specific language impairment", *Journal of Speech, Language and Hearing Research*, Vol. 42, No. 1, pp. 195–205.

Levelt, W.J.M. (1989), *Speaking, from Intention to Articulation*, MIT Press, Cambridge, MA, US.

Levelt, W.J.M. (2001), "Inaugural article: Spoken word production: A theory of lexical access", *Proceedings of the National Academy of Sciences*, Vol. 98, No. 23, pp. 13464–13471.

Luce, P.A. and Pisoni, D.B. (1998), "Recognizing spoken words: The neighborhood activation model", *Ear and Hearing*, Vol. 19, No. 1, pp. 1–36.

McGregor, K.K. (1994), "Use of phonological information in word-finding treatment for children", *Journal of Speech and Hearing Research,* Vol. 37, pp. 1381–1393.

McGregor, K.K. and Appel, A. (2002), "On the relation between mental representation and naming in a child with specific language impairment", *Clinical Linguisitics and Phonetics*, Vol. 16, No. 1, pp. 1–20.

Messer, D. and Dockrell, J.E. (2006), "Children's naming and word-finding difficulties: Descriptions and explanations", *Journal of Speech Language and Hearing Research*, Vol. 49, pp. 309–332.

Montgomery, J.K. (2007), "Evidence based strategies for vocabulary instruction/intervention", in Denti, L. and Guerin, G. (Eds.), *Effective Practice for Adolescents with Reading and Literacy Challenges*. Routledge, Taylor & Francis Group, New York, NY, pp. 25–43.

Morsella, E. and Miozzo, M. (2002), "Evidence for a cascade model of lexical access in speech production", *Journal of Experimental Psychology: Learning, Memory, and Cognition*, Vol. 28, pp. 555–563.

Newman, D. (2010), "Impact and implications of word-finding difficulties in adolescents on listening comprehension assessment", *Communication Disorders Quarterly*, Vol. 31, No. 3, pp. 155–161.

Newman, R.S. and German, D.J. (2002), "Effects of lexical factors on lexical access among typical language-learning children and children with word-finding difficulties", *Language and Speech*, Vol. 43, No 3, pp. 285–317.

Nickels, L. (2002), "Therapy for naming disorders: Revisiting, revising and reviewing", *Aphasiology*, Vol. 16, pp. 935–980.

Ovchinnikova, I. (2007), "Slips of the tongue in children's narratives: Connectionist interpretations", *Psychology of Language and Communication*, Vol. 11, No. 1, pp. 23–41.

Paul, R. (2001), *Language Disorders form Infancy through Adolescence, Second Edition*. Mosby, Philadelphia, PA, US.

Ramus, F. and Szenkovits, G. (2008), "What phonological deficit?", *Quarterly Journal of Experimental Psychology*, Vol. 6, No. 1, pp. 129–141.

Roelofs, A. (2000), "WEAVER++ and other computational models of lemma retrieval and word-form encoding", In Wheeldon, L. (Ed.), *Aspects of Language Production*, Psychology Press, New York, NY, pp. 71–114.

Seiger-Gardner, L. and Schwartz, R.G. (2008), "Lexical access in children with and without specific language impairment: A cross-modal picture–word interference study", *International Journal of Language and Communication Disorders*, Vol. 43, No. 5, pp. 528–551.

Stackhouse, J. and Wells, B. (1997), *Children's Speech and Literacy Difficulties 1: A Psycholinguistic Framework.* Whurr Publishers, London.

Stamatakis, E.A., Shafto, M.A., Williams, G., Tam, P. and Tyler, L.K. (2011), "White matter changes and word finding failures with increasing age", available online at PLoS ONE 6(1):e14496.doi:10.1371/journal.pone.0014496

Thomas, M. (2003), "Multiple causality in developmental disorders: Methodological implications from computational modeling", *Developmental Science*, Vol. 6, No. 5, pp. 537–556.

Vitevitch, M.S. and Sommers, M.S. (2003), "The facilitative influence of phonological similarity and neighborhood frequency in speech production", *Memory and Cognition*, Vol. 31, pp. 491–504.

Wolf, M. and Bowers, P. (2000), "Naming-speed deficits in developmental reading disabilities: An introduction to the special series on the double-deficit hypothesis", *Journal of Learning Disabilities,* Vol. 33, No. 4, pp. 322–324.

20

THE PERSON BEHIND THE WRITTEN LANGUAGE LEARNING DISABILITY

Kerri Wingert, Roxana Del Campo and Virginia Berninger

First, we explain how a research team redirected focus from only diagnosing and treating specific learning disabilities to attending also to the person behind the disability. This switch in focus is situated within the context of current research, policy, and practice issues for specific learning disabilities (SLDs) across research groups, stakeholders, and practitioners. Examples are shared from observations of research participants to illustrate the importance of paying attention to the person with the SLD during instruction and in the context of the person's developmental, educational, medical, family and cultural history. Applications to practice are offered with emphasis on the critical role of the person behind the instruction—the teacher in attending to individual differences in a learner's response to instruction (RTI) and members of the interdisciplinary team who support teachers in this effort, including speech–language pathologists (SLPs), psychologists, and OTs.

Defining and treating SLDs

The aims of the research featured in this chapter are to validate evidence-based definitions and related instruction for three SLDs described in Silliman and Berninger (2011): dysgraphia (impaired letter writing), dyslexia (impaired word decoding [pseudowords], word reading [real words], and spelling), and oral and written language learning disability (OWL LD), also known as specific language impairment (SLI) (impaired morphology and syntax, word finding, discourse processing or production, and/or pragmatics). First, a comprehensive test battery is administered and parents are asked to complete questionnaires and rating scales about developmental, educational, medical and family issues. If these data rule out pervasive or specific developmental disabilities, then learning profiles are described for specific reading and writing skills. Phenotype profiles (behavioral markers of genetic variations) are then described for phenotypes shown in prior research to be related to the reading and writing skills. Second, each student receives 18 sessions of computerized instruction on iPads for the same levels of language used in defining SLDs: (a) *subword* letters; (b) *word* reading and spelling; (c) *syntactic* processing in reading comprehension and syntactic production in written expression; and (d) *discourse* processing while reading or listening to text and taking notes, and discourse production while summarizing read or heard text. Participants complete lessons at work stations in the same room. For many of the computerized learning activities, number of correct responses or total time for completion of specific learning activities is assessed by the computer and computer-generated feedback is provided at the end of many learning activities. This feedback is used to monitor RTI delivered at different levels of language within and across lessons. Only selected RTI data from the first cohort to complete this intervention in an after school program are reported here. Although computerized instruction enhances fidelity of treatment implementation, it also affords an opportunity for teachers to observe the person responding to the instruction. That is, not only instruction but also learner variables, which may co-occur with a disability and vary across learners with the same disability, may affect learning outcomes. These learning variables are discussed next in reference to current issues in the SLD field.

Current SLD issues

Research

Nearly 40 years after the first national special education law in the United States, which defined SLD as an educationally handicapping condition, researchers still do not agree on how to define SLD. It is a difficult task because some learning variables are categorical and some are continuously distributed on one or more dimensions. Also, humans exhibit normal variation on many traits and differentiating normal variation versus true disability is challenging. However, evidence is mounting that some learning disabilities surface in oral language in the preschool years but often then affect written language learning in the school-age years (e.g., Catts, 2013); late talking is one of the best predictors of OWL LD during the school years (Silliman and Berninger, 2011). Other SLDs only surface at the kindergarten–first grade transition when children struggle to name letters, associate sounds in alphabetic principle with them, and write them. Some children have dyslexia and trouble with learning to use the alphabetic principle and other aspects of language to decode and spell words, whereas others have dysgraphia and problems specific to writing the letters (Berninger and Swanson, 2013).

Moreover, not all reading disabilities are the same. Although the earlier studies emphasized word decoding problems, more recent ones focus on reading comprehension problems (see Miller, Cutting, and McCardle, 2013). After considerable research documenting benefits of early intervention for preventing or reducing the severity of reading and writing disabilities, researchers are turning their attention to persisting learning disabilities, despite early intervention, in the upper elementary and middle school grades (e.g., Denton *et al.*, 2013). Likewise, not all writing disabilities are the same—individuals can be impaired in handwriting, spelling, and/or text composing skills (macro-level organization and text length, sentence-level syntax, and lexical diversity) (Wagner *et al.*, 2011).

Progress is being made in understanding the co-occurring conditions in some but not all individuals with SLDs. In the 1970s and 1980s researchers argued about whether reading disability was related to impaired auditory discrimination or phonemic awareness; recent research shows that some individuals have difficulty with early processing of speech sounds (auditory discrimination) and thus encounter subsequent difficulty with reflection about abstract sounds in words corresponding to alphabet letters that make a difference in meaning (phoneme awareness) (e.g., Johnson *et al.*, 2011; Nittrouer and Lowenstein, 2013). Although in the past students who were English Language Learners (ELLs) were thought not to have SLDs, this belief is changing. Research shows that some ELLs have SLDs (e.g., Geva and Massey-Garrison, 2013). Moreover, ADHD has been shown to interfere with social interactions with other students during academic but not social activities (Ogg *et al.*, 2013).

Policy and practices

Policy. For individuals with SLDs, it is the best of times and the worst of times. On the one hand, there is a wealth of research studies and findings. Educational policy requires using evidence-based practices. On the other hand, there is no consensus on how to define SLDs. Categories of eligibility for special education services vary widely across states and even within states.

Practices. Even professional organizations have differing perspectives. For example, the most recent revision of the *Diagnostic and Statistics Manual* (*DSM*, American Psychiatric Association, 2013) recommends that all SLDs be diagnosed under one category, SLD. The most recent official position statement from the school psychologists' organization on identification of SLD (National Association of School Psychologists, NASP [2011]; also see Anderson, 2011) emphasizes the heterogeneity of SLDs and the academic and cognitive deficits in individual students. One way to reconcile these conflicting views is an evidence-based, multi-component model of working memory that supports language learning and is impaired in some way in all SLDs; but different impaired components are associated with different SLDs (Berninger and Swanson, 2013; Silliman and Berninger, 2011). Put another way, there are commonalities as well as specific, instructionally relevant variables across the SLDs. The NASP position statement emphasizes the importance of evidence-based multi-tiered intervention, but does not deal with linking specific instructional interventions to the nature of an individual's SLD. Despite a national, federally sponsored clearinghouse's claims about What Works, it is not clear that the same intervention works for all. A more appropriate question might be What Works for Whom? (Berninger and Dunn, 2012).

Answering this question may require addressing the issue of co-occurring conditions systematically in research. Tables 20.1 and 20.2, based on the first 35 participants to complete the comprehensive assessment and computerized instruction (Cohort 1) in the featured study, provide preliminary evidence for two co-occurring conditions that may be instructionally relevant.

If diagnosed with ADHD, what is the likelihood of dysgraphia? The results in Table 20.1 show that 14 of the 15 (93 percent) students in grades 4 to 9 with ADHD (43 percent of Cohort 1) also met research criteria for dysgraphia (impairment in the first 15 seconds in writing legible letters in order on an alphabet writing task from memory and/or in best or fastest copying a sentence with all the letters of the alphabet). Speech (e.g., articulation or auditory discrimination problems) and aural/oral language problems (e.g., word finding or late onset of multi-word constructions) reported by parents co-occurred with diagnosed ADHD but at a lower rate (40 percent) and only accounted for 17 percent of Cohort 1. Conversely, not all participants with speech and aural/oral language problems had ADHD or dysgraphia. As shown in Table 20.2, of the eight who did (23 percent of Cohort 1), only one might possibly have ADHD, 37.5 percent have dysgraphia, and 37.5 percent have OWL LD. Thus, co-occurring disorders should be considered in practice and research. The RTI data in both tables show that students with ADHD and dysgraphia or OWL LD, and other co-occurring conditions, can respond to instruction organized around levels of language, especially if implemented with teachers monitoring the learners' attention and providing the necessary supports to help the children to focus, switch, and sustain attention and self-monitor as necessary during oral and written language instruction. That is children have to learn to pay attention to language.

Table 20.1 Co-occurring diagnoses, RTI for letter writing (print, cursive, keyboard), and whether medication prescribed for individuals diagnosed with ADHD.

Case	Gender	RTI Letter Writing	Also Dysgraphia[a]	Also Speech Problem/s[a]	Also Oral Language Problems[a]	Also Medical Problems[a]	AD[d]
1	M	Y[f]	Y	Y	N	N	Y
2	M	Y	Y	N	N	Y[b]	Y
3	F	Y	Y	Y	N	N	N
4	F	Y[i]	Y	N	N	N	Y
5	M	N[e]	Y	Y	N	N	Y
6	M	Y	N	N	N	N	Y
7	F	Y	Y	N	N	N	Y
8	M	Y	Y	Y[h]	Y[g]	N	Y
9	M	Y	Y	Y[h]	N	N	Y
10	M	Y	Y	N	N	N	Y
11	M	Y[f]	Y	N	Y[g]	N	Y
12	M	Y[f]	Y	N	N	Y[b,c]	Y
13	M	Y	Y	N	N	N	Y
14	M	N[e]	Y	N	N	N	Y
15	M	Y	Y	N	N	N	Y

(a) Y=Yes N=No; (b) hypothyroidism; (c) asthma; (d) premature; (e) only on oral language; (f) also on oral language; (g) late talking; (h) articulation problems; (i) on spelling and composing not handwriting

Table 20.2 Co-occurring diagnoses and RTI (aural, oral, written language) for individuals diagnosed with speech or oral language disorders.

Case	Gender	RTI	Speech Problem[a]	Oral Language Problem[a]	ADHD[a]	Diagnosis	Medical Diagnosis
1	M	Y[e]	N	Y[h]	N	OWL LD	N
2	M	Y[e]	Y	Y	?	OWL LD	Y[i]
3	M	Y[e]	Y[b]	N	N	Dysgraphia	Y[b]
4	F	Y[f]	Y	Y	N	Dyslexia	Y[j]
5	M	Y[g]	Y[c]	N	N	Dyslexia + Dysgraphia	Y[k]
6	M	Y[f]	Y[d]	Y	N	Dysgraphia	Y[d]
7	F	Y[g]	N	Y	N	Dyslexia	N
8	M	Y[g]	Y	Y	N	OWL LD	N

(a) Y=Yes, N=No; (b) due to 50% hearing loss until tubes inserted and hearing was normal; (c) now stutters and repeats himself; (d) ear infections and vocal cord dysfunction related to confusing speech sounds; tonsils and adenoids removed; sleep apnea; (e) RTI WJ3 Oral Comprehension, CELF4 Sentence Formulation; WJ3 Passage Comprehension; also handwriting, spelling, and word reading; (f) CELF4 Sentence Formulation; handwriting, spelling, composing; (g) handwriting, spelling, composing, and word reading; (h) severe until 2nd birthday; (i) during pregnancy and after birth; (j) tonsils removed; (k) hypothyroidism

Teachers paying attention to learners during instruction and learning activities

Not all attention problems are the same

While students worked on the iPad lessons at individual work stations in a group setting, the first two authors and other lead teachers observed students' attention. Each student wore ear phones to listen to the instructional talk of the "computer teacher," viewed visual displays on the monitor, provided oral or written language responses for prompts, and received auditory or visual feedback. The lead teachers paid attention to whether individual students were visibly engaged (i.e., attending and fully participating) in: (a) listening and learning activities, which varied frequently across lessons; (b) following instructions; and (c) completing learning activities fully and in the correct sequence. Many, but not all, were engaged (e.g., sometimes they doodled, generating scribbles or drawing, or made off-topic comments to the teachers). They did not follow instructions or complete activities in the sequence presented. The following eight vignettes capture observed individual differences in students' abilities to self-regulate their attention during language learning. The names are fictitious but the vignettes illustrate the authentic story of the varied kinds of difficulties students displayed that pose challenges for teachers in implementing evidence-based instruction.

Jason. A very social person, he initially showed more interest in what other students in the room were doing than what he was supposed to be doing. With repeated scaffolding from the lead teacher, he learned to focus just on his own laptop. However, he was not able to complete all of a lesson or do the learning activities in order. At first these problems were attributed to his OWL LD and difficulty in following directions, but closer inspection showed that at times he seemed to "space out" and stare blankly. However, these momentary lapses did not last long and then he would regain his attention. His mother was encouraged to consult with a neurologist about possible absence seizures. According to Batshaw *et al.* (2013), absence seizures are characterized by momentary lapses in attention and are often mistaken for ADHD.

Sean. At times Sean, who also had OWL LD, was very focused and worked well, but other times he would stand up, walk around, and move out of the room to do jumping jack exercises to re-energize. His mother explained that he was born with congenital hypothyroidism but, even with thyroid medicine, had difficulty maintaining sufficient glucose levels to focus fully. However, frequent small snacks could maintain his energy level. So a plan was implemented. Sean had a snack right before beginning the after school program and snack breaks during it. As long as he had the snacks, he was able to focus and complete the lessons; in fact he was a robust treatment responder. See Batshaw *et al.* (2013) for more information about inborn errors of metabolism, such as hypothyroidism, which may interfere with students' self-regulation of attention unless dietary management and thyroid replacement are in place. Three Cohort 1 participants had hypothyroidism at birth or shortly thereafter.

Gordon. Not only could Gordon not focus, but also he distracted all other students working in the same room. He talked loudly and nonstop even though the other students did not reciprocate and asked him to stop disturbing them. The research director talked to Gordon and his mother to set limits because these behaviors interfered with both his and the other students' learning. Gordon, who has dyslexia and dysgraphia, was motivated to continue because he wanted to read and write better. He returned to the next session with a set of Bose earphones, which were recommended by a pilot who uses them to shut out distracting auditory stimuli during flight. Once Gordon used these earphones, he was able to shut out the auditory distractions, stop distracting others, and focus on the computerized instruction. Thus, his attention problems were related to selective attention, the ability to screen out irrelevant auditory stimuli and focusing attention only on what is relevant.

John. During the initial sessions, John, who met research criteria for dysgraphia, complained that he could not understand what the computer teacher was saying through earphones. Because his family had a history of speech problems, the research director referred his mother to a speech and language specialist, but John was found to have normal hearing and no evidence of speech problems related to processing sequential speech sounds (auditory discrimination) or sequential oral-motor difficulties (articulation). However, he had difficulty with attending to instruction and processing the academic register of teacher talk, which requires strategies beyond those used in the informal conversational register (Silliman and Scott, 2009). Indeed, with teacher scaffolding, he began to learn from oral instruction via ear phones. Comparison of John's normed scores from pretest to posttest showed he made significant gains in: (a) phonological skills (nonword repetition) from average to above average, (b) morphological skills on the Comes From task (deciding whether a second word, such as corner or builder, does or does not come from [is derived from] a first word such as corn or build, respectively), from the mean to about 1/3 z-score above the mean; (c) syntax skills from average to above average range; and (d) silent reading comprehension from the average to above average range.

Greg. He had been diagnosed with dysgraphia without signs of SLI but complained that he could not hear what was being said. The volume was turned up but he still could not hear. Greg's mother reported no hearing loss or use of hearing aids, a long-standing history of lisping, and prior refusal to participate in auditory training. However, with time he began to respond to the lessons, which included not only oral instruction but also many opportunities to analyze sounds in heard words and produce sounds in spoken words. His oral language comprehension of sentences improved from average to above average range and oral language expression improved from average to superior range. Also, his overall speed of planning and executing switching speech sounds on the Pa–Ta–Ka task improved from eight to four seconds.

Joe. This boy, with OWL LD (late talker and persisting problems on morphological, syntactic, and orthographic tasks) plus dysgraphia (automatic access, retrieval, and production of letters in alphabetic order when writing the alphabet from memory) required much monitoring to stay on task, even though he had never been diagnosed with ADHD. He had a preschool history of underdeveloped oral language, speech, and gross motor (walking) problems for his age and received ongoing speech therapy. Nevertheless, with the teacher monitoring to stay on task, Joe responded to instruction. His phonological skills (nonword repetition) improved from below the mean to the mean. His morphological skills improved from the below average range to the average range. His syntax skills improved for oral expression from below the mean to above the mean, and written expression from the below average range to the average range. Joe also improved in sentence combining from low average to average range. In addition, Joe was a treatment responder on the handwriting tasks. Unlike John and Greg, Joe's attention problems were related to staying on task for computerized learning activities aimed at all levels of language—subword, word, syntax, and discourse—not to paying attention to the computer teacher's instructional talk heard through the earphones. The teacher prompts plus the opportunity to combine multi-modal learning (listen to the spoken word, tap for each syllable or phoneme you hear, look for the one- or two-letter grapheme in the word, say the phoneme alone and in the word) appeared to help him engage and stay on task for oral and written language learning activities. His gains in oral and written language may be related to his improvement on measures of supervisory attention in verbal working memory for: (a) switching attention (0.2 standard score) and (b) self-monitoring from below the average to average range.

Penny. Although very social and verbal, she had previously been diagnosed at age seven with ADHD and her current self-regulation difficulties interfered with attending to written language learning, interacting with others, and tolerating frustration. She met the research criteria for dyslexia and dysgraphia. Her ADHD interfered with her response to the computerized instruction. To begin with, she would not use the earphones provided for the oral instruction. Rather, she insisted on using her own earphones and listened to music on the web which was of more interest to her. During the course of the intervention her compliance improved greatly after: (a) the second author introduced a behavioral reinforcement program to reward Penny for focusing and staying on task during the computerized lessons; and (b) Penny's physician changed her ADHD medication. By end of the intervention Penny improved on writing and reading skills, but most gratifying was her improvement in supervisory attention skills in verbal working memory. Her focused attention increased from low average to above average range. Her switching attention improved (0.4 standard score). Of concern, however, was her free flight of ideas during her conversations with other students and the teachers and in her written compositions.

Leonard. This boy, who had dysgraphia, sustained a concussion during the intervention, of which he had no memory. He also tended to "space out" at times. A review of his handwriting lessons stored on the server showed that after the concussion he became disorganized and did not always complete activities in the correct sequence. Yet, he showed improvement on normed tests. Thus, it is important not to rely only on test scores but also to observe behaviors during instruction, and talk to students about their perceptions of sports–related concussions.

Synthesis. Underlying reasons for observed attention difficulties may vary from absence seizures to inborn errors of metabolism (congenital hypothyroidism), to difficulty in selective focus to incoming auditory speech stimuli, to difficulty in paying attention to instructional talk in the academic register (see the chapter by Silliman and Wilkinson, this volume), to auditory discrimination or production difficulties, to full blown ADHD (inattentive, hyperactive, and impulsive subtypes), to concussions. Males appear to have more problems with attention during learning activities than females. Monitoring the attention problems of learners and providing supports for supervisory attention of verbal working memory (focusing, switching, sustaining, and self-monitoring) can facilitate RTI (see RTI columns in Tables 20.1 and 20.2).

Not all social emotional problems are the same

Self-concept issues. Many parents reported self-esteem problems of their children due to lack of academic success. However, some reported adverse emotional consequences beyond self-esteem, such as crying and sighing with homework and other assignments that required writing. All parents supported their children's participation in extracurricular activities where they could gain a sense of accomplishment outside academics. These included a variety of sports, music, drama, and art activities. For example, one boy and one girl had starred in plays.

Motivation issues. Research has shown that students avoid learning activities that are difficult for them; and the avoidance factor tends to persist much longer in writing than reading (Hamilton *et al.*, 2013). Work in progress is analyzing whether prior research findings showing a reduction in writing avoidance following systematic, multi-leveled written language instruction can be replicated.

Family issues. In the zest to help students meet high stakes standards, it is important to take the time to listen to the stressors many students and their families face. One participant and his mother had to deal with the sudden loss of his father who had been murdered. Several were dealing with the divorce of their parents. Some parents were struggling financially and trying to manage both working and helping their child with learning difficulties.

Not all medical issues are the same

Several enrolled participants had significant medical issues. One could not focus because of an immune disorder that could lead to death if exposed to viral infections from other children. Another one developed such a severe sleep disorder he could no longer attend school. Another had to be hospitalized for severe anxiety disorder, which ran in the family.

Not all speech, listening, and oral expression problems are the same

Most students who met the research criteria for OWL LD based on test performance in upper elementary and middle school had a preschool history of speech and/or oral language impairments. This pattern is even clearer in the larger sample of students with OWL LD in subsequent cohorts. Dyslexia co-occurred with speech and/or aural/oral language problems affecting phonological problems; and dysgraphia co-occurred with speech and/or aural/oral language problems related to both oral-motor and grapho-motor planning problems.

Not all reading disabilities are the same

Developmental issues. The belief that children learn to read in the first three grades and then read to learn in the upper elementary grades needs to be revised for the twenty-first century. Oral reading should be emphasized in the primary grades, but explicit instruction in silent reading skills across the content areas of the curriculum should be emphasized at the fourth grade transition and thereafter through high school. Many students with SLDs learn to read but need ongoing explicit instruction to continue to develop specific reading skills (word identification, vocabulary meaning, silent reading accuracy and rate, and various reading comprehension skills that are specific to content areas of the curriculum). They also need to integrate reading with writing skills for the goals of studying for tests and writing reports and other assignments.

Reading skills in the reading profile. Some students have ongoing struggles with reading familiar words and decoding unfamiliar words, but others struggle with sentence comprehension and larger units of discourse. Sometimes both accuracy and rate are impaired for any of these skills. Sometimes only rate is affected. Comprehensive assessment should assess each of these skills and translate results into a learning profile that is instructionally relevant for educators.

Not all writing disabilities are the same

Developmental trajectory. Transcription skills are important throughout K-12. Current evidence supports the value of letter production through handwriting in the early stages of learning to write, but also of systematic, explicit instruction in computer tools beginning in the middle grades and thereafter. Even with spell checks that detect typos, systematic, explicit instruction in spelling English, which is a morphophonemic orthography, is necessary to learn the interrelationships of morphology, phonology, and orthography to enable word-specific recognition of correct spelling among spell check choices. For example, one student reported a "computer glitch" because the computer teacher thought that a phoneme could be spelled with more than one letter and the student was surprised that phonemes are often spelled with one or two letters. Another student had an "aha experience" when he realized that the vowel in *pink* and *wink* sounded slightly different than the vowels in *hit* and *did* because of the following nasal consonant, which made the vowel more difficult to separate from the other consonants in the word. Many students reported the morphological awareness activities, which are rarely taught at school, were the most interesting and useful. For example, they learned how to segment words by morphemes, how to transform bases by adding inflectional and derivational suffixes, and how to sort words by morphological—-phonological, morphological–orthographic, and morphological–phonological–orthographic interrelationships. Text generation skills are also important throughout K-12. For example, evidence supports think-alouds that support the flow of ideas and explicit strategies for self-regulated writing.

Writing skills in writing profile. Comprehensive assessment should cover handwriting, spelling, composing various genres, and integrating writing with reading and with listening. Individual Education Plans (IEPs) and treatment plans for communication disorders should pay more attention to the co-occurrence of ADHD and writing problems and develop specialized instruction for both (see Table 20.1 for evidence of co-occurring ADHD and writing problems). Finally, the co-occurrence of handwriting and OWL LD was unexpected, but when they co-occur, instruction and treatment should address both in a coordinated way.

Multilingual and multicultural issues

In an increasingly global world, professionals should find out what languages are spoken in the home of students. In Cohort 1, parents reported that French and English, or Tagalog and English, or Spanish and English, or Swahili, Kileuku, and English were spoken in the home. Children who meet research criteria for SLDs should not be denied specialized instruction just because they are growing up in multilingual homes. Languages spoken in the home and school are not the same as culture. Both cultural and language differences should be taken into account.

Educational applications

Issues related to brain–environmental interactions

Although multi-sensory instruction is often recommended for students with SLDs, the RTI evidence in Table 20.1 shows the effectiveness of instructional approaches that integrate sensory (ears, eye, touch from skin on fingers) and motor (mouth and hands/fingers), with sensory-motor feedback and language, cognitive, and metacognitive (executive functions for supervisory attention) domains. Interventions that tailor strategies to learners' individual profiles for each of these systems and their interrelationships may be more effective in developing the complex functional systems that enables learning (i.e., personalized education, Berninger and Advisory Panel, 2014).

Co-occurring attention and other problems

As shown in Table 20.2, if a child has a diagnosed speech and/or aural/oral language problems, co-occurring ADHD appears to be unlikely. However, if a child has diagnosed ADHD, there is a 40 percent probability of also having a speech and/or aural/oral language disorder. If supported with ongoing analyses in a larger sample, practitioners should pay more attention to co-occurring attention and language learning problems in the preschool years and transition to schooling in both assessment and treatment plans.

Teaching strategies for paying attention to instructional talk

The first two authors found the following strategies helpful in helping students pay attention to computerized instruction.

- Monitor students and gently direct them to focus when they are unable to sustain attention.
- Set long- and short-term goals and involve students in marking progress visibly.
- Create a behavioral intervention plan and reward on-task behavior with praise or points or other developmentally-appropriate rewards.
- Engage in conversations with parents about student performance, using statements like "Today I noticed…" to describe observations.
- Be firm about expectations and remind students about them before the lesson begins. For older students, it is appropriate to discuss the relevance of instructional methods to their specific learning profiles.
- If students seem excessively fidgety, provide an outlet for them to move their fingers or toes in ways that do not distract others.
- Provide breaks and encourage good nutrition.
- Finally, remain positive at all times. Young people want to enjoy learning and be successful.

Interactions between learners and instruction

To date most of the research, policy, and practice in literacy has focused on teachers using evidence-based instruction. Too little attention has been given to the individual learner and how instruction may have to be adapted to individual differences in the learner during the implementation of those evidence-based practices. We need to go beyond assessing RTI to paying attention to how children are responding during instruction and then engage in problem solving to adapt, when necessary, intervention to meet those individual differences. We also need to do more reaching out to parents to learn about a child's developmental, medical, educational, and family history and use that information in problem solving adaptations. That is, we need to pay more attention to the Persons who are the oral and written language learners (OWLs) in and out of school.

Acknowledgments

Preparation of this chapter was supported by HD P50HD071764 from the *Eunice Kennedy Shriver* National Institute of Child Health and Human Development (NICHD) at the National Institutes of Health (NIH).

The authors thank Zac Alstad, Whitney Griffin, Jasmine Niedo, and Jennie Warmouth, who were also lead teachers for the computerized interventions. The first two authors contributed equally to this chapter.

References

American Psychiatric Association (May 27, 2013), *Diagnostic and Statistical Manual of Mental Disorders, 5th Edition*, American Psychiatric Association, Arlington, VA, US.

Anderson, D. (2011), "Identification of students with specific learning disabilities", National Association of School Psychologists, Bethesda, MD, US. Available online: www.k12.wa.us/

Batshaw, M., Roizen, N. and Lotrecchinao, G. (2013), *Children with Disabilities, 7th Edition*, Paul H. Brookes, Baltimore, MD, US.

Berninger, V. and Dunn, M. (2012), "Brain and behavioral response to intervention for specific reading, writing, and math disabilities: What works for whom?", in B. Wong and D. Butler, (Eds.), *Learning about LD, 4th Edition*, Elsevier, Academic Press, pp. 59–89.

Berninger, V. and Swanson, H.L. (2013), "Diagnosing and treating specific learning disabilities in reference to the brain's working memory system", in H. Lee Swanson, K. Harris, and S. Graham, (Eds.), *Handbook of Learning Disabilities, 2nd Edition*, Guilford, New York, US, pp. 307–325.

Berninger, V.W. and Advisory Panel (2014), *Interdisciplinary Frameworks for Schools: Best Professional Practices For Serving The Needs Of All Students*, American Psychological Association, Washington, DC. Companion Websites with Readings and Resources. All royalties go to Division 16 to support these websites and develop future editions.

Catts, H. (2013), "Oral language disorders and reading comprehension", In Miller, B., Cutting, L. and McCardle, P. (Eds.), *Unraveling Reading Comprehension: Behavioral, Neurobiological, and Genetic Components*, Paul H. Brookes, Baltimore, MD, US, pp. 66–77.

Denton, C., Tolar, T., Fletcher, F., Barth, A., Vaughn, S. and Francis, D. (2013), "Effects of Tier 3 intervention for students with persisting reading difficulties and characteristics of inadequate responders", *Journal of Educational Psychology*, Vol. 105, pp. 633–648.

Geva, E. and Massey-Garrison, A. (2013), "A comparison of the language skills of ELLs and monolinguals who are poor decoders, poor comprehenders, or normal readers", *Journal of Learning Disabilities*, Vol. 46, pp. 387–401.

Hamilton, E., Nolen, S. and Abbott, R. (2013), "Developing measures of motivational orientation to read and write: A longitudinal study", *Learning and Individual Differences*. Uploaded to PubMed Central (PMC) http://publicaccess.nih.gov/FAQ.htm#c1 NIHMS ID of your manuscript is NIHMS 485529.

Johnson, E.P., Pennington, B.F., Lowenstein, J.H. and Nittrouer, S. (2011), "Sensitivity to structure in the speech signal by children with speech sound disorder and reading disability", *Journal of Communication Disorders*, Vol. 44, pp. 294–314.

Miller, B., Cutting, L. and McCardle, P. (2013), *Unraveling Reading Comprehension. Behavioral, Neurobiological, and Genetic Components*, Paul H. Brookes, Baltimore, MD, US.

National Association of School Psychologists, NASP (2011), *Identification of Students with Specific Learning Disabilities (Position Statement)*. Bethesda, MD.

Nittrouer, S. and Lowenstein, J. (2013), "Perceptual organization of speech signals with and without dyslexia", *Research in Developmental Disabilities*, Vol. 34, pp. 2304–2325.

Ogg, J., McMahan, M., Dedrick, R. and Mendez, L. (2013), "Middle school students' willingness to engage in activities with peers with ADHD symptoms: A multiple indicators multiple causes (MIMIC) model", *Journal of School Psychology*, Vol. 51, pp. 407–420.

Silliman, E. and Berninger, V. (2011), "Cross-disciplinary dialogue about the nature of oral and written language problems in the context of developmental, academic, and phenotypic profiles", *Topics in Language Disorders*, Vol. 31, pp. 6–23.

Silliman, E. and Scott, C. (2009), "Research-based oral language intervention routes to the academic language of literacy: Finding the right road", in S. Rosenfield and V. Berninger, (Eds.), *Implementing Evidence-Based Academic Interventions in School Settings*, New York: Oxford University Press, pp. 107–145.

Wagner, R.K., Puranik, C.S., Foorman, B., Foster, E., Wilson, L.G., Tschinkel, E. and Kantor, P.T. (2011), "Modeling the development of written language", *Reading and Writing: An Interdisciplinary Journal*, Vol. 24, pp. 203–220.

21

VOCABULARY AND GRAMMATICAL PROFILES AND RELEVANT INTERVENTIONS FOR ADOLESCENTS WITH DOWN SYNDROME

Lizbeth H. Finestack

Down syndrome (DS; Trisomy 21) is the leading known genetic cause of intellectual disability, estimated to occur in 1 of every 737 live births (Parker *et al.*, 2010). Children with DS have an extra copy of all or part of chromosome 21. Most children with DS are identified upon birth. Delays in the communication skills of children with DS are evident early in development (Berglund *et al.*, 2001) and most individuals with DS will continue to experience significant weaknesses in communication into adulthood. Despite the high incident rate of DS and the well-documented weaknesses in language abilities, there is a paucity of empirical evidence examining appropriate language intervention approaches for children with DS, particularly adolescents with DS.

This chapter focuses on what is known regarding the vocabulary and grammatical profiles of adolescents with DS. The chapter begins with a description of the heterogeneity inherent in aspects of the profiles of adolescents with DS. The remainder of the chapter separately discusses the vocabulary and grammatical profiles of adolescents with DS, highlighting relevant heterogeneity in the profiles. After each profile, intervention implications are provided and information is presented from treatment studies involving individuals with DS. The majority of the information provided in this chapter focuses on adolescents with DS who are expressively verbal because most studies of adolescents with DS have included those who are producing utterances with at least two words in spoken language. Thus, readers should be mindful that the information in this chapter derives from a specified subset of adolescents with DS.

Aspects of heterogeneity in adolescent language profiles

When understanding the language profiles of adolescents with DS, it is important to acknowledge that there is tremendous heterogeneity in language development. Some aspects of this heterogeneity are unique to DS, while other aspects are common across all children. There are at least four types of heterogeneity central to understanding the language profiles of adolescent with DS.

First, there is *heterogeneity in the severity of language weaknesses* across individuals with DS. As noted above, the majority of research that has focused on a better understanding of the language profiles of adolescents with DS includes participants who are producing utterances with at least two words. However, not all adolescents with DS are in this stage of language development. For example, we recently conducted a survey of 98 parents with children aged 5 years or greater that have a child with DS (Schmidt and Finestack, 2011). Table 21.1 displays the responses of the parents regarding their child's stage of language development. To mark a reference point, by 5 years of age typically developing children are expected to readily engage in conversation. Based on our survey results, the majority of the children with DS used conversation and 25 percent used complete or almost complete sentences, but did not engage in conversation frequently. However, 23 percent of parents reported that their child typically produced utterances that contained three words or less, with 30 percent of the children with limited communication greater than 10 years of age. Thus, based on the findings from this parent survey, although the majority of adolescents with DS communicate using complete or almost complete utterances, many are likely to have more limited communication.

Second, there is *heterogeneity in the development of receptive (comprehension) and expressive (production) language* within individuals with DS. Differences in the development of receptive and expressive language, when each is compared to development in children with typical development, are prevalent at an early age. In a study of 43 1- to 5-year-old children with DS, Miller (1999) found that the most common language profile (64 percent) yielded comprehension skills commensurate with mental age expectations and expressive language skills significantly below expectations. The next most common profile (34 percent) in this young group comprised comprehension and expressive language skills that were both commensurate with mental age expectations. However, by 36 months of age, all of the children in the study demonstrated significant delays in expressive language. As children with DS age, greater differences between cognitive development, receptive, and expressive language emerge for many individuals. For example, in a study of 11- to 23-year-olds with DS, Abbeduto et al. (2001) found that, for most individuals, both receptive and expressive language abilities were significantly below mental age expectations and that skills in expressive language were significantly weaker than receptive language skills.

Third, within the receptive and expressive domains, *heterogeneity exists across development of vocabulary and grammar*. Researchers have documented that adolescents with DS have difficulties across each of these domains (see Martin et al., 2009). However, the extent of impairment across these domains is variable (Abbeduto et al., 2001; Chapman, 1997; Miller, 1999; Rice et al.,

Table 21.1 Responses of parents of children with DS regarding current stage of language development.

Age Group	Not Using Words or Signs	Single Words or Signs	Utterances with 2–3 Words or Signs	Complete or Almost Complete Sentences	Conversational Language
5–10 Years (*n* = 50)	2	6	8	17	17
11–18 Years (*n* = 32)	0	2	2	9	19
19+ Years (*n* = 16)	0	1	2	0	13
% of Total (*N* = 98)	2	9	12	27	50

2005). Most frequently, this is characterized by vocabulary development that is at or above expectations based on nonverbal mental age and grammatical development that is significantly below mental age expectations (Abbeduto *et al.*, 2003; Chapman *et al.*, 1991; Miller, 1999).

Fourth, for many individuals with DS, *heterogeneity in language performance exists across language contexts*, namely spontaneous and narrative sampling contexts. As in other populations (Wagner *et al.*, 2000; Westerveld *et al.*, 2004), children and adolescents with DS tend to demonstrate stronger expressive language skills in narrative language contexts relative to conversational contexts. For example, in a study of 12- to 21-year-old adolescents with DS, Miles *et al.* (2006) found that the average mean length of utterance (MLU) based on a picture-supported narrative context was significantly greater than the average MLU based on a researcher–participant interview. Similarly, Chapman *et al.* (1998) found that their 5- to 20-year old participants with DS produced significantly more word tokens, more word types, and longer MLUs in narrative samples than conversational samples. However, stronger performance in narrative contexts is likely related to the use of visual supports to elicit samples. Miles *et al.* (2006) compared performance on personal narratives elicited during conversation with no picture supports and fictional narratives elicited using wordless picture books. Although both samples comprised narrative language, the MLUs of the adolescents with DS were longer in the picture-supported narrative context.

In sum, there are significant differences in the severity of language impairment among adolescents with DS and language performance differs across expressive and receptive domains, vocabulary and grammatical skills, and language sampling contexts. The following vocabulary and grammatical profiles highlight the important differences relevant to each of these aspects of heterogeneity.

Vocabulary profile

Measurement variation

The vocabulary profile of adolescents with DS varies largely depending on the assessment measure. When using measures with vocabulary items that increase in difficulty based on the frequency of the target word, such as the *Peabody Picture Vocabulary Test* (Dunn and Dunn, 1997) or the *Expressive Vocabulary Test* (Williams, 2007), adolescents with DS tend to perform at or near nonverbal mental age expectations. This is true for evaluations of both receptive (Chapman *et al.*, 1998; Finestack *et al.*, 2013; Laws and Bishop, 2003; Rosin *et al.*, 1988) and expressive vocabulary skills (Finestack *et al.*, 2013; Laws and Bishop, 2003). In contrast, when receptive vocabulary is assessed using measures with items varying in difficulty based on conceptual complexity, such as the *Test of Auditory Comprehension of Language* (Carrow-Woolfolk, 1999), adolescents with DS are more likely to perform below younger children of similar nonverbal cognitive mental age with typical development (Chapman, 2006; Price *et al.*, 2007).

Similarly, when expressive vocabulary is assessed based on contextualized measures, such as those derived from conversational or narrative language samples, adolescents with DS are more likely to demonstrate vocabulary skills weaker than those of younger mental-aged matched children of typical development (Boudreau and Chapman, 2000; Chapman, 2006; Chapman *et al.*, 1998; Miolo *et al.*, 2005). For example, Chapman *et al.* (1998) found that, based on both narrative and conversational language samples, participants, ages 5 to 20 years with DS, produced fewer words overall and a lower number of different words than the control group of 2- to 6-year-old children with typical development matched for nonverbal mental age. However, there are noteworthy exceptions to this general pattern. For example, when controlling for nonverbal cognitive ability, Roberts *et al.* (2007) found that the mean age-equivalent scores of 4- to 16-year-old boys with DS were significantly lower than the mean age-equivalent scores of 2- to 7-year-old boys with typical development on both the *Peabody Picture Vocabulary Test-III* (Dunn and Dunn, 1997) and the *Expressive Vocabulary Test* (Williams, 1997). Thus, it appears that adolescents with DS have relative strengths in their vocabulary skills when assessed using items varying in assumed frequency of exposure. However, because age-equivalent scores do not reflect equal intervals, the magnitude of this relative vocabulary strength is unknown. In contrast, when vocabulary is assessed using items varying in conceptual complexity or when based on production in complex language contexts, such as oral language samples, these strengths are no longer evident.

Fast-mapping skills

To better understand the vocabulary development of children and adolescents with DS, investigators have examined their fast-mapping skills. Fast-mapping, one of the first steps involved in the process of lexical acquisition (Carey and Bartlett, 1978), occurs when a learner is able to link an unfamiliar name and referent with minimal exposure to either the name or the referent. Children with significant language weaknesses, including children with specific language impairment, demonstrate difficulties with many fast-mapping tasks (Alt *et al.*, 2004; Dollaghan, 1987; Gray, 2003). For example, an early fast-mapping study by Dollaghan (1987) indicated that children as young as 2 years of age possessed fast-mapping learning skills based on comprehension tasks. When compared to peers with typical language development, 4-year-old children with specific language impairment, demonstrated weaknesses in fast-mapping based on production tasks. Given that fast-mapping skills of children with language impairment are weak, it is likely that vocabulary weaknesses of children and adolescents with DS may be due to weaknesses in fast-mapping skills; thus, several researchers have investigated this possibility.

Chapman *et al.* (1990) first compared the fast-mapping skills of children and adolescents with DS to younger children with typical development matched on nonverbal mental age. On both comprehension and expressive tasks related to the learning of a novel word after a single exposure, there were no significant differences between the children and adolescents with DS, ages 5 to 21 years, and the 2- to 6-year-old children with typical development. Both groups performed better on the comprehension task than the production task. On the comprehension task, the adolescents with DS demonstrated significant improvement in task performance from ages 12–16 years (64 percent) to 16–20 years (100 percent), whereas the children with typical development maintained a high level of accuracy (approximately 80 percent) across age groups. In contrast, on the production task, the adolescents with DS did not demonstrate gains in performance across age groups (range = 18 percent to 62 percent), while the children with typical development demonstrated significant improvement in performance from ages 2 years (9 percent) to 6 years (77 percent). Overall, individuals with DS demonstrated fast-mapping skills on par with younger children with similar nonverbal cognitive skills, but this relatively strong performance appears to be limited to simple fast-mapping tasks.

Subsequent examinations of the fast-mapping skills of children and adolescents with DS indicated that, when the experimental fast-mapping task required the learning of more than one novel word or when the novel target word was presented in a more complex narrative context, the performance of individuals with DS deteriorated (Chapman and Abbeduto, 2003; Kay-Raining Bird *et al.*, 2004). Evidence suggests that adolescents with DS benefitted from repeated exposure to target forms as well as prompts to imitate the target forms (Chapman *et al.*, 2006).

Additionally, similar to children with typical development (Imai *et al.*, 2008), adolescents with DS demonstrated more successful learning of nouns than verbs in fast-mapping tasks (McDuffie *et al.*, 2007). This difference was likely found because verb learning requires greater syntactic skills than noun learning for adequate mapping of the phonological form to the referent (Naigles, 1990). As described below, adolescents with DS have weak grammatical skills, which would negatively impact their verb learning. Indeed, studies have demonstrated that syntax comprehension is a significant predictor variable of fast-mapping performance in children with DS (Kay-Raining Bird *et al.*, 2004; McDuffie *et al.*, 2007). The performance of adolescents with DS on fast-mapping tasks is also significantly related to vocabulary comprehension (Chapman *et al.*, 2006). Thus, it appears that some of the vocabulary weaknesses of children and adolescents with DS may be attributed to combined weaknesses in fast-mapping and grammatical abilities.

Implications for intervention

Although there are no known studies specifically investigating the development of authentic vocabulary items by adolescents with DS through targeted interventions, studies examining the vocabulary profiles and fast-mapping skills of adolescents with DS provide a rich source of information to guide vocabulary interventions. Profile information indicates that vocabulary development is likely to be an area of weakness, relative to nonverbal cognitive ability, throughout adolescence for individuals with DS. However, these significant weaknesses may only be evident when assessed on conceptually complex items or within complex narrative contexts. Thus, to fully understand the receptive and expressive vocabulary skills of adolescents with DS, clinicians must carefully select assessments based on item conceptual complexity and testing context. Furthermore, careful consideration must be given to the selection of vocabulary items to target in intervention.

Given that the new Common Core State Standards emphasize general and specific academic vocabulary (National Governors Association Center for Best Practices and Council of Chief State School Officers, 2010), it is likely that school-based clinicians will need to target vocabulary items drawn from academic content areas, such as science and social studies (for further discussion on content area vocabulary, see the Silliman and Wilkinson chapter, this volume). Content-specific vocabulary is conceptually and contextually complex and, therefore, likely to be challenging for adolescents with DS. Also, there is no evidence of a vocabulary growth plateau for adolescents with DS (Chapman *et al.*, 1998). Thus, it is likely that, with consistent intervention and support, the vocabularies of individuals with DS will continue to improve.

Studies examining the fast-mapping skills of children and adolescents with DS offer additional guidance toward intervention approaches to enhance vocabulary acquisition. First, given that individuals with DS show strength in learning high-frequency words and that multiple encounters with novel target words enhance performance on fast-mapping tasks, clinicians will have to increase the frequency of the exposure of target items for adolescents with DS.

Second, similar to other populations, evidence of stronger performance on comprehension fast-mapping tasks than on production tasks reveals that adolescents are likely to comprehend more than expressed and will encode new vocabulary items into their receptive lexicon prior to encoding the item into their expressive lexicon. Thus, to assist production, clinicians will need to assess vocabulary in both domains and aim to help adolescents with DS comprehend vocabulary items that are neither comprehended nor produced and facilitate the advancement of vocabulary items that are accurately comprehended but not expressed.

Third, given that contextual complexity and syntactic comprehension skills contribute to vocabulary learning, clinicians will need to select topics and activities that are relevant to the learner and rich enough to provide contextual cues regarding the meaning and appropriate use of target items. Additionally, it is important that the linguistic context is not too semantically or syntactically complex; otherwise the adolescent would be unable to pull meaning from the context and enhance his/her representation of the target vocabulary item.

Grammatical profiles

Development across language domains and contexts

Studies examining the relationship between vocabulary development and grammatical skills, generally demonstrate that vocabulary skills are significantly stronger than grammatical skills (Abbeduto *et al.*, 2003; Laws and Bishop, 2003). For example, Laws and Bishop (2003) compared transformed z scores derived from receptive and expressive vocabulary, and grammar measures and found that 10- to 19-year-old adolescents with DS had significantly lower scores on measures of grammar than vocabulary. Study results also indicated that the expressive language scores were significantly lower than the receptive scores.

Weaknesses in the grammatical skills of children and adolescents with DS relative to the skills of younger typically developing children with similar nonverbal cognitive abilities are well documented. In the receptive domain, these weaknesses are evident based on norm-referenced standardized measures that typically require respondents to point to the picture that best represents the presented phrase or sentence, which varies in grammatical complexity (Abbeduto *et al.*, 2003; Finestack *et al.*, 2013; Joffe and Varlokosta, 2007; Laws and Bishop, 2003; Miolo *et al.*, 2005; Price *et al.*, 2007). In the expressive domain, in addition to documented weaknesses on standardized probes similar to those described above (Finestack *et al.*, 2013), significant weaknesses relative to mental age expectations were evident based on measures derived from conversational and/or narrative language samples. These included gross grammatical measures such as MLU (Boudreau and Chapman, 2000; Chapman *et al.*, 1998; Finestack *et al.*, 2013; Laws and Bishop, 2003; Price *et al.*, 2008; Rosin *et al.*, 1988) and fine-grained measures such as the Developmental Sentence Scoring (Lee, 1974) and the Index of Productive Syntax (Scarborough, 1990) (Chapman *et al.*, 1998; Finestack and Abbeduto, 2010; Price *et al.*, 2008). Although significant weaknesses existed in both conversational and narrative language, narrative contexts tended to elicit significantly more advanced grammatical skills than conversational contexts (Chapman *et al.*, 1998).

The pattern of significantly impaired grammatical skills compared to mental age expectations has not been uniformly documented across all studies. For example, in a study that included 5- to 21-year-old children and adolescents with DS and 2- to 6-year-old typically developing children matched on nonverbal mental age, Chapman *et al.* (1991) found no significant group differences based on the standardized receptive measure, the Test for Auditory Comprehension of Language (Carrow-Woolfolk, 1985). In other studies (Keller-Bell and Abbeduto, 2007; Thordardottir *et al.*, 2002), no group differences were found between adolescents with DS and younger children with typical or similar nonverbal cognitive abilities on measures of grammatical complexity when derived from expressive narrative samples. Kay-Raining Bird *et al.* (2008) also found no differences between children and adolescents with DS and a younger group of typically developing children matched on reading word identification skills based on the linguistic complexity produced in narrative language samples. However, the individuals with DS produced significantly longer narratives.

The specific areas of grammatical deficits of children and adolescents with DS align closely with the core language deficits of children with SLI who have inconsistent omissions of tense and agreement markings (Eadie *et al.*, 2002; Laws and Bishop, 2003). For example, in the Eadie *et al.* study, which included children with DS and younger children with SLI matched on MLU and cognitive ability, both the DS and SLI groups demonstrated significant weaknesses in their production of inflectional tense forms (i.e., regular past-tense –ed and third person singular –s) relative to typically developing children. There were no significant differences between the DS and SLI groups on these measures.

Implications for intervention

When considering intervention services for adolescents with DS, it is important to be mindful of cross-sectional data by Chapman and colleagues (Chapman *et al.*, 1998; Chapman *et al.*, 2002). These data indicate that, although grammatical and syntactic growth is slow throughout adolescence, the MLU derived from narrative language samples of individuals with DS continues to increase during this period. Moreover, the distribution of the mean number of utterances based on morpheme length (e.g., number of 1-, 2- , and 3-morpheme utterances) mirrors the distribution of younger typically developing children matched on MLU. This suggests that a grammatical developmental ceiling does not exist for adolescents with DS (Chapman *et al.*, 1998). This evidence combined with the profiles of adolescents with DS, which indicate more severe weaknesses in grammatical skills relative to vocabulary, have treatment implications. Language treatments for this population must devote considerable attention to strengthening grammatical skills to improve communication and academic outcomes. Such interventions will likely need to be more intense than those targeting lexical skills due to the severity of the grammatical and syntactic skills of adolescents with DS.

Few studies have examined language treatments for school-aged children with DS despite a clear potential for individuals in this age range to make language gains (Chapman *et al.*, 2002; Chapman *et al.*, 1998; Thordardottir *et al.*, 2002). Studies that have examined grammatical interventions for individuals with DS have been small-scaled, single-subject designs. For example, Camarata *et al.* (2006) conducted a study broadly targeting grammatical and speech intelligibility in six 4- to 8-year-old children with DS. Using grammatical and speech recasts (i.e., adding grammatical or speech information omitted from the child's platform utterance), treatment-induced MLU gains were documented for two of the participants. In another study (Hewitt *et al.*, 2005) involving three adults with DS, grammatical elements, such as the pronoun *I*, third person pronouns, and prepositions, were targeted. The approach included both naturalistic modeling and recasting, as well as drill-based imitation. All three participants demonstrated dramatic increases in their percentage of correct spontaneous productions with this intervention approach. These studies suggest that adolescents with DS are likely to benefit from interventions that use traditional approaches, such as modeling and recasting, to strengthen use of morphological and syntactic forms.

Conclusion

The language profiles of adolescents with DS are heterogeneous such that not all adolescents are in the same stage of language development. Although the majority of parents with adolescents with DS report that their child communicates using complete or almost complete sentences, some parents report that their child communicates using one- or two-word utterances. Heterogeneity also exists in the individual language profiles of adolescents with DS. Specifically, for most individuals with DS, receptive language is stronger than productive language, vocabulary development progresses more quickly than grammatical development, and narrative language sampling contexts yield more complex language skills than conversational contexts. Despite these profile characteristics, it is clear that adolescents experience significant weaknesses in their vocabulary and grammatical skills that are likely to negatively impact their academic success and social well-being. Thus, language intervention services for adolescents with DS are necessary. In our survey of parents with children with DS between the ages of 5 and 19 years (Schmidt and Finestack, 2011), 93 percent of the parents indicated that their child was currently receiving speech–language services. Of these parents, 64 percent indicated that they were generally satisfied with the selection of goals for intervention. Moreover, 79 percent of parents surveyed responded they believed that, because of their speech–language services, their child had made gains, which helped with communication outside of therapy.

Despite the clear need for intervention services to further support the language development of adolescents with DS and preliminary evidence that this population is generally receiving beneficial and satisfactory services, few studies have focused on language interventions for this population. Clinicians are able to draw on information regarding the profiles of adolescents with DS, such as that presented in this chapter. Clinicians may also consult evidence-based treatment findings from other populations, such as children with SLI, to guide intervention services. However, it remains unknown if these approaches maximize the effectiveness of language interventions for adolescents with DS. Thus, it is imperative for clinicians and researchers to continue to improve treatments and to evaluate these approaches to maximize language outcomes and to ensure that adolescents with DS are reaching their greatest potential.

References

Abbeduto, L., Pavetto, M., Kesin, E., Weissman, M.D., Karadottir, S., O'brien, A. and Cawthon, S. (2001), "The linguistic and cognitive profile of Down syndrome: Evidence from a comparison with fragile X syndrome", *Down Syndrome: Research and Practice,* Vol. 7, pp. 9–15.

Abbeduto, L., Murphy, M.M., Cawthon, S.W., Richmond, E.K., Weissman, M.D., Karadottir, S. and O'brien, A. (2003), "Receptive language skills of adolescents and young adults with Down syndrome or fragile X syndrome", *American Journal on Mental Retardation,* Vol. 108, pp. 149–160.

Alt, M., Plante, E. and Creusere, M. (2004), "Semantic features in fast-mapping: Performance of preschoolers with specific language impairment versus preschoolers with normal language", *Journal of Speech, Language, and Hearing Research,* Vol. 47, pp. 407–420.

Berglund, E., Eriksson, M. and Johansson, I. (2001), "Parental reports of spoken language skills in children with Down syndrome", *Journal of Speech, Language, and Hearing Research,* Vol. 44, pp. 179–191.

Boudreau, D.M. and Chapman, R.S. (2000), "The relationship between event representation and linguistic skill in narratives of children and adolescents with Down syndrome", *Journal of Speech, Language, and Hearing Research,* Vol. 43, pp. 1146–1159.

Camarata, S., Yoder, P. and Camarata, M. (2006), "Simultaneous treatment of grammatical and speech-comprehensibility deficits in children with Down syndrome", *Down Syndrome: Research and Practice,* Vol. 11, pp. 9–17.

Carey, S. and Bartlett, E. (1978), "Acquiring a single new word", *Papers and Reports on Child Language Development,* Vol. 15, pp. 17–29.

Carrow-Woolfolk, E. (1985), "Test for Auditory Comprehension of Language-Revised", Allen, TX, US: DLM Teaching Resources.

Carrow-Woolfolk, E. (1999), "Test for Auditory Comprehension of Language-Third Edition", Circle Pines, MN, US: American Guidance Services.

Chapman, R.S. (1997), "Language development in children and adolescents with Down syndrome", *Mental Retardation and Developmental Disabilities Research Reviews,* Vol. 3, pp. 307–312.

Chapman, R.S. (2006), "Language learning in Down syndrome: The speech and language profile compared to adolescents with cognitive impairment of unknown origin", *Down Syndrome: Research and Practice,* Vol. 10, pp. 61–66.

Chapman, R.S. (2003), "Language and communication in individuals with Down syndrome", *International Review of Research in Mental Retardation: Language and Communication in Mental Retardation*, Vol 27, pp. 1–34.

Chapman, R.S., Kay-Raining Bird, E. and Schwartz, S.E. (1990), "Fast mapping of words in event contexts by children with Down syndrome", *Journal of Speech and Hearing Disorders,* Vol. 55, pp. 761–770.

Chapman, R.S., Schwartz, S.E. and Kay-Raining Bird, E. (1991), "Language skills of children and adolescents with Down syndrome: I Comprehension", *Journal of Speech, Language, and Hearing Research*, Vol. 34, pp. 1106–1120.

Chapman, R.S., Seung, H.-K., Schwartz, S.E. and Bird, E.K.-R. (1998), "Language skills of children and adolescents with Down syndrome: II Production deficits", *Journal of Speech, Language, and Hearing Research,* Vol. 41, pp. 861–873.

Chapman, R.S., Hesketh, L.J. and Kistler, D.J. (2002), "Predicting longitudinal change in language production and comprehension in individuals with Down syndrome: Hierarchical linear modeling", *Journal of Speech, Language, and Hearing Research,* Vol. 45, pp. 902–915.

Chapman, R.S., Sindberg, H., Bridge, C., Gigstead, K. and Hesketh, L. (2006), "Effect of memory support and elicited production on fast mapping of new words by adolescents with Down Syndrome", *Journal of Speech, Language, and Hearing Research,* Vol. 49, pp. 3–15.

Dollaghan, C.A. (1987), "Fast mapping in normal and language-impaired children", *Journal of Speech and Hearing Disorders,* Vol. 52, pp. 218–222.

Dunn, L. and Dunn, L. (1997), "Peabody Picture Vocabulary Test-3rd Edition", Circle Pines, MN, US: American Guidance Service.

Eadie, P.A., Fey, M.E., Douglas, J.M. and Parsons, C.L. (2002), "Profiles of grammatical morphology and sentence imitation in children with specific language impairment and Down syndrome", *Journal of Speech, Language, and Hearing Research,* Vol. 45, pp. 720–732.

Finestack, L.H. and Abbeduto, L. (2010), "Expressive language profiles of verbally expressive adolescents and young adults with Down syndrome or fragile X syndrome", *Journal of Speech, Language, and Hearing Research,* Vol. 53, pp. 1334–1348.

Finestack, L.H., Sterling, A.M. and Abbeduto, L. (2013), "Discriminating Down syndrome and fragile X syndrome based on language ability", *Journal of Child Language,* Vol. 40, pp. 244–265.

Gray, S. (2003), "Word-learning by preschoolers with specific language impairment: What predicts success?", *Journal of Speech, Language, and Hearing Research,* Vol. 46, pp. 56–67.

Hewitt, L.E., Hinkle, A.S. and Miccio, A.W. (2005), "Intervention to improve expressive grammar for adults with Down syndrome", *Communication Disorders Quarterly,* Vol. 26, pp. 144–155.

Imai, M., Li, L., Haryu, E., Okada, H., Hirsh-Pasek, K., Golinkoff, R.M. and Shigematsu, J. (2008), "Novel noun and verb learning in Chinese-, English-, and Japanese-speaking children", *Child Development,* Vol. 79, pp. 979–1000.

Joffe, V. and Varlokosta, S. (2007), "Patterns of syntactic development in children with Williams syndrome and Down's syndrome: Evidence from passives and wh-questions", *Clinical Linguistics and Phonetics,* Vol. 21, pp. 705–727.

Kay-Raining Bird, E., Chapman, R. and Schwartz, C.E. (2004), "Fast mapping of words and story recall by individuals with Down syndrome", *Journal of Speech, Language, and Hearing Research,* Vol. 47, pp. 1286–1300.

Kay-Raining Bird, E., Cleave, P.L., White, D., Pike, H. and Helmkay, A. (2008), "Written and oral narratives of children and adolescents with Down syndrome", *Journal of Speech, Language, and Hearing Research,* Vol. 51, pp. 436–450.

Keller-Bell, Y.D. and Abbeduto, L. (2007), "Narrative development in adolescents and young adults with fragile X syndrome", *American Journal on Mental Retardation,* Vol. 112, pp. 289–299.

Laws, G. and Bishop, D.V. (2003), "A comparison of language abilities in adolescents with Down syndrome and children with specific language impairment", *Journal of Speech, Language, and Hearing Research,* Vol. 46, pp. 1324–1339.

Lee, L. (1974), "Developmental Sentence Analysis", Evanston, IL, US: Northwestern University Press.

McDuffie, A.S., Sindberg, H.A., Hesketh, L.J. and Chapman, R.S. (2007), "Use of speaker intent and grammatical cues in fast-mapping by adolescents with Down syndrome", *Journal of Speech, Language, and Hearing Research,* Vol. 50, pp. 1546–1561.

Martin, G.E., Klusek, J., Estigarribia, B. and Roberts, J.E. (2009), "Language characteristics of individuals with Down syndrome", *Topics in Language Disorders,* Vol. 29, pp. 112–132.

Miles, S. (2006), "Sampling context affects MLU in the language of adolescents with Down syndrome", *Journal of Speech, Language, and Hearing Research*, Vol. 49, pp. 325–337.

Miller, J. (1999), "Profiles of language development in children with Down syndrome", In: Miller, J., Leddy, M. and Leavitt, L. (Eds.), *Improving the Communication of People with Down Syndrome*. Baltimore, MD, US: Paul H. Brookes, pp. 11–40.

Miolo, G., Chapman, R.S. and Sindberg, H.A. (2005), "Sentence comprehension in adolescents with Down syndrome and typically developing children: Role of sentence voice, visual context, and auditory-verbal short-term memory", *Journal of Speech, Language, and Hearing Research,* Vol. 48, pp. 172–188.

Naigles, L. (1990), "Children use syntax to learn verb meanings", *Journal of Child Language,* Vol. 17, pp. 357–374.

National Governors Association Center for Best Practices and Council of Chief State School Officers. (2010), "Common Core State Standards: English Language Arts Standards", Washington D.C., US: National Governors Association Center for Best Practices, Council of Chief State School Officers.

Parker, S.E., Mai, C.T., Canfield, M.A., Rickard, R., Wang, Y., Meyer, R.E., Anderson, P., Mason, C.A., Collins, J.S., Kirby, R.S., Correa, A. and National Birth Defects Prevention Network (2010), "Updated National Birth Prevalence estimates for selected birth defects in the United States, 2004–2006", *Birth Defects Research,* Vol. 88, pp. 1008–1016.

Price, J., Roberts, J., Vandergrift, N. and Martin, G. (2007), "Language comprehension in boys with fragile X syndrome and boys with Down syndrome", *Journal of Intellectual Disability Research*, Vol. 51, pp. 318–326.

Price, J., Roberts, J., Hennon, E.A., Berni, M.C., Anderson, K.L. and Sideris, J. (2008), "Syntactic complexity during conversation of boys with fragile X syndrome and Down syndrome", *Journal of Speech, Language, and Hearing Research,* Vol. 51, pp. 3–15.

Rice, M.L., Warren, S. and Betz, S.K. (2005), "Language symptoms of developmental language disorders: An overview of autism, Down syndrome, fragile X, specific language impairment, and Williams syndrome", *Applied Psycholinguistics,* Vol. 26, pp. 7–27.

Roberts, J., Price, J., Barnes, E., Nelson, L., Burchinal, M., Hennon, E.A. *et al.* (2007), "Receptive vocabulary, expressive vocabulary, and speech production of boys with fragile X syndrome in comparison to boys with Down Syndrome", *American Journal on Mental Retardation,* Vol. 112, pp. 177–193.

Rosin, M.M., Swift, E., Bless, D. and Kluppel Vetter, D. (1988), "Communication profiles of adolescents with Down syndrome", *Journal of Childhood Communication Disorders,* Vol. 12, pp. 49–64.

Scarborough, H.S. (1990), "Index of productive syntax", *Applied Psycholinguistics,* Vol. 11, pp. 1–22.

Schmidt, V. and Finestack, L.H. (2011), *Parent perspectives of language services for children with Down syndrome.* Poster presented at the annual meeting of the American Speech-Language, and Hearing Association. San Diego, CA, US.

Thordardottir, E.T., Chapman, R.S. and Wagner, L. (2002), "Complex sentence production by adolescents with Down syndrome", *Applied Psycholinguistics,* Vol. 23, pp. 163–183.

Wagner, R., Nettelbladt, U., Sahlen, B. and Nilholm, C. (2000), "Conversation versus narration in preschool children with language impairment", *International Journal of Language and Communication Disorders,* Vol. 35, pp. 83–93.

Westerveld, M.F., Gillon, G.T. and Miller, J.F. (2004), "Spoken language samples of New Zealand children in conversation and narration", *International Journal of Speech-Language Pathology,* Vol. 6, pp. 195–208.

Williams, K.T. (1997), *Expressive Vocabulary Test,* Circle Pines, MN, US: American Guidance Service.

Williams, K.T. (2007), *Expressive Vocabulary Test-Second Edition,* Circle Pines, MN, US: American Guidance Service.

22

BEYOND THE THEORY OF MIND HYPOTHESIS

Using a causal model to understand the nature and treatment of multiple deficits in Autism Spectrum Disorder

Tiffany L. Hutchins and Patricia A. Prelock

Autism Spectrum Disorder (ASD) is a genetically-based neurobiological disorder defined by deficits in social communication and social interaction, and by restricted, repetitive patterns of behavior, interests, or activities (American Psychiatric Association, 2013). Several influential single-deficit accounts of ASD (theories of executive dysfunction, weak central coherence, and Theory of Mind) have been put forth as candidate explanations for the cognitive mechanisms involved in ASD. In this chapter, we focus on the most prominent single-deficit account: the Theory of Mind Hypothesis (Baron-Cohen, 1995a; Baron-Cohen *et al.*, 1985), which proposes ASD is the result of a foundational impairment in the ability to make accurate inferences about inner mental worlds. A cursory look at the literature reveals wide variability in how Theory of Mind (ToM) and its relation to biological and behavioral functions are understood. Thus, it is important to clarify the concept of ToM to understand autism, develop testable theoretical models, and make informed choices about treatment.

In this chapter, the nature and scope of ToM and its relationships to biological factors and autistic symptoms are roughly sketched using a causal model to integrate research findings. The contributions of executive function and central coherence are briefly discussed and the benefits of a multiple-deficits model for understanding the characteristics of ASD are described. Finally, we demonstrate how causal modeling can be applied in clinical practice and detail some of the strengths and challenges in this approach to intervention.

Causal modeling

The causal modeling approach (detailed by Morton, 2004) provides a graphic representation within a neutral framework from which different views of a developmental disorder can be understood. This approach has three requisite components that correspond to different levels of scientific discourse: biological, behavioral, and cognitive. The role of the environment is also represented and viewed as having extensive contributions across all three levels. The biological (e.g., genes, neurological substrates, brain systems) and behavioral (e.g., lack of imitation and pretend play, pragmatic language deficits) levels are descriptive. It is only with the inclusion of an intervening cognitive level (e.g., impaired face processing, lack of empathy, inability to represent false beliefs) that examination of a range of probabilistic (although not deterministic) causal links from biological to behavioral functions can be modeled (Morton and Frith, 1995).

The causal modeling approach was designed to represent developmental disorders in general and ASD in particular for which a description of functioning at the cognitive level is essential (Frith *et al.*, 1991; Morton and Frith, 1995). As such, causal modeling has two specific advantages for the present purposes. First, it allows for a description of a disorder or an individual case providing a flexible framework for advancing research and clinical practice. Second, causal models can be represented with any required degree of complexity and detail. To construct a causal model, we adhere to the maxims put forth by the developers of this approach, and "start with biology" (Morton and Frith, 1995, p. 359).

ToM at the biological level

Although no specific set of genetic biomarkers is considered as necessary and sufficient to explain the development of ASD, the available genetic and neurological evidence suggests the presence of strong biological bases (e.g., Betancur, 2011; Bowers *et al.*, 2011). The biological bases of ToM (or social cognition more broadly) have been revealed in twin studies (Mazefsky *et al.*, 2008) and neurological and brain imaging studies of typically developing (TD) persons and persons with ASD (Anagnostou and Taylor, 2011; Schultz *et al.*, 2000). This body of literature has implicated genes, hormones, and heritability as well as early brain enlargement (Nordahl *et al.*, 2012; Raznahan *et al.*, 2013), abnormal brain connectivity (Dichter *et al.*, 2012; Vissers *et al.*, 2012), and specific brain structures and regions and complex brain systems (Neuhaus *et al.*, 2010; Pelphrey *et al.*, 2011).

Our description of the biological bases of social-cognitive deficits in ASD is cursory and only provides a sense of the range of biological factors, brain regions, and processes that are implicated in ASD. This heterogeneity of factors gains importance in light of the tremendous individual variation that is found in ASD at the biological level. Further, persons with ASD often present with a diverse set of concomitant medical conditions including, but not limited to, intellectual disability, motor disturbances, seizure disorder, and other psychiatric conditions. Taken together, these findings have led most researchers to conclude that the biological bases of ToM are complex and that disruptions in ToM (and for that matter the presence of the primary deficits that define the diagnostic category of ASD) have no single biological origin (e.g., Happé and Ronald, 2008; Robinson *et al.*, 2012). A graphic representation of this understanding is presented in Figure 22.1 (see the Biological level) where several distinct biological origins (O_1, O_2, O_3) give rise to distinct biological consequences on the brain (Br_1, Br_2, Br_3), which interact to result in distinct biological consequences for brain systems (br_1, br_2, br_3). Of course, the other important lesson from the brain imaging research is that complex capacities employ networks of brain regions that work in concert to solve a range of problems. This foreshadows the difficulty in finding an adequate description of ToM functioning at the cognitive and behavioral levels, understanding the relationships between ToM and other cognitive domains, and determining what constitutes a developmental endpoint versus a developmental foundation of ASD.

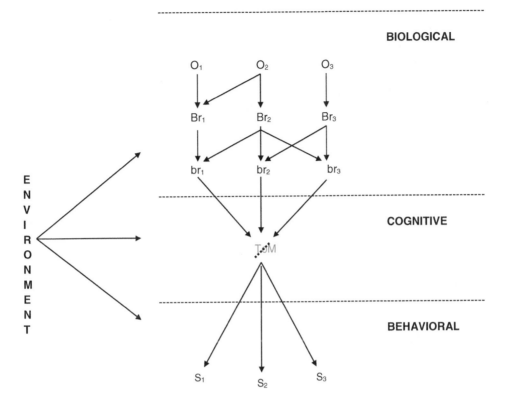

Figure 22.1 A candidate causal model of the ToM hypothesis of ASD developed using the notation of Morton and Frith (1995) where O = a biological origin, Br = biological consequence on the brain, br = biological consequence on a brain system, S = behavioral sign or symptom. At the cognitive level, the slash (dotted line) through ToM indicates a faulty ToM mechanism.

ToM at the cognitive level

Owing to nearly three decades of empirical findings revealing deficits in ToM in ASD, enthusiasm for the ToM hypothesis of ASD has endured. Although differences in the measurement of ToM clearly influence performance (e.g., van Buijsen *et al.*, 2011) research shows that persons with ASD generally underperform TD individuals on assessments of mental states (e.g., Sterck and Begeer, 2010). However, several other cognitive features have been implicated as faulty ToM dimensions in ASD. These include atypical self-concept and self-awareness (Hobson *et al.*, 2006), misperception of biological motion (Gowen *et al.*, 2008), impaired face recognition (e.g., Baron-Cohen, 1995b), and deficits in humor processing (Samson and Hegenloh, 2010), empathy (e.g., Mathersul *et al.*, 2013), and moral reasoning (e.g., Zalla *et al.*, 2011).

ToM has been described as a "slippery concept" that is "difficult to pin down" (Belmonte, 2009, p. 122). Indeed, ToM is a term that "refuses to be corralled" (Astington and Baird, 2005, p. 4) and it is often used interchangeably with terms like 'perspective-taking,' 'social cognition,' 'metacognition,' 'mind-reading,' and 'mentalizing' (e.g., Astington and Baird, 2005; Frith, 2003). Consistent with the tendency toward an expansive definition, we propose that one useful description of ToM is its conceptualization as "a complex and multifaceted construct that reflects the understanding of an interconnected network of mental states" (Hutchins *et al.*, 2012,

p. 327). This broad definition not only mirrors the biological reality involving the diverse brain networks implicated in ASD but has utility for the purposes of causal modeling wherein features can be represented with any required degree of complexity and detail.

Although the nature of ToM accounts vary in their specific proposals (see Morton, 2004 for a contrast of ToM models in ASD), the general idea behind all of them is that the behavioral symptoms of ASD are explained by some disrupted, biologically-based social-cognitive capacity(ies) that need not be conscious or deliberate. When modeling ToM at the cognitive level, one might invoke the notion of ToM when used in its broadest and most inclusive sense in which case it is expressed in the strongest terms in the causal model (Morton and Frith, 1995; see the Cognitive level in Figure 22.1 where a general ToM construct is represented as faulty). Alternatively, one might imagine a granular representation of ToM competencies where specific dimensions or entire ToM systems are represented. This may be particularly useful in modeling ToM for an individual. Although the group experimental data suggest a portrait of pervasive ToM impairments in ASD (e.g., Sterck and Begeer, 2010), disruptions in ToM are not monolithic and ToM is unlikely to be systematically deficient in ASD (Begeer *et al.*, 2010; Gonzalez *et al.*, 2013). Rather, persons with ASD probably pass and fail ToM tasks for different reasons and across different stages of development. Not surprisingly, such complex social-cognitive profiles translate into a set of ToM-related behavioral patterns that also show tremendous individual variation (Scheeren *et al.*, 2012).

ToM at the behavioral level

Although it has some serious limitations (described below), the ToM hypothesis makes intuitive sense and parsimoniously explains the social communication and social interaction deficits that are the defining features of ASD at the behavioral level. Social communication challenges are commonly described for young children with ASD. For example, the communicative acts of children with ASD tend to be more limited in function than those of their TD peers (Wetherby, 1986) (for elaboration on the social interactions of young children with ASD, see the chapter by Longard and Moore, this volume). Verbal children with ASD may exhibit unconventional verbal behavior (e.g., echolalia, perseverative speech; Prelock, 2006; Prizant and Rydell, 1993) and have difficulty modulating their use of prosody and gesture to aid communication. They often experience difficulty selecting and shifting topics appropriately (Church *et al.*, 2000; Prelock, 2006), demonstrate deficits in narrative construction and the use of metaphoric language (Landa, 2000; Tager-Flusberg, 1997), and may appear socially unresponsive due to failures in establishing and maintaining eye contact (Hobson and Lee, 1998). Moreover, when children with ASD are given the opportunity to play, they often withdraw or exhibit less diverse and elaborate functional play than do children with other developmental disabilities (Rutherford and Rogers, 2003). Whatever explanation is provided for social communication difficulties in ASD, it is clear they are a result of some underlying cognitive process that is impacted by a biological vulnerability.

The behavioral manifestations of ToM deficits in ASD show themselves in a variety of ways. This is represented in Figure 22.1 as the presence of distinct behavioral symptoms (S_1, S_2, S_3). Understanding the outward signs of ASD is complex and depends on one's level of analysis and quality of interpretation. For example, one might see an inappropriate social interaction where another might see a child's inability to attend visually to relevant social information, engage in reciprocal social interaction, or imitate in response to a communication partner. Moreover, variability in performance is the norm requiring consideration of multiple factors when explaining the complexity of ASD including what is behind the biological and cognitive processes that lead to the observed behaviors, and what contexts create more difficulty for children with ASD. These challenges to understanding the complex nature of ASD can be addressed using a causal model.

Causal modeling of ToM in ASD

Causal models are constructed using correlational evidence linking biological origin, to psychological constructs, outward signs and symptoms so as to offer a set of *plausible causal links* that can be empirically tested and formally or informally evaluated in clinical contexts. The links initially proposed are not deterministic and provide a means for summarizing large amounts of information so as to give one a view of the state of the science or of an individual case. Causal models are useful in that they may reveal plausible causal links from biological to cognitive to behavioral levels that have not been previously considered and may be worth pursuing. They also help us remember the distinction between cognition and behavior. Researchers and other professionals working in the area of developmental disabilities tend to confuse *descriptions* with *explanations* of challenging behaviors and often offer a vague general explanation (Morton, 2004). For example, in ASD, atypical prosodic patterns are caused by a pragmatic language disorder, absent empathic behavior is caused by a lack of empathy, and poor eye contact is a result of impaired social communication. Because behavioral elements cannot be mapped one-to-one onto the cognitive features they are intended to account for, and despite the fact that *all* psychological tests measure behavior, the causal model requires distinction between observable behaviors at the behavioral level and the putative underlying constructs at the cognitive level (Morton, 2004).

Of course, there are other cognitive features and mechanisms that are crucial in explaining the full set of symptoms observed in ASD. As Morton (2004) noted, when the job is to explain all the symptoms, it is hazardous to choose one underlying process fault (e.g., ToM) and ignore the other symptoms or assume that they derive from the same underlying cognitive dysfunction. Indeed, the remaining symptoms are in as much need of causal explanation as the supposed primary ones. The ToM hypothesis is not special in this regard and so it is necessary to acknowledge the contributing influences of at least two competing (although not necessarily mutually exclusive) theories of ASD that are situated at the cognitive level of discourse: the theories of executive dysfunction and weak central coherence.

Executive function (EF) is traditionally described as a range of higher order functions (e.g., planning, inhibition, working memory), which helps guide flexible, goal-oriented behavior (Pellicano, 2011). EF is often invoked to explain the difficulties observed in ASD in inhibitory control, attentional flexibility, and the presence of repetitive restricted patterns of behavior, interests, and activities that are diagnostic of the condition (American Psychological Association, 2013). Several studies demonstrate a relationship between ToM and EF, however, it is difficult to evaluate the developmental interaction between the two (Hill, 2008). Whether one is a precursor to the other or whether ToM reduces to a more general EF ability remains a matter of debate (see Pellicano, 2011).

Central coherence is a term coined by Frith (2003) to refer to the tendency of the cognitive system to integrate information into meaningful, high-level, gestalt representations. The proposal for a propensity toward weak central coherence (WCC) in ASD has received empirical support demonstrating intact, even superior, performance of individuals with ASD on tasks designed to assess part versus whole processing. Despite its success at explaining aspects of ASD where EF and ToM theories fail, WCC suffers from theoretical difficulties (e.g., WCC is likely neither universal in nor unique to ASD; Pellicano, 2011) leading many to conclude that WCC is an important, but not a primary feature of ASD (Happé *et al.*, 2006; López, 2008).

Cognitive theories of ASD attempt to identify a single deficit underlying the behavioral impairments characteristic of the disorder. However, no single theory has been able to do this causing researchers to advocate for a multiple-deficits model of ASD (Happé *et al.*, 2006; Happé and Ronald, 2008; Hill, 2008; Lind and Williams, 2011; Pellicano, 2011). This movement is consistent with contemporary notions that the heterogeneity in ASD at the biological, cognitive, and behavioral levels is abundant and there is little evidence for the unity of the proposed core areas of impairment. Specifically, Happé and colleagues (Happé *et al.*, 2006; Happé and Ronald, 2008; Robinson *et al.*, 2012) have challenged this assumption by finding evidence for the fractionability of the triad (i.e., deficits in communication, social interaction, and the presence of restricted and repetitive behaviors and interests). This would explain the difficulty in finding any single deficit that can adequately account for the entire syndrome and why only isolated features of the full clinical picture often occur (Happé and Ronald, 2008). An important theoretical and diagnostic implication of a multiple-deficits model is that common deficits seen in ASD need not be specific to the disorder since it is a combination of deficits that is unique (Happé and Ronald, 2008). As represented in Figure 22.2, heterogeneity in brain conditions at the biological level produces multiple deficits at the cognitive level—leading to various symptoms at the behavioral level. An important clinical implication is that when multiple deficits occur, the resulting portrait has a special quality, distinct prognosis, and unique response to intervention.

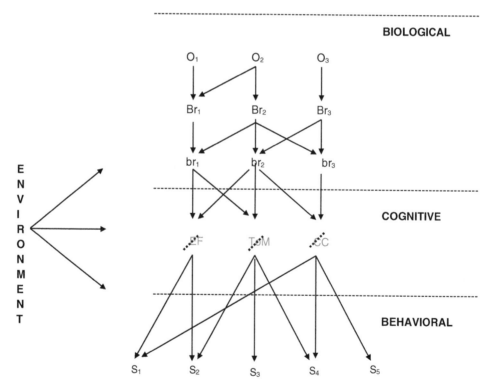

Figure 22.2 A candidate casual model of multiple deficits of ASD developed using the notation of Morton and Frith (1995) where O = a biological origin, Br = biological consequence on the brain, br = biological consequence on a brain system, S = behavioral sign or symptom. EF = executive function, ToM = Theory of Mind, CC = central coherence. Dotted lines represent faulty mechanisms. The environment is also represented (left) and seen as having important influences at the biological, cognitive, and behavioral levels.

Causal modeling for an individual case: Implications for intervention

Causal modeling allows for the modeling of different notions about what may be theoretically primary versus secondary features of ToM in ASD or to ignore this controversy altogether as when making clinical decisions for individual cases. For the purposes of treatment planning, we argue that an assumed secondary feature can be just as vital as a primary feature. This rationale is based on explanations of disorders as the function of interactions between factors at the biological, cognitive, and behavioral levels and the notion that both developmental antecedents (often termed 'precursors' or 'core deficits') *and* consequences may benefit from intervention that affect ultimate developmental endpoints. Although not shown in our graphic representations of causal models, this would take the form of bidirectionality across the three levels of functioning. The clear clinical implication is that, although ToM is situated at the cognitive level, intervention may be targeted at any or all levels of functioning as illustrated below.

Interventions vary in the number and type of ToM dimensions they aim to address. What interventions often fail to consider, however, is the role of context and the influence of the environment (e.g., Joosten *et al.*, 2012) for understanding the complexity of the causal model. Environment is a critical consideration that is reflected in behavior fluctuations and the lack of generalization of intervention effects across contexts (López, 2011). The physical, psychological, and social environments matter in understanding the behaviors observed and the interventions proposed (Cale *et al.*, 2009).

Application of a causal model for a young teen with ASD

Figure 22.3 presents an application of the causal model for a 13-year-old boy, Ethan (pseudonym), with ASD. At the biological level, Ethan was diagnosed with ASD at age 3 years. Recently, his parents reported a seizure disorder where Ethan stares off and seems to forget where he is or what he is doing. He is usually tired and inattentive following these episodes, which occur two to three times a week. At the cognitive level, Ethan recognizes basic emotions (e.g., mad, sad, scared) but has difficulty with more complex emotions (e.g., disappointment, confusion). He passes false belief tasks but fails to understand peer sarcasm. Both his poorly developed emotion-recognition and perspective-taking have implications for social isolation, unsuccessful peer-interactions, and social anxiety. Ethan also has difficulty understanding character intent and internal reactions of characters in the narratives he reads at school, leading to difficulties in reading comprehension—another behavior response to his cognitive process challenges rooted in his neurological differences.

Recently, Ethan's parents and teachers noted an increase in his inattention and difficulty with working memory, which may be contributing to complications at the behavior level as evidenced by Ethan's difficulty following instructions. The environmental context is important here as the management approach for social anxiety has been pharmacological, but the medication prescribed can increase risk for seizures for those who are already biologically vulnerable. Although children with ASD may have EF difficulties, Ethan's challenges in this area seem to be new and may be a result of seizures and/or the increased expectations in middle school for independent learning, planning, and engagement.

This is Ethan's first year in middle school. There is inconsistent support for speech and language services, but there have been two peers trained in peer-mediation techniques and there is an opportunity to capitalize on access to those peers during lunch to foster conversational engagement. This is important given that Ethan lives in a rural community about 10 miles from school and his parents report that this distance has interfered with his ability to 'hang out' with

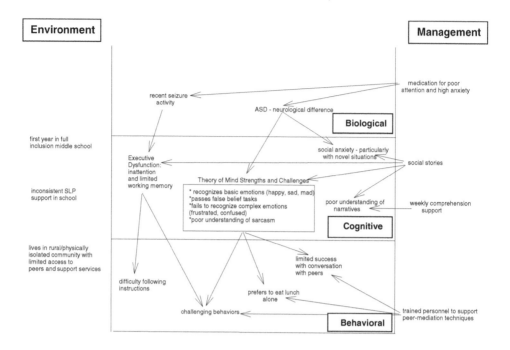

Figure 22.3 Causal model of functioning at the biological, cognitive, and behavioral levels for an individual case ('Ethan'; aged 13 years). Relevant environmental factors are indicated on the left and current and proposed management techniques (i.e., interventions) are indicated on the right.

peers and build positive peer-connections. Given the constellation of features operating on the biological, cognitive, and behavioral level, consultation with the speech–language pathologist might be used to support Ethan's parents and teachers to develop Social Stories™. Developed by Gray (2010), these are personalized short stories that explain the who, what, why, when, and where surrounding challenging situations. Social Stories™ recognize his anxiety, provide a strategy to manage novel situations with peers, and might also build on his ToM strengths involving his ability to identify basic emotions. They also can be used to review social exchanges with peers to increase his understanding of, and expectations for, reciprocity during interaction. Social Stories™ are not only considered an evidence-based intervention for children with ASD (National Autism Center, 2009) but also they are theoretically potent for reducing anxiety, advancing social cognition, and supporting narrative understanding and EF (Reyhnout and Carter, 2011), which are challenge areas for Ethan. As such, Social Stories™ may effectively complement the weekly comprehension support that is available to Ethan in school.

Implications for practitioners

Our approach to address Ethan's challenges reflects our interpretation of the brain conditions, cognitive features, and behavioral consequences that we believe not only describe his current functioning but also have developmental significance. Because our interpretation is surely incomplete and may be faulty, it is imperative that the causal model be evaluated with regard to clinical outcomes. When outcomes are not encouraging, practitioners should seek additional information and propose alternative models. This is a strength of the causal modeling approach, which serves as a neutral framework in which various theories can be represented and compared.

Practitioners trained in the causal modeling approach to clinical practice report that it can be time consuming and complex and that it "demands a lot of background…and theoretical knowledge" (Krol *et al.*, 2006, p. 23). They also report that attention to the different levels demonstrates connections between factors at those levels as well as factors likely to be influenced by treatment. Further, they indicate that causal modeling: a) is especially useful for complex cases; b) helps one to think in an orderly way and generate hypotheses; c) makes comparison of different theories easy; d) forces one to entertain potential causal influences and make explicit the links between features in the client data instead of simply summarizing the data; and e) provides a means to communicate a rationale for treatment decisions (Krol *et al.*, 2006).

In summary, the ToM hypothesis of ASD has endured due to an impressive evidence base and its link to complex biological origins and multiple behavioral consequences. Although it often invoked to explain the social communication and social interaction deficits of ASD, it is inadequate for explaining the full range of signs and symptoms that occur in ASD. Causal modeling is conducive to the notion of multiple deficits and provides a flexible framework for explaining the biological foundations, cognitive processes, and behavioral manifestations of ASD. Causal modeling also integrates environmental factors that can influence our interpretation of what particular behaviors are occurring and how they might be addressed.

References

American Psychiatric Association (2013), *Diagnostic and Statistical Manual of Mental Disorders* (5th ed.), New York: American Psychiatric Association.

Anagnostou, E. and Taylor, M.J. (2011), "Review of neuroimaging in autism spectrum disorders: What have we learned and where we go from here?", *Molecular Autism*, Vol. 2, No. 4, pp. 1–9.

Astington, J.W. and Baird, J.A. (2005), "Introduction: Why language matters", in Astington, J.W. and Baird, J.A. (Eds.), *Why Language Matters for Theory of Mind*, New York, NY: Oxford University Press, pp. 3–25.

Baron-Cohen, S. (1995a), *Mindblindness*, Cambridge, MA, US: MIT Press.

Baron-Cohen, S. (1995b), "Theory of mind and face processing: How do they interact in development and psychopathology?", in S. Baron-Cohen (Ed.), *Developmental Psychopathology: Theory and Methods*, Oxford, UK: John Wiley & Sons, pp. 343–356.

Baron-Cohen, S., Leslie, A. and Frith, U. (1985), "Does the autistic child have a 'theory of mind'?", *Cognition*, Vol. 21, No. 1, pp. 37–46.

Begeer, S., Malle, B., Nieuwland, M. and Keysar, B. (2010), "Using theory of mind to represent and take part in social interactions: Comparing individuals with high-functioning autism and typically developing controls", *Journal of Developmental Psychology*, Vol. 7, No. 1, pp. 104–122.

Belmonte, M.K. (2009), "What's the story behind 'theory of mind' and autism?", *Journal of Consciousness Studies*, Vol. 16, pp. 118–139.

Betancur, C. (2011), "Etiological heterogeneity in autism spectrum disorders: More than 100 genetic and genomic disorders and still counting", *Brain Research*, Vol. 22, pp. 42–77.

Bowers, K., Li, Q., Bressler, J., Avramopoulos, D., Newschaffer, C. and Fallin, M.D. (2011), "Glutathione pathway gene variation and risk of autism spectrum disorders", *Journal of Neurodevelopmental Disorder*, Vol. 3, pp. 132–143.

Cale, S., Carr, E., Blakeley-Smith, A. and Owen-DeSchryver, J. (2009), "Context-based assessment and intervention for problem behavior in children with autism spectrum disorder", *Behavior Modification*, Vol. 33, No. 6, pp. 707–742.

Church, C., Alisanski, S. and Amanullah, S. (2000), "The social, behavioral, and academic experiences of children with Asperger syndrome", *Focus on Autism and Other Developmental Disabilities*, Vol. 15, No. 1, pp. 12–20.

Dichter, G.S., Richey, J.A., Rittenberg, A.M., Sabatino, A. and Bodfish, J.W. (2012), "Reward circuitry function in autism during face anticipation and outcomes", *Journal of Autism and Developmental Disorders*, Vol. 42, pp. 147–160.

Frith, U. (2003), *Autism: Explaining the Enigma* (2nd ed.), Oxford, UK: Blackwell.

Frith, U., Morton, J. and Leslie, A.M. (1991), "The cognitive basis of biological disorder: Autism", *Perspectives on Disease,* Vol. 14, No. 10, pp. 433–438.

Gonzalez, M.L., Baez, S., Torralva, T., Castellano, F.X., Rattazzi, A., Bein, V., *et al.,* (2013), "Cognitive variability in adults with ADHD and AS: Disentangling the roles of executive functions and social cognition", *Research in Developmental Disabilities,* Vol. 34, pp. 817–830.

Gowen, E., Stanely, J. and Maill, R. (2008), "Movement interference in autism spectrum disorder", *Neuropsychologia,* Vol. 46, No. 4, pp. 1060–1068.

Gray, C. (2010), *The New Social Story Book.* Arlington, TX, US: Future Horizons.

Happé, F. and Ronald, A. (2008), "The fractionable autism triad: A review of evidence from behavioural, genetic, and cognitive neural research", *Neuropsycholgoical Review,* Vol. 18, pp. 274–304.

Happé, F., Ronald, A. and Plomin, R. (2006), "Time to give up on a single explanation for autism", *Nature Neuroscience,* Vol. 9, No. 10, pp. 1218–1220.

Hill, E.L. (2008), "Executive functioning in autism spectrum disorder. Where it all fits in the causal model", in McGregor, E., Nunez, M., Cebula, K. and Gomez, J. (Eds.), *Autism: An Integrated View From Neurocognitive, Clinical, and Intervention Research,* Malden, MA, US: Blackwell, pp. 145–165.

Hobson, P., Chidambi, G., Lee, A. and Meyer, J. (2006), "Foundations for self-awareness: An exploration through autism: VII. The place of self in development", *Monographs of the Society for Research in Child Development.* Vol. 72, No. 2, pp. 128–165.

Hobson, R.P. and Lee, A. (1998), "Hello and goodbye: A study of social engagement in autism", *Journal of Autism and Developmental Disorders,* Vol. 28, No. 2, pp. 117–127.

Hutchins, T.L., Prelock, P.A. and Bonazinga, L. (2012), "Psychometric evaluation of the Theory of Mind Inventory (ToMI): A study of typically developing children and individuals with autism spectrum disorder", *Journal of Autism and Developmental Disabilities,* Vol. 42, No. 3, pp. 327–341.

Joosten, A., Bundy, A. and Stewart, E. (2012), "Context influences the motivation for stereotypic and repetitive behavior in children diagnosed with intellectual disability with and without autism", *Journal of Applied Research in Intellectual Disabilities,* Vol. 25, No. 3, pp. 262–270.

Krol, N., Morton, J. and De Bruyn, E. (2006), "Causal modeling: A framework as diagnostic tool", Presentation given at Radboud University, Nijmegen, Netherlands.

Landa, R. (2000), "Social language use in Asperger syndrome and high-functioning autism", in Klin, A., Volkmar, F. and Sparrow, S.S. (Eds.), *Asperger Syndrome,* New York, US: Guilford Press, pp. 125–155.

Lind, S.E. and Williams, D.M. (2011), "Behavioral, biopsychosocial, and cognitive models of autism spectrum disorders", in Matson, J.L. and Sturmey, P. (Eds.), *International Handbook of Autism and Pervasive Developmental Disorders. Autism and Child Psychopathology Series,* New York, US: Springer Science and Business Media, pp. 99–114.

López, B. (2011), "Building the whole beyond its parts: A critical examination of current theories of integration ability in autism", in McGregor, E., Nunez, M., Cebula, K. and Gomez, J. (Eds.), *Autism: An Integrated View From Neurocognitive, Clinical, and Intervention Research,* Malden, MA, US: Blackwell, pp. 104–123.

López, B., Leekam, S.R. and Arts, G.R. (2008), "How central is central coherence? Preliminary evidence on the link between conceptual and perceptual processing in children with autism", *Autism,* Vol. 12, No. 2, pp. 159–171.

Mathersul, D., McDonald, S. and Rushby, J. (2013), "Understanding advanced theory of mind and empathy in high-functioning adults with autism spectrum disorder", *Journal of Clinical and Experimental Neuropsychology,* Vol. 35, No. 6, pp. 655–668.

Mazefsky, C.A., Goin-Kochel, R.P., Riley, B.P. and Maes, H. (2008), "Genetic and environmental influences on symptom domains in twins and siblings with autism", *Research in Autism Spectrum Disorders,* Vol. 2, pp. 320–331.

Morton, J. (2004), *Understanding Developmental Disorders: A Causal Modeling Approach,* Oxford, UK: Blackwell.

Morton, J. and Frith, U. (1995), "Causal modeling: A structural approach to developmental psychopathology", in Morton, J. and Frith, U. (Eds.), *Developmental Psychopathology, Vol. 1: Theory and Methods.* Oxford, UK: John Wiley and Sons, pp. 357–390.

National Autism Center (2009), *The National Standards Report of The National Standards Project—Addressing the Need for Evidence Based Practice Guidelines for Autism Spectrum Disorders.* Randolph, MA, US: National Autism Center.

Neuhaus, E., Beauchaine, T.P. and Bernier, R. (2010), "Neurobiological correlates of social functioning in autism", *Clinical Psychology Review,* Vol. 30, pp. 733–748.

Nordahl, C.W., Scholz, R., Yang, X., Buonocore, M.H., Simon, T., Rogers, S. and Amaral, D.G. (2012), "Increased rate of amygdala growth in children aged 2 to 4 years with autism spectrum disorders", *Archives of General Psychiatry*, Vol. 69, No. 1, pp. 53–61.

Pellicano, E. (2011), "Psychological models of autism: An overview", in Roth, I. and Rezaie, P. (Eds.), *Researching the Autism Spectrum: Contemporary Perspectives*, New York, US: Cambridge University Press, pp. 219–265.

Pelphrey, K., Shultz, S., Hudac, C. and Vander Wyk, B. (2011), "Research review: Constraining heterogeneity: The social brain and its development in autism spectrum disorder", *Child Psychology and Psychiatry*, Vol. 52, No. 6, pp. 631–644.

Prelock, P.A. (2006), *Communication Assessment and Intervention in Autism Spectrum Disorder*, Austin, TX, US: Pro-ed Publishers.

Prizant, B.M. and Rydell, P.J. (1993), "Assessment and intervention considerations for unconventional verbal behavior", in Warren, S.F. and Reichle, J. (Series Eds.) and Reichle ,J. and Wacker (Vol. Eds.), *Communication and Language Intervention Series: Vol. 3. Communicative Alternatives to Challenging Behavior: Integrating Functional Assessment and Intervention Strategies*, Baltimore, MD, US: Paul H. Brookes Publishing, pp. 263–297.

Raznahan, A., Wallace, G., Antezana, L., Greenstein, D., Lenroot, R., Thurm, A., *et al.*, (2013), "Compared to what? Early brain overgrowth in autism and the perils of population norms", *Biological Psychiatry*, Vol. 73, No. 12, pp. 1–14.

Reynhout, G. and Carter, M. (2011), "Social stories™: A possible theoretical rationale", *European Journal of Special Needs*, Vol. 26, No. 3, pp. 367–378.

Robinson, E., Koenen, D., McCormick, M., Munir, K., Hallett, V., Happé, F., Plomin, R. and Ronald, A. (2012), "A multivariate twin study of autistic traits in 12-year-olds: Testing the fractionable autism triad hypothesis", *Behavior Genetics*, Vol. 42, No. 2, pp. 245–255.

Rutherford, M.D. and Rogers, S.J. (2003), "Cognitive underpinnings of pretend play in autism", *Journal of Autism and Developmental Disorders,* Vol. 33, No. 23, pp. 289–302.

Samson, A. and Hegenloh, M. (2010), "Stimulus characteristics affect humor processing in individuals with Asperger syndrome", *Journal of Autism and Developmental Disorders*, Vol. 40, No. 4, pp, 438–447.

Scheeren, A., Koot, H. and Begeer, S. (2012), "Social interaction style of children and adolescents with high-functioning autism spectrum disorder", *Journal of Autism and Developmental Disorders,* Vol. 42, No. 1, pp. 2046–2055.

Schultz, R.T., Gauthier, I., Klin, A., Fulbright, R.K., Anderson, A.W., Volkmar, F., *et al.*, (2000), "Abnormal ventral temporal cortical activity during face discrimination among individuals with autism and Asperger Syndrome", *Archives in General Psychiatry,* Vol. 57, pp. 331–340.

Sterck, E. and Begeer, S. (2010), "Theory of mind: Specialized capacity of emergent property?", *European Journal of Development*, Vol. 7, No. 1, pp. 1–16.

Tager-Flusberg, H. (1997), "The role of theory of mind in language acquisition: Contributions from the study of autism", in Adamson, L. and Romski, M. (Eds.), *Research on Communication and Language Disorders: Contributions to Theories of Language Development*, Baltimore, MD, US: Paul H. Brookes, pp. 133–158.

van Buijsen, M., Hendriks, A., Ketelaars, M. and Verhoeven, L. (2011), "Assessment of theory of mind in children with communication disorders: Role of presentation mode", *Research in Developmental Disabilities*, Vol. 32, pp. 1038–1045.

Vissers, M., Cohen, M. and Geurts, H. (2012), "Brain connectivity and high functioning autism: A promising path of research that needs refined models, methodological convergence, and stronger behavioral links", *Neuroscience and Biobehavioral Reviews*, Vol. 36, No. 1, pp. 604–624.

Wetherby, A.M. (1986), "Ontogeny of communicative functions in autism", *Journal of Autism and Developmental Disorders,* Vol. 16, pp. 295–319.

Zalla, T., Barlassina, L., Buon, M. and LeBoyer, M. (2011), "Moral judgment in adults with autism spectrum disorders", *Cognition*, Vol. 121, No. 1, pp. 115–126.

257

23

LANGUAGE AND THE SPEAKING MIND

Brain in stuttering

Nathan D. Maxfield

Spontaneous speech is typically produced quickly, effortlessly and with little awareness by the speaker of how the process unfolded. Occasional, typical disfluencies are mostly non-disruptive and may even facilitate comprehension. Conversely, some speaker groups face chronic, atypical disfluencies that may impact communication negatively or beyond repair. Understanding how speech production mechanisms function in these groups has implications for informing interventions. This chapter focuses on language ability in people who stutter (PWS).

Whether stuttering and language ability are connected, is a century-old question (see Hall *et al.*, 2007; Newman and Ratner, 2007). Modern-day theories of stuttering also emphasize language contributions (e.g., Perkins *et al.*, 1991; Postma and Kolk, 1993; Wingate, 1988).

Different reasons have been cited for exploring language contributions to stuttering. One, is that stuttering moments often coincide with linguistic phenomena in the speech stream. Second, stuttering onset is often time-locked with a period of significant language development. Third, the psycholinguistic perspective posits that the ability to speak fluently is driven, mechanistically, by the ability to process linguistic information efficiently. This chapter initially focuses on the first two of these points. The remainder discusses real-time language production and its relationship to fluency and, possibly, to stuttering. The final section addresses clinical implications of research to date and future directions in language production research in stuttering.

Language contributions to stuttering: Circumstantial connections

One reason for exploring language contributions to stuttering, is that moments of stuttering coincide, somewhat predictably, with a number of specific linguistic phenomena in the speech stream, albeit somewhat differently in younger versus older child PWS (e.g., Sasisekaran, 2014) and in child versus adult PWS (see Bloodstein and Ratner, 2008). The linguistic distribution of stuttering has been interpreted to suggest ties to decrements in prearticulatory language planning (e.g., Tetnowski, 1998) or in planning speech motor gestures for specific linguistic units (e.g., Howell, 2004). Cross-linguistic investigations of stuttering may shed further light on these different hypotheses (Dworzynski *et al.*, 2003).

Stuttering onset in relation to language acquisition

The onset of stuttering also tends to coincide, developmentally, with a period of exponential language growth (e.g., Yairi, 2004). This has led to investigation about whether child PWS are more prone than typically-fluent speakers (TFS) to language impairments. At least some child PWS have frank language impairments (e.g., Blood *et al.*, 2003). Others are vulnerable to more subtle language impairments, including low-normal performance on norm-referenced tests and inter-test dissociations (Ntourou *et al.*, 2011). Thus, language abilities in child PWS should be evaluated and, if warranted, targeted for intervention (Hall *et al.*, 2007). Nippold (2012) concluded there is currently limited sustainable evidence that PWS, as a group, are more prone to language impairments. Her conclusion was based on methodological limitations of research to date such as failure to control for covariates of language acquisition (e.g., Richels *et al.*, 2013).

Conversely, Seery *et al.* (2007) reviewed evidence that some child PWS had expressive language abilities at or above age-level near stuttering onset. Kloth *et al.* (1995) also reported evidence of age-typical language abilities in some child PWS prior to stuttering onset. Yairi and Ambrose (2005) described longitudinal evidence that children recovered from stuttering were decelerated in language development, perhaps reflecting a 'trade-off' of language ability to allow speech motor skills to develop, while children with persistent stuttering were more likely to have expressive language abilities at or above age-level norms. Nippold (2012) cited similar findings to refute the claim that stuttering restricts language development. Still, some PWS develop linguistic secondary behaviors to cope with stuttering (Vanryckeghem *et al.*, 2004). Dumas (2012) also observed that PWS use a unique discourse style that serves sociolinguistic functions. Thus, experience with stuttering can influence language behavior, albeit in ways not necessarily evident using norm-referenced testing.

There also exists a literature on phonological ability in child PWS. At least some child PWS have frank phonological impairments (e.g., Blood *et al.*, 2003). Some younger child PWS evidence subtle phonological decrements (e.g., Pelczarski and Yaruss, 2014), which may normalize by school age (e.g., Paden and Yairi, 1996). Limited evidence suggests that risk of phonological disorders increases for older child PWS (Morley, 1957). Thus, phonological abilities should also be evaluated in child PWS and, if appropriate, targeted for intervention. However, Sasisekaran (2014) concluded, from her review of literature, that norm-referenced tests of phonological ability have not consistently differentiated PWS versus TFS.

Disfluency patterns in relation to norm-referenced test performance

An important question is how performance on norm-referenced language and phonology tests may relate to patterns of disfluency in children. As TFS acquire language milestones, periods of heightened disfluency are sometimes observed (e.g., Rispoli, 2003), suggesting a link between processes in language growth and disfluency. Similarly, the frequency of normal disfluency, but not of stuttering, correlates with language acquisition status in PWS (e.g., Tumanova *et al.*, 2014; although see Millager *et al.*, 2014). Significant correlations between measures of phonology and stuttering frequency were not detected either (e.g., Louko *et al.*, 1990). Thus, it appears that norm-referenced tests have limited value in predicting the frequency of stuttering-like disfluency in child PWS, perhaps due to limited sensitivity to real-time language production which plays a central role in fluent (and disfluent) speaking.

Real-time language production, fluency and disfluency

The ability to produce speech fluently requires not only that a speaker be linguistically proficient (i.e., possess discourse knowledge) but also able to process linguistic knowledge efficiently. Information processing in language production involves: 1) associating concepts with words in the mental lexicon (lexical-semantic processing); 2) assembling those words into higher-level phrases (grammatical encoding); and 3) retrieving and coordinating the sound and syllable structures of those words (phonological encoding) (see Levelt et al., 1999; Bock and Levelt, 1994; Selkirk, 1984).

These information processing activities operate in several ways to set the stage for fluent speech production (see Levelt, 1989). First, language production operates rapidly. Lexical items are selected, and their grammatical and phonological elements encoded, on the order of hundreds of milliseconds. Second, utterance planning unfolds incrementally. Lexical knowledge is retrieved in incremental units that can be managed by the speaker's processing resources yet encoded into utterances at rates that allow for relatively continuous verbal output over time. Third, different types of linguistic knowledge can be processed simultaneously, allowing different elements of a verbal message (e.g., its meaning, structure and form) to be encoded at least partially in parallel. Finally, utterance planning operates in parallel with speech motor programming and articulation. As one increment of a message is specified, it is articulated by the speaker who – at the same time – rapidly and covertly encodes more message increments. The result is a fluent succession of utterances that emerge, one after another, at rates of several words per second. 'Quality control' in language production is governed by an internal monitor, which checks the surface structure of utterance plans for accuracy and may detect the presence of errors, such as ill-retrieved phonemes. On such occasions, this monitor may signal the speaker to halt speaking and initiate a self-repair, potentially disrupting fluency but preserving accuracy.

Real-time language production in child PWS

The processes outlined above represent what is currently known about real-time language production in adult TFS. Language production in child TFS also seems to involve distinct semantic and phonological processes that can be manipulated with priming (e.g., Jerger et al., 2002). However, semantic and phonological fluency take time to mature, progress at somewhat different rates, and do not reach adult-like status until at least age 16 years (e.g., Kavé et al., 2010). Novel syntactic patterns seem to appear in elicited productions as early as age 3 years (Chang et al., 2006), and children this young also produce adult-like between-word phonological processes (Newton, 2012). Thus, the functional architecture of language production in children seems to resemble that in adults, although one must consider, and control for, the relative state of maturation when investigating language production in child PWS.

Despite the close relationship between real-time language production and fluency, there have been few explicit studies of this process in child PWS. At the level of lexical-semantic processing, child PWS performed more poorly than TFS on norm-referenced tests of word finding (see Pellowski, 2011). Pellowski and Conture (2005) reported naming reaction time (RT) evidence from a semantic picture–word interference task suggesting that PWS (3 to 5 years old) had difficulty resolving competition among semantically-related words on the path to picture naming. Hartfield and Conture (2006) also reported naming RT evidence from a similar task. Findings suggested that PWS (3–5 years) organized and processed lexical-semantic knowledge with greater emphasis on functional relationships between words. The authors proposed that this is a less mature level of lexical-semantic development than emphasizing physical relationships between words, which prevailed in child TFS. Anderson (2008) reported naming RT data that PWS (3–5 years) had weakened semantic–phonological connections in the mental lexicon. Relationships between these effects and stuttering behaviors have yet to be explored.

At the level of grammatical encoding, child PWS and TFS scored comparably on the Developmental Sentence Analysis, but PWS made more grammatical errors (Westby, 1979), pointing to grammatical encoding problems. Anderson and Conture (2004) investigated effects of sentence structure priming on speech production in PWS versus TFS (3–5 years). Results suggested that, without syntactic priming, grammatical encoding was less efficient in PWS, although the impact on stuttering behavior was not explored. Savage and Howell (2008) reported that both child PWS and TFS were more fluent with priming of function words than content words in a sentence priming task, with this effect more pronounced for PWS. One possibility is that, during grammatical encoding without function word priming, child PWS have difficulty calling up modifiers or inflectional elements, with this effect directly impacting fluency.

At the level of phonological encoding, Melnick *et al.* (2003) investigated naming RT in PWS and TFS (3–5 years) in a phonological priming condition. Priming did not disproportionately affect naming RT in the PWS, pointing to typical phonological processing. Similarly, phonological complexity did not correlate with stuttering frequency in younger child PWS (Coalson *et al.*, 2012). Nor did word frequency or phonological neighborhood characteristics disproportionately impact naming RT in older child PWS versus TFS (Ratner *et al.*, 2009). These factors did influence the likelihood of stuttering in the discourse of younger PWS (3–5 years) (Anderson, 2007). Older child PWS were also shown to retain immature, holistic phonological representations of words (Byrd *et al.*, 2007). Performance on implicit phonological tasks also differentiated older child PWS from TFS (Sasisekaran, 2014). Thus, evidence regarding efficiency of phonological processing in child PWS and its impact on stuttering behavior is equivocal.

Real-time language production in adult PWS

Limited evidence also exists on real-time language production in adult PWS. Beginning with lexical-semantic processing, adult PWS responded at least as fast as TFS on word association, but were more variable in the types of associations produced and in the time taken to produce them (Crowe and Kroll, 1991), suggesting that semantic processing operates less consistently. On a word definition task, adult PWS produced more verbose responses but used fewer synonyms (Wingate, 1988). In picture naming, adult PWS produced more naming errors (Newman and Ratner, 2007). Both point to decrements in the activation of words associated with increasingly specific concepts. Naming error patterns (Newman and Ratner, 2007) suggest that target labels are engaged in high competition with (and sometimes lost to) unrelated words and, occasionally, synonymous words in adult PWS; target labels did not seem to receive unusually high competition from distant semantic neighbors, a finding supported by a picture–word inference study (Hennessey *et al.*, 2008). Also noteworthy is evidence of poorer performance of adult PWS versus TFS on a norm-referenced test of word finding (Pellowski, 2011). As with child PWS, relationships between these effects and stuttering behaviors in adult PWS are unknown.

At the level of grammatical encoding, there is limited evidence that adult PWS encounter difficulty encoding verb phrases in discourse (Prins *et al.*, 1997). Tsiamtsiouris and Cairns (2009) investigated grammatical encoding in adult PWS in two experiments. One investigated whether syntactic complexity disproportionately increased speech initiation times in adult PWS versus TFS, separately from the contributions of phonological word length. The second investigated whether sentence structure priming had a disproportionately facilitative effect on speech initiation times in adults PWS versus TFS. Both of these outcomes were observed, suggesting adult PWS may be inefficient in grammatical encoding. Tsiamtsiouris and Cairns (2013) further showed that certain complex sentence types not only increased speech initiation times in adult PWS, but elicited a disproportionately higher rate of disfluencies.

Finally, several primed word production experiments found no evidence of atypical phonological encoding in adult PWS (e.g., Hennessey et al., 2008; Newman and Ratner, 2007). However, implicit phonological tasks produced evidence of phonological processing decrements in adult PWS (e.g., Sasisekaran et al., 2006). Adult PWS were also more prone to stuttering on lower-frequency words (e.g., Newman and Ratner, 2007), pointing to difficulty in phonological code activation (Jescheniak and Levelt, 1994). Increasing cognitive demand also negatively impacted phonological processing efficiency in adult PWS (e.g., Weber-Fox et al., 2004).

Brain electrophysiological correlates of real-time language production in PWS

One factor limiting the sustainability of evidence outlined in the preceding sections was a heavy reliance on behavioral methods to index real-time processing in language production in PWS. For example, RT measures can differ in PWS versus TFS even in the absence of task demands on word retrieval (see Bloodstein and Ratner, 2008). New views also exist about some behavioral psycholinguistic effects. For example, the locus of picture–word inference effects – used to investigate language production in PWS – was recently challenged (Collina et al., 2013).

One advancement has been to use brain event-related potentials (ERPs) to investigate real-time language processing with increasing precision. As described in Meyer et al. (1988), "Because standard behavioral measures obtained through mental chronometry represent the total duration and final output of many processing stages in combination, they do not offer an especially close look at underlying component processes" (p. 41). In contrast, averaged ERP activity can be decomposed into different components, with specific components reliably indexing specific language or cognitive processes (Hagoort and Kutas, 1995). As reviewed in Maxfield et al. (2014), scalp-recorded ERPs have been used to investigate a variety of hypotheses about mechanisms of language production in TFS.

ERP measures are not new in research on stuttering either (see Maxfield et al., 2014). Christine Weber-Fox and colleagues have used ERPs to investigate language processing in PWS, primarily in *receptive* mode (i.e., during word recognition and sentence processing) (e.g., Weber-Fox et al., 2004). Unclear is whether ERP differences observed between PWS and TFS in receptive language processing generalize to language production (see Pickering and Garrod, 2013).

In three recently published experiments, Maxfield et al. (2010; 2012; 2014) began using ERPs to investigate lexical-semantic and phonological processing in adult PWS on the path to picture naming. A main, albeit still tentative, outcome of that research is that PWS atypically heightened focal attention during word retrieval, an effect not evident behaviorally. We likened this effect to center-surround inhibition, a compensatory attentional mechanism for retrieving words poorly represented in the mental lexicon (Dagenbach et al., 1990).

We are excited about the potential for cognitive neuroscience approaches to clarify or extend existing evidence about language production in PWS, including the time-course of language production (e.g., Hennessey et al., 2008) and parallel processing in language production (e.g., Bosshardt, 2006). ERP evidence of over-active internal monitoring of phonological processing in PWS was recently reported (Arnstein *et al.*, 2011). Weber-Fox *et al.* (2013) also demonstrated that ERP correlates of language processing can be used for early detection of children at-risk of stuttering.

Summary, clinical implications, and future directions

Stuttering often coincides with specific linguistic events in the speech stream. Unknown is whether the linguistic loci of stuttering impact mechanisms of sentence processing (see Ferreira and Bailey, 2004). Healey (2010) made recommendations for modifying the verbal output of PWS, based on results of studies of listener recall and perceptions of speech produced by PWS. Understanding from a psycholinguistic perspective how sentences produced by PWS are processed may refine recommendations for modifying verbal output of PWS to optimize listener comprehension.

Existing evidence also suggests that frank language or phonological impairments are present in at least some child PWS. Hall (2004) recommends using a 'scaffolding' approach to enrich language in PWS. She also reviews approaches for enriching lexical-semantic knowledge. Nippold (2004) challenges conventional wisdom that co-occurring fluency and phonological impairments should be treated indirectly, and reviews treatment options.

There is evidence, too, that at least some child PWS have subtle impairments in language or phonological ability. Cognitive interventions such as attentional training programs improve language performance in other populations with subtle language deficits (e.g., Stevens *et al.*, 2008) and may have a place in interventions for stuttering as well (e.g., Nejati *et al.*, 2013). Typically-fluent language production draws on central cognitive resources (e.g., Ferreira and Pashler, 2002), i.e., cognitive resources that support performance in a broad range of activities. Psychologists differentiate three aspects of fluid cognitive processing – speed, working memory and other executive functions – all of which support rapid and fluent language production (e.g., Hussey and Novick, 2012; Kail and Park, 1994). Understanding how these mechanisms support real-time language production in PWS may inform targeted cognitive interventions for stuttering.

Finally, there is evidence of differences in real-time language production in PWS. Much of this evidence originated from language priming studies. Priming methods are used to treat lexical-semantic and grammatical deficits post-stroke (Howard, 2000), and may have a place in interventions for stuttering too. Other interventions may foster phonological encoding during language production in PWS (e.g., McGregor, 1994).

What future research directions might shed additional light on language contributions to stuttering? Relatively little is known about the potential for change (i.e., plasticity) in the language production systems of PWS. This focus seems critical, as the case is built that language intervention is necessary for at least some PWS. Investigating the trajectory of the development, maturation and aging of language production abilities in PWS may also be informative. A large share of intra-individual variability in the cognitive–behavioral system may be attributed to genetic constraints, which are likely to be highest on the two ends of the lifespan (Li *et al.*, 2004). In healthy aging, changes are seen in lexical-semantic, grammatical and phonological aspects of language production (Mortensen *et al.*, 2006). Little is known about these factors and their relationship to fluency and stuttering in aging PWS.

It also seems important to understand the potential for maladaptive plasticity in the language production systems of PWS. For this, it may be useful to compare neural activations in PWS with neural activations of other groups with persistent language impairments. PWS evidence over-activation of right-hemisphere brain regions including frontal operculum, anterior insula, cerebellar vermis and right rolandic region; atypical activations are also seen in basal ganglia (see Ingham *et al.*, 2005). Some of these same patterns are associated with poor recovery from stroke, and have been related to maladaptive functioning of the cognitive system of intention, which plays a role in regulating hemispheric involvement in word retrieval (Crosson, 2008). Unexplored is whether PWS may benefit from intervention aimed at stabilizing functioning of the intention system in word retrieval (Crosson, 2008).

Finally, language contributions to stuttering must be validated in multiple languages. A body of cross-linguistic research in stuttering exists. However, sustainability of findings has been limited by methodological issues (Tsai *et al.*, 2011; Coalson *et al.*, 2013).

References

Anderson, J.D. (2007), "Phonological neighborhood and word frequency effects in the stuttered disfluencies of children who stutter", *Journal of Speech, Language, and Hearing Research*, Vol. 50, pp. 229–247.

Anderson, J.D. (2008), "Age of acquisition and repetition priming effects on picture naming of children who do and do not stutter", *Journal of Fluency Disorders*, Vol. 33, pp. 135–155.

Anderson, J.D. and Conture, E.G. (2004), "Sentence-structure priming in young children who do and do not stutter", *Journal of Speech, Language, and Hearing Research*, Vol. 47, pp. 552–571.

Arnstein, D., Lakey, B., Compton, R.J. and Kleinow, J. (2011), "Preverbal error-monitoring in stutterers and fluent speakers", *Brain and Language*, Vol. 116, pp. 105–115.

Blood, G.W., Ridenour Jr, V.J., Qualls, C.D. and Hammer, C.S. (2003), "Co-occurring disorders in children who stutter", *Journal of Communication Disorders*, Vol. 36, pp. 427–448.

Bloodstein, O. and Ratner, N.B. (2008), *A Handbook on Stuttering*, 6th ed., Thomson-Delmar, New York, NY.

Bock, J.K. and Levelt, W.J.M. (1994), "Language production: Grammatical encoding", in Gernsbacher, M.A. (Ed.), *Handbook of Psycholinguistics*, Academic Press, San Diego, CA, US, pp. 945–984.

Bosshardt, H.G. (2006), "Cognitive processing load as a determinant of stuttering: Summary of a research programme", *Clinical Linguistics and Phonetics*, Vol. 20, pp. 371–385.

Byrd, C.T., Conture, E.G. and Ohde, R.N. (2007), "Phonological priming in young children who stutter: Holistic versus incremental processing", *American Journal of Speech-Language Pathology*, Vol. 16, pp. 43–53.

Chang, F., Dell, G.S. and Bock, K. (2006), "Becoming syntactic", *Psychological Review*, Vol. 113, pp. 234–272.

Coalson, G.A., Byrd, C.T. and Davis, B.L. (2012), "The influence of phonetic complexity on stuttered speech", *Clinical Linguistics and Phonetics*, Vol. 26, pp. 646–659.

Coalson, G.A., Peña, E.D. and Byrd, C.T. (2013), "Description of multilingual participants who stutter", *Journal of Fluency Disorders*, Vol. 38, pp. 141–156.

Collina, S., Tabossi, P. and De Simone, F. (2013), "Word production and the picture-word interference paradigm: The role of learning", *Journal of Psycholinguistic Research*, Vol. 42, pp. 461–473.

Crosson, B. (2008), "An intention manipulation to change lateralization of word production in nonfluent aphasia: Current status", *Seminars in Speech and Language*, Vol. 29, pp. 188–204.

Crowe, K.M. and Kroll, R.M. (1991), "Response latency and response class for stutterers and nonstutterers as measured by a word-association task", *Journal of Fluency Disorders*, Vol. 16, pp. 35–54.

Dagenbach, D., Carr, T.H. and Barnhardt, T.M. (1990), "Inhibitory semantic priming of lexical decisions due to failure to retrieve weakly activated codes", *Journal of Experimental Psychology: Learning, Memory, and Cognition*, Vol. 16, pp. 328–340.

Dumas, N.W. (2012), "More than hello: Reconstituting sociolinguistic subjectivities in introductions among American Stuttering English speakers", *Language and Communication*, Vol. 32, pp. 216–228.

Dworzynski, K., Howell, P. and Natke, U. (2003), "Predicting stuttering from linguistic factors for German speakers in two age groups", *Journal of Fluency Disorders*, Vol. 28, pp. 95–113.

Ferreira, V.S. and Pashler, H. (2002), "Central bottleneck influences on the processing stages of word production", *Journal of Experimental Psychology: Learning, Memory, and Cognition*, Vol. 28, pp. 1187–1199.

Ferreira, F. and Bailey, K.G. (2004), "Disfluencies and human language comprehension", *Trends in Cognitive Sciences*, Vol. 8, pp. 231–237.

Hagoort, P. and Kutas, M. (1995), "Electrophysiological insights into language deficits", *Handbook of Neuropsychology*, Vol. 10, pp. 105–134.

Hall, N.E. (2004), "Lexical development and retrieval in treating children who stutter", *Language, Speech, and Hearing Services in Schools*, Vol. 35, pp. 57–69.

Hall, N., Wagovich, S. and Bernstein Ratner, N. (2007), "Language considerations in childhood stuttering", in Conture, E.G. and Curlee, R. (Eds.), *Stuttering and Related Disorders of Fluency* (3rd ed.), Thieme, New York, NY, pp. 151–167.

Hartfield, K.N. and Conture, E.G. (2006), "Effects of perceptual and conceptual similarity in lexical priming of young children who stutter: Preliminary findings", *Journal of Fluency Disorders*, Vol. 31, pp. 303–324.

Healey, E.C. (2010), "What the literature tells us about listeners' reactions to stuttering: Implications for the clinical management of stuttering", *Seminars in Speech and Language*, Vol. 31, pp. 227–235.

Hennessey, N.W., Nang, C.Y. and Beilby, J.M. (2008), "Speeded verbal responding in adults who stutter: Are there deficits in linguistic encoding?", *Journal of Fluency Disorders*, Vol. 33, pp. 180–202.

Howard, D. (2000), "Cognitive neuropsychology and aphasia therapy: The case of word retrieval", in Papathanasiou, I. (Ed.), *Acquired Neurogenic Communication Disorders: A Clinical Perspective*, Whurr, Philadelphia, PA, US, pp. 76–99.

Howell, P. (2004), "Assessment of some contemporary theories of stuttering that apply to spontaneous speech", *Contemporary Issues in Communication Science and Disorders*, Vol. 31, pp. 122–139.

Hussey, E.K. and Novick, J.M. (2012), "The benefits of executive control training and the implications for language processing", *Frontiers in Psychology*, Vol. 3, pp. 158–172.

Ingham, R.J., Finn, P. and Bothe, A.K. (2005), "Roadblocks' revisited: Neural change, stuttering treatment, and recovery from stuttering", *Journal of Fluency Disorders*, Vol. 30, pp. 91–107.

Jerger, S., Martin, R.C. and Damian, M.F. (2002), "Semantic and phonological influences on picture naming by children and teenagers", *Journal of Memory and Language*, Vol. 47, pp. 229–249.

Jescheniak, J.D. and Levelt, W.J.M. (1994), "Word frequency effects in speech production: Retrieval of syntactic information and of phonological form", *Journal of Experimental Psychology: Learning, Memory, and Cognition*, Vol. 20, pp. 824–843.

Kail, R. and Park, Y.S. (1994), "Processing time, articulation time, and memory span", *Journal of Experimental Child Psychology*, Vol. 57, pp. 281–291.

Kavé, G., Knafo, A. and Gilboa, A. (2010), "The rise and fall of word retrieval across the lifespan", *Psychology and Aging*, Vol. 25, pp. 719–724.

Kloth, S.A.M., Janssen, P., Kraaimaat, F.W. and Brutten, G.J. (1995), "Communicative behavior of mothers of stuttering and nonstuttering high-risk children prior to the onset of stuttering", *Journal of Fluency Disorders*, Vol. 20, pp. 365–377.

Levelt, W.J.M. (1989), *Speaking: From Intention to Articulation*, Bradford, Cambridge, MA.

Levelt, W.J., Roelofs, A. and Meyer, A.S. (1999), "A theory of lexical access in speech production", *Behavioral and Brain Sciences*, Vol. 22, pp. 1–38.

Li, S.C., Lindenberger, U., Hommel, B., Aschersleben, G., Prinz, W. and Baltes, P.B. (2004), "Transformations in the couplings among intellectual abilities and constituent cognitive processes across the life span", *Psychological Science*, Vol. 15, pp. 155–163.

Louko, L.J., Edwards, M.L. and Conture, E.G. (1990), "Phonological characteristics of young stutterers and their normally fluent peers: Preliminary observations", *Journal of Fluency Disorders*, Vol. 15, pp. 191–210.

McGregor, K.K. (1994), "Use of phonological information in a word-finding treatment for children", *Journal of Speech and Hearing Research*, Vol. 37, pp. 1381–1393.

Maxfield, N.D., Huffman, J.L., Frisch, S.A. and Hinckley, J.J. (2010), "Neural correlates of semantic activation spreading on the path to picture naming in adults who stutter", *Clinical Neurophysiology*, Vol. 121, pp. 1447–1463.

Maxfield, N.D., Pizon-Moore, A.A., Frisch, S.A. and Constantine, J.L. (2012), "Exploring semantic and phonological picture-word priming in adults who stutter using event-related potentials", *Clinical Neurophysiology*, Vol. 123, pp. 1131–1146.

Maxfield, N.D., Morris, K., Frisch, S.A., Morphew, K. and Constantine, J. (2014), "Real time processing in picture naming in adults who stutter: ERP evidence", *Clinical Neurophysiology*, Advance online publication.

Melnick, K.S., Conture, E.G. and Ohde, R.N. (2003), "Phonological priming in picture naming of young children who stutter", *Journal of Speech, Language and Hearing Research*, Vol. 46, pp. 1428–1443.

Meyer, D.E., Osman, A.M., Irwin, D.E. and Yantis, S. (1988), "Modern mental chronometry", *Biological Psychology*, Vol. 26, pp. 3–67.

Millager, R.A., Conture, E.G., Walden, T.A. and Kelly, E.M. (2014), "Expressive language intratest scatter of preschool-age children who stutter", *Contemporary Issues in Communication Disorders*, Vol. 41, pp. 110–119.

Morley, M. (1957), *The Development and Disorders of Speech in Childhood*, Livingstone, Edinburgh, UK.

Mortensen, L., Meyer, A.S. and Humphreys, G.W. (2006), "Age-related effects on speech production: A review", *Language and Cognitive Processes*, Vol. 21, pp. 238–290.

Nejati, V., Pouretemad, H.R. and Bahrami, H. (2013), "Attention training in rehabilitation of children with developmental stuttering", *NeuroRehabilitation*, Vol. 32, pp. 297–303.

Newman, R.S. and Ratner, N.B. (2007), "The role of selected lexical factors on confrontation naming accuracy, speed, and fluency in adults who do and do not stutter", *Journal of Speech, Language, and Hearing Research*, Vol. 50, pp. 196–213.

Newton, C. (2012), "Between-word processes in children with speech difficulties: Insights from a usage-based approach to phonology", *Clinical Linguistics and Phonetics*, Vol. 26, pp. 712–727.

Nippold, M.A. (2004), "The child stutters and has a phonological disorder: How should treatment proceed?", in Bothe, A. K. (Ed.), *Evidence-Based Treatment of Stuttering*, Erlbaum, Mahwah, NJ, US, pp. 97–115.

Nippold, M.A. (2012), "Stuttering and language ability in children: Questioning the connection", *American Journal of Speech-Language Pathology*, Vol. 21, pp. 183–196.

Ntourou, K., Conture, E.G. and Lipsey, M.W. (2011), "Language abilities of children who stutter: A meta-analytical review", *American Journal of Speech-Language Pathology*, Vol. 20, pp. 163–179.

Paden, E.P. and Yairi, E. (1996), "Phonological characteristics of children whose stuttering persisted or recovered", *Journal of Speech, Language, and Hearing Research*, Vol. 39, pp. 981–990.

Pelczarski, K.M. and Yaruss, J.S. (2014), "Phonological encoding of young children who stutter", *Journal of Fluency Disorders*, Vol. 39, pp. 12–24.

Pellowski, M.W. (2011), "Word-finding and vocabulary abilities of adults who do and do not stutter", *Contemporary Issues in Communication Disorders*, Vol. 38, pp. 126–134.

Pellowski, M.W. and Conture, E.G. (2005), "Lexical priming in picture naming of young children who do and do not stutter", *Journal of Speech, Language, and Hearing Research*, Vol. 48, pp. 278–294.

Perkins, W.H., Kent, R.D. and Curlee, R.F. (1991), "A theory of neuropsycholinguistic function in stuttering", *Journal of Speech, Language, and Hearing Research*, Vol. 34, pp. 734–752.

Pickering, M.J. and Garrod, S. (2013), "An integrated theory of language production and comprehension", *Behavioral and Brain Sciences*, Vol. 36, pp. 329–347.

Postma, A. and Kolk, H. (1993), "The covert repair hypothesis: Prearticulatory repair processes in normal and stuttered disfluencies", *Journal of Speech, Language, and Hearing Research*, Vol. 36, pp. 472–487.

Prins, D., Main, V. and Wampler, S. (1997), "Lexicalization in adults who stutter", *Journal of Speech, Language, and Hearing Research*, Vol. 40, pp. 373–384.

Ratner, N.B., Newman, R. and Strekas, A. (2009), "Effects of word frequency and phonological neighborhood characteristics on confrontation naming in children who stutter and normally fluent peers", *Journal of Fluency Disorders*, Vol. 34, pp. 225–241.

Richels, C.G., Johnson, K.N., Walden, T.A. and Conture, E.G. (2013), "Socioeconomic status, parental education, vocabulary and language skills of children who stutter", *Journal of Communication Disorders*, Vol. 46, pp. 361–374.

Rispoli, M. (2003), "Changes in the nature of sentence production during the period of grammatical development", *Journal of Speech, Language, and Hearing Research*, Vol. 46, pp. 818–830.

Sasisekaran, J. (2014), "Exploring the link between stuttering and phonology: A review and implications for treatment", *Seminars in Speech and Language*, Vol. 35, pp. 95–113.

Sasisekaran, J., De Nil, L.F., Smyth, R. and Johnson, C. (2006), "Phonological encoding in the silent speech of persons who stutter", *Journal of Fluency Disorders*, Vol. 31, pp. 1–21.

Savage, C. and Howell, P. (2008), "Lexical priming of function words and content words with children who do, and do not, stutter", *Journal of Communication Disorders*, Vol. 41, pp. 459–484.

Seery, C.H., Watkins, R.V., Mangelsdorf, S.C. and Shigeto, A. (2007), "Subtyping stuttering II: Contributions from language and temperament", *Journal of Fluency Disorders*, Vol. 32, pp. 197–217.

Selkirk, E. (1984), *Phonology and Syntax: The Relation between Sound and Structure*. MIT Press, Cambridge, MA, US.

Stevens, C., Fanning, J., Coch, D., Sanders, L. and Neville, H. (2008), "Neural mechanisms of selective auditory attention are enhanced by computerized training: Electrophysiological evidence from language-impaired and typically developing children", *Brain Research*, Vol. 1205, pp. 55–69.

Tetnowski, J.A. (1998), "Linguistic effects on disfluency", in Paul, R. (Ed.), *Exploring the Speech-Language Connection*. Brookes, Baltimore, MD, US, pp. 227–251.

Tsai, P., Lim, V.P., Brundage, S.B. and Ratner, N.B. (2011), "Linguistic analysis of stuttering in bilinguals: Methodological challenges and solutions", *Multilingual Aspects of Fluency Disorders*, Vol. 5, pp. 308–332.

Tsiamtsiouris, J. and Cairns, H.S. (2009), "Effects of syntactic complexity and sentence-structure priming on speech initiation time in adults who stutter", *Journal of Speech, Language, and Hearing Research*, Vol. 52, pp. 1623–1639.

Tsiamtsiouris, J. and Cairns, H.S. (2013), "Effects of sentence-structure complexity on speech initiation time and disfluency", *Journal of Fluency Disorders*, Vol. 38, pp. 30–44.

Tumanova, V., Conture, E.G., Lambert, E.W. and Walden, T.A. (2014), "Speech disfluencies of preschool-age children who do and do not stutter", *Journal of Communication Disorders*, Vol. 49, pp. 25–41.

Vanryckeghem, M., Brutten, G.J., Uddin, N. and Borsel, J.V. (2004), "A comparative investigation of the speech-associated coping responses reported by adults who do and do not stutter", *Journal of Fluency Disorders*, Vol. 29, pp. 237–250.

Weber-Fox, C., Spencer, R., Spruill III, J.E. and Smith, A. (2004), "Phonologic processing in adults who stutter: Electrophysiological and behavioral evidence", *Journal of Speech, Language, and Hearing Research*, Vol. 47, pp. 1244–1258.

Weber-Fox, C., Hampton Wray, A. and Arnold, H. (2013), "Early childhood stuttering and electrophysiological indices of language processing", *Journal of Fluency Disorders*, Vol. 28, pp. 206–221.

Westby, C.E. (1979), "Language performance of stuttering and nonstuttering children", *Journal of Communication Disorders*, Vol. 12, pp. 133–145.

Wingate, M.E. (1988), *The Structure of Stuttering: A Psycholinguistic Analysis*, Springer-Verglag, New York, NY.

Yairi, E. (2004), "The formative years of stuttering: A changing portrait", *Contemporary Issues in Communication Science and Disorders*, Vol. 31, pp. 92–104.

Yairi, E. and Ambrose, N.G. (2005), *Early Childhood Stuttering for Clinicians by Clinicians*. Pro Ed, Austin, TX, US.

24

LINGUISTIC DISRUPTION IN PRIMARY PROGRESSIVE APHASIA, FRONTOTEMPORAL DEGENERATION, AND ALZHEIMER'S DISEASE

Amanda Garcia and Jamie Reilly

Dementia is a non-specific term denoting a neurodegenerative condition that impacts memory, language, and other cognitive functions (Albert *et al.*, 2011; Naik and Nygaard, 2008). Although Alzheimer's Disease (AD) is the most common dementia variant, AD is not synonymous with dementia. Numerous other forms of dementia exist, many with unique profiles of communicative impairment. Clinical neuroscience has made recent strides toward elucidating the molecular and genetic bases of many dementia subtypes. In turn, diagnostic specificity also has seen rapid improvement. A picture of complexity and diversity has since emerged with our improved understanding of the dementia variants.

While diverse in both presentation and underlying pathology, many dementia variants have an element of communicative disruption. Often, such communicative disorders can be highly debilitating for patients. They can be classified based on expressed language impairments or based on histopathology of the brain. This chapter aims to elucidate the difference between these two classification systems. First, we describe typical clusters of language impairment found in patients with neurodegenerative diseases that primarily impact language. That is, we describe the typical presentation of those with Primary Progressive Aphasia, outlining deficits across linguistic domains. We additionally discuss the impact of underlying neuropatholgical conditions on language functioning in certain dementia subpopulations (i.e., Frontotemporal Degeneration and AD). We conclude with a discussion of new directions for cognitive treatment in these specific dementia subtypes.

Primary Progressive Aphasia

There are numerous ways to describe, classify, and categorize the dementias; however, the two dominant classification schemata classify by phenotype (i.e., the outward manifestation of a pathological process) or by pathology (e.g., presence or absence of particular protein inclusions). Primary Progressive Aphasia (PPA) is the best known taxonomy applied to the phenotype of a progressive language loss. Mesulam (1982, 2007) first described PPA as a language-based dementia. The hallmark of this disorder is two years of progressive language impairment in the absence of generalized dementia. PPA is not typically caused by an acute stroke, trauma, or tumor. Rather, PPA is insidious and steadily progressive.

Classifying the pathophysiology of PPA has presented a major challenge. PPA typically occurs during the early stages of an unspecified disease process (e.g., Frontotemporal Degeneration). Thus, patients with PPA do not typically come to autopsy until their language symptoms have evolved into more severe, generalized forms of dementia. The most extensive postmortem confirmation studies to date suggest that approximately two-thirds of PPA cases are caused by Frontotemporal Degeneration (FTD) protein pathology. AD pathology contributes to about 30 percent of PPA cases, with the remainder secondary to other dementias (e.g., Vascular Dementia) (Grossman, 2010; Mesulam *et al.*, 2008).

Three variants of PPA have been described by clusters of symptoms, rather than neuropathology. Gorno-Tempini and colleagues have delineated formal diagnostic criteria for: 1) Nonfluent/Agrammatic PPA; 2) Semantic variant PPA; and 3) Logopenic Progressive Aphasia (Gorno-Tempini *et al.*, 2011). The language impairments of these subtypes are described next and summarized in Table 24.1.

Nonfluent/Agrammatic Progressive Aphasia

Nonfluent/Agrammatic Progressive Aphasia (NFPA) is characterized by atrophy that encompasses both the classical Broca's Area and a more extensive distribution of the left dorsolateral prefrontal cortex (Ash *et al.*, 2009; Gorno-Tempini *et al.*, 2004, 2011). This atrophy

Table 24.1 Overview of linguistic deficits by phenotype and pathology.

	Phenotype Classification			Pathology Classification	
	Nonfluent Progressive Aphasia	Semantic Variant PPA	Logopenic Progressive Aphasia	Frontotemporal Degeneration*	Alzheimer's Disease
Sentence Comprehension	−	−	+	+	−
Single Word Comprehension**	+	−	+	+	+
Naming	−	−	−	+	−
Repetition	−	+	−	+	+
Syntax	−	+	+	+	+
Semantics	+	-	+	+	−
Speech Production	−	+	−	Discourse −	Discourse −
Reading and Writing	−	−	+	+	+

Note. This table outlines generally preserved and impaired linguistic functions in the different conditions, distinguished here by clinical presentation (phenotype) and by neuropathology. The + represents preserved linguistic functions; the − represents impaired linguistic function.

*Note that frontotemporal degeneration resists a clean histopathological translation to outward cognitive impairment. These represent generalizations for behavioral variant FTD.

**Comprehension refers to single-word auditory comprehension.

contributes to a number of linguistic input and output deficits, though impairments are especially striking in production. Agrammatism, for example, manifests in the use of syntactically sparse sentences and the omission of grammatical morphemes and function words (Gorno-Tempini *et al.*, 2011; Grossman, 2012). Reduced grammatical complexity is also evident in conversational speech, wherein patients tend to produce an overabundance of canonical sentence structures (e.g., subject–verb–object) that are peppered with grammatical and morphological errors (Knibb *et al.*, 2009). Non-linguistic cognitive deficits also contribute to their compromised sentence processing. NFPA patients experience impaired executive functioning, which may impact their ability to organize complex grammatical forms and process long-distance dependencies (Ash *et al.*, 2009; Libon *et al.*, 2007).

Effortful speech is clearly the most striking deficit seen in NFPA. Output is marked by frequent pauses, increased effort in production, and overall slowed rate of production (Amici *et al.*, 2006; Gorno-Tempini *et al.*, 2011; Grossman *et al.*, 2012). The presence of agrammatism and a preponderance of semantic naming errors in NFPA (Reilly *et al.*, 2011b) bolster the claim of a supra-motor basis for language disturbance in NFPA: syntax, semantics, and phonology are all higher level linguistic functions.

NFPA is also characterized by linguistic input deficits, specifically in the comprehension of syntactically complex sentences and in detecting syntactic anomalies (Amici *et al.*, 2006, Gorno-Tempini *et al.*, 2011, Grossman and Moore, 2005; Grossman *et al.*, 2005). Impairment in these domains has also been linked to a complex interaction between grammatical and working memory resource deficits (Grossman and Moore, 2005; Grossman *et al.*, 2005). Patients with NFPA typically show comprehension advantages for material presented at the single word level relative to material embedded within discourse.

Semantic variant PPA

In a classic study, Warrington (1975) described a series of patients who showed a selective impairment of semantic memory, now designated as Semantic variant PPA (SvPPA). SvPPA is characterized by primary neurodegeneration of anterolateral portions of the temporal lobes (i.e., neocortex). Cortical atrophy during the early stages of SvPPA is often asymmetric, impacting the left cerebral hemisphere. As the disease progresses, atrophy spreads to homologous right hemisphere structures, engulfing much of the temporal lobes (Lambon Ralph *et al.*, 2001; Mummery *et al.*, 1999, 2000). This distribution of temporal lobe pathology is unique from that of AD in that SvPPA appears to somewhat spare the medial structures (e.g., hippocampus) that are crucial for episodic memory encoding (see Figure 24.1).

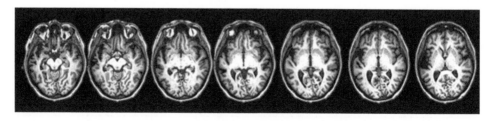

Figure 24.1 MR image of a patient with SvPPA, illustrating temporal lobe degeneration. This figure shows slices of the brain in the axial view, presenting views of the structures in an inferior (i.e., the left) to superior (i.e., the right) manner. These slices demonstrate atrophy of the temporal poles, with relative sparing of more posterior cortices (i.e. decreased volume of cortex in anterior portion of the temporal lobes as demonstrated in the leftmost slices).

The impairment associated with SvPPA tends to be fairly homogeneous across representational modalities (Benedet *et al.*, 2006; Bozeat *et al.*, 2000, 2003; Coccia *et al.*, 2004, Lambon Ralph *et al.*, 1998, 2001, 2010). That is, patients with SvPPA tend to show comparably poor performance for words, pictures, environmental sounds, odors, etc. Such consistency strongly implicates damage to a central semantic store that subserves both verbal and nonverbal cognitive performance. This highly impaired semantic functioning (across verbal and nonverbal modalities) is at odds with seemingly intact functioning across more general cognitive domains. In other words, patients with SvPPA tend to show focal deficits in semantic knowledge with relative preservation of many other cognitive domains (e.g., phonology, perceptual matching, visuospatial functioning) (Reilly *et al.*, 2005, 2007, 2010; Reilly and Peelle, 2008).

SvPPA also is characterized by profound anomia with the presence of frequent omissions and superordinate semantic naming errors (e.g., "animal" for dog). These errors tend to occur, however, in the context of speech that is phonologically, prosodically, and grammatically well formed. Language production is generally fluent, personality is grossly preserved, and many of the automatic, overlearned conversational pleasantries that punctuate casual discussion remain intact. Thus, it can often be quite difficult in casual conversation to detect that anything is "wrong" with a person with SvPPA. Yet, impairments quickly become apparent in discourse when probing basic aspects of word and object knowledge. Language tends to be empty and circumlocutory. As disease severity worsens, such deficits are ever more apparent in nonverbal domains (e.g., pouring detergent into marinara sauce, feeding visitors non-edible plants).

Logopenic Progressive Aphasia

Logopenic Progressive Aphasia (LPA) is characterized by primary thinning of the left temporo-parietal junction, though different aspects of the syndrome have discrete neuroanatomical correlates. Confrontation naming deficits are most associated with atrophy of the inferior-posterior parietal lobe, while sentence repetition deficits are most associated with that of the posterior superior temporal gyrus (Leyton and Hodges, 2013; Rogalski *et al.*, 2011a). As the disease progresses, this atrophy spreads to include the anterior temporal lobe and dorsal frontal cortex/inferior frontal gyri (Rogalski *et al.*, 2011b).

Gorno-Tempini and colleagues (2008) have characterized many of the language comprehension difficulties in LPA as arising from impairments of phonological storage and articulatory rehearsal (Gorno-Tempini *et al.*, 2008). In this way, the slow speech and speech errors observed in these patients can be thought of as qualitatively different from those observed in patients with NFPA. For example, while these patients had decreased speech rate compared to healthy older adults, this slowing can primarily be attributed to word finding problems, false starts, and filled pauses rather than a difficulty with syntactic processing or frank agrammatism (Amici *et al.*, 2006; Wilson *et al.*, 2010). These patients may also express phonological speech errors (Gorno-Tempini *et al.*, 2011). Additionally, their confrontation naming errors primarily result from difficulty with lexical retrieval rather than loss of semantic knowledge, differentiating their performance from that of SvPPA patients. Speech errors produced during discourse also seem to stem from phonological rather than motor errors (Wilson *et al.*, 2010).

Patients with LPA often have difficulty comprehending sentences, regardless of syntactic complexity, and have impaired performance on tasks of sequential commands (Amici *et al.*, 2006; Gorno-Tempini *et al.*, 2008). They additionally show difficulty repeating sentences or phrases, often substituting semantically similar responses for the target. For example, they may say "It looks like nobody is there" for "It looks as if nobody is around" (Gorno-Tempini *et al.* 2008: 1231). Their overall single word repetition, however, is mostly intact (Amici *et al.*, 2006;

Gorno-Tempini *et al.*, 2008; Hodges *et al.*, 2008). Thus, their impairment does not seem to result from impaired speech perception but rather from difficulty maintaining and integrating phonological information.

Histopathological dementia subtypes

We have thus far described several variants of PPA, or syndromes, delineated by a common set of core behaviors (as illustrated in Table 24.1). One might also classify dementia subtypes via histopathological similarities, such as the presence or absence of particular proteins in the brain. The following sections utilize a histopathological classification system to explain linguistic impairments found in dementia patients with different types of neuropathology. Of note, patients with these types of dementia can, and often do, exhibit a variant of PPA. We describe the impact of these pathologies on language functioning that may occur outside of a PPA. These linguistic impairments are also depicted in Table 24.1.

Frontotemporal Degeneration

Frontotemporal Degeneration (FTD) is a non-Alzheimer's pathology linked to abnormal levels of several proteins, including tau, ubiquitin, and TDP-43 (Heutink, 2000, Neumann *et al.*, 2006, Van Deerlin *et al.*, 2007). A distinctive property of FTD is that the pathology tends to produce relatively circumscribed and asymmetric cortical atrophy during its early to middle stages, particularly impacting regions of the frontal and temporal lobes. The location and extent of the associated neurodegeneration mediates the qualitative nature of its associated cognitive impairment. Thus, when FTD impacts posterior frontal lobe structures in the language dominant hemisphere, patients most commonly show NFPA. In contrast, when FTD impacts regions of the temporal lobe, patients may experience SvPPA or LPA. FTD is commonly associated with language disturbance, with the exception of one FTD subtype known as behavioral variant FTD (bvFTD).

In bvFTD, progressive atrophy of anterior portions of the frontal lobes (e.g. orbitofrontal cortex) produces a variety of cognitive difficulties, including personality change, rigidity, apathy, impaired impulse control, and a prominent dysexecutive disorder (Rascovsky *et al.*, 2011). BvFTD is not associated with frank language disturbance. Patients with bvFTD do not experience the profound anomia seen in SvPPA or the speech production difficulties seen in NFPA. Nevertheless, patients with this FTD variant do experience high-level linguistic disruption, impacting macroscale elements of language production. Thus, while the subcomponents of language seem relatively intact (e.g. phonology and syntax), the overall ability to communicate through articulate discourse is impaired. For example, patients with BvFTD have difficulties with cohesion and organization of conversational narratives, with frequent tangents and poor topic maintenance (Ash *et al.*, 2006). Patients with BvFTD have also been reported to show deficits in conversational turn-taking, comprehension of emotional language, and the production and comprehension of emotional prosody (Dara *et al.*, 2012). Thus, bvFTD patients typically exhibit language difficulties that are associated with increased executive load.

Alzheimer's Disease

AD, the most common form of dementia, is among the leading causes of mortality in industrialized nations (Alzheimer's Association, 2012; Attems *et al.*, 2005; Hebert *et al.*, 2001).

The onset of AD is strongly correlated with advanced aging. Although episodic memory impairment is indeed a hallmark of AD, the diagnostic criteria reflect a range of additional impairments that impact language and other cognitive processes that directly support communicative functioning. The most current clinical criteria for diagnosis include: (1) insidious onset; (2) history of cognitive decline; (3) cognitive deficit in learning/recall and one other domain, such as, language, visuospatial, or executive functioning (McKhann *et al.*, 2011).

Language disorders are commonplace in AD. Moreover, subtle linguistic deficits may be detectable during prodromal stages decades before the disease converts to frank dementia (Riley *et al.*, 2005; Verma and Howard, 2012). The early course of AD is characterized by relatively preserved *input* processes critical for the perception of spoken words (e.g., phonological perception, lexical representation, grammar) (Taler and Phillips, 2008). These relatively preserved linguistic domains do, however, exist in the context of more pervasive deficits in working memory, attention, and visuospatial functioning. Thus, language comprehension tasks that tax additional memory and attentional resources (e.g., processing long sentences, processing speech in noise) often elicit comprehension breakdowns in AD (Rochon *et al.*, 1994, 2000; Waters *et al.*, 1998). Such breakdowns highlight the complexity involved in disentangling language versus memory impairment in AD.

Relative to input processing, linguistic output is often profoundly impaired in AD. Patients often have great difficulty naming single words, especially proper nouns and living things (Hodges and Patterson, 1995; Hodges *et al.*, 1992; Reilly *et al.*, 2011a). The root cause of this associated anomia remains highly controversial. One hypothesis is that patients experience a disconnection syndrome wherein impaired retrieval processes slow or prevent access to concepts (e.g., a patient might recognize a dog but fail to retrieve the name, *dog*). Conversely, others have argued that it is the result of fundamentally degraded semantic knowledge (e.g., patients are actively "forgetting" what a dog is). In our own work, we have argued for a dual locus of naming impairment in AD with roots both in degraded semantic content and in active retrieval processes that operate on such content (Reilly *et al.*, 2011a).

Deficits in single word production carry forward and are amplified at the discourse level. Narrative discourse in AD (e.g., "tell me about your day") is characterized by a range of deficits, including diminished mean length of utterance, reduced syntactic complexity, ambiguous pronoun references (e.g., all characters are referred to as "it"), poor information content, and limited global cohesion (Gottschalk *et al.*, 1988; Gottschalk, 1994).

In summary, the pathology of AD produces numerous linguistic disruptions, including anomia, alexia, and aphasia. Some of these language disorders (e.g., long sentence comprehension) arguably emerge secondary to primary memory impairment. Nevertheless, there exists a complex interaction between language and memory loss in AD that resists "clean" root cause assessments. Moreover, variability both between and within patients with AD (e.g., some patients show priming effects, others do not) contribute to the debate regarding why language disorders are present and how we might best intervene to ameliorate such problems.

Concluding remarks

In this chapter, we have presented a necessarily highly selective review, merely scratching the surface of describing a small subset of dementias. This perspective was motivated both by space restrictions but also for a more dubious reason. That is, very little remains known about linguistic disruption associated with most non-Alzheimer's dementia subtypes (Reilly *et al.*, 2010). While communicative impairments are among the most functionally debilitating symptoms of the dementias, we have only a rudimentary understanding of how to effectively treat the complex language impairments these patients experience. Moreover, treatment of dementia is not yet currently mandated as part of the curriculum for speech–language clinical programs in the USA, Australia, and the UK. Consequently, many practitioners apply techniques that may have efficacy for other populations (e.g., stroke aphasia) but have fundamental limitations in the context of a neurodegenerative condition. Thus, dementia presents a very new and pressing frontier for language rehabilitation research. Despite all of the unknowns regarding the potential for language rehabilitation in the dementias, several promising behavioral techniques have begun to emerge, including spaced retrieval training, errorless learning, group reminiscence therapy, and Montessori-based skill learning approaches (Bier and Macoir, 2010; Jelcic *et al.*, 2012; Savage *et al.*, 2013).

Much like the dementia diagnosis, the treatment of dementia can target a variety of either microscale (e.g., cellular) or macroscale (e.g., behavior) processes. Certainly, the optimal treatment for dementia would involve a "cure" that reverses tissue damage and restores neural function. Although this contingency seems unlikely, biomedical research has recently identified several recent protein targets and also developed agents that clear specific protein depositions (e.g., amyloid-b). Another approach involves prevention, through the development of vaccines that would be administered before dementia symptoms evolve. These vaccines would aim to prevent the cascade of microcellular damage associated with the neurodegeneration. Both of these approaches represent the future of dementia management. The present state of dementia treatment involves pharmacological agents that target the downstream effects of brain damage (e.g., depletion of acetylcholine) rather than slowing or reversing such damage. The philosophy of neurorehabilitation for the dementias has followed a parallel course. One argument is that cognitive rehabilitation should pursue compensatory approaches, modifying environmental cues and caregiver interactions to somewhat passively optimize a patient's function. An alternative approach involves working directly with the patient to restore lost functions (e.g., retraining lost face–name associations).

In our own approach to the treatment of progressive language impairment, we have embraced a middle ground between restoration and compensation of function. We argue that *maintenance* of extant cognitive function might prove more effective as a treatment strategy for combatting language loss in a strategic way. Our treatment approach involves intensive semantic training and repeated naming of a small set of carefully crafted items (i.e., a microlexicon) (Reilly, in press). This approach is unique in that it involves training a finite vocabulary and protecting a set of highly salient words against loss rather than retraining forgotten words *ad hoc*. This approach is also novel in that it forgoes treatment generalization in favor of functional naming of a highly constrained personal vocabulary.

In conclusion, the last decade has seen rapid advances in diagnostic specificity along with promising biomarkers that may eventually provide drug targets that slow or ultimately halt the progression of some forms of dementia. Yet, we have much to learn about cognitive–linguistic rehabilitation for the many millions of adults impacted by dementias. This complex societal problem will, therefore, require a multi-pronged attack coordinating prevention with evidence-based management of existing cases.

Acknowledgement

This work was funded by US Public Health Service grants DC010197 and DC013063 from the National Institute on Deafness and Other Communication Disorders.

References

Albert, M.S., Dekosky, S.T., Dickson, D., Dubois, B., Feldman, H.H., Fox, N.C., *et al.*, (2011), "The diagnosis of mild cognitive impairment due to Alzheimer's disease: Recommendations from the National Institute on Aging-Alzheimer's Association workgroups on diagnostic guidelines for Alzheimer's disease", *Alzheimers and Dementia*, Vol. 7, pp. 1–10.

Alzheimer's Association (2012), "2012 Alzheimer's Disease facts and figures", *Alzheimer's Disease and Associated Dementias*, Vol. 8, pp. 158–194.

Amici, S., Gorno-Tempini, M.L., Ogar, J.M., Dronkers, N.F. and Miller, B.L. (2006), "An overview on primary progressive aphasia and its variants", *Behavioural Neurology*, Vol. 17, pp. 77–87.

Ash, S., Moore, P., Antani, S., Mccawley, G., Work, M. and Grossman, M. (2006), "Trying to tell a tale: Discourse impairments in progressive aphasia and frontotemporal dementia", *Neurology*, Vol. 66, pp. 1405–1413.

Ash, S., Moore, P., Vesely, L., Gunawardena, D., Mcmillan, C., Anderson, C., *et al.*, (2009), "Non-fluent speech in frontotemporal lobar degeneration", *Journal of Neurolinguistics*, Vol. 22, pp. 370–383.

Attems, J., Konig, C., Huber, M., Lintner, F. and Jellinger, K.A. (2005), "Cause of death in demented and non-demented elderly inpatients; An autopsy study of 308 cases", *Journal of Alzheimer's Disease*, Vol. 8, pp. 57–62.

Benedet, M., Patterson, K., Gomez-Pastor, I. and Luisa Garcia De La Rocha, M. (2006), "'Non-semantic' aspects of language in semantic dementia: As normal as they're said to be?", *Neurocase*, Vol. 12, pp. 15–26.

Bier, N. and Macoir, J. (2010), "How to make a spaghetti sauce with a dozen small things I cannot name: A review of the impact of semantic-memory deficits on everyday actions", *Journal of Clinical and Experimental Neuropsychology*, Vol. 32, pp. 201–211.

Bozeat, S., Lambon Ralph, M.A., Patterson, K., Garrard, P. and Hodges, J.R. (2000), "Non-verbal semantic impairment in semantic dementia", *Neuropsychologia*, Vol. 38, pp. 1207–1215.

Bozeat, S., Lambon Ralph, M.A., Graham, K.S., Patterson, K., Wilkin, H., Rowland, J., *et al.*, (2003), "A duck with four legs: Investigating the structure of conceptual knowledge using picture drawing in semantic dementia", *Cognitive Neuropsychology*, Vol. 20, pp. 27–47.

Coccia, M., Bartolini, M., Luzzi, S., Provinciali, L. and Lambon Ralph, M.A. (2004), "Semantic memory is an amodal, dynamic system: Evidence from the interaction of naming and object use in semantic dementia", *Cognitive Neuropsychology*, Vol. 21, pp. 513–527.

Dara, C., Kirsch-Darrow, L., Ochfeld, E., Slenz, J., Agranovich, A., Vasconcellos-Faria, A., *et al.*, (2012), "Impaired emotion processing from vocal and facial cues in frontotemporal dementia compared to right hemisphere stroke", *Neurocase*, Vol. 19. pp. 521–529.

Gorno-Tempini, M.L., Dronkers, N.F., Rankin, K.P., Ogar, J.M., Phengrasamy, L., Rosen, H.J., *et al.*, (2004), "Cognition and anatomy in three variants of primary progressive aphasia", *Annals of Neurology*, Vol. 55, pp. 335–346.

Gorno-Tempini, M.L., Brambati, S.M., Ginex, V., Ogar, J., Dronkers, N.F., Marcone, A., *et al.*, (2008), "The logopenic/phonological variant of primary progressive aphasia", *Neurology*, Vol. 71, pp. 1227–1234.

Gorno-Tempini, M.L., Hillis, A.E., Weintraub, S., Kertesz, A., Mendez, M., Cappa, S.F., *et al.*, (2011), "Classification of primary progressive aphasia and its variants", *Neurology*, Vol. 76, pp. 1006–1014.

Gottschalk, L.A. (1994), "The development, validation, and applications of a computerized measurement of cognitive impairment from the content analysis of verbal behavior", *Journal of Clinical Psychology*, Vol. 50, pp. 349–361.

Gottschalk, L.A., Uliana, R. and Gilbert, R. (1988), "Presidential candidates and cognitive impairment measured from behavior in campaign debates", *Public Administration Review*, Vol. 48, March/April, pp. 613–619.

Grossman, M. (2010), "Primary progressive aphasia: Clinicopathological correlations", *Nature Reviews Neurology*, Vol. 6, pp. 88–97.

Grossman, M. (2012), "The non-fluent/agrammatic variant of primary progressive aphasia", *The Lancet Neurology*, Vol. 11, pp. 545–555.

Grossman, M. and Moore, P. (2005), "A longitudinal study of sentence comprehension difficulty in primary progressive aphasia", *Journal of Neurology, Neurosurgery, and Psychiatry*, Vol. 76, pp. 644–649.

Grossman, M., Rhee, J. and Moore, P. (2005), "Sentence processing in frontotemporal dementia", *Cortex*, Vol. 41, pp. 764–777.

Grossman, M., Powers, J., Ash, S., Mcmillan, C., Burkholder, L., Irwin, D. and Trojanowski, J.Q. (2012), "Disruption of large-scale neural networks in non-fluent/agrammatic variant primary progressive aphasia associated with frontotemporal degeneration pathology", *Brain and Language*, Vol. 127, pp. 106–120.

Hebert, L.E., Scherr, P.A., Bienias, D.A. and Evans, D.A. (2001), "Annual incidence of Alzheimer's disease in the United States projected to the years 2000 through 2050", *Alzheimer's Disease and Associated Disorders*, Vol. 15, pp. 169–173.

Heutink, P. (2000), "Untangling tau-related dementia", *Human Molecular Genetics*, Vol. 9, pp. 979–986.

Hodges, J.R. and Patterson, K. (1995), "Is semantic memory consistently impaired early in the course of Alzheimer's disease? Neuroanatomical and diagnostic implications", *Neuropsychologia*, Vol. 33, pp. 441–459.

Hodges, J.R., Salmon, D.P. and Butters, N. (1992), "Semantic memory impairment in Alzheimer's disease: Failure of access or degraded knowledge?", *Neuropsychologia*, Vol. 30, pp. 301–314.

Hodges, J.R., Martinos, M., Woollams, A.M., Patterson, K. and Adlam, A.L. (2008), "Repeat and point: Differentiating semantic dementia from progressive non-fluent aphasia", *Cortex*, Vol. 44, pp. 1265–1270.

Jelcic, N., Cagnin, A., Meneghello, F., Turolla, A., Ermani, M. and Dam, M. (2012), "Effects of lexical-semantic treatment on memory in early Alzheimer Disease: An observer-blinded randomized controlled trial", *Neurorehabilitation and Neural Repair*, Vol. 26, pp. 949–956.

Knibb, J.A., Woollams, A.M., Hodges, J.R. and Patterson, K. (2009), "Making sense of progressive non-fluent aphasia: An analysis of conversational speech", *Brain*, Vol. 132, pp. 2734–2746.

Lambon Ralph, M.A., Graham, K.S., Ellis, A.W. and Hodges, J.R. (1998), "Naming in semantic dementia – What matters?", *Neuropsychologia*, Vol. 36, pp. 775–784.

Lambon Ralph, M.A., Mcclelland, J.L., Patterson, K., Galton, C.J. and Hodges, J.R. (2001), "No right to speak? The relationship between object naming and semantic impairment: Neuropsychological evidence and a computational model", *Journal of Cognitive Neuroscience*, Vol. 13, pp. 341–356.

Lambon Ralph, M.A., Sage, K., Jones, R.W. and Mayberry, E.J. (2010), "Coherent concepts are computed in the anterior temporal lobes", *Proceedings of the National Academy of Sciences USA*, Vol. 107, pp. 2717–2722.

Leyton, C.E. and Hodges, J.R. (2013), "Towards a clearer definition of logopenic progressive aphasia", *Current Neurology and Neuroscience Reports*, Vol. 13, p. 396.

Libon, D.J., Xie, S., Moore, P., Farmer, J., Antani, S., Mccawley, G., *et al.*, (2007), "Patterns of neuropsychological impairment in frontotemporal dementia", *Neurology*, Vol. 68, pp. 369–375.

McKhann, G.M., Knopman, D.S., Chertkow, H., Hyman, B.T., Jack Jr, C.R., Kawas, C.H., *et al.*, (2011), "The diagnosis of dementia due to Alzheimer's disease: Recommendations from the National Institute on Aging-Alzheimer's Association workgroups on diagnostic guidelines for Alzheimer's disease", *Alzheimer's and Dementia*, Vol. 7, pp. 263–269.

Mesulam, M.M. (1982), "Slowly progressive aphasia without generalized dementia", *Annals of Neurology*, Vol. 11, pp. 592–598.

Mesulam, M.M. (2007), "Primary progressive aphasia: A 25-year retrospective", *Alzheimer's Disease and Associated Disorders*, Vol. 21, pp. S8–S11.

Mesulam, M.M., Wicklund, A., Johnson, N., Rogalski, E., Leger, G.C., Rademaker, A., *et al.*, (2008), "Alzheimer and frontotemporal pathology in subsets of primary progressive aphasia", *Annals of Neurology*, Vol. 63, pp. 709–719.

Mummery, C.J., Patterson, K., Wise, R.J.S., Vandenbergh, R., Price, C.J. and Hodges, J.R. (1999), "Disrupted temporal lobe connections in semantic dementia", *Brain*, Vol. 122, pp. 61–73.

Mummery, C.J., Patterson, K., Price, C.J., Ashburner, J., Frackowiak, R.S.J. and Hodges, J.R. (2000), "A voxel-based morphometry study of semantic dementia: Relationship between temporal lobe atrophy and semantic memory", *Annals of Neurology*, Vol. 47, pp. 36–45.

Naik, M. and Nygaard, H.A. (2008), "Diagnosing dementia – ICD-10 not so bad after all: A comparison between dementia criteria according to DSM-IV and ICD-10", *International Journal of Geriatric Psychiatry*, Vol. 23, pp. 279–282.

Neumann, M., Sampathu, D.M., Kwong, L.K., Truax, A.C., Micsenyi, M.C., Chou, T.T., *et al.*, (2006), "Ubiquitinated TDP-43 in frontotemporal lobar degeneration and amyotrophic lateral sclerosis", *Science*, Vol. 314, pp. 130–133.

Rascovsky, K., Hodges, J.R., Knopman, D., Mendez, M.F., Kramer, J.H., Neuhaus, J., *et al.*, (2011), "Sensitivity of revised diagnostic criteria for the behavioural variant of frontotemporal dementia", *Brain*, Vol. 134, pp. 2456–2477.

Reilly, J. and Peelle, J.E. (2008), "Effects of semantic impairment on language processing in semantic dementia", *Seminars in Speech and Language*, Vol. 29, pp. 32–43.

Reilly, J., Martin, N. and Grossman, M. (2005), "Verbal learning in semantic dementia: Is repetition priming a useful strategy?", *Aphasiology*, Vol. 19, pp. 329–339.

Reilly, J., Cross, K., Troiani, V. and Grossman, M. (2007), "Single word semantic judgments in semantic dementia: Do phonology and grammatical class count?", *Aphasiology*, Vol. 21, pp. 558–569.

Reilly, J., Rodriguez, A.D., Lamy, M. and Neils-Strunjas, J. (2010), "Cognition, language, and clinical pathological features of non-Alzheimer's dementias: An overview", *Journal of Communication Disorders*, Vol. 43, pp. 438–452.

Reilly, J., Peelle, J.E., Antonucci, S.M. and Grossman, M. (2011a), "Anomia as a marker of distinct semantic memory impairments in Alzheimer's disease and semantic dementia", *Neuropsychology*, Vol. 25, pp. 413–426.

Reilly, J., Rodriguez, A., Peelle, J.E. and Grossman, M. (2011b), "Frontal lobe damage impairs process and content in semantic memory: Evidence from category specific effects in progressive nonfluent aphasia", *Cortex*, Vol. 47, pp. 645–658.

Reilly, J. (2015), "How to constrain and maintain a lexicon for the treatment of progressive semantic naming deficits", *Neuropsychological Rehabilitation*. doi:10.1080/09602011.2014.1003947.

Riley, K.P., Snowdon, D.A., Desrosiers, M.F. and Markesbery, W.R. (2005), "Early life linguistic ability, late life cognitive function, and neuropathology: Findings from the Nun Study", *Neurobiology of Aging*, Vol. 26, pp. 341–347.

Rochon, E., Waters, G.S. and Caplan, D. (1994), "Sentence comprehension in patients with Alzheimer's Disease", *Brain and Language*, Vol. 46, pp. 329–349.

Rochon, E., Waters, G.S. and Caplan, D. (2000), "The relationship between measures of working memory and sentence comprehension in patients with Alzheimer's disease", *Journal of Speech, Language and Hearing Research*, Vol. 43, pp. 395–413.

Rogalski, E., Cobia, D., Harrison, T.M., Wieneke, C., Thompson, C.K., Weintraub, S. and Mesulam, M.M. (2011a), "Anatomy of language impairments in primary progressive aphasia", *Journal of Neuroscience*, Vol. 31, pp. 3344–3350.

Rogalski, E., Cobia, D., Harrison, T.M., Wieneke, C., Weintraub, S. and Mesulam, M.M. (2011b), "Progression of language decline and cortical atrophy in subtypes of primary progressive aphasia", *Neurology*, Vol. 76, pp. 1804–1810.

Savage, S.A., Ballard, K.J., Piguet, O. and Hodges, J.R. (2013), "Bringing words back to mind – Improving word production in semantic dementia", *Cortex*, Vol. 49, pp. 1823–1832.

Taler, V. and Phillips, N.A. (2008), "Language performance in Alzheimer's disease and mild cognitive impairment: A comparative review", *Journal of Clinical and Experimental Neuropsychology*, Vol. 30, pp. 501–556.

Van Deerlin, V.M., Wood, E.M., Moore, P., Yuan, W., Forman, M.S., Clark, C.M., et al., (2007), "Clinical, genetic, and pathologic characteristics of patients with frontotemporal dementia and progranulin mutations", *Archives of Neurology*, Vol. 64, pp. 1148–1153.

Verma, M. and Howard, R.J. (2012), "Semantic memory and language dysfunction in early Alzheimer's disease: A review", *International Journal of Geriatric Psychiatry*, Vol. 27, pp. 1209–1217.

Warrington, E.K. (1975), "The selective impairment of semantic memory", *Quarterly Journal of Experimental Psychology*, Vol. 27, pp. 635–657.

Waters, G.S., Rochon, E. and Caplan, D. (1998), "Task demands and sentence comprehension in patients with dementia of the Alzheimer's type", *Brain and Language*, Vol. 62, pp. 361–397.

Wilson, S.M., Henry, M.L., Besbris, M., Ogar, J.M., Dronkers, N.F., Jarrold, W., et al., (2010), "Connected speech production in three variants of primary progressive aphasia", *Brain*, Vol. 133, pp. 2069–2088.

25

WORD RETRIEVAL IMPAIRMENT IN ADULT APHASIA

Myrna F. Schwartz, Erica L. Middleton and Roy Hamilton

For speech to be fluent and informative, words must be retrieved in a timely and accurate manner. Aphasia compromises the retrieval of known words in speech and naming, manifesting in lengthy pauses, word-finding struggle and/or speech errors (i.e., paraphasias) which involve substitution of the wrong word or the wrong phonological segments.

The present chapter discusses word retrieval impairment primarily as it relates to the confrontation naming of objects. Naming is the canonical paradigm used to study word retrieval, and there is a large research literature devoted to naming in typical speakers and people with aphasia (PWA). This chapter provides a selective discussion of that literature. The first section describes theoretical approaches to understanding the cognitive architecture of word retrieval and the stages and processes that can go awry in aphasia. Subsequent sections discuss learning models of naming treatment and the emerging science of neuromodulation.

Cognitive processing models of word retrieval

Most of us have experienced the "tip of the tongue" (TOT) state, wherein we have the target word clearly in mind, can describe its meaning, yet are momentarily unable to produce the word's complete phonological form. TOT provides intuitive evidence that the meanings of words are stored and retrieved separately from their phonological form.

This intuition is formalized in cognitive processing models that postulate a mental lexicon with two (or more) levels of representation—one level populated with semantically and syntactically specified words, the other with units of phonological form. The generic box-and-arrow model in Figure 25.1 shows how such a multi-level lexicon might be accessed for naming and other word-processing tasks. Lexical access in naming is deemed a two-step process. The first step involves selection of the semantic-syntactic "word" that best matches the target concept. The second step takes the word as input and outputs the corresponding phonological form units. TOT reflects the state where one has retrieved the target word but has only partial access to its phonology (e.g., number of syllables or initial sound) or no access at all. Errors at Step 1 generate word substitutions, typically one bearing a semantic relation to the target (e.g., cat named as "dog"). Errors at Step 2 yield phonologically-related nonwords or words (e.g., cat named as "dat" or "mat").

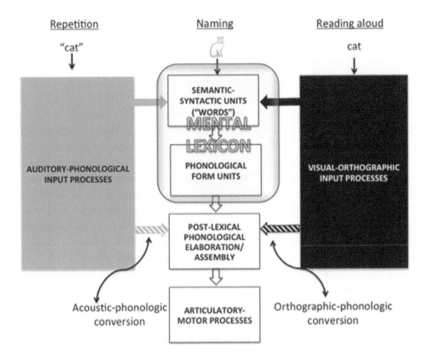

Figure 25.1 A generic account of the functional architecture of picture naming (center path), word repetition (left) and reading aloud (right). Omitted from the naming path are the visual and semantic components that derive the concept from the picture and input it to the lexicon.

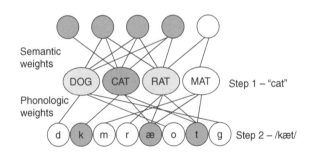

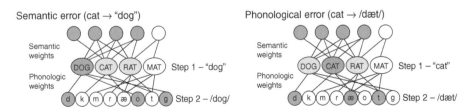

Figure 25.2 Interactive two-step model showing outputs of Step 1 and Step 2 where the target is cat, and the response is correct (top), a semantic error (lower left) and a phonological error (lower right). Shading of units denotes their relative activation strength.

Gary Dell and colleagues developed a two-step model of naming that, when run on the computer, was able to simulate with close precision the individual naming response patterns (proportion of correct responses and five types of naming errors) of large and diverse groups of PWA (Foygel and Dell, 2000; Schwartz *et al.*, 2006). This "interactive two-step model" is shown in Figure 25.2. It features a three-level network of nodes in which those in the middle level stand in one-to-one relation to known words, those above it correspond to semantic features, and those below it to position-specified phonemes (e.g., onset /k/; coda /t/). To formulate a concept is to activate a set of semantic features (e.g., for the concept feline, the features animal, small, pet-like, whiskers). The interconnections between those features and the word node, *cat*, constitutes the lexical-semantic representation. The interconnections between the word *cat* and the phonemes /k//æ//t/ constitute the lexical-phonological representation. Response patterns in aphasia are simulated by weakening the lexical-semantic interconnections (s-weights) or the lexical-phonological interconnections (p-weights) or both. Such connectionist lesions compromise the efficiency of activation spreading, making it more likely that the wrong word will be selected during Step 1, or the wrong phoneme(s) during Step 2. As discussed in Schwartz *et al.* (2006), a strength of this model, and an important reason for its success in fitting error data, is that it allows lesions to impact lexical-semantic and lexical-phonological access independently, thereby providing a natural explanation for why some PWA make more semantic than phonemic errors, while others do the reverse (see Nadeau chapter, this volume, for an alternate model).

The interactive two-step model, like all models, simplifies the true state of affairs. For one thing, the model assumes that semantic errors in naming always derive from weak interconnections between semantic and word representations, where the representation themselves are intact. This assumption is contradicted by evidence that some PWA are prone to semantic errors by virtue of problems with semantic processing *per se* (Hillis *et al.*, 1990). The hallmark of such "core semantic" deficits is that their impact is multi-modal, including semantic errors in both comprehension and production (Jefferies and Lambon Ralph, 2006). In contrast, lesions to s-weights promote semantic errors in production but not necessarily comprehension. A complete account of semantic errors in aphasic naming must acknowledge causal origins within both loci: semantic and lexical-semantic (e.g., Rapp and Goldrick, 2000).

Phonological naming errors also are likely to arise from multiple causes. Figure 25.1 illustrates that phonological information retrieved from the lexicon is operated on by post-lexical-phonological processes that elaborate and/or assemble the sublexical output. Goldrick and Rapp (2007) along with many others consider such post-lexical-phonological processes to be another locus for phonological error production in aphasia, i.e., apart from impaired lexical-phonological retrieval. This idea figures importantly in research on phonological deficits impacting word repetition and word naming (i.e., reading aloud). The fact that healthy adults can effortlessly repeat and read aloud nonwords indicates that, for these tasks, unlike naming, a non-lexical route to production is available. On the other hand, as with naming, performance on these tasks is affected by the lexical and semantic properties of targets (e.g., lexical frequency), indicating the contribution of a lexical route. Figure 25.1 shows a possible configuration of the dual routes in repetition and reading. It can be seen that a lesion affecting lexical retrieval will compromise the lexical route to pronunciation, potentially sparing the non-lexical route. This benefits repetition and reading over naming, for which no non-lexical route exists. On the other hand, the post-lexical-phonological component is a common pathway to articulation for naming, repetition and reading alike, so a lesion here is expected to compromise phonological production similarly on all three tasks (Caplan *et al.*, 1986).

Model-based diagnosis and treatment

Cognitive models of aphasic word retrieval have produced useful diagnostics for determining the locus of the impairment in a PWA. For example, the status of semantic and phonological retrieval can be determined from the profile of different error types in naming. The distribution of semantic errors in naming versus comprehension can indicate whether the deficit resides within semantics or in the lexicon. Comparison of phonological errors across word production tasks can help distinguish a lexical- from a post-lexical-phonological deficit. To enable clinicians to apply such diagnostics, a number of theory-inspired cognitive assessments are available (e.g., Kay *et al.*, 1992). Such tools can be useful for planning treatment programs, on the reasonable assumption that different types of word retrieval impairments call for individualized treatment approaches (Nickels, 2002).

For example, a common method for treating word retrieval is hierarchical cueing, in which the PWA is supplied with phonologic and/or orthographic cues of progressive strength to encourage successful retrieval and production of the name of pictured targets. From the cognitive perspective, one might be particularly inclined to use the cueing approach with PWA who are prone to phonological errors and/or TOT states in naming, and whose post-lexical-phonological encoding is not so impaired that production cannot be successfully cued. On the other hand, with an individual whose naming impairment implicates the semantic system or lexical-semantic retrieval, one might be more inclined to use an approach aimed at strengthening semantic processing (e.g., semantic feature analysis: Boyle, 2010) and/or the semantics-to-words association (e.g., word-to-picture matching).

Small-scale treatment research has investigated the aforementioned phonological and semantic treatments. All have been shown to produce lasting gains on treated items. Generalization to untreated items and/or tasks has been more variable, but results are promising particularly with semantic treatments (Boyle, 2010; Kiran and Bassetto, 2008; see also Best *et al.*, 2013). To date, model-inspired predictions about which type of PWA should benefit from phonological versus semantic treatments have not generally been supported (Lorenz and Ziegler, 2009), though this continues to be an active focus of research (Howard *et al.*, 2006). We are inclined to agree with those who argue that an understanding of who benefits from which treatments and why requires more than a cognitive analysis of the system undergoing treatment; it also requires a model of learning (e.g., Baddeley, 1993).

Learning models of naming treatment

The goal of learning models is to provide a theoretical foundation for clinical decision-making by identifying the properties of a treatment that affect change (i.e., a treatment's "active ingredients"), as well as an understanding of how they do so in a damaged system. Relating a treatment's effects to underlying learning mechanisms is expected to help inform decisions about how to prioritize treatments given a PWA's profile of cognitive and language-based impairment, and how to administer the treatment to maximize its benefits.

A body of research is emerging in response to the need for models of learning to inform neuropsychological treatment. Most relevant to naming treatment in aphasia are two distinct literatures—*errorless learning* and *retrieval practice effects*—that advocate the prioritization of qualitatively different kinds of learning experiences.

Errorless learning

The impetus for the errorless learning (EL) approach is the possibility that naming errors committed by PWA during treatment can be learned, strengthening errors or faulty access procedures. For example, recent research indicates that the dysfunctional retrieval state reflected in TOT can be learned in PWA with naming impairment (Middleton and Schwartz, 2013). The standard form of EL naming treatment involves presenting the object name simultaneously with the depicted object and the patient repeating the name. Commensurate with Hebbian theory (often summarized as "cells that fire together, wire together"), EL treatment may be desirable because it preempts an attempt at retrieving the name (thus avoiding error), and instead only strengthens the association between the correct name and the depicted object (for discussion, see Fillingham *et al.*, 2003).

A number of studies have compared the efficacy of standard EL naming treatment in aphasia with *errorful* (EF) treatments (where naming attempts are permitted and hence, errors are possible) by measuring performance on items given EL or EF naming treatment. For example, in a series of single-subject controlled comparisons, Fillingham *et al.* (2005a; 2005b; 2006) compared standard EL treatment to EF training where phonological cueing (e.g., first letter/ first sound of the target name) was provided to facilitate naming. The general finding across studies was that both EL and EF methods lead to post-therapy gains for most PWA, with neither method emerging as consistently superior. Individual differences analyses showed that PWA who benefitted most from naming therapy were those who performed better on measures of memory, executive function, and monitoring of their own errors. Interestingly, the same factors were predictive of greater benefit from EF relative to EL treatment (Fillingham *et al.*, 2006), suggesting that intact attentional-executive functions and memory abilities may be important for modulating error learning.

McKissock and Ward (2007) also compared EL treatment to EF treatment involving naming without cueing but manipulated whether feedback regarding accuracy, which included provision of the correct name for repetition, was provided. They found no benefit from EF treatment when feedback was withheld, whereas both EL and EF treatment with feedback improved naming for all participants. Compared to EF treatment with feedback, group analyses revealed superior performance in the EL condition immediately post-treatment but not after a three-month delay. To summarize, this literature suggests that both EL and EF forms of treatment are effective for ameliorating naming impairment in aphasia but that feedback may be important to increase EF treatment efficacy.

Retrieval practice

Substantial research has shown retrieval practice (RP) powerfully bolsters learning, particularly when RP is effortful (for a review, see Roediger and Karpicke, 2006). Empirical demonstrations of this effect typically start with initial study of target information followed by an opportunity to recall the information from long-term memory (RP condition) or restudy for an equivalent amount of time (restudy condition). The benefits from RP are demonstrated when the RP condition outperforms the restudy condition on subsequent measures of performance. Remarkably, far superior performance can emerge in the RP condition even though it is at a marked disadvantage in terms of the amount of exposure to target information, demonstrating the power of RP for learning. Standard EL naming treatment, where attempts to retrieve target names from long-term memory are avoided, may be limited in its efficacy because it eschews the potent learning experience of RP.

Important to note, RP has primarily been studied as it relates to learning new concepts, associations, or skills. However, RP is likely relevant to naming rehabilitation because difficulty accessing language-based representations is a common locus of naming impairment in aphasia; and, studies suggest that RP is particularly beneficial for bolstering the associative strength between representations (e.g., Vaughn and Rawson, 2011). Indeed, a recent study has confirmed that RP beneficially impacts naming performance in PWA with mild-to-moderate naming impairment (Middleton *et al.*, 2014). This study involved first presenting depicted objects along with their names to prime the name in long-term memory. After a delay, each item was given one trial of either EL treatment (repetition, where the name was seen/heard at picture onset and repeated) or RP treatment involving either *cued naming* (the name's first sound/letter was presented to facilitate picture naming) or *non-cued naming* (only the picture was presented). *Feedback* was provided at the end of each trial, where the name was provided (seen/heard) for repetition. Similar to prior work, production of target names during training was nearly perfect in the EL condition, and significantly less so in the RP conditions. However, a naming test administered after a one-day delay revealed superior performance in the RP conditions relative to the EL condition, an effect that persisted after one week in the cued naming condition. This result is impressive in that the advantage was obtained with only one training trial per item; and, during training, there was greater exposure to (and production of) the target name in the EL versus RP conditions.

An important and understudied topic concerns how treatment should be scheduled. A fundamental property of RP is that its effects are maximized when retrieval is difficult, but successful, and effort during retrieval is increased when retrieval attempts for an item are distributed (i.e., spaced) over time (e.g., providing a RP opportunity for an item once per session for multiple sessions, rather than providing all RP opportunities for an item within one session). In fact, a broad range of motor and verbal learning experiences (not simply those that involve RP) benefit from spacing. This fact offers a unique perspective on growing interest in treatment *intensity*; work that seeks to delineate the most effective amount and schedule of language therapy. A model of learning based on RP principles would contend that, holding the number and length of treatment sessions constant, administering sessions over several months instead of weeks should be preferred for greater efficacy (for evidence, see Sage *et al.*, 2011).

In summary, learning approaches to rehabilitation strive to elucidate the mechanisms of change that drive various treatments' effects, an important first step in understanding how to design and prioritize treatments. However, each of the learning approaches discussed here has limitations. EL treatment may be limited in its long-term potency because of failure to incorporate opportunities for effortful RP. In turn, research on the application of RP principles to naming impairment is still in its infancy with many unknowns such as how RP principles apply when interventions are administered at a scale approximating conventional speech–language treatments; and, how the effectiveness of RP versus EL treatment and schedule of administration relates to a patient's profile of cognitive–linguistic deficits and personality traits. An exciting possibility is that the field may witness hybridization of the two techniques, where EL training is used early in treatment to achieve a certain initial level of mastery followed by transition to a spaced schedule of RP.

Neuromodulation and naming treatment

As advances in cognitive neuroscience continue to expand our understanding of the neural basis of aphasia and language recovery, the development of neuromodulation technologies, such as transcranial magnetic stimulation (TMS) and transcranial direct current stimulation (tDCS), offer an exciting approach for enhancing recovery in PWA. Evidence suggests that the therapeutic effects of TMS and tDCS are due to their ability to induce beneficial functional changes in the networks that represent language in PWA. Neuroimaging studies indicate that during language tasks, PWA often exhibit increased activity of perilesional left hemisphere areas, as well as regions of the right hemisphere that are homotopic (correspond topographically and anatomically) to left hemisphere language areas (Turkeltaub *et al.*, 2011). Although there is agreement that left hemisphere perilesional activation is likely compensatory with respect to language recovery (Karbe *et al.*, 1998), the role of the right hemisphere remains controversial. One idea is that homotopic right hemisphere areas play a beneficial role (Rosen *et al.*, 2000), while a second hypothesis is that increased right hemisphere activation interferes with aphasia recovery by exerting a transcallosal inhibitory effect on left hemisphere language areas (Crosson *et al.*, 2007).A third notion is that the right hemisphere, while part of a compensatory language network, may have inefficient or "noisy" components (Turkeltaub *et al.*, 2012).

These theories have led to different treatment approaches for PWA using brain stimulation. As we will review below, some studies have focused solely on exciting left hemisphere perilesional areas to facilitate recovery. Others have attempted to increase neural activity in the right hemisphere in an attempt to enhance function in a presumed network of compensatory right hemisphere language areas. Finally, several other investigations have focused on suppressing brain activity in the right hemisphere, based on the notion that its contribution to language recovery may be either inefficient or deleterious.

Brain stimulation techniques

TMS employs a strong electrical current that passes through a coil of wires held above the scalp in order to create a brief time-varying magnetic field, which penetrates the scalp, skull, and meninges unimpeded. This induces an electrical current in underlying cortical neurons that is sufficient to depolarize neuronal membranes and generate action potentials (Rossi *et al.*, 2009). Pulses of TMS can be delivered in a variety of patterns to elicit different effects on cortical activity. Repetitive runs of TMS (rTMS) are used frequently in both cognitive neuroscience and neurorehabilitation research, in part because their effects have been shown to persist at least temporarily after the discontinuation of stimulation. Low frequency rTMS (< 5 Hertz [Hz]) has been associated with decreased cortical excitability following stimulation, whereas high frequency rTMS (≥ 5 Hz) can enhance excitability (Hallett, 2007). In patient populations, persistent changes in performance have been observed after repeated sessions of rTMS (e.g. Naeser *et al.*, 2005), and it is believed that these enduring behavioral changes are likely related to neurophysiologic mechanisms of plasticity, such as long-term potentiation (LTP) and long-term depression (LTD; Chen and Udupa, 2009).

The tDCS procedure is administered by delivering small electrical currents (1–2 milliamperes [mA]) to the scalp using a battery-driven device connected to two surface electrodes (often 5 × 7 cm² or 5 × 5 cm²) soaked in isotonic saline (Nitsche and Paulus, 2000). The electrode that is used to target the brain region to be stimulated is considered the "active" electrode; the other electrode is termed the "reference" or "return" electrode. Currents delivered during tDCS are insufficient to generate action potentials, and instead are believed to incrementally alter neuronal resting membrane potentials. Like TMS, tDCS can alter cortical excitability in predictable ways; anodal tDCS (a-tDCS) is believed to increase cortical excitability while cathodal tDCS (c-tDCS) is thought to decrease cortical excitability (Nitsche and Paulus, 2000). Like TMS, repeated sessions of tDCS show persistent effects on behavior, thought to be related to LTP-like or LTD-like neuroplastic changes (Fritsch *et al.*, 2010).

Neuromodulation treatment results

Many studies involving rTMS in PWA have been predicated on the notion that right hemisphere activity is either inefficient or deleterious to language performance, and have therefore involved inhibitory stimulation of right-sided homologues of left hemisphere language areas. For example, in an influential early investigation, Naeser and colleagues (2005) applied 1 Hz rTMS to the right pars triangularis (homologue of a part of Broca's area) of individuals with chronic non-fluent aphasia. After ten days of stimulation, participants demonstrated improvement in multiple measures of picture naming that persisted for two months, with some benefits persisting for at least eight months. Several other studies have confirmed that repeated inhibition of the right pars triangularis is associated with long-term improvements in naming, spontaneous elicited speech and, less commonly, other language abilities (see Shah *et al.*, 2013 for a recent review). A similar TMS approach appears beneficial in PWA in the subacute phase (e.g. Weiduschat *et al.*, 2011). Moreover, excitatory high frequency rTMS of Broca's area in the left hemisphere has also been associated with improved language performance and a leftward shift of fMRI activity during language tasks (Szaflarski *et al.*, 2011). Low frequency rTMS of the right hemisphere has been employed more often than high frequency rTMS of the damaged left hemisphere, in part to minimize seizure concerns, although seizures have not yet been observed with either approach.

Mounting evidence indicates that tDCS can also enhance recovery in PWA. Monti and colleagues were the first to pair tDCS with speech therapy in patients with chronic aphasia (2008). They found that cathodal left hemisphere stimulation induced transient improvement in naming accuracy and speculated that this may have been due to inhibition of intrahemispheric inhibitory connections within the left hemisphere. By contrast, subsequent studies have shown improvement in naming after anodal left hemisphere stimulation in persons with both fluent and non-fluent aphasia (Shah *et al.*, 2013), while other studies have shown improved language outcomes after inhibitory cathodal stimulation of the right hemisphere (Kang *et al.*, 2011). As with TMS, the benefits of tDCS seem to persist for months following stimulation (Marangolo *et al.*, 2013).

Most investigators have focused on naming ability as the main indicator of treatment efficacy. Some studies have examined other abilities, such as auditory comprehension or repetition, but few have explored how brain stimulation alters the cognitive processes that support language (Medina *et al.*, 2012). Future investigations could produce richer insights by elucidating whether stimulation enhances word retrieval by facilitating access to semantic or lexical representations (or both). Furthermore, as converging evidence in the fields of neurorehabilitation and neuromodulation suggest, the combination of brain stimulation and behavioral rehabilitation is more effective than either in isolation. It will be important in future research to delineate how best to pair the two to modulate learning and optimize recovery of word retrieval impairment in PWA.

Conclusions

The theoretical analysis of aphasia rehabilitation aims to explain how and why rehabilitation works. Towards this aim, research contributes information on each of the many different variables underlying the therapeutic process. Research guided by cognitive models of word retrieval informs our understanding of one variable—*the nature of the impairment*. Research applying principles of learning, such as RP, spaced retrieval, and error learning elucidates *how treatment promotes (or retards) change in the language system*. Finally, studies that use TMS and tDCS in the treatment of word retrieval address the *nature and malleability of neurophysiological recovery*. Although it may be naïve to expect that these distinct research paths will converge any time soon, it is important to maintain this as a future goal and look for possible points of contact wherever they may present.

References

Baddeley, A. (1993), "A theory of rehabilitation without a model of learning is a vehicle without an engine: A comment on Caramazza and Hillis", *Neuropsychological Rehabilitation*, Vol. 3, No. 3, pp. 235–244.

Best, W., Greenwood, A., Grassly, J., Herbert, R., Hickin, J. and Howard, D. (2013), "Aphasia rehabilitation: Does generalisation from anomia therapy occur and is it predictable? A case series study", *Cortex*, Vol. 49, No. 9, pp. 2345–2357.

Boyle, M. (2010), "Semantic feature analysis treatment for aphasic word retrieval: What's in a name?", *Topics in Stroke Rehabilitation*, Vol. 17, No. 6, pp. 411–422.

Caplan, D., Vanier, M. and Baker, E. (1986), "A case study of reproduction conduction aphasia: 1. Word production", *Cognitive Neuropsychology*, Vol. 3, No. 1, pp. 99–128.

Chen, R. and Udupa, K. (2009), "Measurement and modulation of plasticity of the motor system in humans using transcranial magnetic stimulation", *Motor Control*, Vol. 13, No. 4, pp. 442–453.

Crosson, B., McGregor, K., Gopinath, K.S., Conway, T.W., Benjamin, M., Chang, Y.L., *et al.*, (2007), "Functional MRI of language in aphasia: A review of the literature and the methodological challenges", *Neuropsychology Review*, Vol. 17, No. 2, pp. 157–177.

Fillingham, J.K., Hodgson, C., Sage, K. and Lambon Ralph, M.A. (2003), "The application of errorless learning to aphasic disorders: A review of theory and practice", *Neuropsychological Rehabilitation*, Vol. 13, No. 3, pp. 337–363.

Fillingham, J.K., Sage, K. and Lambon Ralph, M.A. (2005a), "Treatment of anomia using errorless versus errorful learning: Are frontal executive skills and feedback important?", *International Journal of Language and Communication Disorders*, Vol. 40, No. 4, pp. 505–523.

Fillingham, J.K., Sage, K. and Lambon Ralph, M.A. (2005b), "Further explorations and an overview of errorless and errorful therapy for aphasic word-finding difficulties: The number of naming attempts during therapy affects outcome", *Aphasiology*, Vol. 19, No. 7, pp. 597–614.

Fillingham, J.K., Sage, K. and Lambon Ralph, M.A. (2006), "The treatment of anomia using errorless learning", *Neuropsychological Rehabilitation*, Vol. 16, No. 2, pp. 129–154.

Foygel, D. and Dell, G.S. (2000), "Models of impaired lexical access in speech production", *Journal of Memory and Language*, Vol. 43, No. 2, pp. 182–216.

Fritsch, B., Reis, J., Martinowich, K., Schambra, H.M., Ji, Y., Cohen, L.G. and Lu, B. (2010), "Direct current stimulation promotes BDNF-dependent synaptic plasticity: Potential implications for motor learning", *Neuron*, Vol. 66, No. 2, pp. 198–204.

Goldrick, M. and Rapp, B. (2007), "Lexical and post-lexical phonological representations in spoken production", *Cognition*, Vol. 102, No. 2, pp. 219–260.

Hallett, M. (2007), "Transcranial magnetic stimulation: A primer", *Neuron*, Vol. 55, No. 2, pp. 187–199.

Hillis, A.E., Rapp, B.C., Romani, D. and Caramazza, A. (1990), "Selective impairment of semantics in lexical processing", *Cognitive Neuropsychology*, Vol. 7, No. 3, pp. 191–243.

Howard, D., Hickin, J., Redmond, T., Clark, P. and Best, W. (2006), "Re-visiting 'semantic facilitation' of word retrieval for people with aphasia: Facilitation yes but semantic no", *Cortex*, Vol. 42, No. 6, pp. 946–962.

Jefferies, E. and Lambon Ralph, M.A. (2006), "Semantic impairment in stroke aphasia versus semantic dementia: A case-series comparison", *Brain*, Vol. 129, pp. 2132–2147.

Kang, E.K., Kim, Y.K., Sohn, H.M., Cohen, L.G. and Paik, N.J. (2011), "Improved picture naming in aphasia patients treated with cathodal tDCS to inhibit the right Broca's homologue area", *Restorative Neurology and Neuroscience*, Vol. 29, No. 3, pp. 141–152.

Karbe, H., Thiel, A. and Weber-Luxenburger, G. (1998), "Reorganization of the cerebral cortex in post-stroke aphasia studied with positron emission tomography", *Neurology*, Vol. 50, p. A321.

Kay, J., Lesser, R. and Coltheart, M. (1992), *PALPA: Psycholinguistic Assessment of Language Processing in Aphasia*, Lawrence Erlbaum Associates Ltd., Hove, UK.

Kiran, S. and Bassetto, G. (2008), "Evaluating the effectiveness of semantic-based treatment for naming deficits in aphasia: What works?", *Seminars in Speech and Language*, Vol. 29, No. 1, pp. 71–82.

Lorenz, A. and Ziegler, W. (2009), "Semantic vs. word-form specific techniques in anomia treatment: A multiple single-case study", *Journal of Neurolinguistics*, Vol. 22, No. 6, pp. 515–537.

Marangolo, P., Fiori, V., Calpagnano, M., Campana, S., Razzano, C., Caltagirone, C. and Marini, A. (2013), "tDCS over the left inferior frontal cortex improves speech production in aphasia", *Frontiers in Human Neuroscience*, Vol. 7, p. 539.

McKissock, S. and Ward, J. (2007), "Do errors matter? Errorless and errorful learning in anomic picture naming", *Neuropsychological Rehabilitation*, Vol. 17, No. 3, pp. 355–373.

Medina, J., Norise, C., Faseyitan, O., Coslett, H.B., Turkeltaub, P.E. and Hamilton, R.H. (2012), "Finding the right words: Transcranial magnetic stimulation improves discourse productivity in non-fluent aphasia after stroke", *Aphasiology*, Vol. 26, No. 9, pp. 1153–1168.

Middleton, E.L. and Schwartz, M.F. (2013), "Learning to fail in aphasia: An investigation of error learning in naming", *Journal of Speech, Language, and Hearing Research*, Vol. 56, No. 4, pp. 1287–1297.

Middleton, E.L., Schwartz, M.F., Rawson, K.A., and Garvey, K. (2014, December 22), "Test-enhanced learning versus errorless learning in aphasia rehabilitation: Testing competing psychological principles", *Journal of Experimental Psychology: Learning, Memory, and Cognition*. Advance online publication. http://dx.doi.org/10.1037/xlm0000091.

Monti, A., Cogiamanian, F., Marceglia, S., Ferrucci, R., Mameli, F., Mrakic-Sposta, S., et al., (2008), "Improved naming after transcranial direct current stimulation in aphasia", *Journal of Neurology, Neurosurgery and Psychiatry*, Vol. 79, No. 4, pp. 451–453.

Naeser, M.A., Martin, P.I., Nicholas, M., Baker, E.H., Seekins, H., Kobayashi, M., et al., (2005), "Improved picture naming in chronic aphasia after TMS to part of right Broca's area: An open-protocol study", *Brain and Language*, Vol. 93, No. 1, pp. 95–105.

Nickels, L. (2002), "Therapy for naming disorders: Revisiting, revising, and reviewing", *Aphasiology*, Vol. 16, No. 10/11, pp. 935–979.

Nitsche, M.A. and Paulus, W. (2000), "Excitability changes induced in the human motor cortex by weak transcranial direct current stimulation", *Journal of Physiology*, Vol. 527, No. 3, pp. 633–639.

Rapp, B. and Goldrick, M. (2000), "Discreteness and interactivity in spoken word production", *Psychological Review*, Vol. 107, No. 3, pp. 460–499.

Roediger, H.L. and Karpicke, J.D. (2006), "The power of testing memory: Basic research and implications for educational practice", *Perspectives on Psychological Science*, Vol. 1, No. 3, pp. 181–210.

Rosen, H.J., Petersen, S.E., Linenweber, M.R., Snyder, A.Z., White, D.A., Chapman, L., et al., (2000), "Neural correlates of recovery from aphasia after damage to left inferior frontal cortex", *Neurology*, Vol. 55, No. 12, pp. 1883–1894.

Rossi, S., Hallett, M., Rossini, P.M. and Pascual-Leone, A. (2009), "Safety, ethical considerations, and application guidelines for the use of transcranial magnetic stimulation in clinical practice and research", *Journal of Clinical Neurophysiology*, Vol. 120, No. 12, pp. 2008–2039.

Sage, K., Snell, C. and Ralph, M.A.L. (2011), "How intensive does anomia therapy for people with aphasia need to be?", *Neuropsychological Rehabilitation*, Vol. 21, No. 1, pp. 26–41.

Schwartz, M.F., Dell, G.S., Martin, N., Gahl, S. and Sobel, P. (2006), "A case-series test of the interactive two-step model of lexical access: Evidence from picture naming", *Journal of Memory and Language*, Vol. 54, No. 2, pp. 228–264.

Shah, P.P., Szaflarski, J.P., Allendorfer, J. and Hamilton, R.H. (2013), "Induction of neuroplasticity and recovery in post-stroke aphasia by non-invasive brain stimulation", *Frontiers in Human Neuroscience*, Vol. 7, p. 888.

Szaflarski, J.P., Vannest, J., Wu, S.W., DiFrancesco, M.W., Banks, C. and Gilbert, D.L. (2011), "Excitatory repetitive transcranial magnetic stimulation induces improvements in chronic post-stroke aphasia", *Medical Science Monitor*, Vol. 17, No. 3, pp. CR132–139.

Turkeltaub, P.E., Messing, S., Norise, C. and Hamilton, R.H. (2011), "Are networks for residual language function and recovery consistent across aphasic patients?", *Neurology*, Vol. 76, No. 20, pp. 1726–1734.

Turkeltaub, P.E., Coslett, H.B., Thomas, A.L., Faseyitan, O., Benson, J., Norise, C. and Hamilton, R.H. (2012), "The right hemisphere is not unitary in its role in aphasia recovery", *Cortex*, Vol. 48, No. 9, pp. 1179–1186.

Vaughn, K.E. and Rawson, K.A. (2011), "Diagnosing criterion-level effects on memory: What aspects of memory are enhanced by repeated retrieval?", *Psychological Science*, Vol. 22, No. 9, pp. 1127–1131.

Weiduschat, N., Thiel, A., Rubi-Fessen, I., Hartmann, A., Kessler, J., Merl, P., et al., (2011), "Effects of repetitive transcranial magnetic stimulation in aphasic stroke: A randomized controlled pilot study", *Stroke*, Vol. 42, No. 2, pp. 409–415.

SECTION IV

Social interactional systems of communication impairments

26

TWO CHALLENGES OF THE ACADEMIC LANGUAGE REGISTER FOR STUDENTS WITH LANGUAGE LEARNING DISABILITIES

Elaine R. Silliman and Louise C. Wilkinson

The academic language register is the "major gatekeeper" (Bailey, 2010, p. 229) through which language and literacy knowledge and skills evolve, providing access to and membership in the greater community of "educated" persons (Silliman and Wilkinson, 2014). Furthermore, from a global perspective less instructional emphasis on the multiple dimensions of the academic language register may be a major reason why US students perform below other nations in mathematics, science, and literacy domains (Hanushek *et al.*, 2014). If this is the case for typically developing students, then this problem is doubly compounded for students with language learning disabilities (LLD) partially because "language knowledge does not 'stick'" (Bishop, 2009, p. 164) in many students with LLD in spite of repeated experience.

The overarching perspective of this chapter, based on Vygotsky's social constructivist theory, is that speaking, listening, reading, and writing are interconnected because they are communicative processes (Wilkinson and Silliman, 2000). What is learned about language, how it is used, and how it changes over time is indivisible from the patterns that students identify and internalize through recurrent, but varied, engagements with their social and linguistic worlds (Beckner *et al.*, 2009; Silliman and Mody, 2008) that extend from family interactions through peer relationships to educational and learner memberships. An assumption therefore is that patterns of engagement also contribute to individual differences in that the scope and variety of experiences, including academic language experiences, differ within family, peer, and educational interactions (Cummins, 2014).

Chapter organization consists of four sections. We first present the key concepts and features of the academic language register. The second section focuses on the academic language register at the macrostructure or discourse level describing challenges for students with LLD, which expository text often presents. The third section details another set of challenges at the microstructure level – the lexical and syntactic features characteristic of the mathematics and science registers – that can block access to learning and engagement for students with LLD. We conclude with the outlines of a new practice model that has potential to bridge the research–practice gap in disciplinary literacy for students with LLD.

Defining the academic language register

Broadly, the academic language register is "the specialized language, both oral and written, of academic settings that facilitates communication and thinking about disciplinary content" (Nagy and Townsend, 2012, p. 92) irrespective of whether this content occurs in educational settings or other mediums that communicate disciplinary ideas (including print publications and digital media). For textbooks, this means that informational density is a main characteristic: a higher proportion of content words and complex clauses are packed into the text than appear in everyday talk. Increased density results in messages conveyed through linguistic layers; that is, "the informational load is in fact even greater than the sum of the individual parts" (Wong Fillmore and Fillmore, 2012, p. 4). Moreover, command of academic language is essential for processing disciplinary content (Cummins, 2013) and for developing the confidence to assume an academic identity (Zwiers and Crawford, 2011).

Interdependence of the everyday and academic language registers

Academic language is comprised of varying text types, subject-specific vocabulary and definitions as well as complex clausal and phrasal constructions and connectives (e.g., *in contrast, otherwise, as a consequence*) (Nippold, 2007; Schleppegrell *et al.*, 2004). Figure 26.1 presents our visualization of this concept. Although there are cross-content, lexical items that are central to teaching and learning, such as *relationship* and *hypothesis*, mastery of academic language is quite content-specific.

Understanding the components of the academic language register relies on considering the interrelationships represented as a continuum in Figure 26.1 (Snow and Uccelli, 2009), beginning in the preschool years and advancing through the high school years and beyond (Berman and Nir, 2010). The roots of academic language knowledge originate in the *everyday language register* of first language acquisition. This register is a description of primary language abilities that reflect face-to-face conversation in family, community, and cultural contexts;

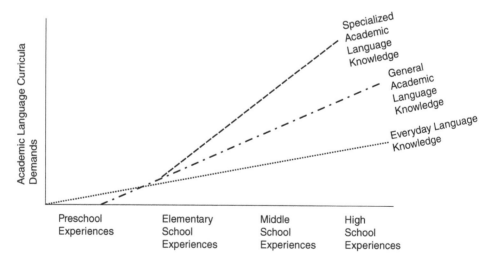

Figure 26.1 A continuum of academic language curricula demands across the school years. Although agreement exists about the three types of language knowledge that comprise the continuum, little is known about the reciprocal influences of general and specialized academic language on more complex development of everyday language.

hence, the attitude (discourse stance) expressed is intended to create and consolidate interpersonal connections (Ravid and Berman, 2006). With sufficient practice, for example, through repeated experiences with shared book reading and longer discourse interactions in the preschool years, the *general academic language register* then germinates and progressively matures. This new knowledge source, which represents more objective discourse attitudes, consists of the overall linguistic and discourse tools necessary to manage reasoning, reading, and writing across disciplinary content areas, such as recognizing and generating various types of expository text, following themes, and decomposing word parts into their roots and affixes (Uccelli *et al.*, in press). *Specialized language registers* for each disciplinary area then develop, starting in early elementary experiences with disciplinary content. Depending on the degree and nature of engagement, the ultimate scope of the specialized registers can enlarge or become smaller (Zwiers, 2008). Unresolved, however, is which aspects of the everyday language register are prognostic of particular academic language skills (Snow and Uccelli, 2009) or even how and in what ways academic language skills in both the oral and print domains influence a more sophisticated everyday language register.

The notion of academic languages

The phrase "academic language" is a misnomer to some extent as there are differing academic languages. Each discipline has their own linguistic and discourse repertoires or their own ways of cultivating "reading, writing, speaking, thinking, and reason" (Fang *et al.*, 2014, p. 302) that students must master, much as encountering a new foreign language. Hence, academic language repertoires will vary as a function of the discipline, topic, and mode of communication (oral or written) (Snow, 2010). The distinctiveness of the academic discourses relates to their shared lexical and syntactic features, including (Snow, 2010): 1) Increased conciseness in word selection to avoid redundancy; 2) a higher frequency of informational words as the means to achieve more concise expression; and 3) syntactic processes that embed complex ideas into fewer words. The result is the co-existence of greater linguistic informativeness with increased complexity.

Academic language development has not been explicitly studied in students with LLD, an odd oversight since "the kinds of knowledge or skills that need to be acquired" (Seidenberg, 2013, p. 345) do not substantively differ from typically developing students. Given the absence of information, one speculation is that students with LLD likely have a less well developed everyday (oral) language register. Underdevelopment can then result in less robust general academic language knowledge, which presents at least two challenges for students with LLD. One challenge encompasses knowledge of organizational variations, or the macrostructures, of expository texts, while the second obstacle focuses on the linguistic, or microstructure, level, particularly the features of lexical and syntactic density in content languages, such as mathematics and science.

The macrostructure level: Expository text organization

Expository (discourse) text, whether oral or written, has received little attention until recently in the LLD literature (Nippold, 2010), unlike narrative text. Whereas narrative texts are action-oriented, stress intentionality, are evaluative, and have a chronological structure usually expressed through a three-part organization (beginning, middle, and end) (Westby, 2005), the macrostructure of expository texts differs in three critical ways. Dissimilarities include (Berman and Nir, 2010; Ravid *et al.*, 2010): 1) a focus on new ideas, opinions, or claims with themes that are not action-oriented or linked to a specific temporal period; 2) an interface between lexical and syntactic complexity; and 3) a more detached discourse stance towards the content being expressed. Moreover, expository texts have a more variable organization even within the same paragraph (Mason and Hedin, 2011) as text purposes shift. This factor can present formidable challenges for reading or writing, even for adolescent students who are typically developing (Nippold and Ward-Lonergan, 2010).

Enhanced concentration on the academic language register inherent to expository texts takes on even greater urgency today in the United States as new educational standards, known as the Common Core State Standards (CCSS; Council of Chief State School Officers [CCSSO] and the National Governors Association [NGA] Center for Best Practices, 2010) are being implemented from kindergarten through high school by a majority of states. The CCSS calls for greater student facility with expository texts in the oral, reading, and writing domains.

Illustrations of descriptive and procedural text development

Tables 26.1 and 26.2 present a contrasting illustration of written expository text development. Brief expository compositions are displayed of two females in Grades 2 and 4, one typically developing (J, age 7;5 years; Table 26.1) and the other with a diagnosed LLD (K, age 9;9 years; Table 26.2). J spontaneously composed her ideas about plants on a computer and the resulting organizational pattern is descriptive; it tells about plant characteristics and features and includes examples through the nominal device of elaborated noun phrases (ENPs). ENPs function semantically to define, identify, and attribute (Fang *et al.*, 2014), which not only creates more complex content but also may be a more characteristic feature of complex writing than are subordinated clauses (Biber *et al.*, 2011). Furthermore, J's description is consistent with the objectivity of expository writing (although not entirely – note her insertion of the personal evaluation "I love plants" on the left side).

Table 26.1 Example of a descriptive (expository) science composition by J, a typically developing female, age 7;5, Grade 2 (reproduced verbatim; all designs, punctuation and spellings are unchanged; underlined portions indicate elaborated noun phrases).

PLANTS

- ❑ Plants start as <u>a seed at the end of the life cycle</u> it turns into <u>a kind of plant</u>.
- ❑ All plants need <u>sunlight, water, and carbon dioxide</u> an order to grow.
- ❑ Some insects drink the pollen <u>from the middle of a flower.</u>
- ❑ Some plants grow <u>fruit and vegetables</u>.
- ❑ They have a life cycle <u>just like people</u>.

I love plants

Table 26.2 Example of a procedural (expository) composition by K, a female, age 9;9, Grade 4, with a diagnosed LLD (reproduced verbatim; punctuation and spellings are unchanged; underlined portion indicates an elaborated noun phrase).

The 1st step is to get <u>a piece of bread</u>. You need bread to make it!!

The 2nd step is to put peanut butter on both sides. You need peanut butter!!

The 3rd step is to put jelly on. Also you need jelly!!

Last is you put them together. Then you eat it!

In contrast to J's authentic product, K was assigned a prompt to complete with pencil and paper, *How would you make a peanut butter and jelly sandwich?* This solicited a procedural pattern of text organization (the ordered steps necessary to complete a task). K is obviously still working through the objective stance of expository writing; note her use of the generalized "*you*," which serves to personalize content (Perera, 1984) as well as the exclamations that follow each of the four steps. Unlike J, who linguistically expressed an evaluation, K utilized a non-linguistic means, the addition of punctuation marks.

These two examples are offered to demonstrate the relationship between knowledge about text macrostructures and the academic language register. From a conceptual perspective, it is obvious that J has begun the process of integrating the expression of ideas with the voice of the academic language register through expository writing. Emerging integration is partially premised on children's differentiation of writing as structurally different from talking (Perera, 1984). In contrast, K, who is two years older, has a basic schema for ordering the components of a familiar activity but still communicates that knowledge with the everyday oral language register, at least for the assigned task.

Further expository text barriers for students with LLD

Other expository text barriers affecting instruction have been identified in the reading disabilities literature. These include (Sáenz and Fuchs, 2002): 1) greater conceptual complexity of expository texts in contrast to narrative texts; 2) the specialized vocabulary of the content area academic languages; and 3) prior knowledge about the content or, alternately, underuse of prior knowledge, both of which can affect the ease or difficulty of inferencing. Combined with variable text structures, these obstacles can result in lower quality mental representations, which influence the comprehension (or composing) of expository texts (Fox, 2009). Although vocabulary knowledge plays a role in content learning, instructional studies have seldom considered other linguistic aspects of expository reading or writing in any depth, such as clausal and phrasal complexity.

The same cannot be said about LLD studies. The few investigations that included expository text primarily considered spoken syntactic complexity (as measured by subordinated clauses) across the age spectrum (for a review of these studies, see Nippold, 2010) and, to a lesser extent, adolescents with LLD (Nippold *et al.*, 2008, 2009). A general pattern for adolescents with LLD was that their oral syntactic complexity increased with spoken expository discourse contrasted with conversational tasks. Scott and Windsor (2000) also examined the written syntactic complexity of 20 preadolescent students through a descriptive text structure (summary of a video). In contrast to those of chronological-aged peers (but similar to those of language-aged matched peers), the written expository summaries of the students with LLD had shorter clauses and contained minimal subordination complexity. In one of the few longitudinal investigations that also went beyond syntax, Dockrell *et al.* (2009) administered a variety of oral and print measures from ages 8 to 16 years. They indirectly examined the expository writing performance of students with LLD through the type of writing task employed, e.g., describing their ideal house, an activity that likely involved a descriptive text organization. In contrast to the multi-dimensional gains of the typically developing participants, results for the participants with LLD showed decreasing synchrony over time among idea generation, vocabulary choices, the complexity of sentence production, spelling accuracy, and handwriting fluency.

The paucity of studies on expository text organization of students with LLD is a major gap that, unless addressed, will likely leave many of these students unprepared for vocational success, much less advancement to higher education. A priority is developing more efficacious interconnections among: 1) the developmental needs of these students in the academic languages; 2) their sustained engagement in disciplinary activities in which the understanding of expository text organization is crucial for both reading and writing achievement; and 3) most critically, the creation of instructional contexts that foster greater access to disciplinary literacy while simultaneously establishing a sense of "identity and empowerment" (Cummins, 2014, p. 4). These same instructional contexts must also take into account the microstructure level or interactions between the lexical and syntactic systems.

The microstructure level: The lexical–syntactic interface

As noted earlier, an overriding feature of both systems in the academic language register is their linguistic complexity, a feature that increases the likelihood that students like K will encounter major obstacles in dealing with expository texts in the content domains. Lexical complexity is defined by two general components (Ravid *et al.*, 2010): 1) lexical density, which is the frequency of content versus function words in a text; and 2) lexical diversity as assessed by the frequency of new lexical items in a text. The syntactic complexity of sentences broadly refers to (Ravid *et al.*, 2010): their length (number of clauses in a sentence), depth (the amount of hierarchical embeddings within clauses), and diversity (varied subordinators within the same sentence). Scott and Koonce (2014) identify other equally important factors affecting complexity. These include the ordering of syntactic elements (whether or not subject–verb–object [SVO] is primary) and the degree of distance between the main subject and the verb phrase. An example of a long distance dependency is *Harold, whose army had just marched across England after fighting an invading group of Norwegians back, was tired and sore* (authors' underline; Scott and Koonce, 2014, p. 285). The notion that "lexical items and syntactic constructions conspire to make a given piece of language more or less 'complex'" (Ravid *et al.*, 2010, p. 126) captures the interdependence between the two systems. Because linguistic complexity is also a trademark of the disciplinary languages, we focus on the languages of mathematics and science because they are the most researched.

The language of mathematics and the lexical–syntactic interface

Aspects of the mathematics register potentially reveal what may be difficult for students learning math, especially those with LLD. For example, mathematics employs a highly technical, precise, and densely structured language, uses technical vocabulary that is uniquely mathematical (e.g., *hypotenuse, sine*), depends on everyday words that are re-designated to reference mathematical concepts (e.g., *length, prove*), and utilizes complex ENPs (e.g. *two trigonometric formulas*).

The fact that some mathematical terms reference different or more precise meanings in the mathematics register than in other contexts (Schleppegrell, 2007) creates another linguistic impediment for many students with LLD. The following exemplifies how meanings specific to the mathematical register must be incorporated into students' lexicons. This Grade 6 sample item draws on ratio concepts and the relationship of unit rates to ratios (Partnership for Assessment of Readiness for College and Careers, PARCC, 2013):

> Mr. Ruiz is starting a marching band at his school. He first does research and finds the following data about other local marching bands (note: these data graphically display the number of brass instrument players and the number of percussion instrument players in each of three bands).

> Part A – Mr. Ruiz realizes that there are X brass instrument players per percussion player (a student must understand that a unit rate has to be determined even though the instructions do not explicitly state this purpose).

> Part B – Mr. Ruiz has 210 students who are interested in joining the marching band. He decides to have 80% of the band be made up of percussion and brass instruments. Use the unit rate you found in Part A to determine how many students should play brass instruments.

Most dictionary definitions of *rate* reference mathematical notions associated with *estimate* (e.g., How do you *rate* your chances of winning the lottery?) or *amount* (What's your average *rate* for the mile run?). The test item uses specialized vocabulary particular to formulating tables of equivalent ratios: *Rate* must be understood relationally as a unit for determining equivalence linkages among two quantities. Students must grasp the arithmetic distinction between *percent* of a quantity as a rate per 100 (i.e., "80% of the band be made up of percussion and brass instruments") and *unit rate* as a quantity realized as a proportion ("Use the unit rate you found in Part A to determine how many students should play brass instruments").

The lexical–syntactic interface is further illustrated by how complicated mathematical processes are often signified by nominalizations (verbs or adjectives converted into nouns), which may be operated on in new ways, for example, *taking the limit of a difference quotient* becomes *the derivative*. Nominalization results in attributing agency to mathematical objects and processes rather than to the people doing the mathematics. Moreover, verbs may act differently compared with other domains where there is a prevalence of doing or thinking verbs. In the mathematics register, relational verbs like *is*, *be*, *have*, and *means* are often used to express relationships between objects and processes. Mathematics also uses conjunctions (e.g., *if… then*) with technical, precise meanings in developing theorems and proofs.

Recent research reveals that students with LLD struggle with the lexical–syntactic components of mathematical language (e.g., Alt *et al.*, 2014; Fazio, 1996, 1999; Mainela-Arnold *et al.*, 2011). However, research has not yet examined whether the content complexity generated, for example, through embedded ENPs, is a barrier to conceptual understanding. Additionally, a mediator variable identified in the word problem skills of students in Grades 2 to 5 with reading and mathematical disabilities is syntactic awareness (Peake *et al.*, in press).

The language of science and the lexical–syntactic interface

At the text level, the language of science is designed to cultivate more interpretive reasoning through explanation, comparison, and description (Bailey and Butler, 2007). These functions are interlocked with the lexical–syntactic interface characterized by conceptual, lexical, and syntactic density. This density is reflected by more technical vocabulary, logical connectives that link to subordinate clauses, complex ENPs, and the passive voice, among other features (Scott and Balthazar, 2010). Consider the following seven sentence excerpt from an expository passage on the life cycle of stars taken from a reading assessment keyed to the upper middle school level (all passages were developed using a readability formula) (Leslie and Caldwell, 2011, p. 360).

(1) Stars begin their life cycle with different masses. (2) A star's mass determines how long its life cycle will last and how it will die. (3) Stars with a mass less than five times that of the sun are called low-mass stars. (4) Most stars are in this group.

(5) A low-mass star begins its life cycle as a main-sequence star. (6) Over a period of billions of years, its supply of hydrogen is slowly changed by nuclear fusion into helium. (7) During this time, the star changes very little.

To begin with, the understanding of stars' life cycles requires conceptual knowledge about the meaning of mass and its transformative relationship to chemical elements and atomic nuclei. This conceptual knowledge then must be applied to discerning the text purpose as garnered from the excerpt's organization, a combination of description in the first paragraph (sentences 1–4) and cause/effect in the second paragraph (sentences 5–7). In terms of language patterns, one outstanding feature is the specialized vocabulary (*mass, low-mass, main-sequence, hydrogen, nuclear fusion, helium*), which must be interconnected with the conceptual knowledge that supports their meaning.

Of interest, there is minimal depth to sentence construction (there are no subordinated clauses); however, sentence 3 contains a long distance dependency (a break between the primary subject *Stars* and the verb phrase *are called*). For sentence processing to operate efficiently, long distance dependencies must be quickly resolved to reduce the burden on working memory (O'Grady, 2005). Inadequate resolution increases the difficulty of predicting plausible syntactic relationships among elements and promotes less appropriate parsing. Both patterns are found in the oral processing of long distance dependency sentences for preteens and adolescents with a known LLD (Hsu *et al.*, 2014; Purdy *et al.*, 2014). Even the two left-branching sentences with longer noun phrases (6 and 7) can further complicate processing because their specific linguistic features must be deconstructed in working memory (Scott and Koonce, 2014).

A third linguistic feature of science language also meshes the lexical and syntactic realms in the frequency with which ENPs appear. Like mathematics, these constructions are relatively common in science texts, especially in the higher grades (Fang and Schleppegrell, 2010). The life cycle excerpt illustrates ENP frequency. Simpler ENPs (head noun pre-modifications) are underlined, while more complex ENPs (head noun post-modifications) are double underlined. In fact, sentences 3 and 6 represent multiple ENP embeddings. For example, the two post-modifying ENPs in sentence 3 (*with a mass less than five times that of the sun*) function to condense information about the head noun (*stars*, the sentence subject) (Fang and Schleppegrell, 2010), so that a semantic relationship is constructed through the linking verb (*are called*) to identify a star subtype (*low-mass stars*). Hence, unpacking just this one sentence for middle school students with LLD assumes that the requisite conceptual and text organization knowledge is accessible to them. If so, they then must apply a flexible repertoire of cognitive and linguistic resources to hold in mind and efficiently manage the syntactic challenge of long distance dependencies while simultaneously uncovering the lexical and semantic relationships embedded in the dense noun phrases inherent to both the languages of mathematics and science.

Summary

Over 15 years ago, Westby *et al.* (1999) issued a prescient call to understand better the cognitive and linguistic demands of scientific literacy for students who were struggling with knowing, doing, and talking science. It still is unknown how the synchrony of the lexical–syntactic interface in the social context of the academic language registers goes awry in LLD, much less in other students who struggle with mathematics and science. There has been some focus on the language-heavy load of mathematics (Alt *et al.*, 2014) for students with LLD and the problems they encounter with incidental learning as the primary means for acquiring scientific meanings (Dockrell *et al.*, 2007). But broad-scale studies have yet to be conducted on how they manage the lexicons and syntax of the academic disciplines, much less how the nature of classroom interactions affects the depth of what they learn.

Conclusion: Reaching towards a new practice model

Speech–language pathologists in the United States have become increasingly familiar with their varied roles in supporting the oral language underpinnings of beginning reading, and, in some cases, reading comprehension. However, the academic language registers, the core of disciplinary literacy, have received less attention.

In this era of new educational standards in the United States, an innovative practice model is called for that integrates the neurocognitive and sociocultural perspectives in order to accomplish three aims (Silliman, 2014; see also Stone, this volume). These are to: 1) interconnect developmental knowledge about expository text organization and the lexical–syntactic interface with appropriate clinical/educational benchmarks; 2) offer a sufficiently utilitarian and collaborative perspective so that communicative processes are integrated into actual disciplinary realms in the school setting; and 3) maintain multilevel and formative assessments of oral–written language system interactions at the word, sentence, and text levels in order to meaningfully inform instruction/intervention, promote student engagement in learning, and support a self-identity as a competent learner.

References

Alt, M., Arizmendi, G.D., Beal, C.R., Nippold, M. and Pruitt-Lord, S. (2014), "The relationship between mathematics and language: Academic implications for children with specific language impairment and English language learners", *Language, Speech, and Hearing Services in Schools*, Vol. 45, pp. 220–233.

Bailey, A.L. (2010), "Implications for assessment and instruction", in M. Shatz and L.C. Wilkinson, (Eds.), *The Education of English Language Learners: Research to Practice*, Guilford Press, New York, NY, pp. 222–247.

Bailey, A.L. and Butler, F.A. (2007), "A conceptual framework of academic English language for broad application to education", in A.L. Bailey, (Ed.), *The Language Demands of School: Putting Academic English to the Test*, Yale University Press, Yale, CT, US, pp. 68–102.

Beckner, C., Blythe, R., Bybee, J., Christiansen, M.H., Croft, W., Ellis, N.C., *et al.*, (2009), "Language is a complex adaptive system: Position paper", *Language Learning*, Vol. 59, Supp. 1, pp. 1–26.

Berman, R.A. and Nir, N. (2010), "The language of expository discourse across adolescence", in M.A. Nippold and C.M. Scott, (Eds.), *Expository Discourse in Children, Adolescents, and Adults*, Psychology Press, New York, NY, pp. 99–121.

Biber, D., Gray, B. and Poopon, K. (2011), "Should we use characteristics of conversation to measure grammatical complexity in L2 writing development?", *TESOL Quarterly*, Vol. 45, pp. 5–35.

Bishop, D.V.M. (2009), "Specific language impairment as a language learning disability", *Child Language Teaching and Therapy*, Vol. 25, pp. 163–165.

Council of Chief State School Officers (CCSSO) and the National Governors Association (NGA) Center for Best Practices. (2010), "*Common Core State Standards Initiative*". Retrieved from www.corestandards.org.

Cummins, J. (2013), "BICS and CALP: Empirical support, theoretical status, and policy implications of a controversial distinction", in M.R. Hawkins (Ed.), *Framing Language and Literacies: Socially Situated Views and Perspectives*, Routledge, New York, pp. 10–23.

Cummins, J. (2014), "Beyond language: Academic communication and student success", *Linguistics and Education*, Vol. 26, pp. 145–154.

Dockrell, J.E., Braisby, N. and Best, R.M. (2007), "Children's acquisition of science terms: Simple exposure is insufficient", *Learning and Instruction*, Vol. 17, pp. 577–594.

Dockrell, J.E., Lindsay, G. and Connelly, V. (2009), "The impact of specific language impairment on adolescents' written text", *Exceptional Children*, Vol. 75, pp. 427–446.

Fang, Z. and Schleppegrell, M.J. (2010), "Disciplinary literacies across content areas: Supporting secondary reading through functional language analysis", *Journal of Adolescent and Adult Literacy*, Vol. 53, pp. 587–597.

Fang, Z., Scheppegrell, M.J. and Moore, J. (2014), "The linguistic challenge of learning across academic disciplines", in C.A. Stone, E.R. Silliman, B.J. Ehren and G.P. Wallach, (Eds.), *Handbook of Language and Literacy: Development and Disorders*, Second edn., Guilford Press, New York, NY, pp. 302–322.

Fazio, B.B. (1996), "Mathematical abilities of children with specific language impairment: A 2-year follow-up", *Journal of Speech and Hearing Research*, Vol. 39, pp. 839–849.

Fazio, B.B. (1999), "Arithmetic calculation, short-term memory, and language performance in children with specific language impairment: A 5-year follow-up", *Journal of Speech, Language, and Hearing Research*, Vol. 42, pp. 420–431.

Fox, E. (2009), "The role of reader characteristics in processing and learning from informational text", *Review of Educational Research*, Vol. 79, pp. 197–261.

Hanushek, E.A., Peterson, P.E. and Woessmann, L. (2014), *Not Just the Problems of Other People's Children: US Student Performance in Global Perspective*, Taubman Center for State and Local Government, Harvard Kennedy School, Cambridge, MA, US.

Hsu, H.J., Tomblin, J.B. and Christiansen, M.H. (2014), "Impaired statistical learning of non-adjacent dependencies in adolescents with specific language impairment", *Frontiers in Psychology*, Vol. 5, www.frontiersin.org/Journal/Abstract.aspx?s=603&name=language_sciences&ART_doi=10.3389/fpsyg.2014.00175.

Leslie, L. and Caldwell, J. (2011), *Qualitative Reading Inventory 5*, Fifth edn., Pearson, Boston, MA, US.

Mainela-Arnold, E., Alibali, M.W., Ryan, K. and Evans, J.L. (2011), "Knowledge of mathematical equivalence in children with specific language impairment: Insights from gesture and speech", *Language, Speech, and Hearing Services in Schools*, Vol. 42, pp. 18–30.

Mason, L.H. and Hedin, L.R. (2011), "Reading science text: Challenges for students with learning disabilities and considerations for teachers", *Learning Disabilities Research and Practice*, Vol. 26, pp. 214–222.

Nagy, W. and Townsend, D. (2012), "Words as tools: Learning academic vocabulary as language acquisition", *Reading Research Quarterly*, Vol. 47, pp. 91–108.

Nippold, M.A. (2007), *Later Language Development: School-Age Children, Adolescents, and Young Adults*. Second edn., Pro-Ed, Austin, TX, US.

Nippold, M.A. (2010), "Explaining complex matters: How knowledge of domain drives language" in M.A. Nippold and C.M. Scott, (Eds.), *Expository Discourse in Children, Adolescents, and Adults*, Psychology Press, New York, pp. 41–61.

Nippold, M.A., Mansfield, T.C., Billow, J.L. and Tomblin, J.B. (2008), "Expository discourse in adolescents with language impairments: Examining syntactic development", *American Journal of Speech-Language Pathology*, Vol. 17, pp. 356–366.

Nippold, M.A., Mansfield, T.C., Billow, J.L. and Tomblin, J.B. (2009), "Syntactic development in adolescents with a history of language impairments: A follow-up investigation", *American Journal of Speech-Language Pathology*, Vol. 18, pp. 241–251.

Nippold, M.A. and Ward-Lonergan, J.M. (2010), "Argumentative writing in pre-adolescents: The role of verbal reasoning", *Child Language Teaching and Therapy*, Vol. 26, pp. 238–248.

O'Grady, W. (2005), *Syntactic Carpentry: An Emergentist Approach to Syntax*, Lawrence Erlbaum, Mahwah, NJ, US.

Partnership for Assessment of Readiness for College and Careers, PARCC (2013) Retrieved from www. parcconline.org/sites/parcc/files/Grade6-ProportionsofInstruments.pdf

Peake, C., Jimenez, J.E., Rodrigue, C., Bisschop, E. and Villarroel, R. (in press; Available online, February, 2014), "Syntactic awareness and arithmetic word problem solving in children with and without learning disabilities", *Journal of Learning Disabilities*. doi: 10.1177/0022219413520183

Perera, K. (1984), *Children's Reading and Writing*, Basil Blackwell, New York, NY.

Purdy, J.D., Leonard, L.B., Weber-Fox, C. and Kaganovitch, N. (2014), "Decreased sensitivity to long-distance dependencies in children with a history of specific language impairment: Electrophysiological evidence", *Journal of Speech, Language, and Hearing Research*, Vol. 57, pp. 1040–1059.

Ravid, D. and Berman, R.A. (2006), "Information density in the development of spoken and written narratives in English and Hebrew", *Discourse Processes*, Vol. 41, pp. 117–149.

Ravid, D., Dromi, E. and Kotler, P. (2010), "Linguistic complexity in school-age text production: Expository versus mathematical discourse" in M.A. Nippold and C.M. Scott, (Eds.), *Expository Discourse in Children, Adolescents, and Adults*, Psychology Press, New York, NY, pp. 123–154.

Sáenz, L.M. and Fuchs, L.S. (2002), "Examining the reading difficulty of secondary students with learning disabilities: Expository versus narrative text", *Remedial and Special Education*, Vol. 23, pp. 31–41.

Schleppegrell, M.J. (2007), "The linguistic challenges of mathematics teaching and learning: A research review", *Reading and Writing Quarterly: Overcoming Learning Difficulties*, Vol. 23, pp. 139–159.

Schleppegrell, M.J., Achugar, M. and Oteiza, T. (2004), "The grammar of history: Enhancing content-based instruction through a functional focus on language", *TESOL Quarterly*, Vol. 38, pp. 67–93.

Scott, C.M. and Windsor, J. (2000), "General language performance measures in spoken and written narrative and expository discourse of school-age children with language learning disabilities", *Journal of Speech, Language, and Hearing Research*, Vol. 43, pp. 324–339.

Scott, C. and Balthazar, C. (2010), "The grammar of information challenges for older students with language impairments", *Topics in Language Disorders*, Vol. 30, pp. 288–307.

Scott, C.M. and Koonce, N.M. (2014), "Syntactic contributions to literacy learning" in C.A. Stone, E.R. Silliman, B.J. Ehren, and G.P. Wallach, (Eds.), *Handbook of Language and Literacy: Development and Disorders*, Second edn., Guilford Press, New York, NY, pp. 283–301.

Seidenberg, M.S. (2013), "The science of reading and its educational implications", *Language Learning and Development*, Vol. 9, pp. 331–360.

Silliman, E.R. (2014), "Integrating oral and written language into a new practice model: Perspectives of an oral language researcher and practitioner", in B. Arfe, J. Dockrell, and V. Berninger, (Eds.), *Writing Development and Instruction in Children with Hearing, Speech, and Oral Language Difficulties*, Oxford, New York, NY, pp. 158–175.

Silliman, E.R. and Mody, M. (2008), "Individual differences in oral language and reading: It's a matter of experience", in M. Mody and E.R. Silliman, (Eds.), *Brain, Behavior, and Learning in Language and Reading Disorders*, Guilford Press, New York, NY, pp. 349–386.

Silliman, E.R. and Wilkinson, L.C. (2014), "Policy and practice issues for students at risk in language and literacy learning: Back to the future", in C.A. Stone, E.R. Silliman, B.J. Ehren, and G.P. Wallach,

(Eds.), *Handbook of Language and Literacy: Development and Disorders*, Second edn., Guilford Press, New York, NY, pp. 105–126.

Snow, C.E. (2010), "Academic language and the challenge of reading for learning", *Science*, Vol. 328, pp. 450–452.

Snow, C.E. and Uccelli, P. (2009), "The challenge of academic language", in D.R. Olson and N. Torrance, (Eds.), *The Cambridge Handbook of Literacy*, Cambridge University Press, New York, NY, pp. 112–133.

Uccelli, P., Barr, C.D., Dobbs, C.L., Galloway, E.P., Meneses, A. and Sanchez, E. (in press), "Core academic language skills (CALS): An expanded operational construct and a novel instrument to chart school-relevant language proficiency in pre-adolescent and adolescent learners", *Applied Psycholinguistics*.

Westby, C., Dezale, J., Fradd, S.H. and Lee, O. (1999), "Learning to do science: Influences of culture and language", *Communication Disorders Quarterly*, Vol. 21, pp. 50–94.

Westby, C.E. (2005), "Comprehending narrative and expository text", in H.W. Catts and A.G. Kamhi, (Eds.), *Language and Reading Disabilities*, Second edn., Pearson, Boston, MA, US, pp. 159–232.

Wilkinson, L.C. and Silliman, E.R. (2000), "Classroom language and literacy learning", in M.L. Kamil, P.E. Mosenthal, P.D. Pearson, and R. Barr, (Eds.), *Handbook of Reading Research*, Lawrence Erlbaum, Mahwah, NJ, US, pp. 337–360.

Wong Fillmore, L. and Fillmore, C.J. (2012), *What does Text Complexity mean for English Learners and Language Minority Students?*, Stanford University Graduate School of Education Understanding Language Project, Stanford, CA, US.

Zwiers, J. (2008), *Building Academic Language: Essential Practices for Content Classrooms*, International Reading Association, Newark, DE, US.

Zwiers, J. and Crawford, M. (2011), *Academic Conversations: Classroom Talk that Fosters Critical Thinking and Content Understandings*, Stenhouse, Portland, ME, US.

27

AFRICAN AMERICAN CHILDREN'S EARLY LANGUAGE AND LITERACY LEARNING IN THE CONTEXT OF SPOKEN DIALECT VARIATION

Nicole Patton Terry, Megan C. Brown and Adrienne Stuckey

Ample basic and applied research indicates the importance of oral language skills in the acquisition of literacy skills. In general, children with good reading and writing skills also have good phonological, morphosyntactic, and semantic knowledge and skills (see, for example, chapters provided by Bahr and Cain in this volume). Thus, it is not surprising that researchers focus on oral language skills while trying to understand why specific groups of children exhibit difficulty with literacy achievement. Such is the case with research on African American children in the United States.

Over the past 40 years, advances in understanding literacy development and instruction have generated little progress in alleviating the academic underachievement of African American children. For example, the most recent report of the National Assessment of Educational Progress (National Center for Education Statistics, NCES, 2013) indicated that 83 percent of African American fourth graders were reading below grade-level expectations, compared to 55 percent of White students. Conversely, 15 percent of African American students and 34 percent of White students were "proficient" readers (NCES, 2013). Unfortunately, these achievement gaps have remained relatively stable over the years, with no substantive indications as to how to resolve them.

Multiple factors are considered predictors of the achievement gap, including socioeconomic, educational, environmental, and family factors (see Washington, Terry, and Seidenberg, 2013 for more extensive discussion). Given the established relationship between oral language and literacy achievement, attention has turned to the unique oral language patterns that many African American children bring to the literacy-learning task. Specifically, many African American children enter school as fluent speakers of African American English (AAE), a nonmainstream, cultural dialect of American English. The chapter's purpose, therefore, is to consider the role of African American children's use of AAE in the acquisition of reading and writing skills. After presenting the literature on child AAE use, findings from recent research on this relationship are reviewed. These findings are then integrated into current theoretical perspectives on the relations between spoken dialect variation and literacy achievement. Finally, questions are posed for future research needed to move both research and practice forward.

Child AAE

American English is characterized by various cultural and regional dialects that generate rule-governed, systematic differences in language production (Wolfram and Schilling-Estes, 2006). AAE is a cultural dialect spoken by most African Americans, irrespective of geographic location, socioeconomic status, age, or gender. Like other nonmainstream American English varieties, AAE is characterized by phonological, morphosyntactic, and semantic differences from mainstream American English (MAE). Comprehensive lists of AAE features have been published elsewhere (see for example Charity, 2008; Green, 2011; Washington and Craig, 2002). Importantly, although each dialect has unique features, AAE and MAE share many overlapping features. However, AAE and MAE vary in their social prestige. Thus, as is true with many other dialects, the overlapping features of AAE and MAE are less stigmatizing than are the nonoverlapping features. As a low-prestige dialect, AAE is often perceived negatively, especially when used in educational contexts.

With respect to literacy learning and achievement among African American children, the pioneering work of Julie Washington and Holly Craig deserves discussion. Many of the initial empirical descriptions of AAE were from adolescent and adult speakers, so these researchers set out to characterize typical and atypical child AAE use and language development. Spanning 15 years, their research program contributed four key findings that inform the study of dialect variation and literacy learning.

Differences in type and frequency of AAE production

African American children produce a wide variety of morphosyntactic and phonological AAE features. Children as young as two years old reliably produce more than 20 morphosyntactic features of AAE (Horton-Ikard, 2002; Jackson and Roberts, 2001; Oetting and McDonald, 2001; Washington and Craig, 1994, 2002). It has been more challenging to reliably characterize children's phonological AAE production, primarily because it is difficult to discern what is developmental and what is dialect-related. Moreover, AAE and MAE share the same consonants, although phonotactic differences between the dialects can result in production frequency differences (Pearson *et al.*, 2009).

Variation in the type of phonological and morphosyntactic features used appears to be minimal across geographic and demographic contexts, supporting the stability of child AAE and its patterns of unique feature usage. However, the frequency with which features are used can vary a great deal among children. In general, higher frequency rates have been reported among children in the Southern US, African American boys, and children from low-income households (Charity, 2007; Craig and Washington, 2002; Washington and Craig, 1998).

Developmental changes in child AAE production

Children's AAE use changes significantly during early schooling, with children shifting from more frequent to less frequent AAE use between preschool and first grade. For example, in a large cross-sectional study, Craig and Washington (2004) found a marked decrease in AAE production between kindergarten and first grade, but not between preschool and kindergarten and not between first and fifth grades. Similar decreases have been found between kindergarten and first grade (Terry and Connor, 2012) and first and second grades (Terry *et al.*, 2012). These changes in dialect use may be associated with developing reading and writing skills, as well as growing language skills.

Discourse context and child AAE use

Production of child AAE is related to the discourse context. Washington, Craig, and Kushmaul (1998) found that 4–6 year olds produced more types of AAE features on a picture description task than a free play task. Connor and Craig (2006) also found that preschoolers varied their amount of AAE production between sentence imitation and story-retell tasks. Both Thompson and colleagues (2004) and Craig and colleagues (2009) found that school-aged children used more AAE on oral tasks (e.g., spoken narrative) than writing or reading tasks (e.g., written narrative). These differences in AAE production may be related to the tasks' implicit expectations for AAE production. A sentence imitation task presupposes MAE production, as the child is expected to repeat the targeted sentence verbatim. Conversely, a story-retell or picture description task does not presuppose use of either dialect. It has been hypothesized that children's awareness of these discourse differences is associated not only with their AAE production in specific contexts, but also their general metalinguistic and linguistic knowledge and academic achievement (Craig *et al.*, 2009; Terry *et al.*, 2012).

Receptive knowledge of both MAE and AAE

Young AAE speakers demonstrate knowledge of both AAE and MAE forms. The aforementioned studies documenting children's varied AAE feature use suggest that children are rarely observed to speak AAE 100 percent of the time. However, what children produce in overt speech is not always indicative of underlying language knowledge or comprehension. In a series of studies focused on phonological knowledge, Terry and colleagues found typically developing African American children between four and eight years old demonstrated knowledge of both nonmainstream and MAE forms (Mansour and Terry, 2014; Terry, 2014; Terry and Scarborough, 2011). For instance, while listening to words, AAE speaking children accepted AAE pronunciations of targets 60 percent of the time and accepted MAE pronunciations 95 percent of the time. On a non-word repetition task, children either produced the target word verbatim or with a correct AAE substitution – a behavior that would not be expected unless children had knowledge of MAE and its phonological substitution rules.

Results like these suggest that African American children have implicit knowledge of both AAE and MAE forms to draw upon while learning to read and write. Yet, emerging evidence suggests that AAE and MAE speakers may differ in the order and rate at which they acquire the sounds and syntactic structures of American English. For instance, Pearson *et al.* (2009) found that school-aged MAE and AAE speakers demonstrated different trajectories in the acquisition of some consonant sounds. For example, while few differences were observed with sounds in the initial position (where MAE and AAE do not differ), several final consonants were mastered earlier by MAE speakers (around fouryears) than AAE speakers (between five to eight years old). The researchers suggested that phonological and syntactic discrepancies between the dialects may come from certain sounds, morphemes, and words being less frequent in AAE than in MAE. Such acquisition differences may have some bearing on lexical knowledge.

In sum, several key findings about child AAE production and use have been reported recently in the literature. In general, researchers have found nuanced relationships between child AAE use and various factors, like discourse type, age, gender, and expressive and receptive knowledge.

Not surprisingly, researchers have observed equally complex and nuanced associations between child AAE production and literacy learning and achievement.

AAE and early language and literacy achievement

Interest in the association between spoken dialect variation and academic achievement is neither novel nor limited to the U.S. Indeed, researchers in many countries with salient and distinct dialects have been grappling with the educational implications of language variation on literacy achievement for years, especially for low-performing students from low-income households (for example, see discussions of Arabic-speaking children in Israel in Saiegh-Haddad, 2003 and Zuzovsky, 2010). In the U.S., African American children are more likely than their White peers to be raised in poverty, to attend low-performing schools, to show persistent patterns of underachievement, and to drop out of high school. Thus, beginning in the 1960s, researchers posited that dialect variation might be a causal factor in the reading underachievement of African American children. Interdisciplinary investigations completed in the last 15 years have been characterized by relatively large sample sizes, sensitive measures of child AAE use, and developmental designs with children who were learning to read and write. Accordingly, these investigations have provided converging evidence of significant associations between children's AAE production and language and literacy skills, including vocabulary, syntax, morphological awareness, phonological awareness, oral narration, decoding, word reading, spelling, reading comprehension, and text composition (e.g., Charity *et al.*, 2004; Craig *et al.*, 2004, 2009; Kohler *et al.*, 2007; Terry and Connor, 2010; Terry *et al.*, 2010). Three trends in the findings across these studies are worth noting.

Improved measures of AAE production

Significant associations have emerged between language and literacy skills and dialect use in part because of advancements in measuring child AAE use. Common measures include: (1) sentence repetition tasks (Charity *et al.*, 2004); (2) dialect density measures (DDM) calculated from spoken language samples (Washington and Craig, 2002); (3) criterion scores from a standardized measure, the *Diagnostic Evaluation of Language Variation, Screening Test* (DELV-S; Seymour *et al.*, 2003); and (4) a percentage dialect variation (DVAR) score derived from the DELV-S (Terry *et al.*, 2010). These measures reliably capture rate of AAE production in children ages 3 to 12 years old and are sensitive to developmental differences in AAE production. These measures also allow conclusions about AAE production to be generalized across studies despite differences in measures.

Relationships between AAE production and literacy skills

Although all significant, the nature of the relationships between AAE production and various language and literacy skills has varied across studies. Researchers have found *negative* linear correlations (e.g., Charity *et al.*, 2004; Mansour and Terry, 2014; Terry, 2006; Terry *et al.*, 2010). Across these studies, children who used more AAE performed more poorly on various language and literacy measures. Conversely, researchers have also found *positive* relationships, in particular with complex syntax (Craig and Washington, 1994) and oral narration (e.g., Curenton and Justice, 2004). Across these studies, children who use more AAE performed well on these language and literacy measures.

Researchers have also observed *indirect* relationships between AAE production and language and literacy skills, especially when using multi-level methodologies. In these studies, children's AAE use explained some of the variance in their reading ability, but much more significant variance was explained by other factors. For example, Terry and colleagues found children's AAE use to be significantly associated with reading skill, but not predictive of it after controlling for other language skills or contextual factors like SES, phonological awareness, and oral vocabulary (Mansour and Terry, 2014; Terry, 2012, 2014; Terry and Connor, 2012; Terry and Scarborough, 2011). Interestingly, in many of these studies, dialect use was predictive of phonological awareness skills, which in turn was predictive of word reading ability. This pattern of results might suggest an indirect relationship between dialect use and reading that is mediated by phonological awareness.

Finally, researchers have also observed *U-shaped* relationships, where children with higher rates of AAE production performed better on various language and literacy measures than children with moderate rates of AAE production (Connor and Craig, 2006; Terry *et al.*, 2010, 2012). In these studies, children who spoke more AAE did not always perform more poorly than children who spoke less AAE. Importantly, in all instances, children who spoke AAE at moderate or high frequency rates still performed more poorly than those who spoke AAE at very low rates. More complex, and arguably more precise, accounts of the relationship between children's AAE use and literacy achievement are likely to emerge as the field continues to adopt more advanced, multi-level methodologies.

Code-switching and literacy outcomes

Change in dialect use may be just as important to consider as frequency of dialect use. Style-shifting or code-switching is a sociolinguistic, pragmatic language phenomenon in which speakers vary their speech style by increasing, decreasing, or substituting features between dialects (Wolfram and Schilling-Estes, 2006). Successful shifting requires some degree of metalinguistic knowledge because speakers would have to understand contextual demands for using a specific dialect and how to adjust their dialect production appropriately for each linguistic context.

African American children appear to shift from producing more to less AAE in school contexts during the early schooling years at the same time they are learning to read and write. Thus, some researchers have hypothesized that change in dialect use at this time is related to literacy learning and achievement. This relationship may be reciprocal. Literacy learning may be a catalyst for change in dialect use and change in dialect use may beget literacy learning, or they may create a feedback loop, where literacy acquisition causes more code-switching, which allows for more literacy acquisition.

Only a handful of studies have examined shifting explicitly, either by observing changes in dialect use over time (Terry *et al.*, 2012; Terry and Connor, 2012) or across contexts (Connor and Craig, 2006; Craig *et al.*, 2009). For example, in one longitudinal study, Terry and colleagues (2012) found that most African American children decreased their AAE use during first grade but not second grade, and that these decreases were associated with greater growth in word reading and passage comprehension. Interestingly, children with stronger oral language skills were more likely to shift from more to less nonmainstream production. With regard to shifting across contexts, Craig and colleagues (2009) found that school-aged African American children produced more AAE forms in spoken than in written narratives. Children with the strongest reading skills demonstrated higher amounts of shifting between oral and written contexts, and children who used more AAE forms in their writing demonstrated lower reading achievement.

In sum, armed with new, more sensitive measures of spoken dialect variation, researchers have provided converging evidence of significant, complex relationships between children's AAE use and language and literacy skills. However, the nature of these relationships is inconsistent, typically varying by methodological approach. Moreover, changes in dialect use appear to be important to consider, especially as research turns to interventions designed to modify children's dialect knowledge and use. These findings are the foundation for three distinct hypotheses about the relationship between dialect variation and literacy learning and achievement.

Three hypotheses on the relationship between dialect variation and literacy achievement

Although it is clear that African American children's spoken dialect use is significantly associated with their language and literacy achievement during early schooling, it is less clear how or why. It is important to uncover the mechanisms through which dialect variation affects how children learn to read and write, as these mechanisms should drive clinical and educational practice. Three primary hypotheses have been posited: teacher bias, linguistic-interference mismatch, and a nascent set of relatively new hypotheses that emphasize linguistic flexibility.

Teacher bias

The first hypothesis, *teacher bias*, suggests that teachers develop low expectations for students who use nonmainstream, stigmatized dialects like AAE, because they generally have negative perceptions of such dialects (e.g., Shields, 1979; Washington and Miller-Jones, 1989). That is, teachers may perceive children who speak AAE to be at-risk, to use disordered or incorrect speech, to be low-achievers, or to have learning difficulties. Such low expectations beget negative or unsupportive interactions, inadequate and inappropriate instruction, and ultimately poor academic achievement. To date, this premise has received little attention in empirical investigations. However, it is plausible, as many studies have reported significant associations between teachers' expectations and student achievement (e.g., Robinson-Cimpian *et al.*, 2014).

Linguistic-interference mismatch

The *linguistic-interference mismatch* hypothesis suggests that differences between spoken AAE and standard written English orthography create confusion during the reading process (e.g., Labov, 1995). For example, a child who says "*col*" and "*rub*" for "*cold*" and "*rubbed*" might be perplexed to find an extra sound represented in the printed words and may misunderstand any associated changes in meaning. Children who speak AAE would encounter many such phonological and morphosyntactic (and even semantic) mismatches while learning to read and write, and certainly many more than children whose speech patterns align more closely to print. Thus, it is speculated that the task of learning to read is more difficult for children who speak AAE, perhaps because AAE speakers have either little or unspecified knowledge of MAE forms or because it may be more difficult to ascertain orthographic regularities if speech patterns vary from print. It may also be that translating between AAE and English orthography strains cognitive processes involved in reading.

Two predictions about the relation between children's spoken AAE use and literacy achievement can be drawn from the mismatch hypothesis: (1) that difficulty learning to read and write is directly related to children's spoken AAE use; and (2) that this difficulty will be greatest for children who speak more AAE than those who do not because they encounter more speech–print mismatches. Findings from the studies reviewed previously provide mixed support for this hypothesis. For example, although multiple studies found that children who used more AAE tended to perform more poorly on various reading, writing, and language measures (e.g., Charity *et al.*, 2004), others found that children who spoke more AAE (and who would presumably encounter the most mismatches) performed better than those who used it only moderately (e.g., Connor and Craig, 2006). Moreover, while significant correlations have been reported, spoken AAE use did not always predict reading outcomes when other known predictors are considered (e.g., Craig *et al.*, 2009; Mansour and Terry, 2014). That is, the relationship between children's AAE use and reading was indirect. Finally, researchers have reported both expressive and receptive MAE knowledge among young AAE speakers, suggesting that children have knowledge of both AAE and MAE forms while learning to read (e.g., Terry and Scarborough, 2011).

An alternate possibility

Such complex and seemingly inconsistent findings gave rise to a group of alternative hypotheses, which are still developing, and may in fact represent a unitary construct. Termed *dialect awareness* (Charity *et al.*, 2004), *dialect shifting-reading achievement* (Craig *et al.*, 2009), and *linguistic awareness– flexibility* (Terry *et al.*, 2010, 2012), proponents all posit that the association between children's AAE use and literacy learning and achievement go beyond speech-print mismatches.

It is worth noting that these researchers emphasize code-switching or style-shifting in understanding the relation between children's dialect use and literacy outcomes. The argument is that simply being an AAE speaker or even a dense AAE speaker does not predict literacy outcomes; rather, lesser AAE production or change in AAE production in contexts that presuppose MAE (like reading or writing standard English orthography) may be better predictors of literacy outcomes. Findings from several studies seem to support this claim (e.g., Craig *et al.*, 2009; Terry *et al.*, 2010, 2012).

Terry and colleagues go further to suggest that this shifting ability may be a linguistic or metalinguistic skill (perhaps in the pragmatic domain) that is akin to other linguistic and metalinguistic skills that are already known to contribute to reading and writing ability (e.g., phonological awareness). Perhaps children's spoken dialect use on specific tasks is a marker indicating their sensitivity to and awareness of language. It could be that this insensitivity is interfering with literacy skills more so than AAE use itself. Findings of better language and literacy performance among children who demonstrated shifting between task contexts seem to support this claim (e.g., Connor and Craig, 2006; Craig *et al.*, 2009; Terry, 2014).

In sum, three primary hypotheses have been suggested to explain the relationship between dialect variation and literacy learning and achievement. In general, these hypotheses vary in their emphasis on speech–print mismatches between MAE and AAE. Importantly, these hypotheses may not be mutually exclusive. For instance, it is plausible that, as children get older and develop more advanced literacy skills, speech–print mismatches become less important to literacy performance than more sophisticated linguistic and metalinguistic skills like style-shifting. Future research can unpack these possibilities.

Conclusions and implications for research and practice

One consistent conclusion emerges from recent research: spoken dialect variation is an important factor to consider in African American children's literacy learning and achievement. The findings presented are exciting and innovative, and encourage harnessing this knowledge to address achievement gaps through changes to instruction and intervention. However, three critical empirical questions must be answered in order to move both research and educational practice forward.

First, researchers should attempt to understand the developmental nature of the relationship between spoken dialect variation and literacy skills. The relation between language and literacy changes over time for all children; thus, it is not surprising that the same is true for the relationship between dialect variation and literacy learning. The interesting question is no longer whether or not children's spoken dialect use is related to literacy learning and achievement. The literature reviewed here suggests that the answer is yes. Rather, the more interesting and timely question is how these factors are related, under what conditions, at what developmental time point, and for whom. Methodological advances, including both statistical and computational modeling, have allowed for more nuanced examinations of how children learn to read and write. Introducing spoken dialect variation as a key variable in these models is sure to produce even more fascinating findings about how young African American children acquire literacy skills and may ultimately clarify which hypothesis is most appropriate for guiding educational and clinical practices.

Second, it will be important to move beyond a focus on language production to include comprehension. Thus far, the majority of studies have used production measures (e.g., sentence imitation, story retells), which reflect only one part of language knowledge. Children may know much more about AAE, MAE, and the relationship between them than can be gleaned from their speech alone. Moreover, children who speak different dialects demonstrate different developmental trajectories in language production that may affect their knowledge and comprehension. It would seem that the effectiveness of interventions designed to improve reading outcomes hinges upon whether students not only speak the targeted dialects but also know and understand them.

Third, the findings amassed thus far support investigations on the effectiveness of dialect-informed instruction in improving literacy achievement. In U.S. contexts, the most commonly cited approach of interest is contrastive analysis, where children are taught to contrast the linguistic characteristics of "home" and "school" or "formal" and "informal" language (e.g., Wheeler and Swords, 2010). Although few empirical studies have been published on such interventions, some recent reports are promising. For example, Wheeler and Swords (2010) published non-experimental accounts of successful writing outcomes for African American children in second–sixth grades who had been taught to use MAE through contrastive analysis. Fogel and Ehri (2000) compared two brief contrastive analysis approaches for African American children in third and fourth grades and found that students who were taught to transform sentences written with AAE grammatical forms into standard English forms outperformed those who were only exposed to text with standard grammatical forms and shown how to apply these forms in writing.

Results like these strongly suggest that dialect-informed instruction that includes both grammar and awareness components can have a robust effect on grammatical writing proficiency. What remains to be determined is whether: (1) the benefits of dialect-informed instruction extend into general writing (or reading) achievement;(2) benefits can be observed among students who are already struggling with literacy skills; (3) instruction should be focused on the phonological, morphosyntactic, and/or semantic aspects of dialects;and (4) instruction should be implemented as interventions for older students who have not demonstrated adequate literacy achievement or as preventions for younger children who have yet to experience literacy failure. Empirical pursuit of these questions, as well as those on development and language knowledge, should guide the next 20 years of research in this area and should produce the knowledge base necessary to address spoken dialect variation in the literacy achievement of African American children.

Acknowledgement

Preparation of this article was supported by NICHD grant R24D075454 (Julie Washington, Nicole Patton Terry, and Mark Seidenberg, PIs).

REFERENCES

Charity, A.H. (2007), "Regional differences in low SES African-American children's speech in the school setting", *Language Variation and Change*, Vol. 19, pp. 281–293.

Charity, A.H. (2008), "African American English: An overview", *Perspectives on Communication Disorders and Sciences in Culturally and Linguistically Diverse Populations*, Vol. 15, pp. 33–42.

Charity, A., Scarborough, H. and Griffin, D. (2004), "Familiarity with school English in African American children and its relation to early reading achievement", *Child Development*, Vol. 75, pp. 1340–1356.

Connor, C. and Craig, H. (2006), "African American preschoolers' language, emergent literacy skills, and use of AAE: A complex relation", *Journal of Speech, Language, and Hearing Research*, Vol. 49, pp. 771–792.

Craig, H.K. and Washington, J.A. (1994), "The complex syntax skills of poor, urban, African American preschoolers at school entry", *Language, Speech, and Hearing Services in Schools*, Vol. 25, pp. 181–190.

Craig, H.K. and Washington, J.A. (2002), "Oral language expectations for African American preschoolers and kindergartners", *American Journal of Speech–Language Pathology*, Vol. 11, pp. 59–70.

Craig, H.K. and Washington, J.A. (2004), "Grade related changes in the production of African American English", *Journal of Speech, Language and Hearing Research*, Vol. 47, pp. 450–463.

Craig, H., Connor, C. and Washington, J. (2004), "Early positive predictors of later reading comprehension for African American students", *Language, Speech, and Hearing Services in Schools*, Vol. 34, pp. 31–43.

Craig, H.K., Zhang, L., Hensel, S.L. and Quinn, E.J. (2009), "African American English-speaking students: An examination of the relationship between dialect shifting and reading outcomes", *Journal of Speech, Language and Hearing Research*, Vol. 52, pp. 839–855.

Curenton, S.M. and Justice, L.M. (2004), "African American and Caucasian preschoolers' use of decontextualized language: Literate language features in oral narratives", *Language, Speech, and Hearing Services in Schools*, Vol. 35, No. 3, pp. 240–253.

Fogel, H. and Ehri, L.C. (2000), "Teaching elementary students who speak Black English to write in standard English: Effects of dialect transformation practice", *Contemporary Educational Psychology*, Vol. 25, pp. 212–235.

Green, L.J. (2011), *Language and the African American Child*, Cambridge University Press: Cambridge, UK.

Horton-Ikard, R. (2002), "Developmental and dialectal influences in early child language", Unpublished doctoral dissertation, University of Wisconsin-Madison, US.

Jackson, S.C. and Roberts, J.E. (2001), "Complex syntax production of African American preschoolers", *Journal of Speech, Language, and Hearing Research*, Vol. 44, pp. 1083–1096.

Kohler, C.T., Bahr, R.H., Silliman, E.R., Bryant, J.B., Apel, K. and Wilkinson, L.C. (2007), "African American English dialect and performance on nonword spelling and phonemic awareness tasks", *American Journal of Speech-Language Pathology*, Vol. 16, pp. 157–168.

Labov, W. (1995), "Can reading failure be reversed: A linguistic approach to the question", in Gadsden, V.L. and Wagner, D.A. (Eds.), *Literacy Among African-American youth: Issues in Learning, Teaching, and Schooling*, Hampton Press, Inc.: Cresskill, NJ, US, pp. 39–68.

Mansour, S. and Terry, N.P. (2014), "Phonological awareness skills of young African American English speakers", *Reading and Writing: An Interdisciplinary Journal*, Vol. 27, pp. 555–569.

National Center for Education Statistics, NCES (2013), "The Nation's Report Card: A first look: 2013 mathematics and reading" (NCES 2014–451), Institute of Education Sciences, US Department of Education, Washington, DC, US, available at http://nationsreportcard.gov.

Oetting, J. and McDonald, J. (2001), "Nonmainstream dialect use and specific language impairment", *Journal of Speech, Language, and Hearing Research*, Vol. 44, pp. 207–223.

Pearson, B.Z., Velleman, S.L., Bryant, T.J. and Charko, T. (2009), "Phonological milestones for African American English-speaking children learning mainstream American English as a second dialect", *Language, Speech, and Hearing Services in Schools*, Vol. 40, pp. 229–244.

Robinson-Cimpian, J.P., Lubienski, S.T., Ganley, C.M. and Copur-Gencturk, Y. (2014), "Teachers' perceptions of students' mathematics proficiency may exacerbate early gender gaps in achievement", *Developmental Psychology*, Vol. 50, No. 4, pp. 262–281.

Saiegh-Haddad, E. (2003), "Linguistic distance and initial reading acquisition: The case of Arabic diglossia", *Applied Psycholinguistics*, Vol. 24, pp. 115–135.

Seymour, H., Roeper, T. and de Villiers, J. (2003), *Diagnostic Evaluation of Language Variation- Screening Test*, Harcourt Assessment, Inc., San Antonio, TX, US.

Shields, P. (1979), "The language of poor black children and reading performance", *Journal of Negro Education*, Vol. 48, pp. 196–208.

Terry, N.P. (2006), "Relations between dialect variation, grammar, and early spelling skills", *Reading and Writing: An Interdisciplinary Journal*, Vol. 19, No. 9, pp. 907–931.

Terry, N.P. (2012), "Examining relationships among dialect variation and emergent literacy skills", *Communication Disorders Quarterly*, Vol. 33, No. 2, pp. 67–77.

Terry, N.P. (2014), "Dialect variation and phonological knowledge: Phonological representations and metalinguistic awareness among beginning readers who speak nonmainstream American English", *Applied Psycholinguistics*, Vol. 35, pp. 155–176.

Terry, N.P. and Scarborough, H.S. (2011), "The phonological hypothesis as a valuable framework for studying the relation of dialect variation to early reading skills", in Brady, S., Braze, D. and Fowler, C. (Eds.), *Explaining Individual Differences in Reading: Theory and Evidence*, Taylor & Francis Group: New York, NY, pp. 97–117

Terry, N.P. and Connor, C.M. (2010), "African American English and spelling: How do second graders spell dialect-sensitive features of words?", *Learning Disabilities Quarterly*, Vol. 33, No. 3, pp. 199–210.

Terry, N.P. and Connor, C.M. (2012), "Changing nonmainstream American English use and early reading achievement from kindergarten to first grade", *American Journal of Speech Language Pathology*, Vol. 21, pp. 78–86.

Terry, N.P., Connor, C.M., Thomas-Tate, S. and Love, M. (2010), "Examining relationships among dialect variation, literacy skills, and school context in first grade", *Journal of Speech, Language, and Hearing Research*, Vol. 53, No. 1, pp. 126–145.

Terry, N.P., Connor, C.M., Petscher, Y. and Conlin, C. (2012), "Dialect variation and reading: Is change in nonmainstream American English use related to reading achievement in first and second grade?", *Journal of Speech, Language, and Hearing Research*, Vol. 55, pp. 55–69.

Thompson, C.A., Craig, H.K. and Washington, J.A. (2004), "Variable production of African American English across oracy and literacy contexts", *Language, Speech, and Hearing Services in Schools*, Vol. 35, pp. 269–282.

Washington, J.A. and Craig, H.K. (1994), "Dialectal forms during discourse of urban, African American preschoolers living in poverty", *Journal of Speech and Hearing Research*, Vol. 37, pp. 816–823.

Washington, J.A. and Craig, H.K. (1998), "Socioeconomic status and gender influences on children's dialectal variations", *Journal of Speech, Language, and Hearing Research*, Vol. 41, pp. 618–626.

Washington, J.A. and Craig, H.K. (2002), "Morphosyntactic forms of African American English used by young children and their caregivers", *Applied Psycholinguistics*, Vol. 23, pp. 209–231.

Washington, V. and Miller-Jones, D. (1989), "Teacher interactions with nonstandard English speakers during reading instruction", *Contemporary Educational Psychology*, Vol. 14, pp. 280–312.

Washington, J., Craig, H. and Kushmaul, A. (1998), "Variable use of African American English across two language sampling contexts", *Journal of Speech, Language, and Hearing Research*, Vol. 41, pp. 1115–1124.

Washington, J.A., Terry, N.P. and Seidenberg, M. (2013), "Language variation and literacy learning", in Stone, C.A., Silliman, E.R., Ehren, B.J. and Wallach, G.P. (Eds.), *Handbook of Language and Literacy, 2nd Edition: Development and Disorders*, Guilford Press, New York, NY, pp. 204–222.

Wheeler, R.S. and Swords, R. (2010), *Code-switching Lessons: Grammar Strategies for Linguistically Diverse Writers*, Heinemann, Portsmouth, NH, US.

Wolfram, W. and Schilling-Estes, N. (2006), *American English*, 2nd edition, Blackwell: Malden, MA, US.

Zuzovsky, R. (2010), "The impact of socioeconomic versus linguistic factors on achievement gaps between Hebrew-speaking and Arabic-speaking students in Israel in reading literacy and in mathematics and science achievements", *Studies in Educational Evaluation*, Vol. 36, pp. 153–161.

28

TREATMENT APPROACHES FOR SECOND LANGUAGE LEARNERS WITH PRIMARY LANGUAGE IMPAIRMENT

Kathryn Kohnert

The focus of this chapter is on treatment for second language learners diagnosed with primary language impairment. Immigrant children who acquire a minority first language (L1) at home are well represented in almost every nation of the world. In the United States, one of every five school children speaks a language other than English at home (U.S. Census Bureau, 2013). Although Spanish is by far the most common, there are more than three hundred other home languages in the U.S. including Cantonese, Hmong, Russian, Somali and Vietnamese. Immigrant children's experience with English, their second language (L2), often begins in early childhood and intensifies with age. To underscore the relevance of both home and community languages, L2 learners are also referred to here as developing bilinguals. Studies consistently show a shift to greater ability in English (L2) with age and experience although the L1 plays an important, complementary, and continuous role in immigrant children's lives (e.g., Kohnert and Bates, 2002; Pham and Kohnert, 2013). As with most monolingual learners, the vast majority of children who learn two languages during childhood are "typical" learners: with appropriate time and experience they become skilled in the languages used consistently in their environments. However, as with single language learners, a subset of developing bilinguals will be challenged in language due to a breach in their internal cognitive–linguistic processing systems.

Primary language impairment or PLI is a high incidence chronic condition affecting an estimated 5 to 7 percent of monolingual children (Tomblin *et al.*, 1997). PLI is referred to in the literature by various names, including specific language impairment (SLI), developmental language disorder, and language-based learning disability. Although there is clear evidence of genetic, neurologic and subtle cognitive correlates, the cause of PLI is unknown (Leonard *et al.*, 2007). PLI is identified on the basis of low language performance in the face of otherwise typical development. Children with PLI show a protracted period of language development, are at high risk for reading and academic failure and, by definition, perform significantly below their age- and experience-matched peers on various measures of language. For children with PLI, effective treatment is viewed as essential to improve language and, by extension, academic, social, emotional and vocational outcomes. It is generally believed that rates of PLI are similar in monolingual and bilingual children. Therefore, all else being equal, we can reasonably predict that 5 to 7 percent of L2 learners will have PLI for which treatment is needed to ameliorate negative long-term effects.

This chapter has three main sections. In the first section I present general characteristics of L2 learners with PLI. The second section reviews studies that directly investigate treatment effects in developing bilinguals with PLI. In the final section, options are discussed for moving available research into clinical actions followed by a brief discussion of research needs.

Bilingual learners with PLI

There are five basic findings that guide practical understanding of bilingual learners with PLI. First, for bilingual learners with PLI, both languages are affected. Although the precise cause of PLI is not known, it is presumed due to child internal factors, either specific to language or in more general cognitive mechanisms, interacting with language-learning demands. The weakness in the child's underlying cognitive–linguistic system manifests in both the L1 and L2 of dual-language learners. For this chronic, developmental condition, it is not the case that one language may be spared while the other is impaired.

Second, available evidence indicates that dual-language learners with PLI do not fare worse than monolingual children with PLI, all else being equal. That is, monolingual children with PLI learn and process one language less efficiently than their typically developing monolingual age peers. Bilingual children with PLI are less efficient in two languages, as compared to unaffected peers with similar cultural, linguistic and educational experiences. However, dual-language learners with PLI are apparently no more impaired than their monolingual peers with PLI, all else being equal (Armon-Lotem, 2010; Kohnert and Ebert, 2010; Windsor *et al.*, 2010). Bilingual environments do not seem to exacerbate the underlying condition.

Third, bilingual learners with developmental PLI have the same social contexts as typically developing bilingual children. These social contexts, including opportunities to use language for diverse, meaningful purposes and the social prestige associated with each language, affect children's proficiency and preferences for L1 and L2 (Kohnert and Pham, 2010). The common finding for typically developing school-age bilingual learners in the U.S. is that skills in a home language plateau or increase slowly alongside a rapid upward trajectory in English. This differential L1–L2 growth pattern results in greater proficiency in English, the L2, by early to mid-childhood for typically developing bilinguals (Kohnert and Bates, 2002; Pham and Kohnert, 2013; Sheng *et al.*, 2011). For children with PLI, the L2 is acquired slowly due to the underlying impairment and the L1, which is less developed than that of their unaffected peers at the time L2 is introduced, is vulnerable and subject to decline in the absence of robust support (e.g., Ebert *et al.*, in press; Jacobson and Walden, 2013).

The fourth finding that guides practical understanding of bilingual PLI is that the condition cannot be identified based on monolingual standards, in either the L1 or the L2 (e.g., Kohnert, 2010; Kohnert *et al.*, 2009). Rather, the determination of what constitutes impairment in the combined language system is done with reference to peers with similar language-learning experiences. Bilingual learners with PLI have a history of delayed acquisition in both languages and perform significantly below their typically developing bilingual peers in various areas of language comprehension and production, including lexical-semantics, grammar, and discourse (Ebert *et al.*, in press; Jacobson and Walden, 2013; Sheng *et al.*, 2012). School-age L2 learners with PLI also perform more poorly than their unaffected bilingual age peers on some language processing and dynamic assessment tasks, including nonword repetition, rapid automatic naming, and word learning (e.g., Windsor *et al.*, 2010). To identify PLI in bilingual learners, legal and professional mandates require the collection of data in both languages using various measures and interpreting this information with respect to the child's experiences in the L1 and L2 (see Kohnert, 2013 for clinical assessment information).

The fifth finding that supports clinical understanding of developing bilingual learners with PLI relates to nonlinguistic cognitive skills. Although PLI is defined by significantly lower than expected language ability, the PLI profile includes subtle processing inefficiencies that extend to the general cognitive domain. Research clearly demonstrates three main areas of cognitive processing weakness in monolingual children with PLI; sustained/selective attention, speed of information processing and working memory (Ebert and Kohnert, 2011; Kohnert *et al.*, 2009; Leonard *et al.*, 2007; see also the Montgomery *et al.* chapter, this volume). Bilingual children with PLI demonstrate the same subclinical cognitive processing weaknesses as monolingual children with PLI. It is unclear if these well-documented, albeit subtle, cognitive processing weaknesses are causally related to the more obvious lags in language or simply correlated. Cognitive theories of language and the Limited Processing Capacity view of PLI (Leonard *et al.*, 2007) hypothesize that subtle weaknesses in attention, processing speed, and working memory form a core part of PLI and directly contribute to the more obvious language impairment (Kohnert and Ebert, 2010). If this is the case, consideration of basic cognitive processing skills along with language would be indicated in PLI treatment.

In summary, bilingual learners with PLI have significant delays in the acquisition and use of two languages, comparable to the challenges monolingual children with PLI face in one language. Subtle inefficiencies in basic cognitive systems are part of the PLI profile. PLI in bilingual learners is identified with respect to standards for dual-language learners with similar experiences; within-child differences in L1 and L2 proficiency levels are expected.

Evidence: Peer-reviewed treatment studies of bilingual PLI

Behavioral treatment is planned action intended to produce a positive effect or favorably alter the course of a disorder or condition. Interventionists train specific communicative or cognitive behaviors through skilled manipulation of selected stimuli. This training is intended to help children with PLI acquire skills which will ultimately support long-term functional language outcomes. Treatment studies focus on specific training protocols and measure response to this training in terms of discrete treatment effects.

Eight peer-reviewed studies that directly investigate treatment outcomes in bilingual learners with PLI are summarized in Table 28.1. These studies vary in methodology and research objectives. Four of the studies use single-subject experimental design (Ebert *et al.*, 2012; Perozzi, 1985; Pham *et al.*, 2011; Thordardottir *et al.*, 1997), one compares outcomes between two participant groups (Perozzi and Sanchez, 1992), and three studies are randomized clinical trials (Ebert *et al.*, 2014; Pham *et al.*, in press; Restrepo *et al.*, 2013). Half of these studies investigate direct treatment effects (Perozzi, 1985; Perozzi and Sanchez, 1992; Restrepo *et al.*, 2013; Thordardottir *et al.*, 1997) and half investigate generalized effects or improvements that go beyond items and tasks directly included in training activities (Ebert *et al.*, 2012 and 2014; Pham *et al.*, 2011 and in press). One study investigates the extent to which generalized effects are maintained three months after the discontinuation of treatment (Pham *et al.*, in press). All study participants have PLI, range in age from 4 to 11 years and live in the U.S. where English is the majority language of the broader community. Participants in six of the studies are children learning Spanish as their L1; exceptions are Pham *et al.* (2011) and Thordardottir *et al.*, (1997).

Table 28.1 Treatment studies of bilingual learners with PLI.

Study	Design	Number of Participants with PLI (Age)	Languages	Treatment Conditions
Perozzi, 1986	SSED	2 (4 to 5 yrs)	Spanish; English	English Vocabulary; Bilingual Vocabulary
Perozzi and Sanchez, 1992	Group	38* (1st grade)	Spanish; English	English Vocabulary; Bilingual Vocabulary
Thordardottir et al., 1997	SSED	1 (4 yrs)	Icelandic; English	English Vocabulary; Bilingual Vocabulary
Pham et al., 2011	SSED	1 (4 yrs)	Vietnamese; English	English Vocabulary; Bilingual Vocabulary
Ebert et al., 2012	SSED	2 (7 and 8 yrs)	Spanish; English	Nonlinguistic Cognitive Processing (speed, attention)
Restrepo et al., 2013	RCT	202 (4 to 5 yrs)	Spanish; English	English Vocabulary; English Math; Bilingual Vocabulary; Bilingual Math
Ebert et al., 2013	RCT	59 (5 to 11 yrs)	Spanish; English	English Language; Bilingual Language; Nonlinguistic Cognitive Processing
Pham et al., 2014	RCT	48 (5 to 11 yrs)	Spanish; English	English Language; Bilingual Language; Nonlinguistic Cognitive Processing

Note: SSED = Single Subject Experimental Design; RCT = Randomized Clinical Trial; * indicates participants in Perozzi and Sanchez, 1992 were classified as "low language." It is unclear if participants met the clinical definition of PLI.

Vocabulary

The focus in five of the eight studies is vocabulary (Perozzi, 1985; Perozzi and Sanchez, 1992; Pham *et al.*, 2011; Restrepo *et al.*, 2013; Thordardottir *et al.*, 1997), both in training and as the dependent variable to determine treatment success. The key question is whether participants learn English more efficiently when training is administered only in English (monolingual condition) as compared to training administered in both the child's languages (bilingual condition). Importantly, training time for each condition is the same. That is, bilingual training divides the allotted treatment time between two languages; monolingual training devotes the entire time to English vocabulary training.

In a very large randomized clinical trial, Restrepo and colleagues (2013) divided 202 bilingual preschoolers with PLI (age 4;0–5;4) into four different treatment conditions: English vocabulary, Spanish–English vocabulary, English math or bilingual math training. Interventionists were trained bilingual graduate students and children were grouped for training sessions. For the two groups of children assigned to vocabulary training (i.e., English-only or bilingual), post-training performance was comparable on English vocabulary words and better than the two groups assigned to the math conditions. In addition, participants assigned to the bilingual vocabulary training condition outperformed all others on Spanish vocabulary words. Although this study was limited to treatment effects on trained vocabulary items, results clearly indicate that dual-language support does not take away from English-learning and that bilingual learners with PLI benefit from dual-language training. Findings replicate and extend previous bilingual PLI vocabulary treatment studies.

Pham and colleagues used single case experimental design to investigate vocabulary learning and generalization in monolingual and bilingual conditions (Pham *et al.*, 2011). The participant was a 4-year-old boy with PLI learning Vietnamese (L1) and English (L2). What was unique in this study was that training stimuli and procedures were developed by a bilingual (Vietnamese–English) speech–language pathologist but implemented by an English-only speaking paraprofessional using computer interface. Researchers found that bilingual (Vietnamese–English) and monolingual (English-only) training conditions yielded comparable gains in English vocabulary comprehension. The bilingual condition also improved the child's Vietnamese vocabulary and his attention to therapeutic activities in English (Pham *et al.*, 2011). This study demonstrated the utility of technology and strategic partnerships to address clinician–client language mismatch to support bilingual development in children with PLI.

Cognition and language

As noted in the previous section, substantial evidence points to the presence of subtle weaknesses in attention, speed of processing and working memory in children with PLI. If these cognitive processes are both modifiable and contribute directly to the language deficits that characterize PLI, then training some basic cognitive skills could generalize to improvement in both languages in bilingual PLI. To test this premise, Ebert and colleagues trained processing speed and sustained selective attention in two Spanish–English bilingual children with PLI (Ebert *et al.*, 2012). The study followed a single-subject multiple baseline design, with both repeated measures and standardized language tasks as pre- and post-treatment outcome measures. The interventionist was a monolingual English-speaking speech–language pathologist. Results showed that both participants made significant gains in nonlinguistic cognitive processing skills, measuring speed and sustained attention as well as on several language measures in Spanish and English. This finding of cross-domain generalization, with positive effects on language resulting from nonlinguistic cognitive processing training, was consistent with a previous study with two monolingual English speakers with PLI (Ebert and Kohnert, 2009). Cross-domain generalization in the opposite direction is also conceivable. That is, treating language skills could result in improved cognitive processing skills.

In a recent randomized clinical trial, Ebert *et al.* (2014) investigated generalized treatment effects for 59 school-age (5;6 to 11;3 years) Spanish–English learners with moderate to severe PLI. Participants were randomly assigned to one of three different treatment conditions. The three treatment conditions were English-only, bilingual (Spanish and English), and nonlinguistic cognitive processing. There was also a deferred treatment condition. Participants in each of the three active treatment conditions received a six week course of intensive training administered by either monolingual or bilingual speech–language pathologists. Children were in pairs or triads for treatment sessions. For all three treatment conditions, procedures were a combination of computer and interactive activities which used different training stimuli and targets. In the English-only treatment condition, training activities focused on increasing English vocabulary, grammar, and listening comprehension. In the bilingual treatment condition, activities trained vocabulary, grammar and listening comprehension in both Spanish and English in the same session. In the nonlinguistic cognitive processing treatment condition, training activities were designed to build attention and response speed using nonlinguistic auditory and visual stimuli (e.g., lights, sounds). The types of procedures, length and intensity of training were constant across the three treatment conditions. Pre- and post-treatment assessments measured generalized change in a wide variety of English, Spanish and nonlinguistic cognitive processing skills. Analyses examined generalized treatment effects within each condition as well as comparative changes in generalized skills between the assigned treatment conditions.

Participants in each of the three treatment conditions demonstrated positive training effects (Ebert *et al.*, 2014). That is, all participants improved on the stimuli and tasks used in training. However, the main study purpose was to identify potential generalized effects. Results showed some generalization within each condition on standardized, criterion referenced, and experimental tasks. Participants in the English-only treatment improved their performance on several English measures and participants in the bilingual treatment improved their performance on several measures in Spanish (L1) and English (L2). Children assigned to the nonlinguistic cognitive processing condition improved performance on untrained cognitive processing measures. There was also evidence of some bidirectional cross-domain generalization. For example, participants in the nonlinguistic cognitive processing treatment improved performance on some English and Spanish measures and English-only treatment participants made significant improvements on some basic cognitive processing measures. There was limited generalization from L2 (English treatment) to Spanish. Indeed, Spanish (L1) treatment effects were smaller than those in English for participants in all three treatment conditions. In terms of relative change, the English-only condition resulted in greater treatment effects in English and the bilingual condition yielded more improvement in Spanish. However, head-to-head comparisons between treatment conditions yielded few statistically significant differences in generalized treatment effects.

In a follow-up study, researchers investigated whether generalized treatment effects from the randomized clinical trial with school-age children with PLI were maintained three months after treatment had been discontinued (Pham *et al.*, in press). Participants were 48 children with PLI from the original study (Ebert *et al.*, 2014). Investigators re-administered each Spanish, English, and cognitive test measures three months after completion of the experimental treatments. Hierarchical linear models were calculated for each measure using pre-treatment testing, post-treatment testing, and follow-up test scores to estimate change trajectories and compare outcomes between treatment conditions. A main finding was that participants assigned to each treatment condition – English-only, bilingual, and nonlinguistic cognitive processing – either maintained skills or showed some generalized improvement at follow-up testing. For English outcome measures, there were comparable, positive rates of change for participants in the English-only and bilingual conditions.

In summary, combined treatment studies with L2 learners with PLI show that bilingual treatment does not detract from outcomes in English (L2), the language of the majority community for study participants. In addition, bilingual treatments advance skills in the L1. It is also the case that many different treatment strategies promote learning in bilingual learners with PLI. There is also some evidence of generalized treatment effects across languages and cognitive–linguistic domains under certain therapeutic conditions, although generalized effects are by no means ubiquitous. By design, experimental treatment studies employ a narrow set of procedures, measure effects objectively, and attempt to control the influence of factors external to the prescribed treatment. In contrast, treatment plans implemented in clinical and educational settings are multi-pronged and designed to promote interactions among home, school and clinical activities. An effective treatment plan will incorporate several direct and indirect strategies and foci implemented simultaneously.

Clinical extensions and research needs

Monolingual children with PLI need one language to be successful in their different communicative environments; bilingual children with PLI need two languages. When the child's internal cognitive–linguistic system is weak, more, not fewer, opportunities in L1 (as well as L2) are needed. The reality is, however, that minority L1 learners with disabilities generally receive fewer instructional opportunities in the L1 than their typically developing minority L1 peers (Zehler *et al.*, 2003). This is due, in part, to the significant mismatch between the languages spoken by children with PLI and the professionals who serve them. Consider that about 5 percent of the 134,100 speech–language pathologists in the U.S. are proficient in a language other than English; Spanish is the other language for just under half of these bilingual professionals (American Speech, Language, Hearing Association [ASHA] 2012; U.S. Bureau of Labor Statistics, 2014). Over 20 percent of the nation's estimated 332 million people speak a language other than English at home; Spanish is the "other than English" home language for about 37 million U.S. residents (U.S. Census Bureau, 2013). Extrapolating from these figures, the conservative ratio of Spanish–English bilingual speech–language pathologists to Spanish L1 speakers in the U.S. is 1 to 11,000 as compared to a ratio of roughly 1 to 2,500 among the general U.S. population. Proportionally the mismatch is far greater for Cantonese, Hmong, Korean, Russian, Somali, or Vietnamese speakers. Distributional limitations further complicate matters as the handful of Vietnamese- or Cantonese-speaking professionals may not be in the same geographic region as the individuals in need of their bilingual clinical services. Given the extent of the potential mismatches between clinician and child languages, indirect methods for supporting L1 as well as expanded roles for bilingual professionals are needed.

Professional strategies to bridge a language gap

The evidence points to several strategies monolingual clinicians can employ to promote skills in the L1 as well as the L2 in bilingual learners with PLI. First, clinicians may enlist additional partners in the process. Restrepo *et al.* (2013) trained bilingual graduate students to administer vocabulary treatment in Spanish and English. In clinical and educational settings, speech–

language pathologists may recruit bilingual paraprofessionals, high school students, family members, cultural liaisons, college students in service learning programs, or other community partners. With training and supervision, these bilingual surrogates may provide authentic language practice opportunities and administer certain aspects of a multi-pronged treatment program in the L1. Monolingual clinicians may collaborate with heritage or foreign language teachers, English as Second Language (ESL) educators, and bilingual speech–language pathologists to develop stimuli and tasks.

Second, speech–language pathologists may use technology to provide diverse learning opportunities in the L1. In the bilingual treatment condition, Ebert *et al.* (2014) used computer programs developed for vocabulary learning and selected exercises from the foreign language-learning software, Rosetta Stone (2005), as part of their Spanish training protocol. In Pham *et al.* (2011), a monolingual paraprofessional used bilingual software to train vocabulary comprehension in Vietnamese and English. These studies demonstrate that a monolingual clinician's careful vetting and judicious use of technology and computer programs can provide diverse learning and practice opportunities in the home language. Although the number of apps, software and internet resources are greatest for Spanish, educational materials can be found for many other languages (Kohnert, 2013; Kohnert and Derr, 2012).

A third strategy monolingual clinicians may employ to enhance skills in the L1 of bilingual learners with PLI is to incorporate tasks designed to shore up the cognitive underpinning or correlates of all languages. Ebert and colleagues (Ebert and Kohnert, 2009; Ebert *et al.*, 2012, 2014) trained nonlinguistic cognitive processing tasks exclusively, then measured generalized effects to language to test hypothesized cross-domain associations. Clinically, the recommendation is to supplement, not supplant, language activities with additional emphasis on the cognitive processes used in the service of language. Activities that focus on sustained or selective attention, processing speed, and working memory are many and varied. Some are multi-leveled activities designed specifically to be used with clients with cognitive or communication impairments (e.g., Scarry-Larkin and Price, 2007); others are commercially available as games or general cognitive enhancement activities (see Kohnert, 2013 for discussion). When used therapeutically, the clinician explicitly links procedures and purpose to increase the child's "buy-in" and understanding. Language is used in tandem with each aspect of the activities to maximize communicative outcomes. Some of these activities may also be used with bilingual partners as the basis for social interaction in the L1.

Home practice or extension activities were not included in the experimental treatment studies reviewed, likely because they would confound interpretation of results related to the main research questions. However, it may be possible for monolingual clinicians to develop home practice programs combining various training procedures to promote L1 use and enhance generalization across settings and languages. For example, home programs may direct children and family members to translate key words or concepts from English into the L1, using all resources available, to create a bilingual dictionary or audio journal. Picture books from the clinical setting may be copied for home use with older siblings or parents as partners to encourage reinforcing the same story across languages. (See Kohnert, 2013 for additional discussion of treatment strategies.)

Bilingual/language-matched professionals: Expanded roles

Bilingual speech–language pathologists are operationally defined by ASHA (1989) as those professionals who have "near-native proficiency" in two or more languages. Although the percentage of bilingual speech–language pathologists has increased in recent years, the language gap between professionals and the broader population will likely persist for the foreseeable future. As such, some expansion of professional roles for bilingual speech-language pathologists is indicated. For example, bilingual professionals may use telepractice as a technique to mentor colleagues long-distance or to work directly with bilingual family members or older children with PLI (Pham, 2012).

Bilingual professionals may also develop treatment materials in other languages (cf. Pham *et al.*, 2011), provide educational programs to families which would support home practice in L1, and monitor treatment outcomes in the L1 for children with PLI. To maximize clinicians' time as well as improve treatment outcomes, professionals may treat bilingual children with PLI in pairs or small groups rather than individually. The randomized clinical trials with bilingual children with PLI were successful in providing training to participants in small group settings (Ebert *et al.*, 2014; Restrepo *et al.*, 2013). The grouping of bilingual children for language and cognitive training may support outcomes by encouraging camaraderie and competition among participants as well as provide additional opportunities to use L1 (Kohnert, 2013).

Research needs

Although the amount and quality of research on L2 learners with PLI has increased exponentially over the past decade, the reality is that high quality treatment studies with developing bilinguals are relatively few. Randomized clinical trials are considered the "gold standard" of treatment efficacy evidence (Oxford Centre for Evidence-Based Medicine, 2001). Yet these types of studies are extraordinarily resource intensive and may not yield definitive answers regarding which treatment is best overall or for a particular child (Ebert *et al.*, 2014; Gillam *et al.*, 2008; see Kohnert, 2013 for discussion). Single case experimental designs are likely the most expeditious way to develop a highly credible and robust treatment literature on bilingual individuals with PLI.

To date, research questions addressed in bilingual PLI treatment studies have been at the macro level: Does bilingual treatment enhance or interfere with gains in English? Does English (L2) training result in improved L1 skills? Does cognitive treatment generalize to improved performance in one or two languages? Can a monolingual interventionist enhance skills in the L1 and the L2 using bilingual software? Studies have provided first-pass answers to these essential questions. The few but high quality bilingual PLI treatment studies provide a firm foundation for moving forward with more nuanced questions.

To improve treatment efficacy with bilingual children with PLI, it is essential to understand the specific factors that promote or limit generalization within and across languages. The transfer of treatment gains from one language to the other as well as from cognition to language is likely constrained by several factors including the child's developmental stage, severity of impairment, attained level of skill in each language, the particular aspect of language considered and, critically, the type of training procedures used (Kohnert, 2010). Additional research in this area is essential as it lies at the heart of educational and clinical treatment issues.

References

American Speech, Language, Hearing Association, ASHA (1989), "Bilingual service provider database", available at: www.asha.org/forms/bilingual-service-provider-form/ (accessed 13 January 2014).
American Speech, Language, Hearing Association, ASHA (2012), "Demographic profile of ASHA members providing bilingual services", available at www.asha.org/uploadedFiles/Demographic-Profile-Bilingual-Spanish-Service-Members.pdf (accessed 13 January 2014).

Armon-Lotem, S. (2010), "Instructive bilingualism: Can bilingual children with specific language impairment rely on one language in learning a second one?", *Applied Psycholinguistics*, Vol. 31, pp. 253–260.

Ebert, K.D. and Kohnert, K. (2009), "Efficacy of nonlinguistic cognitive intervention for school-aged children with language impairment", *Clinical Linguistics and Phonetics*, Vol. 23, pp. 647–664.

Ebert, K.D. and Kohnert, K. (2011), "Sustained attention in children with primary language impairment: A meta-analysis", *Journal of Speech, Language, and Hearing Research*, Vol. 54, pp. 1372–1384.

Ebert, K.D., Rentmeester-Disher, J. and Kohnert, K. (2012), "Nonlinguistic cognitive treatment for bilingual children with primary language impairment", *Clinical Linguistics and Phonetics*, Vol. 26, pp. 485–501.

Ebert, K.D., Kohnert, K., Pham, G., Disher, J. and Payesteh, B. (2014), "Three treatments for bilingual children with primary language impairment: Examining cross-linguistic and cross-domain effects", *Journal of Speech, Language, and Hearing Research*, Vol. 57, pp. 172–186.

Ebert, K.D., Pham, G. and Kohnert, K. (2014), "Lexical profiles of bilingual children with primary language impairment", *Bilingualism: Language and Cognition*, Vol. 17, pp. 766–783.

Gillam, R.B., Loeb, D.F., Hoffman, L.M., Bohman, T., Champlin, C.A., Thibodeau, L. *et al.* (2008), "The efficacy of Fast ForWord Language intervention in school-age children with language impairment: A randomized controlled trial", *Journal of Speech, Language, and Hearing Research*, Vol. 51, pp. 97–119.

Jacobson, P.F. and Walden, P.R. (2013), "Lexical diversity and omission errors as predictors of language ability in the narratives of sequential Spanish–English bilinguals: A cross-language comparison", *American Journal of Speech-Language Pathology*, Vol. 22, pp. 554–565.

Kohnert, K. (2010), "Bilingual children with primary language impairment: Issues, evidence and implications for clinical actions", *Journal of Communication Disorders*, Vol. 43, pp. 456–473.

Kohnert, K. (2013), *Language Disorders in Bilingual Children and Adults*, 2nd edn., Plural, San Diego, CA, U.S.

Kohnert, K. and Bates, E. (2002), "Balancing bilinguals II: Lexical comprehension and cognitive processing in children learning Spanish and English", *Journal of Speech, Language, and Hearing Research*, Vol. 45, pp. 347–359.

Kohnert, K. and Ebert, K.D. (2010), "Beyond morphosyntax in developing bilinguals and specific language impairment", *Applied Psycholinguistics*, Vol. 31, pp. 303–310.

Kohnert, K. and Pham, G. (2010), "The process of acquiring first and second languages", in Shatz, M. and Wilkinson, L. (Eds.), *Preparing to Educate English Language Learners*, Guilford, New York, NY, pp. 48–66.

Kohnert, K. and Derr, A. (2012), "Language intervention with bilingual children", in Goldstein, B. (Ed.), *Bilingual Language Development and Disorders in Spanish-English Speakers*, 2nd edn., Brookes, Baltimore, MD, U.S., pp. 337–363.

Kohnert, K., Windsor, J. and Ebert, K. (2009), "Primary or 'specific' language impairment and children learning a second language", *Brain and Language*, Vol. 109, pp. 101–111.

Leonard, L., Ellis Weismer, S., Miller, C.A., Francis, D.J., Tomblin, J.B. and Kail, R.V. (2007), "Speed of processing, working memory, and language impairment in children", *Journal of Speech, Language, and Hearing Research*, Vol. 50, pp. 408–428.

Oxford Centre for Evidence-Based Medicine. (2001), "Levels of evidence and grades of recommendation", available at: www.Cebm.net/levels_of_evidence.asp (accessed 13 January 2014).

Perozzi, J.A. (1985), "A pilot study of language facilitation for bilingual, language-handicapped children: Theoretical and intervention implications", *Journal of Speech and Hearing Disorders*, Vol. 50, pp. 403–406.

Perozzi, J.A. and Sanchez, M.C. (1992), "The effect of instruction in L1 on receptive acquisition of L2 for bilingual children with language delay", *Language, Speech, and Hearing Services in Schools*, Vol. 23, pp. 348–352.

Pham, G. (2014), "Addressing less common languages via telepractice: a case example with Vietnamese", *Perspectives on Culturally and Linguistically Diverse Populations*, Vol. 19, pp. 77–84.

Pham, G. and Kohnert, K. (2013), "A longitudinal study of lexical development in children learning Vietnamese and English", *Child Development*, Vol. 85, pp. 767–782.

Pham, G. and Kohnert, K. (2014), "A longitudinal study of lexical development in children learning Vietnamese and English", *Child Development*, Vol. 85, No. 2, pp. 767–782.

Pham, G., Kohnert, K. and Mann, D. (2011), "Addressing clinician-client mismatch: Language intervention with a bilingual Vietnamese-English preschooler", *Language, Speech and Hearing Services in School*, Vol. 42, pp. 408–422.

Pham, G., Ebert, K.D. and Kohnert, K. (in press), "Bilingual children with primary language impairment: Three months after treatment", *International Journal of Language and Communicative Disorders*.

Restrepo, M.A., Morgan, G. and Thompson, M. (2013), "The efficacy of vocabulary intervention for dual language learners with language impairment", *Journal of Speech, Language, and Hearing Research*, Vol. 56, pp. 748–765.

Rosetta Stone (2005), Spanish (Latin America, Version 2) [Computer software]. Arlington, VA, U.S.: Author.

Scarry-Larkin, M. and Price, E. (2007), *LocuTour Multimedia Attention and Memory: Volume II* (computer software), Learning Fundamentals, San Luis Obispo, CA, U.S.

Sheng, L., Lu, Y. and Kan, P.F. (2011), "Lexical development in Mandarin-English bilingual children", *Bilingualism: Language and Cognition*, Vol. 14, pp. 579–587.

Sheng, L., Peña, E.D., Bedore, L.M. and Fiestas, C.E. (2012), "Semantic deficits in Spanish-English bilingual children with language impairment", *Journal of Speech, Language, and Hearing Research*, Vol. 55, pp. 1–15.

Thordardottir, E. (2010), "Towards evidence-based practice in language intervention for bilingual children", *Journal of Communication Disorders*, Vol. 43, pp. 523–537.

Thordardottir, E., Ellis Weismer, S. and Smith, M. (1997), "Vocabulary learning in bilingual and monolingual clinical intervention", *Child Language Teaching and Therapy*, Vol. 13, No. 3, pp. 215–227.

Tomblin, J.B., Records, N.L., Buckwalter, P., Zhang, X., Smith, E. and O'Brien, M. (1997), "Prevalence of specific language impairment in kindergarten children", *Journal of Speech, Language, and Hearing Research*, Vol. 40, pp. 1245–1260.

U.S. Bureau of Labor Statistics (2014), "Occupational Outlook Handbook", available at: www.bls.gov/ooh/Healthcare/Speech-language-pathologists.htm (accessed 13 January 2014).

U.S. Census Bureau (2013), "State and County Quick Facts", available at http://quickfacts.census.gov/qfd/states/00000.html (accessed 13 January 2014).

Windsor, J., Kohnert, K., Lobitz, K. and Pham, G. (2010), "Cross-language nonword repetition by bilingual and monolingual children", *Journal of Speech-Language Pathology*, Vol. 19, pp. 298–310.

Zehler, A., Fleischman, H., Hopstock, P., Stephenson, T., Pendzick, M. and Sapru, S. (2003), *Policy report: Summary of findings related to LEP and SPED-LEP students* (Report submitted to U.S. Department of Education, Office of English Language Acquisition, Language Enhancement, and Academic Achievement of Limited English Proficient Students). Development Associates, Arlington, VA, U.S.

29

SECOND LANGUAGE LITERACY LEARNING AND SOCIAL IDENTITY

A focus on writing

Robin L. Danzak

When I go to Puerto Rico I wanna like, demostrarle a everyone like, I like this country, I like speaking and everything. My friend's like, "Oh now you going to be gringa and everything," and I'm like, "Yeah, but I'm going to be bilingüe because I going to speak two language." I feel good.

Nina (a pseudonym), bilingual student in Grade 6

Within the dynamic and complex context of today's schools, writing can serve as a means to engage students in collaboration, real-world application, and self-expression. Additionally, learning to construct effective texts supports students' development of academic language, the key to their empowerment in the world of schooling. This chapter explores the connections between writing and identity for bilingual students, defined here as students who have a need to utilize more than one language in their daily lives (Kohnert, 2008). For bilingual students in the U.S., the mastery of spoken and written academic English is critical, as it remains the language of power in this country (Hakuta, 2011; Nieto, 2010).

To illustrate the relationship between identity and bilingual writing, the research and theories discussed in this chapter are applied to the case of Nina and her emerging bilingual writing. Nina is a recently arrived, Puerto Rican student attending an English for Speakers of Other Languages (ESOL) program at a public middle school in Florida. She has not been identified as having a language learning disability; nonetheless, due to limited experience with English, she struggles with academic language including lexical and syntactic complexity, spelling, and text structure.

Questions explored in the chapter include how to understand the strengths and challenges of Nina's bilingual text composition in relationship to her identity as a bilingual student and writer, and the type of writing theory that might best frame this process. To address this inquiry, current trends in writing research in general and bilingual writing in particular are reviewed, with an emphasis on shifting frameworks and hybrid models, followed by challenges and new directions for bilingual writing assessment. Next, Nina and the project in which she participated are described. Finally, new paradigms and their practice implications are applied to Nina's bilingual writing and identity.

Changing paradigms in writing research

The worlds of communication, education, and socialization are changing rapidly and therefore, so are literacies. As new technologies and ways to learn and interact emerge, new literacies are required to participate in them (e.g., see Castek *et al.*, 2011, regarding skills involved in online literacies), inspiring new ways of thinking about how and why we learn and apply reading and writing practices in our daily lives. In this light, and relevant to this chapter, theories of writing appear to be shifting from more dichotomous to more inclusive, hybrid models.

Blending frames: The integration of cognitive and sociocultural writing models

Previous approaches to writing research tended to align either with a cognitive–constructivist or a sociocultural framework (for elaboration, see the Stone chapter, this volume). Early cognitive frameworks focused on the writer's memory, attention, organization, knowledge of the topic, and writing strategies as these affected the stages of planning, translating, and reviewing (Bereiter and Scardamalia, 1987; Flower and Hayes, 1981). More recently, Hayes and Berninger (2014) proposed a three-tiered framework of cognitive processes that are integrated in writing: a) the resource level, involving general cognitive resources including working and long-term memory, attention, and reading skills; b) the process level, focusing on the text composition process – brainstorming, transcribing, and evaluating – as well as the task environment; and c) the control level, emphasizing task initiation, goal-setting, and writing schemas.

In contrast to cognitive approaches, sociocultural frameworks emphasized writing as a social practice, inseparable from its historical, sociocultural, and political contexts (Fisher, 2012; Moll *et al.*, 2001). Sociocultural frameworks, including new literacy theories (Street, 1993), also consider the role of societal and linguistic power structures in literacy practices. Along these lines, a critical literacy framework, stemming from critical pedagogy (Freire, 1998; Freire and Macedo, 1987), views literacy as a vehicle to empower individuals to question, critique, and overcome social injustices (Johnson and Rosario-Ramos, 2012; Luke, 2012). In summary, on the continuum from cognitive to sociocultural writing theories, the former emphasize text generation, processing, procedural facilitation, and goals, while the latter focus on literacy practices, context, variation, power, and justice.

As an alternative to this dichotomous perspective, writing researchers have begun to acknowledge the value of blended or hybrid approaches. For example, González and Hunt-Gómez (2011) introduced a "metasociocognitive model" for writing development that integrates cognitive, emotional, and sociocultural aspects of text composition. This model addresses metacognitive components (procedural, declarative, and conditional knowledge), self-control of emotions, extrinsic and intrinsic motivation, and creative capacity; all viewed as integrated with cultural identity and self-concept. Thus, writing was framed as both a cultural tool and a contributor to the author's cultural identity. An example of how this hybrid perspective might be applied to research is Serna's (2009) qualitative study that examined bilingual, Grade 4 students' incorporation of linguistic and cultural resources in the context of a process writing instructional approach. Similarly, the study in which Nina took part examined the outcomes of systematic writing strategy instruction within the framework of a critical literacy project. Both of these examples integrate, to some extent, cognitive and sociocultural views of writing.

In another hybrid model, Chandrasegaran (2013) proposed a "socio-cognitive approach" to support bilingual students' development of expository essays, a challenge for many due to the incorporation of content knowledge, logical reasoning, and academic English. With these obstacles in mind, Chandrasegaran (2013) explored the impact of a socio-cognitive instructional strategy that integrated idea generation, planning, and goal development strategies (based on Flower and Hayes, 1981) with sociocultural approaches such as using authentic text models and understanding text purpose, genre, and organization. This model was implemented with 137 bilingual, secondary school students (age 15 years) in English language classes in Singapore. After 14 weeks of the socio-cognitive intervention, pre- and post-intervention essays were scored holistically in the areas of stance support and topicality. Significant improvements were found in both areas in the post-instruction essays. Study limitations included a single pre/post measure and lack of a control group or qualitative data; however, this inquiry suggested the hybrid model has potential for integrating cognitive processes with social practices and cultural contexts in genre-based writing instruction.

Given the challenges of bilingual writers and the power of academic English, it is important to investigate how to best support bilingual students in expository writing development. However, new theories are needed to underpin this developing hybrid research domain.

New directions in conceptualizing bilingual writing

The current bilingual language and literacy model is often criticized for being driven by an English-centric, monolingual perspective that perceives literacy as unidirectional and limits understanding of multilingual writers' resources (e.g., Canagarajah, 2006a). To overturn the monolingualist paradigm, Canagarajah (2006a) proposed a "negotiation model" (p. 590): rather than focusing on one language or the other as a distinct entity, the paramount notion is that multilingual writers "shuttle between" languages and texts.

The negotiation model reflects a translingual conceptualization of literacy, describing languages "not as something we have or have access to but as something we do" (Lu and Horner, 2013, p. 27). In this vein, the negotiation model is a dynamic, process-oriented framework for examining multilingual writing that highlights the writer's versatility rather than stability in either language, and agency rather than passivity in the writing process. Canagarajah (2006a) recommends that multilingual students be taught writing conventions, but should also understand that the rules are dynamic and can be modified or abandoned to express personal interest, identity, and values.

One way that multilinguals can bend the rules is by "code meshing," defined as "a strategy for merging local varieties with Standard Written English in a move toward gradually pluralizing academic writing" (Canagarajah, 2006b, p. 586). Code meshing, more specific than the notion of translanguaging (García, 2009) described below, is the integration of a variety of vernacular, colloquial, and world Englishes, as well as standard/academic English, in writing.

More generally, García (2009) proposed a framework of translanguaging to describe the (oral and written) linguistic behaviors of bilinguals. Like Canagarajah's (2006a) shuttling metaphor, translanguaging can be described as the fluid, strategic mobilization of linguistic resources across communicative contexts; that is, the "*multiple discursive practices* in which bilinguals engage in order to *make sense of their bilingual worlds*" (García, 2009, p. 45, author's italics). Translanguaging both challenges the monolingualist perspective and supports what Paris (2012) terms culturally sustaining pedagogy, an approach that "seeks to perpetuate and foster – to sustain – linguistic, literate, and cultural pluralism as part of the democratic project of schooling" (p. 95). Nina, for example, demonstrates translanguaging and code meshing when she applies a text-planning strategy in Spanish, and then composes a persuasive essay in English by blending more oral, colloquial forms with emerging academic features.

Considering the unique and varied experiences and abilities of bilingual students, as well as the continued need for more research in this area, the ways that we understand and investigate bilingual writing can benefit from novel, hybrid frames of inquiry and more inclusive, new directions in how bilingual writing is defined and observed. However, to apply these innovative conceptualizations to pedagogy and research, hybrid approaches to assessment are also needed.

Hybrid frames for the assessment of bilingual writing

Many questions arise in considering how to appropriately assess bilingual writing. For example, what types of writing should be used to evaluate a bilingual student's academic language skills? What can be learned about bilingual students' identities through their writing and its assessment? Finally, how might the work of a bilingual student, like Nina, who uses translanguaging and code meshing in writing, be adequately and practically assessed in a classroom context? Three approaches are discussed.

Academic literacies approach

Dutro and colleagues (2013) critiqued the notion that standardized writing scores can adequately reflect students' text composition capabilities inside and outside the classroom. Arguing that high-stakes testing sets up a binary and artificial notion of competence (i.e., proficient vs. not-proficient), these authors applied a framework of positioning theory and an academic literacies perspective to inquire into the written texts, writing practices, discourse on writing, and writing identities of four diverse students attending Grades 4 and 5 in an urban, public school over one year. Although the authors only identified one of the participants as bilingual, all were designated with hyphenated ethnic identities (e.g., Mexican-American), indicating potential multilingual home/community contexts.

The academic literacies perspective contends that school writing is necessarily situated in classroom culture, students' social relationships, experiences, cultural resources, and learner identities. Within this framework, the positioning lens provides a means to explore how the students use written language and classroom discourse to position themselves and be positioned, offering a more holistic, hybrid assessment of their writing. Specifically, texts composed for both district- and state-level standardized tests were reassessed in conjunction with the district/state proficiency scores, classroom observations, student interviews, and teacher comments about each student. Ultimately, the authors contended that institutionalized views of writing – i.e., views based on test scores – extract students from more authentic discourses that incorporate identities, lived experiences, and sociocultural contexts into students' development as writers and their written products. This is particularly the case for bilingual students, like Nina, who may use "non-standard" linguistic and text-organization practices as they are developing their academic English language proficiencies.

Mixed methods approach

Similarly framed in a biliteracy approach, Butvilofsky and Sparrow (2012) used mixed methods (i.e., the integration of both quantitative and qualitative data and analyses) to explore the application of a Spanish–English biliterate writing rubric as utilized by teachers of bilingual students in Grades 1–5. The purpose was to examine and identify potential issues in training teachers to apply this approach in the real-life classroom context of emerging biliteracy. The authors contended that teachers of bilingual students must learn to effectively assess students' writing in both Spanish and English to avoid making assumptions about their students' abilities and development based on monolingual norms.

Meaning-making approach

From a different perspective, and emphasizing the dialogic and multimodal processes of academic text composition, Bunch and Willett (2013) proposed a meaning-making approach to support and assess content-area academic writing of bilingual students in middle school. Such an approach shifts the focus from "skills discourses" (p. 142) that stress grammar, mechanics, and native speaker norms to "meaning-making resources" (p. 142) (the representation of ideas, experiences, and relationships) and their social purposes. The meaning-making framework was applied to students' persuasive writing in seventh grade social studies. Forty-one essays were coded for five meaning-making devices: a) reference to curriculum content; b) reference to other texts; c) expression of beliefs relevant to the historical context; d) presentation of the writer's personal stance; and e) use of idioms, similes, metaphors, etc. to enrich the writing.

Bunch and Willett (2013) found that, in addition to applying the traditional, five-paragraph essay structure, the students referenced a wide range of texts to support the arguments developed in their writing, including curricular materials and primary and secondary sources, and also utilized stock phrases, similes, and metaphors to express meaning and engage the reader. These findings suggest that, with preparation and support, bilingual students can successfully integrate multiple texts into language, genre, and discourse features to create meaning and enhance their academic text composition skills.

In summary, writing composed by bilingual students, whether produced in the context of one language or in an environment that promotes translanguaging practices, is never truly monolingual in nature and should not be viewed as such. Thus, it would be beneficial to approach bilingual writing from a flexible, dynamic perspective that includes the production of authentic texts and the application of hybrid assessments that consider both academic language skills and meaning-making resources (e.g., Bunch and Willett, 2013) employed by the student.

New paradigms and Nina's writing

Meet Nina

Nina, an outgoing and loquacious girl in Grade 6 (age 11.9 years), was born in Puerto Rico and attended Grades 1–5 there. Before Grade 6, Nina's family moved to Florida, where the primary language of her schooling shifted from Spanish to English. At school, Nina used both languages to communicate with friends and teachers. Her persuasive writing, which shifted from primarily Spanish to primarily English over the course of the project, demonstrated growth in English vocabulary and text organization, but also struggled with sentence structure and spelling.

The project

Data from Nina were collected as part of a project that explored critical literacy and persuasive writing strategy instruction for bilingual students in middle school (Danzak, 2012). Thirty-five students in Grades 6–8 ESOL classes researched topics in immigration and developed multimedia projects to present at a school/community event. Simultaneously, the students participated in six weeks of persuasive writing strategy instruction with STOP and DARE (Harris *et al.*, 2008). STOP, a planning strategy, stands for: Suspend judgment, Take a side, Organize ideas, and Plan more as you write. Students learned to create two-column planning sheets to brainstorm and prioritize arguments for and against issues. DARE, which provides a way to organize persuasive texts, represents: Develop a topic sentence, Add supporting ideas, Reject arguments from the other side, and End with a conclusion. For an additional six weeks, students continued using STOP and DARE while also receiving instruction on sentence and text revision, sentence structure, sentence combining, and vocabulary development.

Before and after each six-week period, the participants composed persuasive texts on immigration issues: a) pre-project, "English only," regarding a fictitious, proposed law requiring that immigrants to the U.S. learn English within one year; b) mid-project "Letter" to a major supermarket chain persuading them to participate in the Fair Food Program in support of Florida farmworkers; c) mid-project "Dream Act," on a proposed law that would facilitate higher education and a path to citizenship for undocumented students; d) mid-project-revised; and e) post-project, on the Children's Act for Responsible Employment, "CARE Act," a proposed law that would modify labor regulations to protect children working in agriculture.

In addition, interviews were conducted with nine focal participants (three in each grade), including Nina, who were selected to represent variation in their number of years living in the U.S. and their observed writing abilities. Interviews discussed the students' reactions to the immigration project and the utility of the strategies taught, and their feelings about writing and its potential to inspire social change. Nina used a combination of English and Spanish in her written texts and interview.

A hybrid approach to Nina's writing

Nina's writing is explored here through a multi-faceted, translingual, resource-based assessment that takes into account three factors: a) Nina's strategic deployment of Spanish and English resources; b) select elements of Bunch and Willett's (2013) meaning-making approach; and c) Nina's application of STOP and DARE (Harris *et al.*, 2008), as demonstrated in examples used to illustrate the first two factors. Nina's response to the project and her identity as a writer, expressed in her interview, are also considered.

Similarly to the participants in the Bunch and Willett (2013) study, Nina's writing was scored with a holistic measure based on Florida's standardized writing assessment (Florida Department of Education, 2011). On this measure, all of Nina's texts received a holistic score of 1 (out of 6). This score indicated that the topic was minimally addressed; nominal organization patterns were demonstrated; minimal development of support was offered; and challenges with word choice, sentence structure, spelling, and mechanics were obvious. These scores alone would indicate that Nina's writing was of poor quality and did not improve in spite of an engaging curriculum and instruction in persuasive writing strategies. However, a closer look suggests that Nina's academic English and writing did in fact mature during the project.

Linguistic resources
Nina considers herself bilingual and stated that she used English and Spanish with equal frequency. However, she rated her oral language abilities to be stronger in Spanish, with reading and writing proficiency equal in both languages. In her interview, which is an excellent example of translanguaging, she explained:

> When I see new vocabulario en inglés I'm like, "What happened here?" Like, I would think that here speak Spanish. Then, cuando yo fui aprendiendo más y más y más, yo vi palabras diferentes que yo iba a buscar en el diccionario.

Using both languages in this excerpt, Nina described the initial shock of hearing new words in English followed by "learning more and more and more" in part by looking up words in the dictionary. It is clear that Nina's oral English is still emerging; however, she has a strong desire to learn and incorporate it to the extent that she is able in conversational and academic contexts.

In her writing, Nina planned and composed "English only" and "Letter" entirely in Spanish. For the mid-point, "Dream Act" essay, she mixed languages to plan (using STOP) and attempted to compose completely in English. In the "for" column of her planning paper, Nina listed two arguments in favor of the Dream Act: a) "Porque Dream Act ayuda a las personas que no tienen papeles" [Because Dream Act helps people that do not have papers]; b) "Because the Dream Act want to help to the others person." These are not separate arguments, but rather a translation of the same basic argument. In her essay, Nina incorporated this as a supporting idea (DARE), but did not develop the argument: "I think they are doing a good job because they help a other person" and later, "I am very praud of Dream Act they save the person who no have paper." However, in her revision of this essay, Nina achieved a clearer understanding of the Dream Act in an informative topic sentence: "Dream Act help the undocumented student to go college." Use of the more precise term, "undocumented student" also represents a lexical development for Nina as, in the first draft, she referenced "others person" and "person who have no paper."

For the post-project essay, Nina again made use of both languages in her planning. This time, however, she listed separate arguments rather than translating a single one: 1) "Children need to help them parents for they may have clothe"; and 2) "los niños enpiensan en diferentes edades" [the children begin (to work) at different ages]. Her final essay also included more lexically specific terms and phrases, such as "Care Act protect children. Care Act be responsable."

These examples suggest that, over the course of the project, Nina experienced growth in her vocabulary (use of more specific lexical items) and overall persuasive text structure (increased use of supporting ideas), suggesting an emerging integration of linguistic and cognitive processes. However, Nina still requires instruction to acquire more complex English syntax and spelling patterns. Her shift from dominant-Spanish to dominant-English in planning and composing also suggests an increase in competence and confidence with English. However, Nina continued to utilize Spanish as a tool for text planning, a translanguaging practice that served to express content knowledge and appropriate application of the STOP strategy.

Meaning making

Because of Nina's emerging English language and struggles with academic text production, it was sometimes unclear whether she had understood the immigration issues presented. However, in her interview, it became evident that Nina had indeed comprehended the key issues discussed, and had become very passionate about their related injustices. For example, when invited to speak freely about her reaction to the project, she was able to synthesize the challenges of being an undocumented immigrant with the inability to attend higher education (Dream Act), the need to work in agriculture to earn an unacceptable wage (Fair Food Program), and the possibility that children of undocumented parents join their parents in the fields to support the family (CARE Act). She stated:

> Quiero ayudar más, aunque sean los niños de así que no trabajen... lo único que quiero es que, aunque sea les den papeles... para que ellos puedan trabajar en uno de estos, y para que estudien más [I want to help more, that the children like that do not work... the only thing I want is that, whatever happens, they get papers, so that they can work in something, and so they can study more].

Glimmers of this understanding and Nina's strong feelings about the issues are also reflected in her writing when examined with the three categories from Bunch and Willett's (2013) meaning-making approach: a) drawing on curriculum and content; b) invoking generally circulating beliefs; and c) getting personal (Bunch and Willett, 2013, p. 149).

Drawing on curriculum and content

Nina included the largest number of statements specific to the course content ($n = 6$) in the final essay on the CARE Act. For example, she included the fact that children are not able to work at age 11 years, but that they can work on a farm at age 12. She also concluded the essay with, "Care Act want to help children for they have school and work at the same time," a solid summary of the bill's purpose that also serves the "End with a conclusion" component of the DARE strategy.

Generally circulating beliefs

Nina again incorporated the greatest number of these beliefs ($n = 7$) in the CARE Act essay. For example, she suggested that parents (and children) would prefer that their children attend school rather than work: "The parent not want that the children work in one farm. Because the children want to be in the school all the hours." The incorporation of generally circulating beliefs supports the composing step, "Add supporting ideas" in the DARE strategy. In general, Nina's supporting ideas offered some understanding of the content; however, they were not well developed. Another example comes from her Dream Act-Revised essay, where she wrote, "When the undocumented student no have papers for pay $350 or more for go to school." Perhaps she meant to express the generally circulating belief that undocumented students pay higher tuition than residents because they are considered out-of-state or international students; however, Nina did not explain or elaborate beyond this single sentence.

Getting personal

Nina used the most personal statements in the mid-project Dream Act essay ($n = 13$), frequently incorporating metacognitive and affective statements such as, "I think, I feel so good about, I am proud of, I don't feel like," throughout the text and its revision. However, in the final, CARE Act essay, Nina was more straightforward in her language choices: "Care Act protect children. Care act be responsible.... The children want to be protected." The only personal element included in this text was the more convincing, metacognitive statement, "I know that the children dont want to work in the farm" (author's emphasis). Nina's diminishing reliance on personal belief statements demonstrates growth in her expository production, as a more impersonal – rather than subjective – stance reflects a closer approximation to academic writing (Chang and Schleppegrell, 2011).

In conclusion, while standardized scores did not reflect Nina's growth as a bilingual writer, the translingual, resource-based assessment demonstrated that she was in fact developing her academic English language skills and persuasive text composition. This assessment, which incorporated quantitative and qualitative data and explored both cognitive and sociocultural aspects of writing and identity, also suggested that Nina had understood the curriculum content on immigration and had become passionate about the issues. Related to these points, her writing reflected increasing self-confidence and, along with the interview, a growing sense of empowerment in using literacy as a means to social change. She stated:

> Yeah, we got a lot of power.... nosotros como estudiantes estamos demostrando a diferentes personas que nosotros queremos que ellos [migrant farmworkers] tengan más comida y

todo [… we as students are demonstrating to different people that we want them to have more food and everything].

Perhaps most importantly, Nina came to identify herself as a writer:

> But now I, like, I write A LOT. … In my house, like, every day. In Puerto Rico I never do that, never. Like, I just write a sentence. My teacher's like, "write a paragraph," a sentence. And then here I write like, a paragraph, then, like, a lot.

The future of writing: It is all bilingual

This chapter explored new theories and assessments for bilingual writing. Applying a translingual, resource-based approach, it examined Nina's emerging social identity as a competent writer as framed through her budding persuasive texts. Just as classrooms and literacies have become more diverse, multimodal, and multilingual, so have the frameworks and practices for understanding and evaluating writing, including the writing of bilingual texts.

The application of novel, hybrid paradigms and a translingual, resource-based assessment to Nina's writing and interview data demonstrated how she strategically activated her (Spanish and English) linguistic resources while learning and identifying with academic content, participating in writing strategy instruction, planning and composing persuasive texts and, finally, reflecting on the overall project and its impact on her as a bilingual writer. Through translanguaging and code-meshing practices, Nina revealed her development as an emerging user of academic English, a persuasive writer, and an empowered student eager to engage in literacy practices that could potentially contribute to social change. Of course, she has only begun the long journey toward becoming a competent writer of academic English, but Nina will continue to benefit from instruction that combines specific writing/language strategies with authentic literacy practices that motivate her to write in a way that embraces her unique linguistic and cultural resources.

Hybrid frameworks and inclusive, resource-based approaches to literacy instruction and assessment should also be considered when working with students with language learning disabilities (LLD) as, similar to bilingual students, children with LLD often struggle with acquiring the features of academic English writing (Simon-Cereijido and Gutiérrez-Clellen, 2014). Overall, as new literacies blossom in global learning and communicative contexts, ways to understand bilingual writing development – and bilingual identities – become paramount. When hybrid-, dual-, and multi- become the norm, in that their designations become invisible or obsolete, this aim will ultimately be achieved.

References

Bereiter, C. and Scardamalia, M. (1987), *The Psychology of Written Composition*. Lawrence Erlbaum, Hillsdale, NJ, U.S.

Bunch, G.C. and Willett, K. (2013), "Writing to mean in middle school: Understanding how second language writers negotiate textually-rich content-area instruction", *Journal of Second Language Writing*, Vol. 22, No. 2, pp. 141–160.

Butvilofsky, S.A. and Sparrow, W.L. (2012), "Training teachers to evaluate emerging bilingual students' biliterate writing", *Language and Education*, Vol. 26, pp. 383–403.

Canagarajah, A.S. (2006a), "Toward a writing pedagogy of shuttling between languages: Learning from multilingual writers", *College English*, Vol. 68, pp. 589–604.

Canagarajah, A.S. (2006b), "The place of world Englishes in composition: Pluralization continued", *College Composition and Communication,* Vol. 57, No. 4, pp. 586–619.

Castek, J., Zawilinski, L., McVerry, G., O'Byrne, I. and Leu, D.J. (2011), "The new literacies of online reading comprehension: New opportunities and challenges for students with learning difficulties", in Wyatt-Smith, C., Elkins, J., and Gunn, S. (Eds.), *Multiple Perspectives on Difficulties in Learning Literacy and Numeracy,* Springer Press, New York, NY, pp. 91–110. Retrieved from www.newliteracies.uconn.edu/pubs.html

Chandrasegaran, A. (2013), "The effect of a socio-cognitive approach to teaching writing on stance support moves and topicality in students' expository essays", *Linguistics and Education,* Vol. 24, pp. 101–111.

Chang, P. and Schleppegrell, M. (2011), "Taking an effective authorial stance in academic writing: Making the linguistic resources explicit for L2 writers in the social sciences", *Journal of English for Academic Purposes,* Vol. 10, pp. 140–151.

Danzak, R.L. (2012), "BUT IT'S JUST ONE CENT! Middle school ELLs practice critical literacy in support of migrant farmworkers", *Journal of Literacy and Social Responsibility,* Vol. 5, pp. 158–176.

Dutro, E., Selland, K. and Bien, A.C. (2013), "Revealing writing, concealing writers: High stakes assessment in an urban elementary classroom", *Journal of Literacy Research,* Vol. 45, pp. 99–141.

Fisher, R. (2012), "Teaching writing: A situated dynamic", *British Educational Research Journal,* Vol. 38, pp. 299–317.

Florida Department of Education (2011), "2012 Florida Comprehensive Assessment Test (FCAT), Writing: Grade 8 persuasive calibration scoring guide", available at http://sharepoint.leon.k12.fl.us/tdc/external/Shared%20Documents/Writing%20Assessments%20Documents/2012%20FCAT%20Writing%20Calibration%20Scoring%20Guides/Grade%208%202012%20Calibration%20Guides/G8%20Persuasive%20Calibration%20Guide.pdf (accessed 1 September 2013).

Flower, L. and Hayes, J.R. (1981), "A cognitive process theory of writing", *College Composition and Communication,* Vol. 32, pp. 365–387.

Freire, P. (1998), *Teachers as Cultural Workers: Letters to Those Who Dare to Teach,* Westview Press, Boulder, CO, U.S.

Freire, P. and Macedo, D. (1987), *Literacy: Reading the Word and the World,* Bergin & Garvey, Westport, CT, U.S.

García, O. (2009), *Bilingual Education in the 21st Century: A Global Perspective,* Wiley-Blackwell, Malden, MA, U.S.

González, R.A. and Hunt-Gómez, C.I. (2011), "Written communication intercultural model: The social and cognitive model", *The International Journal of Interdisciplinary Social Sciences,* Vol. 6, pp. 19–38.

Hakuta, K. (2011), "Educating language minority students and affirming their social rights: Research and practical perspectives", *Educational Researcher,* Vol. 40, pp. 163–174.

Harris, K.R., Graham, S., Mason, L.H. and Friedlander, B. (2008), *Powerful Writing Strategies for All Students,* Paul H. Brookes, Baltimore, MD, U.S.

Hayes, J.R. and Berninger, V.W. (2014), "Cognitive processes in writing: A framework", In B. Arfé, J. Dockrell, and V.W. Berninger, (Eds.), *Writing Development in Children with Hearing Loss, Dyslexia or Oral Language Problems: Implications for Assessment and Instruction,* Oxford University Press, New York, NY, pp. 3–15.

Johnson, L.R. and Rosario-Ramos, E.M. (2012), "The role of educational institutions in the development of critical literacy and transformative action", *Theory Into Practice,* Vol. 51, pp. 49–56.

Kohnert, K. (2008), *Language Disorders in Bilingual Children and Adults,* Plural Publishing, San Diego, CA, U.S.

Lu, M.Z. and Horner, B. (2013), "Translingual literacy and matters of agency", in Canagarajah, A.S. (Ed.), *Literacy as Translingual Practice: Between Communities and Classrooms,* Routledge, New York, NY, pp. 26–38.

Luke, A. (2012), "Critical literacy: Foundational notes", *Theory Into Practice,* Vol. 51, pp. 4–11.

Moll, L., Saez, R. and Dworin, J. (2001), "Exploring biliteracy: Two case examples of writing as a social practice", *Elementary School Journal,* Vol. 101, No. 4, pp. 435–449.

Nieto, S. (2010), *Language, Culture, and Teaching: Critical Perspectives* (2nd edn.), Routledge, New York, NY.

Paris, D. (2012), "Culturally sustaining pedagogy: A needed change in stance, terminology, and practice", *Educational Researcher,* Vol. 41, pp. 93–97.

Serna, C. (2009), "Autores bilingües/bilingual authors: Writing within dual cultural and linguistic repertoires". *Education,* Vol. 130, pp. 78–95.

Simon-Cereijido, G. and Gutiérrez-Clellen, V.F. (2014), "Bilingual education for all: Latino dual language learners with language disabilities", *International Journal of Bilingual Education and Bilingualism,* Vol. 17, pp. 235–254.

Street, B. (1993), "Introduction: The new literacy studies", in Street, B. (Ed.), *Cross-cultural Approaches to Literacy,* Cambridge University Press, Cambridge, UK, pp. 1–21.

30

CONTINUITIES IN THE DEVELOPMENT OF SOCIAL COMMUNICATION

Triadic interactions and language development in children with autism spectrum disorder

Julie Longard and Chris Moore

During the first few years of life, children's ability to communicate undergoes remarkable transformations. From birth, infants are active participants in their social world and they quickly develop the ability to share attention and communicate with meaningful eye contact, facial expressions, gestures, and vocalizations, which eventually develop into more complex forms of verbal language. It is thought that such prelinguistic and linguistic forms of communication are developmentally related because they share a common social interactive structure (Bates, 1979; Moore, 2013). This interactive structure is often termed "triadic" because it involves a dyad composed of the child and their caregiver, along with a third object of interest which shapes the social interaction, such as an amusing toy or interesting object of conversation. The triadic interactive structure is illustrated in Figure 30.1.

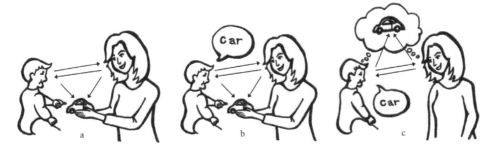

Figure 30.1 Triadic interactions involve a dyad composed of the child and their caregiver, along with a third object of interest, such as an amusing toy or interesting object of conversation, which shapes the social interaction. Early triadic interactions often involve preverbal communication regarding a present object (a), followed by verbal communication about a present object (b), and develop into verbal communication about a non-present or abstract object of interest (c). In order to successfully communicate about a non-present or abstract object, both communication partners must have a shared mental representation of the object of conversation.

This chapter discusses the similarities, or "developmental homology", in the structure of early social interactions and later language development. We follow Moore's (2013) argument that although early social interaction and later language development appear to be different behaviourally, they are structurally and functionally homologous. The homology exists in the common triadic structure in which interaction involves either a concrete or abstract object of interest. This construal suggests that atypical social development, such as is seen in children with Autism Spectrum Disorder (ASD), may adversely impact the development of these triadic interactive structures. As a result, children with ASD often have difficulties with early triadic social interactions as well as later language development. In this chapter, we provide a summary of the homologous development of early triadic interactions and later language development in children with ASD, drawing on examples from relevant research and providing suggestions for future research where the gaps are most evident.

Prelinguistic triadic interactions

Infants engage in social interactions from early in the first year; however, after approximately 6 months of age, they develop the visual and motor coordination to engage with objects in their environment (Moore, 2006). Infants can then begin to engage in more complex triadic interactions, which involve an interplay between two social partners and a third object or idea of interest; for example, a playful interaction between a mother, child, and toy. Triadic interactions are the developmental product of two earlier ways in which infants interact with their worlds: "shared engagement" and "joint attention". Shared engagement requires that both partners are attending toward one another and are actively attempting to elicit a response from the other to enhance the quality of the interaction. In typical development, infants are highly motivated to engage with caregivers and these episodes of shared engagement tend to be strongly and positively emotionally charged. In contrast, joint attention is the simultaneous sharing of attention toward an object by both infant and caregiver. In triadic interactions, both shared engagement and joint attention come together, in that infants become able to use joint attention as a complement to shared engagement. Interactions begin to focus around an object of joint attention, so that infants will try to affect their interactive partner's behaviour toward the object of common interest. Difficulties with triadic interaction in children with ASD may stem from difficulties establishing shared engagement or joint attention or both.

Shared engagement

Typically developing children

Episodes of shared engagement between infants and caregivers require that both social partners direct their attention toward one another. Positive affect is an intrinsically motivating way to secure shared engagement between social partners, and is therefore central to social engagement. Smiling is one of the first social behaviours displayed by infants. Between ages 1 and 2 months, infants' first smiles in response to social stimuli often begin to emerge (Messinger and Fogel, 2007). As development proceeds, positive affect is elicited by progressively more complex sources of stimulation (Sroufe and Waters, 1976). For example, young infants may smile in response to simple social stimuli such as their caregiver's face or voice, whereas older infants may require more complex social interaction such as a game of peek-a-boo to elicit smiling. This allows infants to regulate the amount of social stimulation they are receiving. Shared engagement can help children attain object goals (e.g., increasing smiling toward a caregiver to prolong triadic engagement with a toy of interest) or social goals (e.g., laughing with a caregiver to express pleasure in the current social engagement). Two different types of triadic communicative gestures ("protoimperative" and "protodeclarative"; Bates *et al.*, 1975) are used to attain these different goals. In combination with eye contact, affective expressions, and vocalizations, protoimperative gesturing (such as pointing) is used to attain instrumental goals such as requesting an out of reach object. On the other hand, protodeclarative gesturing (such as showing) is used to attain social goals such as commenting on objects for the sake of social interaction.

Children with ASD

Children with ASD often demonstrate atypical shared engagement (see also chapter by Hutchins and Prelock, this volume). They show less positive affect during episodes of triadic interaction than their typically developing and developmentally delayed peers (Kasari *et al.*, 1990). Children with ASD also show decreased social interest and motivation to interact in social settings. They demonstrate difficulties initiating social gaze compared to typically developing children and other children with developmental disabilities (e.g., Charman *et al.*, 1997). They also tend to prefer familiar objects and show less interest in people compared to typically developing children and children with Down's syndrome (e.g., Adamson *et al.*, 2010, 2012).

According to parental interviews, children with ASD demonstrate limited social engagement and reportedly do not show, give, or point to objects, or follow pointing with their gaze as frequently as children matched on chronological and developmental age (Wimpory *et al.*, 2000). Since children with ASD share less positive affect with social partners and show less interest in interacting with people, they have fewer opportunities for shared engagement, which helps to connect children with their social world and affords them invaluable learning opportunities. Therefore, if children with ASD are participating in fewer instances of shared engagement, this may have significant consequences for their communicative development.

Joint attention

Typically developing children

Joint attention involves the simultaneous sharing of attention toward an object or idea by both infant and caregiver. Like shared engagement, this form of triadic interaction can also help children attain object goals (e.g., protoimperative looking or pointing to request an out of reach object) or social goals (e.g., protodeclarative showing or giving a toy to facilitate social interaction). Eye gaze provides a simple way to establish joint attention with a social partner. This social behaviour undergoes remarkable development over the first year and a half of life:

- 3–6 months: Infants begin to follow an adult's gaze (Moore, 2008).
- 12 months: Infants use an adult's gaze to determine where to look in a scene (Moore, 2008) and they alternate their gaze between an adult and an object of interest. Gestures such as pointing begin (Bates *et al.*, 1975).
- 12–18 months: Communication involving pointing and other gestures during triadic interaction drastically increases (Desrochers *et al.*, 1995).

Interestingly, in a large sample of typically developing and developmentally delayed infants, initiation of joint attention at ages 12 and 18 months predicted language development at age 24 months, when cognitive abilities were controlled for (Mundy *et al.*, 2007). These findings highlight the relationship between early prelinguistic and later linguistic development, both of which rely on a similar underlying triadic structure of interaction.

Children with ASD

Children with ASD are known to have difficulties initiating joint attention and often fail to respond to their social partners' efforts to establish joint attention (see Bruinsma *et al.*, 2004; Meindl and Cannella-Malone, 2011). In fact, a lack of joint attention during the first year of life is among the key indications of ASD (Baron-Cohen *et al.*, 1992). In children with ASD, initiating joint attention is significantly impaired in comparison to typically developing children, whereas the ability to respond to joint attention is less severely impaired (e.g., MacDonald *et al.*, 2006). Perhaps correspondingly, children with ASD also show difficulties using protodeclaratives to serve a social purpose, while their ability to use protoimperatives to serve an instrumental purpose is relatively intact (e.g., Baron-Cohen, 1989). For example, children with ASD use fewer conventional gestures, such as pointing; however, they use more unconventional gestures, such as using an adult's hand as a tool to get an out of reach object (e.g., Stone *et al.*, 1997). Together, these findings suggest that children with ASD are able to respond to bids for joint attention made by social partners and initiate joint attention when social interaction is required to serve a functional purpose. However, children with ASD are less likely to initiate joint attention for the sake of social interaction.

Although there is a great deal of heterogeneity in the development of individual children with ASD, many children with ASD show delays in the development of a variety of social skills, which are required to engage in successful triadic interactions with a social partner. Such delays may impact the development of later language, as a lack of opportunities for social engagement may limit important language learning opportunities. A longitudinal study on the relationship between early joint attention skills and later language development in children with ASD found that children with ASD showed deficits in joint attention compared to children with developmental delays matched on mental and verbal age (Mundy *et al.*, 1990). Additionally, this study found that joint attention skills, and not early language or cognitive skills, predicted later language development in children with ASD.

In summary, the development of triadic interaction appears to follow a gradual time course in which a number of complex social skills, including eye gaze, affect, gestures, and preverbal vocalizations, are coordinated in order to establish joint attention and shared engagement with a social partner. Between ages 6 and 18 months, typically developing children increasingly engage in triadic interactions with their caregivers (Bakeman and Adamson, 1984). However, children with ASD show atypical shared engagement and joint attention. In fact, young children with ASD show such considerable impairments in joint attention, that these behaviours can be used to distinguish children with ASD from individuals who do not have ASD and can aid in the diagnosis of this developmental disorder (Mundy and Vaughan, 2002). The development of prelinguistic triadic interactions, including shared engagement and joint attention are developmentally homologous to later linguistic interactions, as they share a common underlying triadic structure and social communicative function.

Linguistic triadic interactions

As typical communicative development progresses through late infancy, children's triadic interactions begin to be mediated by language, in addition to eye contact, affect, and gestures. The first prelinguistic triadic interactions focus on concrete objects, and so also do the first triadic interactions that are mediated by language. However, the development of language allows later triadic interactions to centre around more complex and abstract ideas, such as objects that are not immediately present, past or future events, and mental states. Language is both representational and conventional, in that it allows for the discussion of absent objects and abstract ideas and requires a shared understanding by the speaker and listener. In a conversation, the speaker and listener must share their attention to the referent of a word or phrase. In this way, later language mirrors the same triadic structure that is seen in prelinguistic triadic interactions (see Figure 30.1 for an illustration of this homologous structure).

In this section, we discuss the development of first words, first phrases, and more complex linguistic constructions in typically developing children and children with ASD, recognizing that the acquisition of language is highly heterogeneous in children with ASD (e.g., Tager-Flusberg *et al.*, 2005) and also variable in typically developing children (e.g., Fenson *et al.*, 1994). As we proceed, we keep in mind that increasingly complex language development retains a homologous structure to earlier prelinguistic triadic interactions, in that they all involve social interaction between two communicative partners, centred around a shared object or idea of interest.

First words

Typically developing children

Children generally acquire language through early triadic social interactions with their caregivers in natural settings (e.g., Carpenter *et al.*, 1998). Triadic interactions provide the contexts within which children are able to connect words with meanings (Tomasello, 2003). For typically developing children, first words often emerge at approximately age 12 months, and by age 18 months, children understand that words are symbols for objects (Tomasello, 2003). Children's first words are usually nouns that name objects in their immediate environment, such as names for their caregivers, familiar food, and favourite toys. These first words allow children to communicate about the objects around them, establish joint attention, and facilitate shared engagement, or both simultaneously.

There are primarily two kinds of first words: those that serve to establish joint attention through naming the object or event that is the focus of the interaction, and those that serve to organize the interaction by facilitating the child's interests, whether object-oriented or socially motivated, in joint engagement (Tomasello, 2003). For example, a child may say "cookie" allowing her to establish joint attention with her caregiver toward a cookie. Alternatively, a child may say "more" while pointing to a cookie, thereby attempting to influence the partner's behaviour within the triadic interaction. As language skills develop throughout the second year of life, children become able to represent referents that extend beyond objects in their immediate environment. Children move from naming present objects only to also naming non-present objects, actions, and even abstract ideas (e.g., Akhtar and Tomasello, 1996; Ganea *et al.*, 2007). Triadic interactions between children, caregivers, and symbolic or abstract objects that are not immediately present, require a shared representation of the abstract object of interest, and this is where the representational properties of words have a natural advantage over nonlinguistic means of establishing joint attention.

Children with ASD

Many children with ASD demonstrate significant delays in their early language development, and approximately 1 in 4 remain non-verbal (Tager-Flusberg *et al.*, 2005). In contrast to typically developing children, who acquire their first words at about 12 months, children with ASD acquire their first words much later, at an average age of approximately 38 months (Howlin, 2003). In addition to delays in their first words, children with ASD generally show less vocal imitation and engage in unusual vocalizations (e.g., Chawarska and Volkmar, 2005).

Although evidence is sparse, it appears that children with ASD may not acquire words through triadic interaction in the same way as typically developing children. Baron-Cohen *et al.* (1997) compared word learning in children with ASD to typically developing and developmentally delayed children in contexts that involved joint attention. They found that approximately 3 in 4 typically developing children and 3 in 4 children with developmental delays were able to learn a new word for a new object based on the direction of the speaker's eye gaze; however, only about 1 in 4 children with ASD were able to make this association. These findings provide evidence that children with ASD do not acquire new words through joint attention as readily as their peers. It is possible that children with ASD show significant delays in their early language acquisition because they have fewer opportunities to engage in word learning through triadic interactions with their caregivers, given that young children with ASD show impairments in shared engagement and joint attention to representational objects. Whereas novel word acquisition may occur differently in children with ASD, there is essentially no research on how children with ASD actually use their first words. Therefore, an important area for future research on language acquisition in children with ASD is to examine whether these children are using their first words in a functional manner in order to establish joint attention and facilitate shared engagement.

First phrases

Typically developing children

Children typically begin to combine single words into phrases between approximately ages 18 and 24 months (Fenson *et al.*, 1994). Once they master the ability to use single words for both establishing joint attention and facilitating shared engagement, they can then combine these two functions into phrases that are used both for establishing the focus of joint attention – the topic – and for facilitating shared engagement in a "lexicalized triadic structure" (Moore, 2013, p. 64). This differentiated use of words in early combinations is often seen in the so-called "pivot" grammars (Braine and Bowerman, 1976; Tomasello, 2003).

In this two-word stage of language development, one word – the pivot – serves a shared engagement function (e.g., as a requestive or indicative/declarative) and is combined with a range of other words, which are used to establish the topics of joint attention. For example, utterances such as "more" or "again" are often used to facilitate shared engagement, whereas nouns that label objects in the environment such as "milk" or "toy" are often used to establish joint attention. Thus, children may say "more milk" or "toy again". Other word combinations might express a comment on an object or event to elicit a social interaction, for example "yummy milk" or "fun toy". Such pivot words provide information on the object of joint attention in the form of a comment to stimulate further social interaction, such as eliciting a further comment by the caregiver. This is similar to adult conversation, in which both partners discuss a topic of interest, within a triadic structure homologous to earlier triadic interactions.

Children with ASD

Although detailed distributional analyses of the first word combinations of children with ASD are lacking, it appears that children with ASD commonly do not follow the typical developmental pattern for early word combinations. Instead of creatively combining single words to make new word combinations, children with ASD often demonstrate the use of rote phrases; and they exhibit much more "echolalia", which involves immediate or delayed repetition of phrases (Tager-Flusberg and Calkins, 1990). Echolalia can be communicative, but a reliance on such rote phrases diminishes opportunities for children to flexibly produce new phrases and advance their social communication skills. Additionally, children with ASD tend to use phrases to request or protest as opposed to indicate, and rarely use questions to obtain information (e.g., Chiang and Carter, 2008; Thurm *et al.*, 2007). The tendency of children with ASD to produce utterances for the sake of requesting rather than indicating may reflect a focus on using language to fulfil personal needs rather than using language to facilitate social interaction. If children with ASD are not frequently using questions to obtain information, this will limit their knowledge of the world, thus children with ASD who ask fewer questions also show decreased academic and social abilities (e.g., Koegel *et al.*, 1999). However, very little is known about how children with ASD use early word combinations in order to construct their first phrases. Therefore, further research is required to understand how early word combinations are used in this population.

Complex language

Typically developing children

The distinction between using words to establish the shared topic and to comment or contribute new information provides an organizing structure for much typical language development from age 2 years (Moore, 2013). More complex language generally retains the triadic structure of earlier communication, in that a shared topic of conversation is the focus for additional comment, which then acts to facilitate shared engagement. The topic of conversation may be an object in the child's immediate environment (such as a toy in the child's hand), or a more abstract topic (such as an activity the child engaged in at daycare yesterday). Both partners in a conversation continually build on the previous turn by taking the preceding utterance as the topic and then adding further comment in order to have a meaningful reciprocal conversation involving shared engagement and joint attention.

Topic-comment structures are inherent in both simple phrases and complex discourses. In order for a successful conversation to take place, a variety of complex linguistic skills are required, including presupposition, turn-taking, topic management, and handling breakdown and repair. These linguistic skills generally fall under the rubric of pragmatics, which describes the ways in which speakers use the various components of language to preserve or clarify the topic-comment structure.

Children with ASD

Pragmatics is an area of language that commonly causes considerable difficulty for children with ASD. These children show difficulties carrying on conversations with others, partly because they have difficulty preserving the pre-established topic of joint attention. They tend to change the topic of conversation without notice more frequently than their typically developing peers (Lam and Yeung, 2012). This tendency reveals a lack of faithfulness to topic-comment structure. Additionally, using social context to understand the meaning of a phrase is often difficult for children with ASD (see Loukusa and Moilanen, 2009). Individuals with ASD are less responsive to cues from their communication partner (e.g., Paul *et al.*, 2009; Tager-Flusberg and Anderson, 1991). They also tend to show difficulties taking turns in conversation as well as answering questions and responding to comments appropriately (Capps *et al.*, 1998). Together, these difficulties with pragmatics can make it exceptionally difficult for children with ASD to communicate with others. Some high-functioning individuals with ASD may develop advanced language skills; however, due to difficulties with pragmatics, many individuals with ASD have difficulty carrying on a conversation.

Conclusions and future research directions

In this chapter, we surveyed the development of early communication in typically developing children and children with ASD. In line with previous accounts (Moore, 2013; Tomasello, 2003), we assumed that earlier social behaviours in the form of prelinguistic triadic interactions are homologous to later complex language, as they have a similar structure and function. In this way, communication in its various manifestations can be seen as increasingly complex homologous forms of triadic interaction. ASD can be conceptualized as involving an impairment in triadic interaction, which leads to impairments in various aspects of communication, including facets of prelinguistic communication, and use of words, phrases, and complex linguistic constructions to establish and facilitate triadic interaction through joint attention and shared engagement.

Research has clearly established that children with ASD have difficulty with both early triadic interactions and aspects of later complex language, such as pragmatics. However, little attention has been paid to how children with ASD use their first words and phrases and the extent to which these initial utterances are used to establish and maintain joint attention and shared engagement. Prospective research that has focused on the early identification of ASD using standardized language assessments has been invaluable in categorizing differences between children with and without ASD; however, it has shed little light on the development of early triadic language in children with ASD. According to the proposed model of language development, it would be valuable to study how children with ASD use their first words and phrases.

Additionally, previous research indicates that the more frequently children engage in joint attention earlier in life, the larger their expressive vocabulary will be later in life (e.g., Markus *et al.*, 2000; Tomasello and Todd, 1983; Tomasello *et al.*, 1986). Future research could attempt to use intervention approaches to investigate if early training in prelinguistic triadic interactions can impact later language development in children with ASD. Such research is particularly relevant for young children with ASD, who have difficulty initiating joint attention and shared engagement. Preliminary research in this area is beginning to lay the groundwork for further research. Kasari *et al.* (2010) studied the efficacy of a caregiver-mediated intervention to help young children with ASD develop their shared engagement skills. Similarly, Lawton and Kasari (2012) investigated the efficacy of a teacher-mediated intervention to help children with ASD develop their joint attention skills. Both treatment studies showed promising improvements in skills related to prelinguistic triadic interactions.

In sum, prelinguistic triadic interactions and later linguistic interactions are developmentally homologous and atypical social development may adversely impact the development of these forms of communication. The fundamental difficulties with social communication in ASD may reflect basic impairments in the triadic structure that underlies both prelinguistic and linguistic communication.

References

Adamson, L.B., Bakeman, R., Deckner, D.F. and Nelson, P.B. (2012), "Rating parent-child interactions: Joint engagement, communication dynamics, and shared topics in autism, Down syndrome, and typical development", *Journal of Autism and Developmental Disorders*, Vol. 42, No. 12, pp. 2622–2635.

Adamson, L.B., Deckner, D.F. and Bakeman, R. (2010), "Early interests and joint engagement in typical development, autism, and Down syndrome", *Journal of Autism and Developmental Disorders*, Vol. 40, No. 6, pp. 665–676.

Akhtar, N. and Tomasello, M. (1996), "Two-year-olds learn words for absent objects and actions", *British Journal of Developmental Psychology*, Vol. 14, pp. 79–93.

Bakeman, R. and Adamson, L.B. (1984), "Coordinating attention to people and objects in mother-infant and peer-infant interaction", *Child Development*, Vol. 55, pp. 1278–1289.

Baron-Cohen, S. (1989), "Perceptual role taking and protodeclarative pointing in autism", *British Journal of Developmental Psychology*, Vol. 7, No. 2, pp. 113–127.

Baron-Cohen, S., Allen, J. and Gillberg, C. (1992), "Can autism be detected at 18 months?: The needle, the haystack, and the CHAT", *The British Journal of Psychiatry*, Vol. 161, pp. 839–843.

Baron-Cohen, S., Baldwin, D.A. and Crowson, M. (1997), "Do children with autism use the speaker's direction of gaze strategy to crack the code of language?", *Child Development*, Vol. 68, No. 1, pp. 48–57.

Bates, E. (1979), "The emergence of symbols", *Cognition and Communication in Infancy*. New York: Academic Press.

Bates, E., Camaioni, L. and Volterra, V. (1975), "The acquisition of performatives prior to speech", *Merrill-Palmer Quarterly*, Vol. 21, No. 3, pp. 205–226.

Braine, M. and Bowerman, M. (1976), "Children's first word combinations", *Monographs of the Society for Research in Child Development*, Vol. 41, No. 1, pp. 1–104.

Bruinsma, Y., Koegel, R.L. and Koegel, L.K. (2004), "Joint attention and children with autism: A review of the literature", *Mental Retardation and Developmental Disabilities Research Reviews*, Vol. 10, No. 3, pp. 169–175.

Capps, L., Kehres, J. and Sigman, M. (1998), "Conversational abilities among children with autism and children with developmental delays", *Autism*, Vol. 2, No. 4, pp. 325–344.

Carpenter, M., Nagell, K. and Tomasello, M. (1998), "Social cognition, joint attention, and communicative competence from 9 to 15 months of age", *Monographs of the Society for Research in Child Development*, Vol. 63, No. 4, pp. 1–176.

Charman, T., Swettenham, J., Baron-Cohen, S., Cox, A., Baird, G. and Drew, A. (1997), "Infants with autism: An investigation of empathy, pretend play, joint attention, and imitation", *Developmental Psychology*, Vol. 33, No. 5, pp. 781–789.

Chawarska, K. and Volkmar, F.R. (2005), "Autism in infancy and early childhood", *Handbook of Autism and Pervasive Developmental Disorders*, Vol. 1, No. 3, pp. 223–246.

Chiang, H.M. and Carter, M. (2008), "Spontaneity of communication in individuals with autism", *Journal of Autism and Developmental Disorders*, Vol. 38, pp. 693–705.

Desrochers, S., Morissette, P. and Marcelle, R. (1995), "Joint attention: Its origins and role in development", In Moore, C. and Dunham, P.J. (Eds.), *Two Perspectives on Pointing in Infancy* (pp. 85–101). Hillsdale, NJ, US: Lawrence Erlbaum Associates.

Fenson, L., Dale, P.S., Reznick, J.S., Bates, E., Thal, D.J. and Pethick, S.J. (1994), "Variability in early communicative development", *Monographs of the Society for Research in Child Development*, Vol. 59, No. 5, pp. 1–172.

Ganea, P.A., Shutts, K., Spelke, E. and DeLoache, J.S. (2007), "Thinking of things unseen: Infants' use of language to update object representations", *Psychological Science*, Vol. 18, No. 8, pp. 734–739.

Howlin, P. (2003), "Outcome in high-functioning adults with autism with and without early language delays: Implications for the differentiation between autism and Asperger syndrome", *Journal of Autism and Developmental Disorders*, Vol. 37, pp. 3–13.

Kasari, C., Gulsrud, A.C., Wong, C., Kwon, S. and Locke, J. (2010), "Randomized controlled caregiver mediated joint engagement intervention for toddlers with autism", *Journal of Autism and Developmental Disorders*, Vol. 40, No. 9, pp. 1045–1056.

Kasari, C., Sigman, M., Mundy, P. and Yirmiya, N. (1990), "Affective sharing in the context of joint attention interactions of normal, autistic, and mentally retarded children", *Journal of Autism and Developmental Disorders*, Vol. 20, No. 1, pp. 87–100.

Koegel, L.K., Koegel, R.L., Shoshan, Y. and McNerney, E. (1999), "Pivotal response intervention II: Preliminary long-term outcome data", *Journal of the Association for Persons with Severe Handicaps*, Vol. 24, No. 3, pp. 186–198.

Lam, Y.G. and Yeung, S. (2012), "Towards a convergent account of pragmatic language deficits in children with high-functioning autism: Depicting the phenotype using the Pragmatic Rating Scale", *Research in Autism Spectrum Disorders*, Vol. 6, No. 2, pp. 792–797.

Lawton, K. and Kasari, C. (2012), "Teacher-implemented joint attention intervention: Pilot randomized controlled study for preschoolers with autism", *Journal of Consulting and Clinical Psychology*, Vol. 80, No. 4, pp. 687–693.

Loukusa, S. and Moilanen, I. (2009), "Pragmatic inference abilities in individuals with Asperger syndrome or high-functioning autism: A review", *Research in Autism Spectrum Disorders*, Vol. 3, No. 4, pp. 890–904.

MacDonald, R., Anderson, J., Dube, W.V., Geckeler, A., Green, G., Holcomb, W., *et al.* (2006), "Behavioral assessment of joint attention: A methodological report", *Research in Developmental Disabilities*, Vol. 27, No. 2, pp. 138–150.

Markus, J., Mundy, P., Morales, M., Delgado, C. and Yale, M. (2000), "Individual differences in infant skills as predictors of child-caregiver joint attention and language", *Social Development*, Vol. 9, No. 3, pp. 302–315.

Meindl, J.N. and Cannella-Malone, H.I. (2011), "Initiating and responding to joint attention bids in children with autism: A review of the literature", *Research in Developmental Disabilities*, Vol. 32, No. 5, pp. 1441–1454.

Messinger, D. and Fogel, A. (2007), "The interactive development of social smiling", *Advances in Child Development and Behaviour*, Vol. 35, pp. 328–366.

Moore, C. (2006), *The Development of Commonsense Psychology*. Mahwah, NJ, US: Lawrence Erlbaum Associates.

Moore, C. (2008), "The development of gaze following". *Child Development Perspectives*, Vol. 2, pp. 66–70.

Moore, C. (2013), "Homology in the development of triadic interaction and language", *Developmental Psychobiology*, Vol. 55, pp. 59–66.

Mundy, P., Block, J., Delgado, C., Pomares, Y., Van Hecke, A.V. and Parlade, M.V. (2007), "Individual differences and the development of joint attention in infancy", *Child Development*, Vol. 78, No. 3, pp. 938–954.

Mundy, P., Sigman, M. and Kasari, C. (1990), "A longitudinal study of joint attention and language development in autistic children", *Journal of Autism and Developmental Disorders*, Vol. 20, No. 1, pp. 115–128.

Mundy, P. and Vaughan, A. (2002), "Joint attention and its role in the diagnostic assessment of children with autism", *Assessment for Effective Intervention*, Vol. 27, No. 1–2, pp. 57–60.

Paul, R., Orlovski, S.M., Marcinko, H.C. and Volkmar, F. (2009), "Conversational behaviors in youth with high-functioning ASD and Asperger syndrome", *Journal of Autism and Developmental Disorders*, Vol. 39, No.1, pp. 115–125.

Sroufe, L.A. and Waters, E. (1976), "The ontogenesis of smiling and laughter: A perspective on the organization of development in infancy", *Psychological Review*, Vol. 83, pp. 173–189.

Stone, W.L., Ousley, O.Y., Yoder, P.J., Hogan, K.L. and Hepburn, S.L. (1997), "Nonverbal communication in two- and three-year-old children with autism", *Journal of Autism and Developmental Disorders*, Vol. 27, pp. 677–696.

Tager-Flusberg, H. and Anderson, M. (1991), "The development of contingent discourse ability in autistic children", *Journal of Child Psychology and Psychiatry*, Vol. 32, No. 7, pp. 1123–1134.

Tager-Flusberg, H. and Calkins, S. (1990), "Does imitation facilitate acquisition of grammar?: Evidence from the study of autistic, Down's syndrome, and normal children", *Journal of Child Language*, Vol. 17, pp. 591–606.

Tager-Flusberg, H., Paul, R. and Lord, C. (2005), "Language and communication in autism", In Volkmar, F.R., Paul, R., Klin, A. and Cohen, D. (Eds.), *Handbook of Autism and Pervasive Developmental Disorders, Vol. 1: Diagnosis, Development, Neurobiology, and Behavior* (3rd ed.) (pp. 335–364). Hoboken, NJ, US: John Wiley and Sons.

Thurm, A., Lord, C., Lee, L.-C. and Newschaffer, C. (2007), "Predictors of language acquisition in preschool children with autism spectrum disorders", *Journal of Autism and Developmental Disabilities*, Vol. 37, pp. 1721–1734.

Tomasello, M. (2003), *Constructing a Language: A Usage-based Theory of Language Acquisition*, Cambridge, MA, US: Harvard University Press.

Tomasello, M. and Todd, J. (1983), "Joint attention and lexical acquisition style". *First Language*, Vol. 4, No. 12, pp. 197–211.

Tomasello, M., Mannle, S. and Kruger, A.C. (1986), "The linguistic environment of one- to two-year-old twins", *Developmental Psychology*, Vol. 22, No. 2, pp. 169–176.

Wimpory, D.C., Hobson, R.P., Williams, J. and Nash, S. (2000), "Are infants with autism socially engaged?: A study of recent retrospective parental reports", *Journal of Autism and Developmental Disorders*, Vol. 30, No. 6, pp. 525–536.

31

EMOTIONAL INTELLIGENCE AND TREATMENT OUTCOMES IN CHILDREN WITH LANGUAGE IMPAIRMENT

Bonnie Brinton and Martin Fujiki

Five-year-old Troy is receiving intervention for language impairment (LI). He has brought four small toy lizards to show to his speech–language pathologist (SLP). Troy and his SLP talk about the lizards and complete their intervention activities. At the conclusion of the session, the SLP talks with Troy's mom. During the adults' conversation, Troy makes his lizard "bite" the SLP. The SLP responds with an exaggerated startled look, says "OH!" and makes a second lizard bite Troy. Troy giggles and makes his lizard bite the SLP once more. Again, the SLP reacts with obvious surprise. As the reciprocal game continues, Troy laughs harder and harder in response to, and in anticipation of, the SLP's reaction. Troy's mother reflects, "It's so nice to hear Troy laugh. He doesn't laugh like that very often. The only time he laughs like that is when he watches the little bear brothers in the movie, *Brave*."

What does this incident tell us about Troy? Despite the fact that Troy has a good rapport with his SLP and is compliant and cooperative in interaction, his mother has rarely observed such moments of emotional engagement and sharing in any social context. Troy has recognized his SLP's facial expression of surprise, he has subsequently anticipated the emotional reaction his actions will elicit, and he has shared his own emotional response (laughing) with his SLP. Such exchanges are commonplace for typically developing children who are considerably younger; however, Troy evidently lacks the social and emotional knowledge to support his full participation in these kinds of interactions. In addition to his language deficits, his difficulties with social and emotional learning can be expected to constrain his ability to communicate, to relate to others, and to acquire academic skills.

In this chapter we discuss social and emotional learning with a focus on emotional intelligence. We then consider internal and external factors that influence emotional intelligence in typical development as well as ways to facilitate social and emotional learning in children with LI.

Social and emotional learning

Social and emotional learning (SEL) is a term used to refer to the processes by which children learn to "understand and manage emotions, set and achieve positive goals, feel and show

345

empathy for others, establish and maintain positive relationships, and make responsible decisions" (Collaborative for Academic, Social, and Emotional Learning [CASEL], 2012, p. 4). In recent years there has been increasing awareness of the critical role that SEL plays in academic and personal development. SEL is instrumental in developing a sense of self, an understanding of one's emotions, and the ability to reflect on one's experience. SEL supports the ability to appreciate the experience of others and to anticipate and understand the emotional reactions of others in given situations. SEL also facilitates learning to regulate one's own emotions and to cooperate with others. SEL is vital in interacting in social contexts and in establishing and maintaining relationships. It is also important in maintaining readiness and motivation to learn, in understanding stories, in comprehending literature, and in interpreting past and present events. As such, SEL plays a major role in a child's social, cognitive, and academic growth. To understand the scope and influence of SEL in a child's development, it is helpful to consider the concept of emotional intelligence.

What is emotional intelligence?

Multiple definitions of the term, emotional intelligence, exist in the academic literature and popular press. Emotional intelligence is "the ability to perceive and express emotions, to understand and use them, and to manage emotions so as to foster personal growth" (Salovey *et al.*, 2008, p. 535). This conception of emotional intelligence represents an integrative abilities model that focuses on the capabilities that contribute to emotionally competent behavior. Mayer *et al.* (2011) separate emotional abilities into four general branches (from Table 26.1, Mayer *et al.*, 2011, p. 532). Each branch categorizes specific abilities.

The four branches of emotion

The first branch, the perception and expression of emotion, includes the ability to perceive and recognize one's own emotions, to express emotions, and to read the expression of other's emotions through facial expression and voice (e.g., to recognize that a particular facial expression conveys sadness, another happiness). Additionally, the perception and expression of emotion includes the ability to identify sincere expressions of emotion (e.g., telling if a smile is genuine).

Assimilating emotion in thought is the second branch. It involves the use of emotions to facilitate performance in tasks or activities. For example, an artist may capitalize on an emotional state to facilitate creativity, or a student may use a conscious fear of failing a test to focus studying.

The third branch, understanding and analyzing emotion, involves sophisticated processes that go beyond simple recognition. For instance, understanding that one may simultaneously experience conflicting emotions is categorized here (e.g., happiness at winning a contest and sadness for a friend who lost). Additionally, understanding emotion includes the knowledge that one emotion may blend into another, as when an individual's initial anger at a friend's betrayal subsequently evolves into sadness. It also includes the understanding of complex emotions such as guilt.

Lastly, the regulation of emotion includes the ability to "monitor and regulate emotions to promote emotional and intellectual growth" (Mayer *et al.*, 2011, p. 532). Regulation may involve decreasing or increasing the intensity of emotion (i.e., an individual who has just experienced a robbery may need to calm down before reporting it accurately. A child who dreads doing homework may need to elevate emotions to complete the task). Additionally, emotion regulation may be internal, as in the case of a child who closes her eyes to keep from being too frightened during a scary movie. It may also be external, as when a parent holds a crying child to provide comfort. Infants and toddlers are heavily dependent upon external regulation, whereas older children are better able to regulate their own emotions. It should be noted, however, that older children, adolescents, and even adults may rely on external regulation (e.g., an individual who turns to a spouse for comfort after a difficult day at work) (Thompson, 1994).

Other ways of organizing emotional intelligence

Although various researchers organize the specific components that comprise emotional intelligence differently, many of the same elements are found across organizational frameworks. For example, Gignac (2010) summarized work reviewing ability-based inventories of emotional intelligence and identified five general abilities present in all of the inventories examined. These included, "Recognizing and Expressing Emotions, Understanding Emotions (External), Emotions to Direct Cognition, Emotional Management (Self and Others), and Emotional Control" (p. 310). In her discussion of emotional competence (a concept similar to emotional intelligence), Denham (1998) described many of the same abilities organized within three general categories of expressing, understanding, and regulating emotion.

It is important to recognize that these aspects of emotional intelligence are not independent of each other. The expression of emotion is interconnected with understanding and regulation. For example, talking about the emotion one is feeling not only contributes to the expression of that emotion; it also allows one to reflect on one's experience of emotion and enhances one's understanding of emotion. For example, talking about negative emotion can help a child become aware that the experience of emotion need not be tied to the present context (e.g., reflecting on and reliving a frightening experience from the past). This awareness may also contribute to more effective regulation of emotion and behavior (Harris, 2008).

Emotional intelligence and development

In the following sections we consider factors that influence the development of emotional intelligence. Some of these factors are intrinsic to the child and others are extrinsic (in the environment). Although our primary focus is on adult talk to children about emotions, we first comment on within-child factors.

The influence of within-child factors

As children develop emotion competence, varying intrapersonal abilities and characteristics come into play. Factors important in emotional learning include temperament, cognitive ability, and language level (Denham *et al.*, 2007). For example, an active, high-strung child may have more difficulty regulating emotion than a child with a more easy-going temperament. A child with greater social cognitive resources may be better able to understand how others feel given a particular situation and adapt accordingly. Even though intrinsic dispositions and abilities influence development in many ways, there is growing evidence that parents and other adults play an important role in helping children learn about emotions.

The influence of caretakers and other important adults

As Thompson (2011) noted, adult input about emotion colors children's earliest perceptions and expectations of other people as well as the nature of their social interactions. Because these exchanges are repeated numerous times a day, they provide a connection between the infant and other individuals. This connection is influential in several important areas of development including attachment, self-concept, and aspects of social cognition such as theory of mind (see also the Hutchins and Prelock chapter, this volume, for further discussion on theory of mind). This adult influence on emotional development can be characterized in three specific ways. First, children learn from adult models as they observe caregivers managing their own emotions. Children also learn as caregivers react and respond to the child's expression of emotion. A third way in which adults influence children's emotional intelligence is by providing direct instruction, or "coaching" about emotion (Denham *et al.*, 2007). There is considerable evidence that adults influence the emotional intelligence of children by both modeling the experience of emotion and by reacting to the child's emotions (see Cole and Tan, 2007; Denham *et al.*, 2007 for review). Of particular interest for present purposes is the influence of caretaker talk on the development of emotionally intelligent behavior.

The influence of conversations about emotion

In younger children, parental talk about emotions is related to higher levels of emotion knowledge (Denham and Auerbach, 1995; Dunn *et al.*, 1991) and better emotion regulation (Brown and Dunn, 1992; Gottman *et al.*, 1997). The sophistication of caregiver talk about emotions is also linked to children's level of social skill (Zahn-Waxler *et al.*, 1993). One of the most effective ways that caregivers and other influential adults teach children about emotion is to talk about emotional experiences. It is important to remember, however, that simply talking about emotion is not enough. Conversation aimed at changing the child's emotional behavior is less effective than talk that focuses on helping children to understand the experience of emotion (Denham *et al.*, 2007; Eisenberg *et al.*, 1998). Thus, it is more effective to comment, "You are crying about your homework. You must feel frustrated," than to say, "Quit crying and finish your homework." Similarly, not all talk about regulating emotions is equally effective. Two useful "talking" strategies about emotion regulation are: (a) talk that focuses on taking another's point of view (e.g., "Kelly is going to the dentist. Kelly is scared of the dentist. Kelly feels scared."); and (b) talk that helps the child see the consequences of behavior (e.g., "You took Kent's toy. Kent is crying. Kent is upset because you took his toy."). Conversely, strategies that either avoid or discourage the discussion of emotions, or that minimize the experience of emotions, are counterproductive (Denham *et al.*, 2007).

Children continue to learn about emotion as they enter school. Similar to their younger peers, school aged children learn about emotions from interactions with other people. In addition, older children may receive direct instruction about emotions in more structured contexts. In some cases, this instruction may be integrated into the school curriculum. Research examining the effectiveness of these types of programs is presented in a later section.

In summary, the development of emotional intelligence is influenced both by factors within the child, such as temperament, and by factors in the environment, such as instruction about emotion from other people. Caretakers and other important adults can play influential roles in the development of emotional intelligence. Conversations that guide children to understand their own emotions as well as the emotions experienced by others are of particular value.

Emotional intelligence in children with LI

Children with LI experience difficulties with multiple aspects of SEL. Some of these difficulties are apparent in the perception and expression of emotion as well as in the understanding and analysis of emotion. For example, children with LI are not as adept as their typically developing peers at recognizing emotion expressed by facial expression or vocal prosody (Boucher *et al.*, 2000; Fujiki *et al.*, 2008). They have more difficulty inferring emotions that others may experience in specific contexts (Ford and Milosky, 2003; Spackman *et al.*, 2006) and in dissembling the expression of emotion to accommodate the feelings of others (Brinton *et al.*, 2007). In addition, children with LI have difficulty with emotion regulation, particularly in gearing up emotion to participate in interactions and accomplish tasks (Fujiki *et al.*, 2002). LI can limit SEL in less direct ways as well. For example, language deficits can restrict children's ability to learn about emotion from the input of parents and caregivers. Children with LI may find it difficult to take advantage of parental input regarding how to express, understand, and regulate emotions. Language problems also limit children's ability to describe emotions they experience and to gain important feedback regarding those emotions.

Limitations in SEL put children with LI at risk for social problems including social withdrawal (Fujiki *et al.*, 1999; Fujiki *et al.*, 2001), difficulty working cooperatively with others (Brinton *et al.*, 2000), and problems in negotiation and conflict resolution (Horowitz *et al.*, 2005; Marton *et al.*, 2005; Timler, 2008). In addition, individuals with LI often experience victimization and loneliness (Conti-Ramsden and Botting, 2004; Fujiki *et al.*, 1996). As a result, children with LI too often exist on the periphery of the classroom community and are left on the outskirts of work and play groups.

Difficulties with SEL not only limit a child's full participation in school and play contexts, they also inhibit a child's learning academic concepts and skills. As Pellitteri (2006) noted, "Emotions influence information processing and cognitive organization as well as motivation and social relations" (p. 168). Emotion regulation facilitates the drive and focus necessary to accomplish difficult and time consuming learning tasks. The perception, understanding, and analysis of emotion are essential to comprehending not only complex literature but even the simplest of stories and virtually all social, historical and political events. For children with LI, difficulties with SEL combine with language processing deficits (receptive and/or expressive) to put them at considerable academic and social risk.

Facilitating SEL development

Integration into the educational curriculum

There is growing support for the idea that SEL should be an integral part of the educational curriculum for all children. As Durlak and colleagues (2011) noted, "...schools have an important role to play in raising healthy children by fostering not only their cognitive development but also their social and emotional development" (p. 406). Accordingly, many school programs have been developed to foster SEL. Studies examining the efficacy of these programs have revealed that systematic, well-conceived programs can be highly successful at reducing negative behavior and promoting social and academic learning. Durlak and colleagues performed a meta-analysis of 213 studies evaluating school-based SEL programs involving 270,034 students. The programs evaluated were implemented on a school-wide basis. Over half of the studies (56 percent) involved elementary school students, with the remainder involving middle school (31 percent) and high school students (13 percent). Results indicated that the children and adolescents in these programs made significantly greater positive gains than did controls on outcome assessments that included measures of emotional abilities, emotional and behavioral difficulties, and social behavior. In addition, measurable gains were also noted in academic skills and achievement. Successful programs were characterized by four factors (Durlak *et al.*, 2011): (a) a sequenced set of activities designed to achieve specific goals; (b) a focus on specific social and emotional skills; (c) active learning opportunities; and (d) at least one component of the program dedicated to social skills.

An example of a SEL program that has been widely adapted by schools is Emotionally Literate Schools (Brackett *et al.*, 2009). This program is based on the idea "that personal, social, and intellectual functioning improves by teaching children and adults how to recognize, understand, label, express, and regulate emotions" (p. 331). The authors use the acronym RULER to refer to these emotional abilities. The program emphasizes the importance of emotional intelligence not just to students, but to teachers, administrators, parents, and other stakeholders. Emotionally Literate Schools consists of detailed, carefully structured plans that focus on readiness, implementation, and sustainability. The classroom lessons on the abilities represented by RULER are designed to be integrated into the academic curriculum in a wide range of subject areas including history, science, math, and music.

The results of a randomized control trial involving 62 schools provided evidence for the efficacy of the Emotionally Literate Schools program (Rivers *et al.*, 2013). After the first year of the study, comparisons with students in control classrooms revealed better relationships between teachers and students, more independence and less victimization by students, and more sensitivity to student interests by teachers (Brackett and Rivers, in press). In the second year, changes were noted on a range of parameters including the emotional and instructional support provided to students, as well as classroom organization (Hagelskamp *et al.*, 2013). The Emotionally Literate Schools program provides a good illustration of a successful SEL program and highlights the importance of the specific abilities that contribute to emotional intelligence.

SEL interventions for children with LI

Although the efficacy of carefully designed instruction in SEL has been illustrated for typically developing children, the picture is not so clear for children with language and learning impairments. Studies investigating interventions to facilitate emotional development are relatively rare, but some investigations have considered the development of social skills. To illustrate, Kavale and Mostert (2004) performed a meta-analysis of 53 studies of social skill interventions for children with learning disabilities (a population that overlaps with children with LI), but found only modest effects. Gerber *et al.* (2012) reported the results of an evidence-based systematic review of treatment programs designed to address social communication skills in children with LI between the ages of 6 and 11 years. Only eight studies were found between 1975 and June, 2008. Treatment programs primarily targeted pragmatic and social behaviors. All were considered exploratory in nature, but results were encouraging enough to warrant a recommendation for further study.

Adams *et al.* (2012) reported the results of a randomized controlled trial of a carefully designed intervention program for children with complex pragmatic communication needs (including children with manifestations of LI and/or ASD). Treatment consisted of components that addressed understanding social context and emotion cues, understanding the thoughts of others, managing aspects of conversation, and several other pragmatic and language abilities. Children in the treatment group demonstrated gains in teacher and parent perceptions of pragmatic behavior. Raters blind to group membership also documented gains in conversational skill. This work demonstrated the challenges and complexities, as well as the possibilities, of intervention programs designed to address aspects of SEL in children with deficits in social communication.

Programmatic considerations for children with LI

Effective programs designed to enhance SEL in a general school population share certain characteristics. They have an organized sequence of instruction, they involve active learning on the part of children, and they focus on specific skills and behaviors (Durlak *et al.*, 2011). In addition, the most effective programs are not limited to specific "lessons" or activities targeting social and emotional behaviors. Rather, instruction and practice opportunities are integrated into the school curriculum and culture. Pellitteri (2006) advised, "Every academic task and social interaction can be an opportunity to facilitate emotional awareness in students" (p. 168).

These characteristics are equally important in designing interventions to support SEL in children with LI. In addition, like all educational programming for children with disabilities, treatment must be adjusted to meet the specific needs and capabilities of individuals. Likewise, it is very likely that treatment programs need to be ongoing over an extended period of time. Sustainable, meaningful gains can rarely be expected from fragmented, cursory, or short-term interventions (Adams *et al.*, 2012; Fujiki *et al.*, 2013).

When planning for children with LI, it can be challenging to determine how to focus treatment on areas of SEL that may be most important. In designing treatment, it can be helpful to consider the following overlapping questions: (a) What behaviors or abilities will enhance this child's ability to establish and maintain positive relationships with others; and (b) What behaviors or abilities will contribute to the efficacy of the child's comprehensive educational program? Research suggests that the most pressing SEL needs of children with LI include emotion regulation and emotion understanding.

Emotion regulation

As indicated previously, many children with LI have trouble regulating their emotions to gear up even for common activities. As a result, they may demonstrate internalizing behaviors, particularly reticent withdrawal. Teachers often report that these children frequently do little or nothing even when there are several activities in which they might be involved. In addition, they may be hesitant to enter work or play groups and lack strategies to join ongoing activity. Without intervention and support, children with LI may never be fully included in classroom and learning contexts. Helping children with LI regulate their emotions to be more proactive in seeking interaction and learning opportunities may be essential to their academic growth.

Although internalizing behaviors have been noted most often in children with LI, many of these children experience considerable frustration and may act out or become aggressive when things become particularly difficult. These externalizing episodes can damage positive relationships and hinder the ability to function in the classroom (Brinton *et al.*, 2000). Children with LI may benefit from carefully designed interventions to help them utilize both internal and external strategies to compose themselves and solve problems in tense situations.

Emotion understanding

Many aspects of emotion understanding can be particularly problematic for children with LI and can seriously limit their social and academic development. Areas that may require particular attention include the ability to recognize, identify (label), and express their own emotions and to understand that others may experience different emotions in the same situations. Treatment goals and activities can be designed to help children attend to and recognize a range of facial expressions of emotions, not just in line drawings and pictures, but on real faces in real contexts.

Children with LI may need help recognizing and interpreting other emotion cues including those expressed in prosody and innuendo. Many children with LI need support to help them link eliciting events to the emotions others experience as well as to anticipate emotions that events might elicit in others (e.g., "Celia is scared of dogs. There is a big dog in a yard. How will Celia feel when she sees that dog?").

Children with LI can be expected to require support in making social and emotional inferences in order to understand interpersonal classroom dynamics, to comprehend stories, and to interpret events. The demands on children's social and emotional knowledge increase dramatically as they encounter more abstract literature and complex social, historical, and political issues. In addition, children with LI may need intervention designed to help them express their own emotions appropriately in order to achieve positive social goals. Many individuals with LI may require support throughout their school years.

Conclusion and future research directions

For many children with language-learning impairments, limitations in various aspects of SEL may well block the efficacy of their overall academic programs. If not addressed, these limitations can undermine children's social development, inclusion in the classroom community, literacy acquisition, and other academic growth.

Research suggests that classroom experience and implicit teaching are insufficient to help children with LI develop the social and emotional knowledge they need to be successful learners. Rather, explicit, integrated, and systematic instruction and intervention in the most important aspects of SEL are warranted. Although preliminary work is promising, additional research is needed to investigate how to design and implement intervention for children with LI. It will be critical to consider how best to integrate instruction facilitating the social and emotional growth of these children within intervention programs that address their complex language and academic needs. As Bernard (2006) advised, "Be aware that the road to raising the achievement of all young people is paved not only with quality academic programs, but also with quality social-emotional-motivational programs" (p. 116).

References

Adams, C., Locktron, E., Freed, J., Gaile, J., Earl, G., McBean, K., *et al.*, (2012), "The social communication intervention project: A randomized controlled trial of the effectiveness of speech and language therapy for school-age children who have pragmatic and social communication problems with or without autism spectrum disorder", *International Journal of Language and Communication Disorders*, Vol. 47, pp. 233–244.

Bernard, M.E. (2006), "It's time we teach social-emotional competence as well as we teach academic competence", *Reading and Writing Quarterly*, Vol. 22, pp. 103–119.

Boucher, J., Lewis, V. and Collis, G.M. (2000), "Voice processing abilities in children with autism, children with specific language impairments, and young typically developing children", *Journal of Child Psychology and Psychiatry*, Vol. 41, pp. 847–857.

Brackett, M.A. and Rivers, S.E. (in press), "Transforming students' lives with social and emotional learning", In Pekrun, R. and Linnenbrink-Garcia, L. (Eds.), *Handbook of Emotions in Education*, Routledge, London. http://ei. yale. edu/wp-content/uploads/2013/09/Transforming-Students'-Lives-with-Social-and-Emotional-Learning. pdf

Brackett, M.A., Patti, J., Stern, R., Rivers, S.E., Elbertson, N.A., Chisholm, C. and Salovey, P. (2009), "A sustainable, skill-based approach to building emotionally literate schools", Hughes, M., Thompson, H.L. and Bradford Terrell, J. (Eds.), *Handbook for Developing Emotional and Social Intelligence: Best Practices, Case Studies and Strategies*, Pfeiffer/John Wiley and Sons, San Francisco, CA, US, pp. 329–358.

Brinton, B., Fujiki, M., Montague, E.C. and Hanton, J.L. (2000), "Children with language impairment in cooperative work groups: A pilot study", *Language, Speech, and Hearing Services in Schools*, Vol. 31, pp. 252–264.

Brinton, B., Spackman, M.P., Fujiki, M. and Ricks, J. (2007), "What should Chris say? The ability of children with specific language impairment to recognize the need to dissemble emotions in social situations", *Journal of Speech, Language, and Hearing Research*, Vol. 50, pp. 798–811.

Brown, J.R. and Dunn, J. (1992), "Talk with your mother or your sibling? Developmental changes in early family conversations about feelings", *Child Development*, Vol. 63, pp. 336–349.

Cole, P.M. and Tan, P.Z. (2007), "Emotion socialization from a cultural perspective", In Grusec, E. and Hastings, P. (Eds.), *Handbook of Socialization: Theory and Research*, Guilford Press, NY, US, pp. 516–542.

Collaborative for Academic, Social, and Emotional Learning (2012), *CASEL Guide: Effective social and emotional learning programs: Preschool and elementary school edition*, Downloaded Aug. 24, 2013 from http://casel. org/guide/download-the-2013-guide/

Conti-Ramsden, G. and Botting, N. (2004), "Social difficulties and victimization in children with SLI at 11 years of age", *Journal of Speech, Language, and Hearing Research*, Vol. 47, pp. 145–161.

Denham, S. (1998), *Emotional Development in Young Children*, Guilford Press, NY, US.

Denham, S.A. and Auerbach, S. (1995), "Mother-child dialogue about emotions and preschoolers' emotional competence", *Genetic, Social, and General Psychology Monographs*, Vol. 121, pp. 313–337.

Denham, S.A., Bassett, H.H. and Wyatt, T. (2007), "The socialization of emotional competence", In Grusec, E. and Hastings, P. (Eds.), *Handbook of Socialization: Theory and Research*, Guilford Press, NY, US, pp. 614–637.

Dunn, J., Brown, J. and Bearsdall, L. (1991), "Family talk about feeling states and children's later understanding of others' emotions", *Developmental Psychology*, Vol. 27, pp. 448–455.

Durlak, J.A., Weissberg, R.P., Dymicki, A.B., Taylor, R.D. and Schellinger, K.B. (2011), "The impact of enhancing students' social and emotional learning: A meta-analysis of school-based universal interventions", *Child Development*, Vol. 82, pp. 405–432.

Eisenberg, N., Cumberland, A. and Spinard, T.L. (1998), "Parental socialization of emotion", *Psychological Inquiry*, Vol. 9, pp. 241–273.

Ford, J.A. and Milosky, L.M. (2003), "Inferring emotional reactions in social situations: Differences in children with language impairment", *Journal of Speech, Language, Hearing Research*, Vol. 46, pp. 21–30.

Fujiki, M., Brinton, B. and Clarke, D. (2002), "Emotion regulation in children with specific language impairment", *Language, Speech and Hearing Services in Schools*, Vol. 33, pp. 102–111.

Fujiki, M., Brinton, B., Isaacson, T. and Summers, C. (2001), "Social behaviors of children with language impairment on the playground: A pilot study", *Language, Speech and Hearing Services in Schools*, Vol. 32, pp. 101–113.

Fujiki, M., Brinton, B., McCleave, C., Anderson, V. and Chamberlain, J. (2013), "A social communication intervention to increase the production of validating comments", *Language, Speech, and Hearing Services in Schools*, Vol. 44, pp. 3–19.

Fujiki, M., Brinton, B., Morgan, M. and Hart, C.H. (1999), "Withdrawn and sociable behavior of children with specific language impairment", *Language, Speech, and Hearing Services in Schools*, Vol. 30, pp. 183–195.

Fujiki, M., Brinton, B. and Todd, C. (1996), "Social skills of children with specific language impairment", *Language, Speech, and Hearing Services in Schools*, Vol. 27, pp. 195–202.

Fujiki, M., Spackman, M.P., Brinton, B. and Illig, T. (2008), "The ability of children with language impairment to understand emotion conveyed by prosody in a narrative passage", *International Journal of Language and Communication Disorders*, Vol. 43, pp. 330–345.

Gerber, S., Brice, A., Capone, N.C., Fujiki, M. and Timler, G.R. (2012), "Language use in social interactions of school-age children with language impairments: An evidence-based systematic review of treatment", *Language, Speech, and Hearing Services in Schools*, Vol. 43, pp. 235–249.

Gignac, G. (2010), "Seven-factor model of emotional intelligence as measured by Genos EI: A confirmatory factor analytic investigation based on self- and rater-report data", *European Journal of Psychological Assessment*, Vol. 26, pp. 309–316.

Gottman, J., Katz, L.F. and Hooven, C. (1997), *Meta-Emotion: How Families Communicate Emotionally*, Erlbaum, Mahwah, NJ, US.

Hagelskamp, C., Brackett, M.A., Rivers, S.E. and Salovey, P. (2013), "Improving classroom quality with the RULER approach to social and emotional learning: Proximal and distal outcomes", *American Journal of Community Psychology*, Vol. 51, pp. 530–543.

Harris, P.L. (2008), "Children's understanding of emotion", In Lewis, M., Haviland-Jones, J. and Feldman Barrett, L. (Eds.), *Handbook of Emotions*, 3rd edn., Guilford Press, NY, US, pp. 320–331.

Horowitz, L., Jansson, L., Ljungberg, T. and Hedenbro, M. (2005), "Behavioural patterns of conflict resolution strategies in preschool boys with language impairment in comparison with boys with typical language development", *International Journal of Language and Communication Disorders*, Vol. 40, pp. 431–454.

Kavale, K.A. and Mostert, M.P. (2004), "Social skills interventions for individuals with learning disabilities", *Learning Disability Quarterly*, Vol. 27, pp. 31–43.

Marton, K., Abramoff, B. and Rosenzweig, S. (2005), "Social cognition and language in children with specific language impairment", *Journal of Communication Disorders*, Vol. 38, pp. 143–162.

Mayer, J., Salovey, P., Caruso, D. and Cherkasskiy, L. (2011), "Emotional intelligence", In Sternberg, R. and Kaufman, S. (Eds.), *The Cambridge Handbook of Intelligence*, Cambridge University Press, Cambridge, UK, pp. 528–549.

Pellitteri, J. (2006), "Emotionally intelligent interventions for students with reading disabilities", *Reading and Writing Quarterly*, Vol. 22, pp. 155–171.

Rivers, S.E., Brackett, M.A., Reyes, M.R., Elbertson, N. and Salovey, P. (2013), "Improving the social and emotional climate of classrooms: A clustered randomized controlled trial testing the RULER approach", *Prevention Science*, Vol. 14, pp. 77–87.

Salovey, P., Detweiler-Bedell, B.T., Detweiler-Bedell, J.B. and Mayer, J.D. (2008), "Emotional intelligence", In Lewis, M., Haviland-Jones, J. and Feldman Barrett, L. (Eds.), *Handbook of Emotions*, 3rd edn., Guilford Press, NY, US, pp. 533–547.

Spackman, M.P., Fujiki, M. and Brinton, B. (2006), "Understanding emotions in context: The effects of language impairment on children's ability to infer emotional reactions", *International Journal of Language and Communication Disorders*, Vol. 41, pp. 173–188.

Thompson, R. (1994), "Emotion regulation: A theme in search of definition", *Monographs of the Society for Research in Child Development*, Vol. 59, Issues 2–3, pp. 25–52.

Thompson, R. (Published online: 1 April 2011), "The emotionate child", In Cicchetti, D. and Roisman, G.I. (Eds.), *Minnesota Symposia on Child Psychology: The Origins and Organization of Adaptation and Maladaptation*, John Wiley and Sons, Hoboken, NJ, US, pp. 13–53.

Timler, G.R. (2008), "Social knowledge in children with language impairments: Examination of strategies, predicted consequences, and goals in peer conflict situations", *Clinical Linguistics and Phonetics*, Vol. 22, pp. 741–763.

Zahn-Waxler, C., Ridgeway, D., Denham, S., Usher, B. and Cole, P.M. (1993), "Pictures of infants' emotions: A task for assessing mothers' and young children's verbal communications about affect", In Ende, R., Osofsky, J. and Butterfield, P. (Eds.), *The IFEEL Pictures: A new instrument for interpreting emotions*, International Universities Press, Madison, CT, US, pp. 217–236.

32

SOCIAL PARTICIPATION AND APHASIA

Madeline Cruice

This chapter covers social participation for researchers and practitioners who work with individuals with aphasia and their family members. It considers social participation with reference to a range of theoretical frameworks and models, and synthesizes the evidence base in networks, activities, relationships and predictors of social participation. Formal assessments and informal measures or approaches for collecting information are presented, including assessment of environmental factors that may facilitate or hinder participation. Finally, the chapter content covers different approaches to rehabilitation as well as long-term support.

Frameworks and models for considering social participation with aphasia

Social participation can be defined as life participation in social contexts. It is broader than the construct of "*communicative participation*" defined as "taking part in life situations where knowledge, information, ideas, or feelings are exchanged" (Eadie *et al.*, 2006, p. 309) and can take any form of speaking, listening, reading, writing, or nonverbal means of communication, providing it involves a communicative exchange in a social context. Social participation is a wider more-encompassing construct, with the primary emphasis on social engagement and exchange, which may be influenced by the person and the environment and includes interactions between the person and others in various environments. It is also distinct from broader "*life participation*," which includes activities relating to home and household management, and activities pertaining to work or education. Social participation can be understood by considering the following theoretical frameworks or models of disability.

International Classification of Functioning, Disability and Health (ICF)

The ICF is a classification system for health and disability for adults (World Health Organization, WHO, 2001, www.who.int/classifications/icf/en/). It considers functioning on body, individual and societal levels, and considers health in terms of functions and structures as well as activities and participation, within a personal and environmental context. The ICF is now widely considered a relevant framework for rehabilitation practice, and allied health practitioners globally ascribe to the conceptual underpinning of impairments, activity limitations, and participation restrictions.

Of the nine Activities and Participation domains, Community, Social and Civic Life, is the most relevant and outlines actions and tasks required to participate in an organized social life outside the person's family. It includes engaging in community life (e.g., charitable organizations), religious or spiritual activities, organizations and practices, and most importantly, any form of recreation and leisure (e.g., sports, crafts, socializing). Simmons-Mackie and Kagan (2007) suggested participation restrictions would likely present for people with aphasia in the form of "minimal engagement in social life via conversations, no longer participates in preferred leisure activities, [and] restrictions in making and keeping friends" (p. 246), reminding practitioners of the importance of considering social participation.

Equally relevant is the section on Environmental Factors. It includes features that can be either a facilitator or barrier of activity and participation, such as assistive products and technology for culture, recreation and sport (e.g., a hearing induction loop in a concert hall), or attitudes of family, the public, and health professionals. Such a framework encourages the clinician to think about relevance and importance in broad assessment and management.

Living with Aphasia: Framework for Outcome Measurement (A-FROM)

The A-FROM is a non-prescriptive conceptual framework for measuring outcomes in life areas impacted by the language and communication disability of aphasia (Kagan et al., 2008). It draws on the WHO ICF and other values-based approaches (see Life Participation Approach to Aphasia below), but has the advantage over the ICF of being visually and conceptually more accessible to clients and clinicians, and more person-centered. It also explicitly considers quality of life.

Framework for Therapy for Living with Aphasia

The Framework for Therapy for Living with Aphasia (Pound et al., 2000) outlines six interconnected goal areas for intervention with people with aphasia including: (1) enhancing communication, (2) identifying and dismantling barriers to social participation, (3) adaptation of identity, (4) promoting a healthy psychological state, (5) promoting autonomy and choice, and (6) health promotion/illness prevention. Whilst one goal explicitly targets social participation, others also have relevance (i.e., identity is shaped through social interactions). Furthermore, the framework addresses the person with aphasia as a social being: first as an individual, and then surrounded by and as a member of their immediate social context, being part of different communities (such as work, neighborhood, and religious community), and then as a citizen of society.

Other relevant approaches and philosophies

The frameworks above consider a person with aphasia holistically and incorporate social participation differently. The ICF and A-FROM both emphasize the person with aphasia; although the A-FROM more clearly encourages consideration within society, and is informed by the Social Model of Disability (Byng and Duchan, 2005), which is often cited as relevant when considering clinical practice that addresses the broader consequences of impaired linguistic functioning. In its true form, the Social Model of Disability sees disability as a socially created phenomenon whereby people with aphasia experience difficulties because of disabling barriers and identity (Pound et al., 2000), in turn affecting social participation. (For a more in-depth account of the Social Model of Disability, see Byng and Duchan, 2005.) Two other approaches are frequently mentioned when considering social participation with aphasia. These are described next.

The Life Participation Approach to Aphasia (LPAA) is a philosophical statement of values and ideas about service provision for people with aphasia and all those affected by it (Chapey *et al.*, 2008). It originates from North America, and explicitly addresses life participation and goals in assessment, treatment and outcome evaluation. Use of this approach requires the clinician to acknowledge an expanded clinical role that might include one as "coach" or "problem solver," which is different from the traditional roles of diagnostician and therapist. Furthermore, the emphasis on all those affected means clinicians may be working with family members, friends, and work colleagues.

Consistent with the LPAA, the Social Approach to Aphasia has the explicit goal of "promot[ing] membership in a communicating society and participation in personally relevant activities for those affected by aphasia" (Simmons-Mackie, 2008, p. 290). By emphasizing healthy, active living, it recognizes that communication is a social act, and disrupted communication is socially significant with social consequences. The approach is underpinned by nine principles, all of which are relevant, but the three critical areas address: (1) communication as a social need (e.g., gossiping over a drink) as well as in message exchange (e.g., buying a ticket to a gallery); (2) communication in authentic, relevant and natural contexts; and (3) natural interaction and social consequences. Whilst the LPAA is broad, the Social Approach is more focused on communication using a social frame of reference.

Synthesis of current evidence

There is a growing evidence base, both for individuals with aphasia and their family members/ relatives that can be broadly clustered into areas relating to networks, activities, relationships, and predictors. Much of the research describes the negative impact of aphasia on social participation and a small field of qualitative research that considers living successfully. These areas are reviewed below.

Impact of aphasia

People with aphasia report difficulties speaking in general, and specifically speaking in group situations because of the number of speakers, pace of conversation, and increase in memory requirements (Le Dorze and Brassard, 1995). These difficulties clearly lead to increases in frustration, irritation, anxiety and fatigue for both people with aphasia and their family members, and in turn, can lead to loss and change in social contacts and activities within and beyond family. Other consequences, such as employment reductions, physical changes, and increased family member responsibilities, are likely to further reduce social participation.

Social networks and activities

Social networks describe the number and type of people in one's social circle, and are influenced by one's social activities. Research shows that people with aphasia have significantly smaller social networks when compared to their peers, and, in particular, fewer acquaintances, strangers and friends (Cruice *et al.*, 2006; Davidson *et al.*, 2008). Similarly, research reveals people's social activities are restricted (particularly leisure activities, such as clubs, classes, sports and craft groups), with people participating mostly in everyday chores and routines or activities within the home (Code, 2003; Cruice *et al.*, 2006; Davidson *et al.*, 2008; Natterlund, 2010).

Recent research has focused on what people with aphasia consider important in *living successfully with aphasia*. Activities or "doing things" were of central importance, and included a diverse range of hobbies and interests (e.g., walking, fishing, traveling), going to the gym, work or educationally related activities (volunteering and going to university), and activities related to household management. Activities provide people with aphasia with a sense of independence, achievement, purpose, pleasure, and well-being, and stimulate the brain (Brown *et al.*, 2010). Finally, evidence suggests it is not the number or nature of the social activity that is important, but rather the sense of engagement (Dalemans *et al.*, 2010).

Social relationships

Meaningful relationships provide support, acceptance and understanding, social companionship, and opportunity for caring for others (Brown *et al.*, 2010). However, aphasia affects and disrupts the basics of everyday communication, limiting communication with others, and reduces satisfaction with relationships (Davidson *et al.*, 2008). This often means less communication with friends, acquaintances, and strangers (Brown *et al.*, 2010; Grohn *et al.*, 2012). Friendship is a core domain for everyday communication (Davidson *et al.*, 2008) and participation in activities (leisure and educational) is linked to everyday communication with friends and well-being (Cruice *et al.*, 2006). Because friendships do not follow prescribed roles, friends need to show more initiative in engaging with individuals with aphasia, which can be challenging.

Impact on families' social participation

Family members of people with aphasia have reported negatively altered recreational activities and social lives (Grawburg *et al.*, 2013). Almost all family members reported changes to their leisure activities, hobbies and sports, many going out less often, participating in fewer social activities, and taking fewer vacations. This is likely caused by the increased household and caregiving responsibilities incurred with a relative with aphasia (Grawburg *et al.*, 2013). On the positive side, some family members replaced previous activities with new ones that could be jointly undertaken with the person with aphasia. For some, socializing increased as the family member visited more often (Grawburg *et al.*, 2013).

Predictors of social participation

Severity of *functional communication ability* (not impairment) is significantly associated with social participation (Code, 2003; Cruice *et al.*, 2003), specifically activities, networks, support, and positive relationships with other people (Cruice *et al.*, 2003), and in turn are relevant for psychological well-being (Cruice *et al.*, 2003). Quite separate from language and aphasia, sensory functioning and health are associated with activities and networks, and are thus important to consider (Cruice *et al.*, 2003). Research shows that age, severity, physical disability and transportation influence social participation. People who were older, had more severe aphasia and had a hemiplegia, spent significantly less time outside their homes (Code, 2003). People with aphasia with a family member or partner who drove had more independence, freedom and opportunities for social participation (Code, 2003; Natterlund, 2010).

People with aphasia have reported a range of external environmental factors that hinder their community participation (Howe *et al.*, 2008). These include: (1) uninformed, negative or impatient attitudes; (2) physical aspects, such as dealing with complicated or unfamiliar equipment, machines, and noise; (3) a general lack of public knowledge, services and policies that support aphasia; (4) procedures that rely heavily on communication (e.g., automated phone banking); (5) limited finances; and (6) a lack of transport (Howe *et al.*, 2008). People with aphasia have also reported factors that facilitate their community participation: (1) time and patience in conversations and exchanges; (2) knowledge that someone has had a stroke and information about communication difficulties; and (3) a supportive environment with clear signage, educated and trained staff, and machines and systems that are accessible for people with aphasia (Howe *et al.*, 2008).

In summary, aphasia has a predominantly negative effect on communication and interactions, which in turn affects relationships with family, friends, and the wider community, who are largely unskilled at knowing how to accommodate aphasia and its communication breakdowns. These factors converge to negatively impact people's activities and participation, resulting in a much less rich social life, and possibly loneliness and isolation. Participating in activities and having meaningful relationships are core to living successfully and should inspire clinicians to prioritize these aspects in intervention.

Assessing social participation in aphasia

Most commonly used assessments within speech–language pathology address language impairment and functional communication dis/ability (Verna *et al.*, 2009). There are relatively few measures designed for assessing social participation in aphasia (Eadie *et al.*, 2006). Whilst many new assessments include social participation, they often evaluate general communication dis/ability, emotions, and severity of impairment as well. Subsequently, the clinician can either: (1) use these broader measures but consider the relatively limited information that may be gained; (2) use measures specific for stroke and aphasia (see Stroke Social Network Scale, Table 32.1); (3) use measures originally intended for other clinical groups, such as brain injury, but are applicable to individuals with aphasia; or (4) use more informal measures and methods extracted from previous research studies. Before expanding on points 2–4, it is worth stating that as a general guide in rehabilitation, any assessment/measurement/appraisal and discussion of participation should: (1) involve the person themselves; and (2) consider barriers and facilitators within the environment (Madden *et al.*, 2013; Simmons-Mackie and Kagan, 2007). The "environment should be considered as an independent component capable of influencing integration and, therefore, as a potential focus of intervention, regardless of [one's] preferred model" (Garcia, 2008, p. 353). Assessing the impact of environmental factors on social participation is easier said than done, as most measures separately evaluate participation and environment (Madden *et al.*, 2013). Regardless of how difficult it is to gather information from the person with aphasia, clinicians should strive to gather the individual's own views, as family members and friends do not reliably and predictably rate the aphasic person's social functioning (Cruice *et al.*, 2005).

Formal measures

A comprehensive assessment of social participation in aphasia would involve assessment of the person's: (1) activities; (2) contacts or relationships, achieved through some form of network analysis; and (3) clear examination of environmental factors. When considering social participation, quality is a better indicator than quantity. How someone feels in terms of satisfaction and importance is usually more important than the number of activities they do. Formal measures and informal measures and approaches are available for use (see Tables 32.1 and 32.2 for specifics). All measures are best administered in an oral and written format, maximizing the person's comprehension opportunities, with a qualified speech-language pathologist (SLP).

Table 32.1 Formal measures of social participation and the environment.

Assessment/Measure	Target Population	Items and Content	Relevant aphasia studies
Stroke Social Network Scale (SSNS) Northcott and Hilari (2013)	People with and without aphasia after stroke	19 items Satisfaction with social network, children, relatives, friends and groups	Northcott and Hilari (2013)
Community Integration Questionnaire (CIQ) www.tbims.org/combi/index.html	Brain injury	15 items Home, social, and education/vocational or other productive activities outside the home	Dalemans, De Witte, Beurskens, Van Den Heuvel, and Wade (2010)
Participation Objective Participation Subjective (POPS) Brown et al. (2004) www.tbims.org/combi/index.html	Brain injury	26 items Recreation and Civic Life, and Interpersonal Interactions and Relationships; each item is evaluated objectively and subjectively	Matos et al. (2010)
Craig Hospital Inventory of Environmental Factors (CHIEF) Harrison-Felix (2001) www.tbims.org/combi/index.html	Brain injury	Explores barriers to participating in social, recreational and civic activities, as well as work, school, home, and to what degree the barrier presents a problem	None known
Measure of the Quality of the Environment (MQE) Fougeyrollas et al. (1999) www.indcp.qc.ca/	Disabilities	Explores minor, medium and major obstacles and facilitators that affect people accomplishing their daily activities (or may exert no influence at all)	None known

Table 32.2 Informal measures and methods of social participation in aphasia.

Measure	Items and Content	Method	Notes
Social Activities Checklist (SOCACT) Cruice (2002)	20 items Measures leisure, informal and formal social activities. 2 additional items (satisfaction and barriers).	Checklist of social activities based on existing tools and research in the stroke, community, and mental health literature (see Cruice, 2002). Administration of checklist using supported-interview style.	Records range of social activities undertaken, frequency of each activity (weekly, fortnightly, monthly, rarely, not at all, and not applicable), social activity partners, overall satisfaction, and barriers. Designed for people with and without aphasia.
Social Network of Aphasia Profile (SNAP) Code (2003)	Undetermined Measures type, place, purpose, and partner in social activities.	7-day Diary People with aphasia and their relatives (mainly partners) record information on who they saw, where they saw them, and why they saw them. This is then discussed with the clinician.	Diary provides valuable information on places visited in the community and reasons for visiting, and who people with aphasia spent time with and for how long. The SNAP's author was especially interested in hours spent *outside* the person's home; however, it may be equally useful to document visits that occur within someone's home, especially if there are significant mobility difficulties for the client and/or their family members.
Communicative Profiling System (CPS) Simmons-Mackie and Damico (2001)	Undetermined Captures the client's authentic communicative experience and establishes what the client does in daily life, their social relationships (extent and quality) and their views about their aphasia.	Ethnographic interview (client and clinician), journal or diary kept by person and/or partner, and a form of social network analysis (completed with clinician).	Identifies key life activities for the client prior to the onset of aphasia, at the start of intervention, and post-intervention outcomes; and a graphic depiction of social networks pre and post can reveal changes in social participation. Requires the clinician to be skilled in ethnographic interviewing.
Social Network Map Antonucci and Akiyama (1987)	Undetermined Records information on perceived closeness, number and type/relationship of social contacts, as well as the type and frequency of social contacts.	Three concentric circles (layers) represent different levels of closeness to the respondent. Client records names of people who are important to them in their life at that current time across the circles. Clinician asks a series of questions about each of the named contacts in the network, such as relationship (e.g., sibling), type of social contact (e.g., speak over Skype) and frequency (e.g., monthly).	Is based on the convoy model, which refers to a protective layer/s of others who surround an individual throughout the course of life, providing and receiving social support, enabling the individual to negotiate life's challenges. See Cruice et al. (2006) for use with people with aphasia.

Three formal measures of social participation exist (see Table 32.1), although the most appropriate measure to date may be the Stroke Social Network Scale (Northcott and Hilari, 2013) designed specifically for people with and without aphasia after stroke. This scale has good psychometrics and uses various design features that increase its accessibility, including white space, larger font size, keyword bolding, and reduced linguistic complexity of items and response format. Regarding environmental factors (see Table 32.1), the two measures could be used with appropriate caution for people with aphasia to help identify environmental supports and barriers. For example, densely written information that is not simplified and altered to accommodate acquired dyslexia and aphasia can be a barrier to reading about social activities and events in one's local community.

Using existing participation measures enables practitioners to collect reliable information from clients. However, clinicians must exercise caution in doing so, considering whether the questions or items are relevant for clients, both on a personal level (i.e., it is irrelevant to ask someone about independence in cooking if this was never their role) and on a cultural level, as measures are not always cross-culturally equivalent (Stevelink and Brakel, 2013). A further consideration in using a formal participation measure is that judgments about what is relevant and important to the respondent have already been made when the test items were devised. Qualitative research undertaken with adults with a range of disabilities reveals that participation to them means "active and meaningful engagement/being part of, choice and control, access and opportunity… personal and societal responsibilities, having an impact and supporting others, and social connection, inclusion and membership" (Hammel *et al.*, 2008, p. 1445). Whilst these perspectives are not usually reflected in the existing standardized assessments, they can be considered through the informal methods or approaches below.

Informal measures and methods

Interviews and observations are one recommended way of assessing participation with aphasia (Simmons-Mackie and Kagan, 2007) to explore "who a person interacts with, what they do, where they go" (p. 247). These assessments determine what has changed for the person, what they desire in terms of participation, and can be structured using several informal measures and methods (Table 32.2). Those discussed here include the Social Activities Checklist (SOCACT: Cruice, 2002), the Social Network of Aphasia Profile (SNAP: Code, 2003), the Communicative Profiling System (CPS: Simmons-Mackie and Damico, 2001), and a gerontological approach called Social Network Mapping (see Antonucci and Akiyama, 1987).

The first three instruments draw on life activities, which are fundamentally important as they provide mechanisms for experiencing our identity and self-worth in the world, as well as giving us something to talk about (Lyon *et al.*, 1997). The SOCACT, CPS, and SNAP have different advantages. The SOCACT is structured and easy to administer in a clinical session, and can be used longitudinally for the same client or for comparisons across clients. The CPS is more flexible, focused around the person and can be used to map change in life activities and social networks, and pre- and post-intervention. The SNAP is a diary format, giving clients total freedom to record their actual activities. Diaries are particularly valuable information gathering tools. It is good practice to ask clients and family members to record information from their home context to assist in intervention, goal planning, and evaluation. Furthermore, individuals' own views (recorded in participant logs) can be more insightful than formal assessments at revealing true change after treatment (Lyon *et al.*, 1997). Finally, the Social Network Map is useful for its graphic representation and may have potential in demonstrating change from intervention. Completing this measure can be communicatively challenging but this can be aided by interviewing the person with aphasia in the home environment, where there may be easy access to photographs of people, and family members who can assist in naming the different social contacts.

To conclude, whilst the majority of clinicians in the USA and Australia conduct outcome assessment after aphasia intervention, most of the outcomes capture language and functional communication and less than 10 percent of clinicians collect life participation assessments (Simmons-Mackie *et al.*, 2005; Verna *et al.*, 2009). Robust outcome assessment tools of social participation are needed so practitioners can demonstrate they are meeting national health and professional agendas that emphasize participation in life situations as functional outcomes of intervention (Simmons-Mackie *et al.*, 2005). Furthermore, the *World Report on Disability* recommends the use of robust data collection tools to meet the international need for accurate statistics on disability (Madden *et al.*, 2013; World Health Organization, 2011).

Treatment

Therapy approaches in rehabilitation may be broadly classified as either addressing conversation, communication and social participation of the person with aphasia, or addressing the broader environmental context (see Table 32.3). Most of the frameworks and models outlined earlier draw on both. Following the Social Approach to Aphasia, a SLP could implement any of the following: conversation therapy, communication partner training or conversational coaching, compensatory strategy training, group therapy, and self-advocacy projects (Simmons-Mackie, 2008), as well as counseling and psychological support for people with aphasia and family members. Following the LPAA, treatment would target training of communication partners and reducing barriers to make environments and settings more accessible (Chapey *et al.*, 2008). The Framework for Therapy for Living with Aphasia encourages self-advocacy groups, conversation groups, but particularly emphasizes provision of accessible information, environmental modifications, educational and training packages, and campaigning (Pound *et al.*, 2000). The A-FROM promotes individuals' engagement in relevant and authentic life situations, typically addressing Participation *and* Activity elements of the ICF, e.g., enhancing friendships by increasing participation in conversations. Sometimes, it is important to target more life activities, either for its own merit or as a means of finding meaningful contexts for people to develop and enhance their communication skills (Simmons-Mackie and Damico, 2001), acknowledging that "life experiences provide something to talk about" (Lyon *et al.*, 1997, p. 695).

Intervention can also focus on reducing the environmental barriers and increasing the communicative support for clients with aphasia. This would involve: (1) educating others about aphasia and its consequences; (2) training family members and friends, and ward and hospital staff in supported conversation skills so they can communicate with the person with aphasia; and (3) developing communication resources or alternative and augmentative communication supports with the person with aphasia and the family/staff (Lyon *et al.*, 1997; Simmons-Mackie and Damico, 2001; Simmons-Mackie and Kagan, 2007).

Long-term support is essential for individuals and family members living with chronic aphasia, and community services and organizations (affiliated with or separate from speech–language pathology) typically provide this. Internationally renowned organizations include the Aphasia Center of California (http://aphasiacenter.net/), the Aphasia Institute (www.aphasia. ca/), and Connect – the communication disability network – (www.ukconnect.org/) amongst others. Such organizations provide a range of activities, training, and services to people with aphasia, their family members and friends, workplaces and the general public.

Table 32.3 Intervention approaches that target increased social participation of people with aphasia.

Interventions that target conversation and/or social participation

---

Conversation therapy for the person with aphasia

Conversational coaching (includes the communication partner)

Compensatory training in strategies

Script training and scaffolding

Conversation groups

Group therapy

Self-advocacy work (projects and groups)

Interventions that target the environment

These interventions focus on reducing the environmental barriers by increasing the communicative support for clients with aphasia

- supported conversation partner training of others, including family members and friends, training ward and hospital staff (sometimes also referred to more broadly as communication partner training), and

- collaboratively developing communication resource or alternative and augmentative communication supports

Provision of accessible information

Education of others about aphasia to address ignorance, lack of awareness and attitudes

Campaigning to raise awareness

Engaging with these organizations significantly improves people's quality of life and well being (Hoen *et al.*, 1997; Mumby and Whitworth, 2012; Van der Gaag *et al.*, 2005). People value the support, information, and practical help that are provided (Mumby and Whitworth, 2012), and, often, the confidence gained through engaging with such organizations leads to gains in independence and community participation (Mumby and Whitworth, 2012; Van der Gaag *et al.*, 2005). National aphasia associations, such as www.aphasia.org/ and www.aphasia.org.au/, also play an important role as a primary source of information and support. Local stroke and aphasia or communication support groups typically provide regular opportunities for people to socialize, engage with local community, and continue living well with aphasia.

In summary, relevant treatments to improve social participation may be framed around conversation therapies, group therapy, and self-advocacy. Appropriate interventions also involve making modifications to the environment, including training of communication partners, increasing accessibility, education, and raising awareness about aphasia. Long-term support made available through community support groups is essential for enabling people with aphasia and their families to live well with aphasia.

Conclusion

Focusing on social participation with people with aphasia acknowledges that the acquired language impairment has far-reaching consequences on the relationships, daily life, and social lives of the person with aphasia and those who surround them. Our role involves working collaboratively with the person with aphasia and their relevant family members and others to negotiate and agree on the direction and purposes of treatment. We must be mindful that some clients will prioritize social participation more than others prioritize it. Similarly, we must realize that terminology itself can be a barrier, and people with aphasia talk about being engaged, involved, and belonging (Dalemans *et al.*, 2010) rather than socially participating. Prioritizing social participation does not preclude other relevant treatment approaches; rather they can be used in conjunction, and clinicians often combine several approaches in practice (Verna *et al.*, 2009). Ultimately, emphasizing social participation enables clinicians to work more directly on aspects that are important to people's quality of life, and achieve a maximal impact of intervention.

References

Antonucci, T. and Akiyama, H. (1987), "Social networks in adult life and a preliminary examination of the convoy model", *Journal of Gerontology*, Vol. 42, pp. 519–527.

Brown, K., Worrall, L., Davidson, B. and Howe, T. (2010), "Snapshots of success: An insider perspective on living successfully with aphasia", *Aphasiology*, Vol. 24, pp. 1267–1295.

Brown, M., Dijkers, M.P.J.M., Gordon, W.A., Ashman, T., Charatz, H. and Cheng, Z. (2004), "Participation objective, participation subjective: A measure of participation combining outsider and insider perspectives", *Journal of Head Trauma Rehabilitation*, Vol. 19, pp. 459–481.

Byng, S. and Duchan, J. (2005), "Social model philosophies and principles: Their applications to therapies for aphasia", *Aphasiology*, Vol. 19, pp. 906–922.

Chapey, R., Duchan, J., Elman, R., Garcia, L., Kagan, A., Lyon, J. and Simmons-Mackie, N. (2008), "Life-participation approach to aphasia: A statement of values for the future", in R. Chapey, (Ed.), *Language Intervention Strategies in Aphasia and Related Neurogenic Communication Disorders, 5th Edition*. Lippincott, Williams & Wilkins, Baltimore, Maryland, US, pp. 279–289.

Code, C. (2003), "The quantity of life for people with chronic aphasia", *Neuropsychological Rehabilitation*, Vol. 13, pp. 379–390.

Cruice, M. (2002), "Communication and quality of life in older people with aphasia and healthy older people", Unpublished doctoral dissertation. Division of Speech Pathology, University of Queensland, Australia. Submitted 09/2001 and conferred 04/2002.

Cruice, M., Worrall, L., Hickson, L. and Murison, R. (2003), "Finding a focus for quality of life with aphasia: Social and emotional health, and psychological well-being", *Aphasiology*, Vol. 17, pp. 333–353.

Cruice, M., Worrall, L., Hickson, L. and Murison, R. (2005), "Measuring quality of life: Comparing family members' and friends' ratings with those of their aphasic partners", *Aphasiology*, Vol. 19, pp. 111–129.

Cruice, M., Worrall, L. and Hickson, L. (2006), "Quantifying aphasic people's social lives in the context of non-aphasic peers", *Aphasiology*, Vol. 20, pp. 1210–1225.

Dalemans, R., de Witte, L., Wade, D. and Van Den Heuvel, W. (2010), "Social participation through the eyes of people with aphasia", *International Journal of Language and Communication Disorders*, Vol. 45, pp. 537–550.

Davidson, B., Howe, T., Worrall, L., Hickson, L. and Togher, L. (2008), "Social participation for older people with aphasia: The impact of communication disability on friendships", *Topics in Stroke Rehabilitation*, Vol. 15, pp. 325–340.

Eadie, T., Yorkston, K., Klasner, E., Dudgeon, B., Deitz, J., Baylor, C. and Miller, R. (2006), "Measuring communicative participation: A review of self-report instruments in speech-language pathology", *American Journal of Speech-Language Pathology*, Vol. 15, pp. 307–320.

Fougeyrollas, P., Noreau, L., St-Michel, G. and Boschen, K. (1999), *Measure of the Quality of the Environment, Version 2.0*. International Network of the Disability Creation Process, Lac St-Charles, Quebec, Canada.

Garcia, L. (2008), "Focusing on the consequences of aphasia: Helping individuals get what they need", in R. Chapey (Ed.), *Language Intervention Strategies in Aphasia and Related Neurogenic Communication Disorders, 5th Edition*. Lippincott, Williams & Wilkins, Baltimore, Maryland, US, pp. 349–375.

Grawburg, M., Howe, T., Worrall, L. and Scarinci, N. (2013), "A qualitative investigation into third-party functioning and third-party disability in aphasia: Positive and negative experiences of family members of people with aphasia", *Aphasiology*, Vol. 27, pp. 828–848.

Grohn, B., Worrall, L.E., Simmons-Mackie, N. and Brown, K. (2012), "The first 3-months post-stroke: What facilitates successfully living with aphasia?", *International Journal of Speech-Language Pathology*, 14 4: 390–400. doi: 10.3109/17549507.2012.692813

Hammel, J., Magasi, S., Heinemann, A., Whiteneck, G., Bogner, J. and Rodriguez, E. (2008), "What does participation mean? An insider perspective from people with disabilities", *Disability and Rehabilitation*, Vol. 30, pp. 1445–1460.

Harrison-Felix, C. (2001), "The Craig Hospital Inventory of Environmental Factors", *The Center for Outcome Measurement in Brain Injury*. www.tbims.org/combi/chief (accessed August 21, 2013).

Hoen, B., Thelander, M. and Worsley, J. (1997), "Improvement in psychological well-being of people with aphasia and their families: Evaluation of a community-based programme", *Aphasiology*, Vol. 11, pp. 681–691.

Howe, T., Worrall, L. and Hickson, L. (2008), "Interviews with people with aphasia: Environmental factors that influence their community participation", *Aphasiology*, Vol. 22, pp. 1092–1120.

Kagan, A., Simmons-Mackie, N., Rowland, A., Huijbrets, M., Shumway, E., McEwen, S., *et al.*, (2008), "Counting what counts: A framework for capturing real-life outcomes of aphasia intervention", *Aphasiology*, Vol. 22, pp. 258–280.

Le Dorze, G. and Brassard, C. (1995), "A description of the consequences of aphasia on aphasic persons and their relatives and friends, based on the WHO model of chronic diseases", *Aphasiology*, Vol. 9, pp. 239–255.

Lyon, J.G., Cariski, D., Keisler, L., Rosenbek, J., Levine, R., Kumpula, J., Ryff, C., *et al.*, (1997), "Communication partners: Enhancing participation in life and communication for adults with aphasia in natural settings", *Aphasiology*, Vol. 11, No. 7, pp. 693–708. doi: 10.1080/02687039708249416

Madden, R., Fortune, N., Cheeseman, D., Mpofu, E. and Bundy, A. (2013), "Fundamental questions before recording or measuring functioning and disability", *Disability and Rehabilitation*, Vol. 35, pp. 1092–1096.

Matos, M., Jesus, L., Cruice, M. and Gomes, A. (2010), "Portuguese translation and adaptation of the Communication Disability Profile (CDP) and the Participation Objective, Participation Subjective (POPS) tools", in *Proceedings of the 28th World Congress of the International Association of Logopedics and Phoniatrics* (IALP 2010), Athens, Greece, pp. 60–63.

Mumby, K. and Whitworth, A. (2012), "Evaluating the effectiveness of intervention in long-term aphasia post-stroke: The experience from CHANT (Communication Hub for Aphasia in North Tyneside)", *International Journal of Language and Communication Disorders*, Vol. 47, pp. 398–412.

Natterlund, B. (2010), "A new life with aphasia: Everyday activities and social support", *Scandinavian Journal of Occupational Therapy*, Vol. 17, pp. 117–129.

Northcott, S. and Hilari, K. (2013), "Stroke Social Network Scale: Development and psychometric evaluation of a new patient-reported measure", *Clinical Rehabilitation*, Vol. 27, pp. 823–833.

Pound, C., Parr, S., Lindsay, J. and Woolf, C. (2000), *Beyond Aphasia: Therapies for Living with Communication Disability*. Speechmark Publishing Ltd: Bicester, Oxon, UK.

Simmons-Mackie, N. (2008), "Social approaches to aphasia intervention", in R. Chapey (Ed.), *Language Intervention Strategies in Aphasia and Related Neurogenic Communication Disorders, 5th Edition*. Lippincott, Williams & Wilkins, Baltimore, Maryland, US, pp. 246–268.

Simmons-Mackie, N. and Damico, J. (2001), "Intervention outcomes: A clinical application of qualitative methods", *Topics in Language Disorders*, Vol. 21, pp. 21–36.

Simmons-Mackie, N. and Kagan, A. (2007), "Application of the ICF in aphasia", *Seminars in Speech and Language*, Vol. 28, pp. 244–253.

Simmons-Mackie, N., Threats, T. and Kagan, A. (2005), "Outcome assessment in aphasia: A survey", *Journal of Communication Disorders*, Vol. 38, pp. 1–27.

Stevelink, S. and Brakel, W. (2013), "The cross-cultural equivalence of participation instruments: A systematic review", *Disability and Rehabilitation*, Vol. 35, pp. 1256–1268.

Van der Gaag, A., Smith, L., Davis, S., Moss, B., Cornelius, V., Laing, S. and Mowles, C. (2005), "Therapy and support services for people with long-term stroke and aphasia and their relatives: A six-month follow-up study", *Clinical Rehabilitation*, Vol. 19, pp. 372–380.

Verna, A., Davidson, B. and Howe, T. (2009), "Speech-language pathology services for people with aphasia: A survey of current practice in Australia", *International Journal of Speech-Language Pathology*, Vol. 11, pp. 191–205.

World Health Organization. (2011), *World Report on Disability*. WHO Press, Switzerland.

33

BILINGUALISM AND APHASIA

Mira Goral

It is no longer the case that one needs to justify the study of bilinguals: more than half of the world's population uses more than one language to communicate daily (Ansaldo *et al.*, 2008; Fabbro, 2001; Grosjean, 2012). Understanding the brain's ability to process two or more languages and the consequences brain damage may have on such processes has become the focus of a growing number of research studies. One source of evidence about the neuronal representation and processing of multiple languages in the brain is the study of speakers of more than one language who acquire aphasia. Clinically, understanding the patterns of impairment and recovery in bilingual aphasia has practical implications for assessment and rehabilitation.

Bilinguals are individuals who use more than one language on a regular basis, because they live in a bilingual (or multilingual) community or family or in border areas, or because they emigrated from one country or community to another (the general term "bilinguals" is used hereto refer to bilingual and multilingual speakers). Clinicians, therefore, are likely to encounter bilingual individuals among their clients, including bilinguals who have aphasia, a language impairment resulting from acquired brain damage. Bilingual individuals with aphasia require the adjustment of typical clinical procedures of assessment and treatment; they may also offer insight into the workings of language in the brain.

In this chapter I review the theoretical questions that have guided the neurolinguistic study of bilingualism and the answers that may be found in the study of aphasia. I then discuss clinical studies of assessment and treatment of bilingual individuals with aphasia, highlight their implications for clinicians, and outline future research directions.

Theoretical considerations

As scientists strive to understand how language is organized and processed in the human brain, data obtained from the study of aphasia have been fundamental to neurolinguistic investigation. The natural question, then, regarding people who use more than one language is how multiple languages are organized in a single brain. And just as instances of aphasia have advanced our understanding of brain–language relations, so have instances of aphasia in bilinguals informed our understanding of the organization of multiple languages in the brain.

Models of bilingual representation

Childhood bilinguals acquire and use two languages automatically and effortlessly, similar to how monolingual children acquire their first language. But those who learn a second language after their first language had been acquired may experience the process of learning and using the second language as a conscious and explicit act. It has been suggested that, whereas implicit (procedural) memory systems are engaged in the acquisition and use of a person's first language, it is explicit (declarative) memory systems that underline second language learning (Paradis, 1994; Ullman, 2001). This hypothesis would be consistent with the postulation of separate neuronal networks for the first versus a second language (Giussani *et al.*, 2007). An alternative approach is the convergence hypothesis (Abutalebi, 2008; Green, 1998), which suggests that all languages of a bilingual are processed by the same neuronal networks, and there is no separation of systems. Under the convergence hypothesis, what allows bilinguals to separate their languages and alternate between them is a control mechanism: a cognitive ability to activate and inhibit each language, associated with its own neuronal networks that may be domain-general or language-specific. Furthermore, the convergence hypothesis postulates a shared language "repertoire" whereas the explicit–implicit systems hypothesis assumes separate "stores", at least for certain linguistic domains (e.g., phonology, syntax).

Research studies that aim to address these hypotheses have examined language behaviors of healthy bilinguals under monolingual versus bilingual task presentations. Psycholinguistic evidence from studies of neurotypical bilinguals supports the convergence theory in that a growing number of experimental data (behavior as well as electrophysiological) show that the languages of bilinguals are always active and ready for selection and that bilinguals engage in processes of inhibition that allow them to select the right word at the right time (de Groot *et al.*, 2000; Kroll *et al.*, 2006; Misra *et al.*, 2012). As well, data from neuroimaging studies with bilingual individuals have accumulated since the first PET and fMRI studies were conducted with bilinguals, starting in the last decades of the twentieth century. These findings are varied and, often, can be interpreted as supporting either of the opposing views, depending on the researchers' focus or bias (e.g., small activation differences between languages can be highlighted as differences or minimized in the context of large overlap; see, for example, Giussani *et al.*, 2007). A review of those studies is beyond the scope of this chapter; for recent reviews of psycholinguistic evidence see Altarriba and Gianico (2003); Dijkstra (2005); Kroll *et al.* (2008, 2012) and of neuroimaging studies see Indefrey (2006); Obler *et al.* (2007); Sebastian *et al.* (2011); Vaid and Hull (2002). The inconsistencies in the findings reported in these literatures may result, in part, from the heterogeneity of the subject population studied. Indeed, several variables have been found to determine whether overlapping activation patterns are likely to be found.

Several key variables have emerged as influencing factors in the psycholinguistic study of response latencies and intrusion errors (during tasks such as picture naming, lexical decision, and oral reading) and in the neurolinguistic study of brain activation during bilingual language processing as captured by neuroimaging techniques. These variables include age of language acquisition, levels of language proficiency, and sociolinguistic considerations of language use and status.

For example, differential activation loci were found for later learners or dominant bilinguals but not for highly proficient early learners during a grammaticality-judgment task in a fMRI study (Wartenburger *et al.*, 2003). As well, during a picture-naming task, when participants were instructed to name the picture in one of their languages given a cue, evidence for greater inhibition of the more dominant language was observed for bilinguals who were more proficient

368

in one of their languages (Costa and Santesteban, 2004; Meuter and Allport, 1999) and when their less-dominant language was the dominant language spoken in the environment (Linck *et al.*, 2009). Thus, conclusions from studies that support separate or shared representations may be specific to the type of populations examined.

Evidence from bilingual aphasia

Evidence from aphasia should be able to provide a straightforward answer to the question of overlapping versus diverging language representation. If the languages of a bilingual share the same neuronal networks, a single focal brain lesion should affect both languages, whereas if there are separate brain regions responsible for each language – within the language-dominant hemisphere or across the two hemispheres – a selective language impairment would be found. Early reports, however, described both types of results: parallel (or comparable) impairment in all languages of a bilingual, and non-parallel impairment in which the languages appeared affected to different degrees (Albert and Obler, 1978; Paradis, 1983).

It has been argued that the majority of bilinguals experience parallel impairment (e.g., Fabbro, 2001). That is, proficient bilinguals prior to the stroke demonstrate comparable impairment in their two languages following the stroke (e.g., de Diego Balaguer *et al.*, 2004). As well, bilinguals who were dominant in one of their languages prior to their strokes will have better abilities in their pre-stroke stronger language than in the pre-stroke weaker one, maintaining the same relative proficiency in their languages (e.g., Kiran and Roberts, 2010, participant 3). These cases of parallel impairment can be taken as supporting evidence for overlapping representation of multiple languages. Yet, the fascinating cases of non-parallel patterns published in the literature, perhaps with even greater frequency than cases of parallel impairment, have piqued the interest of aphasiologists and neurolinguists, leading to a number of hypotheses regarding the reasons underlying a relative sparing of one language and not the other.

Ribot (1882) hypothesized that the earliest acquired language would be more resistant to impairment, consistent with Freud's (1891) idea of the importance of the mother tongue. Pitres (1895) suggested that the language most used at the time prior to the aphasia onset would prevail. In the early twentieth century Minkowski (1983) emphasized the importance of attitude and motivation to the recovery of one language or another. Paradis and colleagues demonstrated that selective accessibility can alternate between the two languages (Paradis *et al.*, 1982). Some of these earlier reports did not include systematic testing or long-term data, nor did they have the advantage of later developed neuroimaging tools. Nevertheless, they documented instances in which one language was relatively spared and one language was affected by a single lesion, suggesting that these languages had differential underlying representations.

Consistent with differential representation, Gloning and Gloning (1983) proposed that a later-learned language would engage right hemisphere regions and predicted more instances of crossed aphasia – aphasia following a right hemisphere stroke – in bilinguals than in monolinguals. While promising, evidence for greater right hemisphere involvement in the processing of later-learned languages of bilinguals did not receive great support either from aphasia data or from early studies of the bilingual brain (Vaid and Hull, 2002).

The lack of clear increased prevalence of crossed aphasia in bilinguals and the existence of a variety of impairment (and recovery) patterns, including bilinguals' alternating accessibility to their languages, pointed researchers back to the assumption of largely overlapping brain regions for multiple languages. But the curious patterns of selective accessibility together with evidence for unintentional language mixing (Fabbro *et al.*, 2000; Perecman, 1984) promoted the idea articulated by Green and Abutalebi (2008) to account for the variable data. They hypothesized that multiple languages are subserved by virtually overlapping brain networks and that other networks are responsible for processes of control, allowing – when intact – for smooth language selection by engaging mechanisms of activation and inhibition. Such a view can account for all patterns of impairment: parallel, because the same networks subserve all languages; and non-parallel, because impaired mechanisms of selection can result in apparent selective impairment.

Thus, evidence from aphasia in bilingual speakers points to a complex picture, supporting current theories of bilingual processing. Parallel patterns of impairment following a single lesion are consistent with the convergence hypothesis of bilingual representation, and non-parallel patterns of impairment and recovery are consistent with processes of language selection via mechanisms of activation and inhibition. The precise manner in which variables, such as age of acquisition, language proficiency, and language use interact in these processes is yet to be explicated.

Clinical implications

The answers to the theoretical questions posed above may have strong implications for clinical practice. Comprehensive assessment in bilingual aphasia could reveal degrees and patterns of impairment, which in turn can inform choices regarding rehabilitation.

Assessment

General tests
The assessment of bilinguals with aphasia can be quite challenging. Obstacles include limited availability of tools, examiners, and scoring and interpretation procedures, as well as a dearth of information regarding pre-stroke levels of language proficiency and language use. Aphasia batteries and tests have been developed in a number of different languages and a number of tests that were developed in one language have been translated and adapted to additional languages. However, few of these measures have been explicitly designed to test bilinguals. As a result, the comparability of the versions of the same test in different languages is not typically established, nor are there systematic normative data for bilingual performance. One exception is the Bilingual Aphasia Test (BAT; Paradis and Libben, 1987), which was specifically developed to provide a comparable battery in multiple languages. The test is available today (at no cost) in more than 50 languages (www.mcgill.ca/linguistics/research/bat/). Moreover, one of its sections specifically addresses translation abilities between common language pair combinations (e.g., Arabic–French, Spanish–English, Cantonese–Mandarin). Despite some limitations, such as a small number of items in certain subsections, the BAT has been successfully used in research studies (see for example recent special issues of the *Journal of Neurolinguistics* and *Clinical Linguistics and Phonetics*), as well as in clinical practice.

Tests of naming ability
In addition to the BAT, several tests to assess anomia in bilingual individuals are now available (for a review of Spanish–English bilinguals, see Muñoz, 2012) and normative data have started to accumulate for tests such as the Object and Action Naming Battery (OANB; Druks and Masterson, 2000) (e.g., Edmonds and Donovan, 2012) and the Boston Naming Test (BNT; Kaplan *et al.*, 2001) (e.g., Gollan *et al.*, 2007; Roberts *et al.*, 2002). Interesting findings have emerged when performance of bilinguals in their two languages is compared. For example, Spanish–English bilinguals who acquire Spanish at home and English in early childhood at school or from peers typically perform better on the BNT in English than in Spanish even when

they rate their Spanish as their dominant language (e.g., Kohnert *et al.*, 1998). Furthermore, bilinguals' scores on the naming test are higher when the number of pictures named in either language is considered than when the score in each language alone is calculated. However, this difference seems to be meaningful in the bilinguals' non-dominant language, but not in their dominant language (Gollan and Silverberg, 2001).

Tests of syntactic ability

Few studies have focused on patterns of impaired syntactic processing across the languages of bilinguals with aphasia. Available evidence suggests that in this domain, a common finding is that of comparable qualitative impairment in two languages that share grammatical structures (Miozzo *et al.*, 2010). For example, de Diego Balaguer and colleagues (2004) have observed the same dissociation of relatively spared regular verb morphology and relatively impaired irregular verb morphology in two different individuals in both their highly proficient Spanish and Catalan, two languages that share verb morphology (but also have some structural differences). A similar pattern was also reported for a highly proficient German–English bilingual (Cholin *et al.*, 2007). Faroqi-Shah and Waked (2010) confirmed a relatively greater impairment in verbs than in nouns in bilinguals with aphasia, similar to the pattern previously reported for monolinguals with aphasia.

Scoring procedures

Even when the comparability of the tests used in different languages is established, scoring procedures pose another challenge for assessment of bilinguals generally and of bilinguals with aphasia particularly. Bilinguals who typically switch between their languages may do so during testing even if the examiners use only one language, and, consequently, correct responses in the non-target language(s) may need to be considered. Cross-language influences, such as borrowed words, foreign pronunciation of cognate words, and awkward syntactic structures that transfer from one language to another comprise special types of errors. The extent to which such errors originate from pre-stroke levels of language proficiency as opposed to aphasia-related impairment needs to be appraised.

Other considerations

Another great challenge that a clinician may face is determining the pre-stroke levels of proficiency in each of a bilingual's languages. There are thorough questionnaires available, which are useful (e.g., Part A of the BAT; Muñoz *et al.*, 1999), but a caution is that information on proficiency primarily comes from self-report. Self-assessment has proven to be a relatively reliable measure of proficiency, but given inter-individual variability, self-rating can only approximate overall levels of ability (Lindman, 1977; Gollan *et al.*, 2012; Muñoz and Marquardt, 2003). Additional practical considerations include: a) concern for the order of testing; b) whether to test both or all languages on the same day; c) whether the examiner should be a monolingual of each language or a person from the same community of speakers; and d) whether testing in all languages should nevertheless be completed with the aid of interpreters if there are no clinicians who are sufficiently proficient in the language in question (e.g., Ansaldo *et al.*, 2008). Limitations here include the tendency of interpreters to "help" the person who is being tested and thus improve their responses (American Speech–Language–Hearing Association, 1985).

Treatment

The central question regarding treatment in bilingual aphasia has been which language should be treated. Decisions can be guided by practical considerations, such as availability of clinicians in a minority language, the preference expressed by the person with aphasia or the caregivers, and the language that may be most useful in daily interactions. As well, theory-driven research evidence may facilitate the decision about language choice. Specifically, information about the degree to which treatment in one language can benefit the untreated language(s) is critical for such decisions (for a similar issue with bilingual children, see the Kohnert chapter, this volume).

A growing body of detailed studies informs us about the effects of treatment in the first versus the second language of bilinguals and about the degree to which treatment benefits carry over to the untreated languages. The findings to date portray a mixed, complex picture (see reviews in Faroqi-Shah *et al.*, 2010; Kohnert and Peterson, 2012). Because bilingual people with aphasia vary greatly in their language history, use, and proficiency, and in their language impairments, generalizing from individual cases should be done with caution. Nevertheless, several patterns can be discerned from the data available, pending additional and supporting research findings. Evidence points to cross-language carry over, dependent on language proficiency, language use, and language similarities. It is possible that treating both (or all) languages is most beneficial for bilinguals with aphasia (Ansaldo *et al.*, 2008), but little systematic research on the efficacy of mixed treatment has been published to date. Most research studies report on the effects of treatment conducted in one of the bilingual's languages.

Language proficiency

Treatment in a bilingual's first or dominant language has been shown to be effective in bilinguals who demonstrate comparable abilities in their two languages, yielding improvement in the first, treated language as well as in the untreated, secondary language (Edmonds and Kiran, 2006; Junqué *et al.*, 1989). Treatment in a bilingual's second language is beneficial to improve skills in the treated language, and benefit may transfer to the untreated language (e.g., Goral *et al.*, 2010; Miertsch *et al.*, 2009). Positive treatment transfer may be found particularly when the proficiency in both languages is comparably high (e.g., Edmonds and Kiran, 2006; Kiran and Roberts, 2010, participant 4; Marangolo *et al.*, 2009). However, recent evidence suggests that when the treated second language presents lower proficiency than the untreated first language, the first (untreated) language does not benefit from the treatment (Kiran and Roberts, 2010, participant 1; Miller Amberber, 2012) or, under certain circumstances, even demonstrates temporary negative effects (Abutalebi *et al.*, 2009). This negative effect on the stronger language is consistent with psycholinguistic findings of the inhibition of the more dominant language during processing of a weaker one, discussed above (Goral *et al.*, 2013).

Language use

In addition to language status and language proficiency, patterns of language use influence cross-language treatment effects. For example, switching between two languages within the same conversation or the same utterance may be a manifestation of impairment (Perecman, 1984), but could also be a useful strategy (Ansaldo *et al.*, 2010; Goral *et al.*, 2006) that resembles typical patterns of communication among bilinguals (e.g., Myers-Scotton, 1993). Moreover, the language spoken in the environment may benefit more from treatment than when treatment is given in a language that is not the one spoken around the person with aphasia (Abutalebi *et al.*, 2009; Goral *et al.*, 2012).

Language similarities

Finally, treating language domains that are shared between the languages in question can yield benefits in both the treated and untreated languages, as suggested in several studies that have found that only shared aspects benefited from cross-language generalization. This has been demonstrated for the lexical domain (Kohnert, 2004) and for morphosyntax (Goral *et al.*, 2010).

Many people with aphasia report having been advised to select only one language for communication following their stroke to maximize recovery; yet there is no clear research evidence to support this decision. Individuals who have had the opportunity to receive treatment in multiple languages have expressed their satisfaction, even excitement, with the prospect of resuming the use of multiple languages. Such ethnographic considerations contribute to clinical decisions (e.g., Centeno, 2007), as do cultural considerations, including the custom of mixing two languages in bilingual conversations and patterns of language use by the critical communication partners of the person with aphasia (e.g., Battle, 1998).

Concluding remarks and future research directions

The systematic investigation of assessment tools and procedures in bilingual aphasia and of within- and between-language treatment effects informs clinicians and caregivers and facilitates decisions about optimal care for bilingual individuals with aphasia. Many questions are still in need of answers, especially amid great inter-individual variability and the multitude of influencing variables. Further examination of the variables that have been identified thus far in the literature can help determine the degree to which each factor and the interaction of factors influence impairment and rehabilitation. Future studies that expand on those published to date, adding participants and language combinations can provide answers to such questions.

Fertile grounds for future study include the investigation of multiple individuals with similar language histories on the one hand, and investigations of multiple individuals with differing language histories on the other hand. Thus, for example, controlling for language proficiency and varying order of acquisition or frequency of language use in one set of studies and controlling order of acquisition and varying the other variables in another can help isolate the contribution of each of these variables to impairment and recovery in aphasia.

Theoretically, understanding the interplay of these critical variables can help test and develop theories of brain networks that support language processing and the adjustments that may take place following lesions. One such avenue is the examination of brain changes following behavioral treatment using functional neuroimaging with individuals with aphasia. Recent studies have begun to address questions of neuronal networks' reorganization that is associated with aphasia recovery in monolinguals (e.g., Berthier *et al.*, 2011) and in bilinguals (e.g., Meinzer *et al.*, 2007). Furthermore, evidence from bilingual aphasia may help resolve current controversies regarding the roles of age of language acquisition and language proficiency in language representation and activation (e.g., Finkbeiner *et al.*, 2006; Hartsuiker and Costa, 2008; Kroll *et al.*, 2006). Indeed, bidirectional communication between theory and practice in bilingual aphasia has the promise of informing clinical practices and advancing scientific investigation.

References

Abutalebi, J. (2008), "Neural aspects of second language representation and language control", *ActaPsychologica*, Vol. 128, pp. 466–478.

Abutalebi, J., Rosa, P.A.D., Tettamanti, M., Green, D.W. and Cappa, S.F. (2009), "Bilingual aphasia and language control: A follow-up fMRI and intrinsic connectivity study", *Brain and Language*, Vol. 109, pp. 141–156.

Albert, M.L. and Obler, L.K. (1978), *The Bilingual Brain: Neuropsychological and Neurolinguistic Aspects of Bilingualism*. Orlando, Florida, US: Academic Press.

Altarriba, J. and Gianico, J. (2003), "Lexical ambiguity resolution across languages: A theoretical and empirical review", *Experimental Psychology*, Vol. 50, pp. 159–170.

American Speech–Language–Hearing Association. (1985), Clinical management of communicatively handicapped minority language populations [Position Statement]. Available from www.asha.org/policy

Ansaldo, A.I., Marcotte, K., Scherer, L. and Raboyeau, G. (2008), "Language therapy and bilingual aphasia: Clinical implications of psycholinguistic and neuroimaging research", *Journal of Neurolinguistics*, Vol. 21, pp. 539–557.

Ansaldo, A.I., Saidi, L.G. and Ruiz, A. (2010), "Model–driven intervention in bilingual aphasia: Evidence from a case of pathological language mixing", *Aphasiology*, Vol. 24, pp. 309–324.

Battle, D.E. (1998), *Communication Disorders in Multicultural Populations*. Boston, MA, US: Butterworth-Heinemann.

Berthier, M.L., García-Casares, N., Walsh, S.F., Nabrozidis, A., Ruíz de Mier, R.J., Green, C., *et al.*, (2011), "Recovery from post-stroke aphasia: Lessons from brain imaging and implications for rehabilitation and biological treatments", *Discovery Medicine*, Vol. 12, pp. 275–289.

Centeno, J.G. (2007), "Considerations for an ethnopsycholinguistic framework for aphasia intervention", in A. Ardila and E. Ramos, (Eds.), *Speech and Language Disorders in Bilinguals*. New York: Nova Science, pp. 213–234.

Cholin, J., Goldberg, A.M., Bertz, J.W., Rapp, B. and Miozzo, M. (2007), "The nature of the processing distinction between regular and irregular verbs: Evidence from an English–German bilingual aphasic speaker", *Brain and Language*, Vol. 103, pp. 61–62.

Costa, A. and Santesteban, M. (2004), "Lexical access in bilingual speech production: Evidence from language switching in highly proficient bilinguals and L2 learners", *Journal of Memory and Language*, Vol. 50, pp. 491–511.

de Diego Balaguer, R., Costa, A., Sebastián-Galles, N., Juncadella, M. and Caramazza, A. (2004), "Regular and irregular morphology and its relationship with agrammatism: Evidence from two Spanish-Catalan bilinguals", *Brain and Language*, Vol. 91, pp. 212–222.

de Groot, A.M., Delmaaret, P. and Lupker, S.J. (2000), "The processing of interlexical homographs in translation recognition and lexical decision: Support for non-selective access to bilingual memory", *The Quarterly Journal of Experimental Psychology*, Vol. 53A, No. 2, pp. 397–428.

Dijkstra, T. (2005), "Bilingual word recognition and lexical access" in J.F. Kroll and A.M.B. De Groot, (Eds.), *Handbook of Bilingualism: Psycholinguistic Approaches*. New York, Oxford University Press; pp. 179–201.

Druks, M. and Masterson, J. (2000), *An Object and Action Naming Battery*. Hove, UK: Psychology Press.

Edmonds, L.A. and Kiran, S. (2006), "Effect of semantic naming treatment on crosslinguistic generalization in bilingual aphasia", *Journal of Speech, Language and Hearing Research*, Vol. 49, pp. 729–748.

Edmonds, L.A. and Donovan, N. (2012), "Item-level psychometrics and predictors of performance for Spanish/English bilingual speakers on an Object and Action Naming Battery", *Journal of Speech-Language-Hearing Research*, Vol. 55, pp. 359–381.

Fabbro, F. (2001), "The bilingual brain: Bilingual aphasia", *Brain and Language*, Vol. 79, pp. 201–210.

Fabbro, F., Skrap, M. and Aglioti, S. (2000), "Pathological switching between languages after frontal lesions in a bilingual patient", *Journal of Neurology, Neurosurgery and Psychiatry*, Vol. 68, pp. 650–652.

Faroqi-Shah, Y. and Waked, A.N. (2010), "Grammatical category dissociation in multilingual aphasia", *Cognitive Neuropsychology*, Vol. 27, pp. 181–203.

Faroqi-Shah, Y., Frymark, T., Mullen, R. and Wang, B. (2010), "Effect of treatment for bilingual individuals with aphasia: A systematic review of the evidence", *Journal of Neurolinguistics*, Vol. 23, pp. 319–341.

Finkbeiner, M., Gollan, T.H. and Caramazza, A. (2006), "Lexical access in bilingual speakers: What's the (hard) problem?", *Bilingualism: Language and Cognition*, Vol. 9, pp. 153–166.

Freud, S. (1891), *ZurAuffassung der Aphasien* (translated to English as On Aphasia by E. Stengel, 1953), New York: International University Press.

Giussani, C., Roux, F.-E., Lubrano, V., Gaini, S.M. and Bello, L. (2007), "Review of language organization in bilingual patients: What can we learn from direct brain mapping?", *Acta Neurochirurgica*, Vol. 149, pp. 1109–1116.

Gloning, I. and Gloning, K. (1983), "Aphasia in polyglots contribution to the dynamics of language disintegration as well as to the question of the localization of these impairments", in M. Paradis, (Ed.), *Readings on Aphasia in Bilinguals and Polyglots*. Montreal, Canada: Marcel Didier, pp. 681–716.

Gollan, T.H. and Silverberg, N.B. (2001), "Tip-of-the-tongue states in Hebrew–English bilinguals", *Bilingualism: Language and Cognition*, Vol. 4, pp. 63–83.

Gollan, T.H., Fennema-Notestine, C., Montoya, R.I. and Jernigan, T.L. (2007), "The bilingual effect on Boston Naming Test performance", *Journal of the International Neuropsycholgical Society*, Vol. 13, pp. 197–208.

Gollan, T.H., Weissberger, G.H., Runnqvist, E., Montoya, R.I. and Cera, C.M. (2012), "Self-ratings of spoken language dominance: A Multilingual Naming Test (MINT) and preliminary norms for young and aging Spanish–English bilinguals", *Bilingualism: Language and Cognition*, Vol. 15, pp. 594–615.

Goral, M., Levy, E.S., Obler, L.K. and Cohen, E. (2006), "Lexical connections in the multilingual lexicon", *Brain and Language*, Vol. 98, pp. 235–247.

Goral, M., Levy, E.S. and Kastl, R. (2010), "Cross-language treatment generalisation: A case of trilingual aphasia", *Aphasiology*, Vol. 24, No. 2, pp. 170–187.

Goral, M., Rosas, J., Conner, P.S., Maul, K.K. and Obler, L.K. (2012), "Effects of language proficiency and language of the environment on aphasia therapy in a multilingual", *Journal of Neurolinguistics*, Vol. 25, pp. 538–551.

Goral, M., Naghibolhosseini, M. and Conner, P.S. (2013), "Asymmetric inhibitory treatment effects in multilingual aphasia", *Cognitive Neuropsychology*, Vol. 30, pp. 564–577.

Green, D.W. (1998), "Mental control of the bilingual lexico-semantic system", *Bilingualism: Language and Cognition*, Vol. 1, pp. 67–81.

Green, D.W. and Abutalebi, J. (2008), "Understanding the link between bilingual aphasia and language control", *Journal of Neurolinguistics*, Vol. 21, pp. 558–576.

Grosjean, F. (2012), *Bilingual: Life and Reality*. Cambridge, MA, US: Harvard University Press.

Hartsuiker, R.J. and Costa, A. (2008), "Bilingualism: Functional and neural perspectives", *Acta Psychologica*, Vol. 128, pp. 413–415.

Indefrey, P. (2006), "A meta-analysis of hemodynamic studies on first and second language processing: Which suggested differences can we trust and what do they mean?", *Language Learning*, Vol. 56, pp. 279–304.

Junqué, C., Vendrell, P. and Vendrell-Brucet, J. (1989), "Differential recovery in naming in bilingual aphasics", *Brain and Language*, Vol. 36, pp. 16–22.

Kaplan, E., Goodglass, H. and Weintraub, S. (2001), *Boston Naming Test*. Philadelphia, PA, US: Lippincott Williams and Wilkins.

Kiran, S. and Roberts, P.M. (2010), "Semantic feature analysis treatment in Spanish–English and French–English bilingual aphasia", *Aphasiology*, Vol. 24, pp. 231–261.

Kohnert, K. (2004), "Cognitive and cognate-based treatments for bilingual aphasia: A case study", *Brain and Language*, Vol. 91, pp. 294–302.

Kohnert, K. and Peterson, M. (2012), "Generalization in bilingual aphasia treatment" in M.R. Gitterman, M. Goral and L.K. Obler, *Aspects of Multilingual Aphasia*. Bristol, UK: Multilingual Matters, pp. 89–105.

Kohnert, K.J., Hernandez, A.E. and Bates, E. (1998), "Bilingual performance on the Boston Naming Test: Preliminary norms in Spanish and English", *Brain and Language*, Vol. 65, pp. 422–440.

Kroll, J.F., Bobb, S. and Wodniecka, Z. (2006), "Language selectivity is the exception, not the rule: Arguments against a fixed locus of language selection in bilingual speech", *Bilingualism: Language and Cognition*, Vol. 9, pp. 119–135.

Kroll, J.F., Bobb, S.C., Misra, M., Guo, M. and Guo, T.M. (2008), "Language selection in bilingual speech: Evidence for inhibitory processes", *Acta Psychologica*, Vol. 128, pp. 416–430.

Kroll, J.F., Dussias, P.E., Bogulski, C.A. and Valdes-Kroff, J. (2012), "Juggling two languages in one mind: What bilinguals tell us about language processing and its consequences for cognition", in B. Ross, (Ed.), *The Psychology of Learning and Motivation*. San Diego: Academic Press, Vol. 56, pp. 229–262.

Linck, J.A., Kroll, J.F. and Sunderman, G. (2009), "Losing access to the native language while immersed in a second language: Evidence for the role of inhibition in second-language learning", *Psychological Science*, Vol. 20, pp. 1507–1515.

Lindman, R. (1977), "Self-ratings and linguistic proficiency in bilingual subjects", *Language and Speech*, Vol. 20, pp. 325–332.

Marangolo, P., Rizzi, C., Peran, P., Piras, F. and Sabatini, U. (2009), "Parallel recovery in a bilingual aphasic: A neurolinguistic and fMRI study", *Neuropsychology*, Vol. 23, pp. 405–409.

Meuter, R.F. and Allport, A. (1999), "Bilingual language switching in naming: Asymmetrical costs of language selection", *Journal of Memory and Language*, Vol. 40, pp. 25–40.

Meinzer, M., Obleser, J., Flaisch, T., Eulitz, C. and Rockstroh, B. (2007), "Recovery from aphasia as a function of language therapy in an early bilingual patient demonstrated by fMRI", *Neuropsychologia*, Vol. 45, pp. 1247–1256.

Miertsch, M., Meisel, J.M. and Isel, F. (2009), "Non-treated languages in aphasia therapy of polyglots benefit from improvement in the treated language", *Journal of Neurolinguistics*, Vol. 22, pp. 135–150.

Miller Amberber, A. (2012), "Language intervention in French-English bilingual aphasia: Evidence of limited therapy transfer", *Journal of Neurolinguistics*, Vol. 25, pp. 588–614.

Minkowski, M. (1983), "A clinical contribution to the study of polyglot aphasia especially with respect to Swiss-German", in M. Paradis, *Readings on Aphasia in Bilinguals and Polyglots*. Montreal, Canada: Marcel Didier, pp. 205–232.

Miozzo, M., Costa, A., Hernandez, M. and Rapp, B. (2010), "Lexical processing in the bilingual brain: Evidence from grammatical/morphological deficits", *Aphasiology*, Vol. 24, pp. 262–287.

Misra, M., Guo, T., Bobb, S.C. and Kroll, J.F. (2012), "When bilinguals choose a single word to speak: Electrophysiological evidence for inhibition of the native language", *Journal of Memory and Language*, Vol. 67, pp. 224–237.

Muñoz, M. (2012), "Anomia in bilingual speakers of Spanish and English", in M.R. Gitterman, M. Goral and L.K. Obler. *Aspects of Multilingual Aphasia*. Bristol, UK: Multilingual Matters, pp. 69–88.

Muñoz, M.L. and Marquardt, T.P. (2003), "Picture naming and identification in bilingual speakers of Spanish and English with and without aphasia", *Aphasiology*, Vol. 17, pp. 1115–1132.

Muñoz, M.L., Marquardt, T.P. and Copeland, G. (1999), "A comparison of the codeswitching patterns of aphasic and neurologically normal bilingual speakers of English and Spanish", *Brain and Language*, Vol. 66, pp. 249–274.

Myers-Scotton, C. (1993), *Duelling Languages: Grammatical Structure in Codeswitching*, Oxford, England: Oxford University Press.

Obler, L.K., Hyun, J-M., Conner, P.S., O'Connor, B. and Anema, I. (2007), "Brain organization of language in bilinguals", in A. Ardila and E. Ramos, (Eds.), *Speech and Language Disorders in Bilinguals*. New York: Nova Science Publishers, pp. 21–46.

Paradis, M. (1983), *Readings on Aphasia in Bilinguals and Polyglots*. Montreal, Canada: Marcel Didier.

Paradis, M. (1994), "Neurolinguistic aspects of implicit and explicit memory: Implications for bilingualism", in N. Ellis (Ed.), *Implicit and Explicit Learning of Second Language*. London: Academic Press, pp. 393–419.

Paradis, M. and Libben, G. (1987), *The Assessment of Bilingual Aphasia*, Hillsdale, NJ, US: Lawrence Erlbaum Associates.

Paradis, M., Goldblum, M.C. and Abidi, R. (1982), "Alternate antagonism with paradoxical translation behavior in two bilingual aphasic patients", *Brain and Language*, Vol. 15, pp. 55–69.

Perecman, E. (1984), "Spontaneous translation and language mixing in a polyglot aphasic", *Brain and Language*, Vol. 23, pp. 43–63.

Pitres, A. (1895), "Etude sur l'aphasie", *Revue de Médecine*, Vol. 15, pp. 873–899.

Ribot, T. (1882), *Disease of Memory* (English trans.), London: Kegan Paul, Trench and Co.

Roberts, P.M., Garcia, L.J., Desrochers, A. and Hernandez, D. (2002), "English performance of proficient bilingual adults on the Boston Naming Test", *Aphasiology*, Vol. 16, pp. 635–645.

Sebastian, R., Laird, A., Kiran, A. and Kiran, S. (2011), "Meta-analysis of the neural representation of first language and second language", *Applied Psycholinguistics*, Vol. 32, pp. 799–819.

Ullman, M.T. (2001), "The neural basis of lexicon and grammar in first and second language: The declarative/procedural model", *Bilingualism: Language and Cognition*, Vol. 4, pp. 105–122.

Vaid, J. and Hull, R. (2002), "Re-envisioning the bilingual brain using functional neuroimaging: Methodological and interpretive issues" in F. Fabbro, (Ed.), *Advances in the Neurolinguistics of Bilingualism: Essays in Honor of Michel Paradis*. Udine, Italy: Forum, pp. 315–355.

Wartenburger, I., Heekeren, H.R., Abutalebi, J., Cappa, S.F., Villringer, A. and Perani, D. (2003), "Early setting of grammatical processing in the bilingual brain", *Neuron*, Vol. 37, pp. 159–170.

SECTION V

Reaching toward systems interdependence

34

INTERACTION OF MOTOR AND LANGUAGE FACTORS IN THE DEVELOPMENT OF SPEECH PRODUCTION

Meredith Saletta, Allison Gladfelter, Janet Vuolo and Lisa Goffman

Traditionally, researchers have investigated the development of the speech, language, and limb motor systems separately; these components were thought to be modular elements of human development and processing (e.g., Fodor, 1983). Past researchers have spoken of "the developmental non-convergence of two independent systems: an audio-motor system and a... syntactic-semantic system" (Fay and Butler, 1968, p. 370). The developmental psychologist Vygotskiĭ, in his study of the genetics of thought and speech, also concluded that these two systems mature separately and converge at a later point, with the development of the action preceding that of the word (Vygotskiĭ, 1962).

More recently, it has become apparent that at least components of the speech, language, and limb motor systems are in fact inter-related. As Zelaznik and Goffman express (2010), "language production, whether spoken, signed, or written, is a motor activity" (p. 383). In this chapter, we explore several aspects of the relationship between language and motor skill. These aspects include: (1) conceptual models; (2) neural underpinnings; (3) methodological procedures, which index the interaction between language and motor processes; (4) typical development of language and motor interactions both in infants and children; and (5) developmental disorders, which are defined in relation to these standard modular distinctions, but which in fact reveal a great deal of interactivity. We conclude with a brief discussion of implications for intervention and future research.

Models of speech and language production

Language production and speech motor control models both have a common goal – to understand how speech is produced – but this has been difficult to accomplish without a unified theory. Language and motor components have classically been treated as independent from each other, and most models address adult production rather than taking a developmental approach. Language processing is generally placed at a higher level than speech motor processing (but see Articulatory Phonology, Browman and Goldstein, 1992, for an exception), with a unidirectional flow from language to movement (Levelt *et al.*, 1999). In models of speech production and motor control, the articulatory motor system is treated as independent from linguistic levels. However, those interested in speech production components elaborate conceptual, syntactic, lexical, and phonological levels (Levelt *et al.*, 1999) and only sparsely detail articulatory preparation and implementation. Conversely, models of speech motor control delineate levels of articulatory preparation and output, yet pay little attention to how specific linguistic targets interact with speech output (Barlow *et al.*, 2010).

Several recent investigators have proposed models attempting to integrate language and motor control (Goffman, 2010; Hickok, 2014; Smith and Goffman, 2004; Tourville and Guenther, 2011). One of the most influential speech motor control models is Directions Into Velocities of Articulators (DIVA), a computational neural network model of speech acquisition and production (Guenther and Vladusich, 2012; Tourville and Guenther, 2011). In this model, the sensory representation of a speech sound and the motor program for that sound are linked via the speech sound map where neurons are sequentially activated by higher-level prefrontal cortex regions, which are responsible for the phonological encoding of an utterance (Guenther and Vladusich, 2012). DIVA specifies how motor, somatosensory, and auditory information are processed while infants acquire speech, but does not delineate how the linguistic properties of words (e.g., semantics, syntax, prosody) influence learning.

Goldrick and colleagues (e.g., Rapp and Goldrick, 2006) have proposed a linguistic processing model with increased interactivity among lexical, phonological, phonetic, and motor processing levels. These researchers conclude that slips of the tongue have a lexical bias; that is, this type of erroneous output is more likely to be a real word than another type of error. Their data suggest that lexical factors, not just motor factors, are implicated in the production of speech errors (Goldrick *et al.*, 2011; McMillan *et al.*, 2009). Smith and Goffman (Goffman, 2010; Smith and Goffman, 2004) apply a developmentally-based modification of the Levelt model (see Figure 34.1) to explain interactions seen across domains (for an application of the Levelt model to interactions between language production and stuttering, see Maxfield, this volume). A crucial component of this developmental model is that, as illustrated in Figure 34.1, there are bi-directional interactions between cognition and action and components of language and articulatory processing. For example, there is now evidence for linkages between lexical-semantic and articulatory processing (Heisler *et al.*, 2010). In addition, in models of language disorders that implicate procedural learning deficits (e.g., Ullman and Pierpont, 2005), sequencing and timing are directly related to syntactic processing. These and other potential bi-directional interactions are illustrated in Figure 34.1.

Neural underpinnings of speech, language, and motor processing

Advances in neuroscience have further supported the notion that motor, language, and speech processing areas in the brain overlap and interact with one another. Broca's area, comprised of Brodmann's areas (BA) 44 and 45, is located just anterior to the primary motor cortex in the posterior portion of the left inferior frontal gyrus. Although considered the language production center of the brain, multiple studies have found that Broca's area is also involved in performing and perceiving actions that have a sequential and hierarchical organization. For example, Fazio and colleagues (2009) demonstrated that patients with lesions to BA44 were impaired in their ability to sequence pictures of actions performed by humans (e.g., a person reaching for a water bottle) but not in their ability to sequence physical events without human involvement (e.g., a bicycle falling over). These findings suggest that, as consistent with embodied cognition (see the Duff *et al.* chapter for elaboration, this volume), patients with damage to Broca's area are unable to map actions performed by humans onto their own motor system.

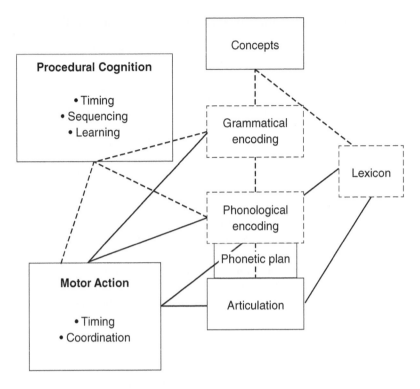

Figure 34.1 Developmental model that illustrates how cognition (dotted lines) and action (solid lines) interact with language and articulation. Crucial linkages may be observed between procedural cognition (e.g., sequencing and timing) and grammatical encoding, as hypothesized within the framework of the procedural deficit hypothesis. An additional well-documented interface is between the lexicon and articulation. Models of interactivity are increasingly prominent.

In the language domain, the high prevalence of subject–object–verb and subject–verb–object word order, which account for approximately 89 percent of all of the world's languages, may have been derived from the sequential and hierarchical organization of Broca's area (Kemmerer, 2012). These word orders express how actions unfold over time: an animate agent acts on an inanimate patient to change its state. Broca's area is therefore involved with not only how actions are performed and perceived, but also with how they are conceptualized and symbolically expressed through language.

In addition to Broca's area, along with their well-established roles in the motor system, the cerebellum and basal ganglia have been implicated in both linguistic and cognitive skills (Vicari *et al.*, 2003). For example, imaging studies indicate that there may be functional and anatomical abnormalities of the cerebellum in individuals with dyslexia (Pernet *et al.*, 2009). In addition, as reported in primary and review sources, brain regions such as the basal ganglia have been associated with procedural learning deficits commonly experienced by individuals with dyslexia, specific language impairment (SLI), or other types of language impairment (Doyon, 2003; Nicolson and Fawcett, 2007; Ullman and Pierpont, 2005).

Language and motor interactions in infants and toddlers

Already within the first months of life, infants begin to temporally coordinate the direction of their gazes, facial expressions, and vocalizations to communicate (Colonnesi *et al.*, 2012). Links between speech and limb motor development are perhaps most evident in the co-occurrence of rhythmic limb movements (e.g., shaking and banging) and reduplicated babbling (e.g., rhythmic production of "bababab") observed at approximately seven months of age (Ejiri and Masataka, 2001; Thelen, 1979).

In their Frame-Content Model, MacNeilage and Davis (2001) proposed that speech evolved through rhythmic action. According to this model, rhythmic oscillations of the jaw (i.e., alternating openings and closings) during chewing form the *frame* for the production of syllables. The *content* is the consonants and vowels overlaid on that syllabic frame. These rhythmic oscillations provide the structure for an infant's earliest canonical syllables, and, eventually, his or her first words. This hypothesis is not without controversy. Electromyographic analyses of oral musculature and articulatory kinematics reveal different patterns of coordinated motor activity for non-speech activities, such as chewing, than for speech activities (e.g., Green *et al.*, 1997; Moore and Ruark, 1996), suggesting a dissociation between chewing and speech.

As infants move beyond the babbling period and develop first words, relationships are observed between vocabulary size and oral motor skill. For example, Alcock and Krawczyk (2010) found correlations between simple oral movements, such as pursing or spreading lips, and spoken vocabulary and grammatical complexity in 21-month-olds, even when cognitive abilities and socioeconomic status were controlled. To investigate the developmental link between oral motor skills and language, Nip *et al.* (2011) collected lip and jaw movements longitudinally in 9- to 21-month-olds. Again, associations between motor and language skills emerged, regardless of age. It appears that language production and speech motor skill are linked during children's earliest productions of words.

Gestures also reveal early language and limb motor interactions. Deictic gestures, such as pointing, appear at approximately eight to ten months and guide joint attention (Zinober and Martlew, 1985), which facilitates object–word correspondences (Bates *et al.*, 1979). As first words are produced, so too emerge recognitory gestures, or prototypical actions showing recognition of an object's meaning, such as putting an empty cup to the lips (Iverson, 2010). As toddlers transition from single words to two-word combinations, an intermediary step is combining a single word with a gesture. These gesture–word combinations (e.g., reaching arms toward mother and saying "mama") convey the same meanings as a child's earliest two-word combinations (Iverson and Goldin-Meadow, 2005). Manual gestures appear to be fundamentally linked to the advancement of language.

One particular manual gesture is thought to lay the social foundation of language learning, the "showing" of objects to adults. Early locomotor abilities are bi-directionally linked with these object showing behaviors in infants as they transition from crawling to walking (Karasik *et al.*, 2011). Walkers are more likely to access objects at a distance, carry objects, and share objects with their mother than crawlers who prefer reaching and sharing objects while remaining stationary. However, crawlers who attempt to access distant objects, carry objects, and share objects learn to walk more readily. Locomotion and communication develop in tandem.

Given the developmental evidence for the interactivity of the language and motor systems, it should come as no surprise that developmental delays in motor skills often coincide with, or even predict, language impairments in young children. One striking example of language and motor interdependence is in the specific profile of language and motor deficits observed in children with autism spectrum disorder (ASD). Studies show differences in the language and motor performance of infants and toddlers with ASD:

1. Five- to 14-month-old infants at high risk for developing ASD showed attenuated increases in rhythmic arm movements at the time of their reduplicated babble onset compared to infants without ASD (Iverson and Wozniak, 2007).
2. These same infants at risk for ASD subsequently presented with delayed language at their 18-month follow-up (Iverson and Wozniak, 2007).
3. Object play and joint attention skills in infants at risk for developing ASD predicted their communication skills at ages three to seven years (Poon *et al.*, 2012).
4. 14-month-olds at risk for ASD also showed fewer non-verbal requesting behaviors, such as pointing (Yirmiya *et al.*, 2006).

These data reveal how, in children with ASD, language and motor systems are related in early development (also see Longard and Moore 2015, this volume).

Language and speech motor interactions in children

With the emergence of methodologies that integrate linguistics and motor control, multiple interactions have been reported across language and speech motor domains. A major finding is that, as language capacities mature, articulatory variability simultaneously decreases (Smith and Zelaznik, 2004). Even in the face of increased articulatory variability, children's speech movement patterns generally reveal the same linguistic distinctions as adults. At the segmental level, investigators have shown that very young children just acquiring a voicing contrast do not show differences in the amplitude, duration, or velocity of movement across voiced and voiceless consonants (Grigos *et al.*, 2005). However, slightly older children (aged four to seven years) demonstrate distinct profiles in the patterning of lip movements while producing a similar voicing contrast (e.g., [p] vs. [b]). Also at the segmental level, but now considering coarticulatory effects, both five-year-old children and adults produce lip rounding (originating from the vowel [u]) that extends over an entire seven-syllable sentence (Goffman *et al.*, 2008). Segmental distinctions emerge in the face of a more variable speech motor system, in this case revealing a disassociation between motor skill and language category.

A locus of interaction is in the lexical-articulatory domain (e.g., Baese-Berk and Goldrick, 2009; McMillan *et al.*, 2009). Typically developing children aged four to six years show decreases in articulatory variability when a novel phonetic string (e.g., "mofpum") is assigned a visual referent (Heisler *et al.*, 2010). However, articulatory variability does not change if the same type of phonetic string is not provided with a visual referent. These results reveal a direct connection between lexical status and articulatory variability. Variability only decreases when a novel phonetic string acquires referential status, or becomes a word.

Furthermore, children produce increasingly variable articulatory movements in long and syntactically complex sentences compared to short and syntactically simple ones (MacPherson and Smith, 2013; Maner *et al.*, 2000). For example, children are more variable when they produce the phrase "Buy Bobby a puppy" embedded in a longer sentence ("Buy Bobby a puppy if he wants one") than in isolation (Maner *et al.*, 2000). Another line of evidence shows that articulatory variability is influenced when the production load is increased by changing the task to involve sentence generation rather than simple repetition (Brumbach and Goffman, 2014). As illustrated in Figure 34.2, variability increases in retrieval compared with imitation contexts. Overall, processing demands related to lexical status, sentence length, sentence complexity, and retrieval influence articulatory variability.

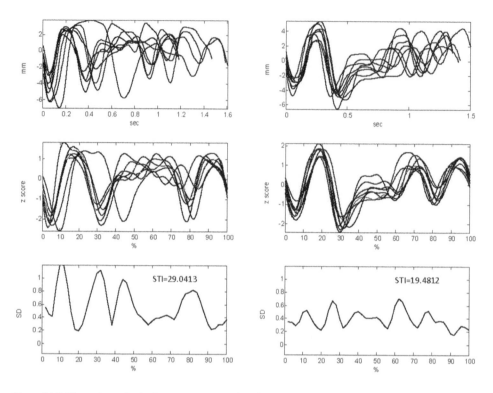

Figure 34.2 Illustration of articulatory movement data during a sentence retrieval (left panels) and a sentence imitation (right panels) task. The top panels show multiple productions of lower lip movement in real time and amplitude. The middle panels show the same records now time- and amplitude-normalized, to reveal the underlying patterning of movement. The bottom panels show the variability of these records, which are the standard deviations obtained at 2 percent intervals. These standard deviations are summed to determine the spatiotemporal index (STI) – a value which quantifies an individual's articulatory stability across multiple productions of a given utterance. A higher STI indicates increased articulatory variability.

Test cases for interactivity: Developmental speech, language, and motor disorders

Language and speech motor systems interact in infants and children with typical development. Many disorders are defined on the basis of deficits in one area, but upon deeper inspection actually involve both language and motor systems. This is true of disorders of higher-order language and phonological processes, including SLI and developmental dyslexia; disorders of motor planning, including childhood apraxia of speech; and disorders of limb motor execution, including developmental coordination disorder. While in most cases these are diagnoses of exclusion – that is, the problem is diagnosed only in the absence of explanatory factors such as neurological compromise or severe environmental deprivation – it is actually the case that many children with these disorders demonstrate concomitant (although sometimes subclinical) deficits in both the language and motor domains.

Specific language impairment

Children with SLI have significant deficits in language, yet typical performance on measures of non-verbal cognition, oral motor skill, and hearing (e.g., Leonard, 2014; for a different perspective, see the Montgomery *et al.* chapter, this volume). While SLI has historically been defined as a modular deficit that is specific to language, it has become apparent that other deficits exist, specifically in gross and fine motor skill (reviewed in Hill, 2001; Zelaznik and Goffman, 2010). For instance, these children perform more slowly on a peg moving task (Bishop and Edmundson, 1987) and are less able to imitate gestures, such as brushing their teeth and saluting (Hill *et al.*, 1998). Children with SLI also demonstrate speech motor deficits (Goffman, 1999, 2004). For example, they show more variable articulatory movements in multi-movement sequences (Brumbach and Goffman, 2014) along with relatively poor control of the small and short movements associated with unstressed syllables (Goffman, 2004). Explanations for these more generalized motor and learning deficits in SLI are varied and often non-specific, ranging from general maturational delays or co-morbidity, to more specific hypotheses regarding deficits in procedural learning (Tomblin *et al.*, 2007; Ullman and Pierpont, 2005).

Developmental dyslexia

Developmental dyslexia is "characterized by difficulties with accurate and/or fluent word recognition and by poor spelling and decoding abilities... [that are] unexpected in relation to other cognitive abilities and the provision of effective classroom instruction" (Lyon *et al.*, 2003, p. 2). Classically, dyslexia has been considered as a high-level linguistic deficit in the phonological system. Recent studies have revealed associated motor deficits (Haslum and Miles, 2007), particularly in the automatic performance of learned skills or in the coordination of multiple actions (Nicolson and Fawcett, 2011). This deficit in learned behaviors underlies impairments beyond the phonological system, and implicates deficits in motor skill and balance in individuals with dyslexia.

Researchers have identified several specific aspects of motor skill which are impaired in children with developmental dyslexia. In particular, children demonstrate deficits in their performance on continuous tapping tasks (Geuze and Kalverboer, 1994) and bi-manual tasks which involve precise timing (Wolff *et al.*, 1990). Moe-Nilssen and colleagues (2003) found that walking speed, cadence, and trunk accelerations (as a measure of balance control during walking) correctly classified between 70–85 percent of individuals with dyslexia. In summary, there seems to be a pattern to the array of impaired and spared motor abilities in children with dyslexia (see also the Wingert *et al.* chapter, this volume, for more information).

Childhood apraxia of speech

Childhood apraxia of speech (CAS) is a "neurological childhood (pediatric) speech sound disorder in which the precision and consistency of movements underlying speech are impaired in the absence of neuromuscular deficits" (American Speech–Language–Hearing Association [ASHA], 2007, pp. 4–5). Primary speech symptoms include: "inconsistent errors on consonants and vowels in repeated productions of syllables or words, lengthened and disrupted coarticulatory transitions between sounds and syllables, and inappropriate prosody, especially in the realization of lexical or phrasal stress" (ASHA, 2007, p. 5).

Although the primary deficit in CAS is considered one of motor speech planning and programming (Grigos and Kolenda, 2010), children with this disorder often present with other limb motor and language deficits. In the limb motor domain, children with CAS have below average manual dexterity skills (Lewis *et al.*, 2004), and lower timing precision in manual tasks (Peter and Stoel-Gammon, 2008). There is also general agreement that children suspected of having CAS have significant language deficits (ASHA, 2007) including problems with receptive and expressive language, phonological awareness, letter knowledge, reading, and spelling (Lewis *et al.*, 2004; McNeill *et al.*, 2009). Some studies also report continuing difficulties in language and motor domains despite improvements in speech articulation (e.g., Lewis *et al.*, 2004; Stackhouse and Snowling, 1992). Despite the fact that CAS is considered a motor speech disorder, this diagnosis is clearly not limited to speech production deficits. Impairments in both limb motor and language in addition to speech development point to interactivity among these domains.

Developmental coordination disorder

Developmental coordination disorder (DCD) is a neurodevelopmental disorder characterized by the child's experience of movement difficulties (American Psychiatric Association, 2013). According to Barnhart and colleagues (2003), "Children's difficulties in coordination can result from a combination of one or more impairments in proprioception, motor programming, timing, or sequencing of muscle activity" (p. 723). Conceptually, DCD can be described as the profile which is the reverse of those with SLI, dyslexia, and CAS. That is, the latter diagnoses typically result from impairments specific to language, whereas the diagnosis of DCD results from impairments specific to limb motor output. But like these other disorders, the deficit in DCD is not exclusively confined to limb motor deficits; in fact, many children with DCD also experience concomitant difficulties in language and/or speech motor output (Visser, 2003).

While some authors maintain that the populations of children with language impairment and DCD differ sharply, and that any similarities are only superficial (Kaplan *et al.*, 1998), many researchers suggest otherwise. According to Hill (2001), it is inaccurate to categorize children into discrete groups of language, motor, or attentional impairments. Rather, "these impairments tend to co-occur in developmentally disordered children, and... those with highly specific deficits are the exception rather than the rule" (p. 150). In fact, Hill and colleagues (1998) found that children diagnosed with language impairment also met the criteria for DCD at a rate nearly ten times that of the general population.

Similar to the disorders mentioned above, the cerebellum has been implicated in both the language and motor difficulties in DCD. Soft neurological signs, which include aspects of motor performance appropriate for a younger child (O'Hare and Khalid, 2002), poor postural control, timing deficits (Geuze, 2005), and poor motor adaptation (Ghez and Thach, 2000) may all be present and at least partially explained by cerebellar dysfunction (Zwicker *et al.*, 2009). Furthermore, Hill *et al.* (1998) discovered that three groups of children (those with DCD, SLI, and younger controls) demonstrated weak hand lateralization and tended to use the non-preferred hand to reach across the body's midline. This evidence indicated that both clinical groups may experience atypical lateralization. Because the development of a consistent hand preference in children with typical development is due to the maturation of their motor performance, atypical lateralization may be caused by children's motor immaturity or dysfunction (Bishop, 1990).

Conclusion

We have presented evidence from typical and atypical development for the interactivity of language and motor skills. This has been documented by numerous behavioral and a small number of neuroanatomical and neuroimaging studies, and described in relation to the development of children from infancy through adolescence. These findings about language and motor interactions influence both theoretical accounts, and clinical assessment and intervention practices. Theoretically, we must move beyond the traditional modular models described in the beginning of this chapter. Interactivity ultimately influences approaches to diagnosis and treatment. For example, in early identification, perhaps performance on motor tasks is a strong predictor of developmental outcome. Similarly, treatment goals for children classically viewed in terms of their primary deficits (e.g., SLI, dyslexia, CAS, ASD, and DCD) may cross language and motor domains in specific and yet to be determined ways. While the link between language and motor skills is well documented, more empirical work is necessary to expand our knowledge regarding this interaction.

Acknowledgment

This work was supported by the National Institutes of Health (National Institute of Deafness and other Communicative Disorders) grant DC04826.

References

Alcock, K.J. and Krawczyk, K. (2010), "Individual differences in language development: Relationship with motor skill at 21 months", *Developmental Science*, Vol. 13, No. 5, pp. 677–691.

American Psychiatric Association (2013), *Diagnostic and Statistical Manual of Mental Disorders: DSM-5*, 5th ed., Washington, DC: American Psychiatric Association.

American Speech–Language–Hearing Association (2007), "Childhood Apraxia of Speech [Technical Report]", www.asha.org/policy/TR2007-00278/

Baese-Berk, M. and Goldrick, M. (2009), "Mechanisms of interaction in speech production", *Language and Cognitive Processes*, Vol. 24, No. 4, pp. 527–554.

Barlow, S.M., Lund, J.P., Estep, M. and Kolta, A. (2009), "Central pattern generators for orofacial movements and speech", *Handbook of Mammalian Vocalization: An Integrative Neuroscience Approach*, Vol. 19, pp. 351–369.

Barnhart, R.C., Davenport, M., Epps, S.B. and Nordquist, V.M. (2003), "Developmental coordination disorder", *Physical Therapy*, Vol. 83, No. 8, pp. 722–731.

Bates, E., Benigni, L., Bretherton, I., Camaioni, L. and Voterra, V. (1979), *The Emergence of Symbols: Cognition and Communication in Infancy*, New York: Academic Press.

Bishop, D.V.M. (1990), *Handedness and Developmental Disorder*, Hove, UK: Lawrence Erlbaum Associates Ltd.

Bishop, D.V.M. and Edmundson, A. (1987), "Specific language impairment as a maturational lag: Evidence from longitudinal data on language and motor development", *Developmental Medicine and Child Neurology*, Vol. 29, pp. 442–459.

Browman, C.P. and Goldstein, L. (1992), "Articulatory Phonology – An Overview", *Phonetica*, Vol. 49, No. 3–4, pp. 155–180.

Brumbach, A. and Goffman, L. (2014), "Interaction of language processing and motor skill in children with specific language impairment", *Journal of Speech, Language, and Hearing Research*, Vol. 57, pp. 158–171.

Colonnesi, C., Zijlstra, B.J.H., van der Zande, A. and Bogels, S.M. (2012), "Coordination of gaze, facial expressions and vocalizations of early infant communication with mother and father", *Infant Behavior and Development*, Vol. 35, No. 3, pp. 523–532.

Doyon, J. (2003), "Distinct contribution of the cotrico-stiratal and cortico-cerebellar systems to motor skill learning", *Neuropsychologia*, Vol. 41, pp. 352–362.

Ejiri, K. and Masataka, N. (2001), "Co-occurrence of preverbal vocal behavior and motor action in early infancy", *Developmental Science*, Vol. 4, No. 1, pp. 40–48.

Fay, W.H. and Butler, B.V. (1968), "Echolalia, IQ, and developmental dichotomy of speech and language systems", *Journal of Speech and Hearing Research*, Vol. 11, No. 2, pp. 365–371.

Fazio, P., Cantagallo, A., Craighero, L., D'Ausilio, A., Roy, A.C., Pozzo, T., Calzolari, F., Granieri, E. and Fadiga, L. (2009), "Encoding of human action in Broca's area", *Brain*, Vol. 132, pp. 1980–1988.

Fodor, J.A. (1983), *The Modularity of Mind: An Essay on Faculty Psychology*, Cambridge, MA, US: MIT Press.

Geuze, R.H. (2005), "Postural control in children with developmental coordination disorder", *Neural Plasticity*, Vol. 12, No. 2–3, pp. 183–196.

Geuze, R.H. and Kalverboer, A.F. (1994), "Tapping a rhythm: A problem of timing for children who are clumsy and dyslexic?", *Adapted Physical Activity Quarterly*, Vol. 11, pp. 203–213.

Ghez, C. and Thach, W. (2000), "The cerebellum", in Kandel, E.R., Schwartz, J.Z. and Jessel, T.M., (Eds.), *Principles of Neural Science*. 4th ed., New York, NY: McGraw Hill, pp. 832–852.

Goffman, L. (1999), "Prosodic influences on speech production in children with specific language impairment and speech deficits: Kinematic, acoustic, and transcription evidence", *Journal of Speech Language and Hearing Research*, Vol. 42, No. 6, pp. 1499–1517.

Goffman, L. (2004), "Kinematic differentiation of prosodic categories in normal and disordered language development", *Journal of Speech Language and Hearing Research*, Vol. 47, No. 5, pp. 1088–1102.

Goffman, L. (2010), "Dynamic interaction of motor and language factors in development in normal and disordered development", in Maassen, B., Lieshout, P.H.H.M. v., Kent, R. and Hulstijn, W., (Eds.), *Speech Motor Control: New Developments in Applied Research*, Oxford, UK: Oxford University Press, pp. 137–152.

Goffman, L., Smith, A., Heisler, L. and Ho, M. (2008), "The breadth of coarticulatory units in children and adults", *Journal of Speech Language and Hearing Research*, Vol. 51, No. 6, pp. 1424–1437.

Goldrick, M., Baker, H.R., Murphy, A. and Baese-Berk, M. (2011), "Interaction and representational integration: Evidence from speech errors", *Cognition*, Vol. 121, No. 1, pp. 58–72.

Green, J.R., Moore, C.A., Ruark, J.L., Rodda, P.R., Morvee, W.T. and Van Witzenburg, M.J. (1997), "Development of chewing in children from 12 to 43 months: Longitudinal study of EMG patterns", *Journal of Neurophysiology*, Vol. 77, No. 5, pp. 2704–2716.

Grigos, M.I. and Kolenda, N. (2010), "The relationship between articulatory control and improved phonemic accuracy in childhood apraxia of speech: A longitudinal case study", *Clinical Linguistics and Phonetics*, Vol. 24, No. 1, pp. 17–40.

Grigos, M.I., Saxman, J.H. and Gordon, A.M. (2005), "Speech motor development during acquisition of the voicing contrast", *Journal of Speech Language and Hearing Research*, Vol. 48, No. 4, pp. 739–752.

Guenther, F.H. and Vladusich, T. (2012), "A neural theory of speech acquisition and production", *Journal of Neurolinguistics*, Vol. 25, No. 5, pp. 408–422.

Haslum, M.N. and Miles, T.R. (2007), "Motor performance and dyslexia in a national cohort of 10-year-old children", *Dyslexia*, Vol. 13, No. 4, pp. 257–275.

Heisler, L., Goffman, L. and Younger, B. (2010), "Lexical and articulatory interactions in children's language production", *Developmental Science*, Vol. 13, No. 5, pp. 722–730.

Hickok, G. (2014), "The architecture of speech production and the role of the phoneme in speech processing", *Language, Cognition and Neuroscience*, Vol. 29, pp. 2–20.

Hill, E.L. (2001), "Non-specific nature of specific language impairment: A review of the literature with regard to concomitant motor impairments", *International Journal of Language and Communication Disorders*, Vol. 36, No. 2, pp. 149–171.

Hill, E.L., Bishop, D.V.M. and Nimmo-Smith, I. (1998), "Representational gestures in developmental coordination disorder and specific language impairment: Error-types and the reliability of ratings", *Human Movement Science*, Vol. 17, No. 4–5, pp. 655–678.

Iverson, J.M. (2010), "Developing language in a developing body: The relationship between motor development and language development", *Journal of Child Language*, Vol. 37, No. 2, pp. 229–261.

Iverson, J.M. and Goldin-Meadow, S. (2005), "Gesture paves the way for language development", *Psychological Science*, Vol. 16, No. 5, pp. 367–371.

Iverson, J.M. and Wozniak, R.H. (2007), "Variation in vocal-motor development in infant siblings of children with autism", *Journal of Autism and Developmental Disorders*, Vol. 37, No. 1, pp. 158–170.

Kaplan, B.J., Wilson, B.N., Dewey, D. and Crawford, S.G. (1998), "DCD may not be a discrete disorder", *Human Movement Science*, Vol. 17, No. 4–5, pp.471–490.

Karasik, L.B., Tamis-LeMonda, C.S. and Adolph, K.E. (2011), "Transition from crawling to walking and infants' actions with objects and people", *Child Development*, Vol. 82, No. 4, pp. 1199–1209.

Kemmerer, D. (2012), "The cross-linguistic prevalence of SOV and SVO word orders reflects the sequential and hierarchical representation of action in Broca's area", *Language and Linguistics Compass*, Vol. 6, No. 1, pp. 50–66.

Leonard, L.B. (2014), *Children with Specific Language Impairment*, 2nd ed., Cambridge, MA, US: The MIT Press.

Levelt, W.J.M., Roelofs, A. and Meyer, A.S. (1999), "A theory of lexical access in speech production", *Behavioral and Brain Sciences*, Vol. 22, No. 1, pp. 1–75.

Lewis, B.A., Freebairn, L.A., Hansen, A.J., Iyengar, S.K. and Taylor, H.G. (2004), "School-age follow-up of children with childhood apraxia of speech", *Language Speech and Hearing Services in Schools*, Vol. 35, No. 2, pp. 122–140.

Lyon, G.R., Shaywitz, S.E. and Shaywitz, B.A. (2003), "Defining dyslexia, comorbidity, teachers' knowledge of language and reading: A definition of dyslexia", *Annals of Dyslexia*, Vol. 53, pp. 1–14.

McMillan, C.T., Corley, M. and Lickley, R.J. (2009), "Articulatory evidence for feedback and competition in speech production", *Language and Cognitive Processes*, Vol. 24, No. 1, pp. 44–66.

MacNeilage, P.F. and Davis, B.L. (2001), "Motor mechanisms in speech ontogeny: Phylogenetic, neurobiological and linguistic implications", *Current Opinion in Neurobiology*, Vol. 11, No. 6, pp. 696–700.

McNeill, B.C., Gillon, G.T. and Dodd, B. (2009), "Phonological awareness and early reading development in childhood apraxia of speech (CAS)", *International Journal of Language and Communication Disorders*, Vol. 44, No. 2, pp. 175–192.

MacPherson, M.K. and Smith, A. (2013), "Influences of sentence length and syntactic complexity on the speech motor control of children who stutter", *Journal of Speech Language and Hearing Research*, Vol. 56, No. 1, pp. 89–102.

Maner, K.J., Smith, A. and Grayson, L. (2000), "Influences of utterance length and complexity on speech motor performance in children and adults", *Journal of Speech Language and Hearing Research*, Vol. 43, No. 2, pp. 560–573.

Moe-Nilssen, R., Helbostad, J.L., Talcott, J.B. and Toennessen, F.E. (2003), "Balance and gait in children with dyslexia", *Experimental Brain Research*, Vol. 150, No. 2, pp. 237–244.

Moore, C.A. and Ruark, J.L. (1996), "Does speech emerge from earlier appearing oral motor behaviors?", *Journal of Speech and Hearing Research*, Vol. 39, No. 5, pp. 1034–1047.

Nicolson, R.I. and Fawcett, A.J. (2007), "Procedural learning difficulties: Reuniting the developmental disorders?", *Trends in Neurosciences*, Vol. 30, No. 4, pp. 135–141.

Nicolson, R.I. and Fawcett, A.J. (2011), "Dyslexia, dysgraphia, procedural learning and the cerebellum", *Cortex*, Vol. 47, No. 1, pp. 117–127.

Nip, I.S.B., Green, J.R. and Marx, D.B. (2011), "The co-emergence of cognition, language, and speech motor control in early development: A longitudinal correlation study", *Journal of Communication Disorders*, Vol. 44, No. 2, pp. 149–160.

O'Hare, A. and Khalid, S. (2002), "The association of abnormal cerebellar function in children with developmental coordination disorder and reading difficulties", *Dyslexia*, Vol. 8, pp. 234–248.

Pernet, C., Andersson, J., Paulesu, E. and Demonet, J.F. (2009), "When all hypotheses are right: A multifocal account of dyslexia", *Human Brain Mapping*, Vol. 30, No. 7, pp. 2278–2292.

Peter, B. and Stoel-Gammon, C. (2008), "Central timing deficits in subtypes of primary speech disorders", *Clinical Linguistics and Phonetics*, Vol. 22, No. 3, pp. 171–198.

Poon, K.K., Watson, L.R., Baranek, G.T. and Poe, M.D. (2012), "To what extent do joint attention, imitation, and object play behaviors in infancy predict later communication and intellectual functioning in ASD?", *Journal of Autism and Developmental Disorders*, Vol. 42, No. 6, pp. 1064–1074.

Rapp, B. and Goldrick, M. (2006), "Speaking words: Contributions of cognitive neuropsychological research", *Cognitive Neuropsychology*, Vol. 23, No. 1, pp. 39–73.

Smith, A. and Goffman, L. (2004), "Interaction of motor and language factors in the development of speech production", in Maasen, B., Kent, R., Peters, H., Lieshout, P. v. and Hulstijn, W., (Eds.), *Speech Motor Control in Normal and Disordered Speech*, Oxford: Oxford University Press, pp. 225–252.

Smith, A. and Zelaznik, H.N. (2004), "Development of functional synergies for speech motor coordination in childhood and adolescence", *Developmental Psychobiology*, Vol. 45, No. 1, pp. 22–33.

Stackhouse, J. and Snowling, M. (1992), "Barriers to literacy development in two cases of developmental verbal dyspraxia", *Cognitive Neuropsychology*, Vol. 9, pp. 273–299.

Thelen, E. (1979), "Rhythmical stereotypes in normal human infants", *Animal Behaviour*, Vol. 27 (Aug), pp. 699–715.

Tomblin, J.B., Mainela-Arnold, E. and Zhang, X. (2007), "Procedural learning in adolescents with and without specific language impairment", *Language Learning and Development*, Vol. 3, No. 4, pp. 269–293.

Tourville, J.A. and Guenther, F.H. (2011), "The DIVA model: A neural theory of speech acquisition and production", *Language and Cognitive Processes*, Vol. 26, No. 7, pp. 952–981.

Ullman, M.T. and Pierpont, E.I. (2005), "Specific language impairment is not specific to language: The procedural deficit hypothesis", *Cortex*, Vol. 41, No. 3, pp. 399–433.

Vicari, S., Marotta, L., Menghini, D., Molinari, M. and Petrosini, L. (2003), "Implicit learning deficit in children with developmental dyslexia", *Neuropsychologia*, Vol. 41, No. 1, pp. 108–114.

Visser, J. (2003), "Developmental coordination disorder: A review of research subtypes and comorbidities", *Human Movement Science*, Vol. 22, pp. 479–493.

Vygotskiĭ, L.S. (1962), *Thought and Language*, Massachusetts Institute of Technology, Cambridge, MA, US: MIT Press.

Wolff, P.H., Michel, G.F., Ovrut, M. and Drake, C. (1990), "Rate and timing precision of motor coordination in developmental dyslexia", *Developmental Psychology*, Vol. 26, No. 3, pp. 349–359.

Yirmiya, N., Gamliel, I., Pilowsky, T., Feldman, R., Baron-Cohen, S. and Sigman, M. (2006), "The development of siblings of children with autism at 4 and 14 months: Social engagement, communication, and cognition", *Journal of Child Psychology and Psychiatry*, Vol. 47, No. 5, pp. 511–523.

Zelaznik, H.N. and Goffman, L. (2010), "Generalized motor abilities and timing behavior in children with specific language impairment", *Journal of Speech Language and Hearing Research*, Vol. 53, No. 2, pp. 383–393.

Zinober, B. and Martlew, M. (1985), "Developmental-changes in 4 types of gesture in relation to acts and vocalizations from 10 to 21 months", *British Journal of Developmental Psychology*, Vol. 3(Sep), pp. 293–306.

Zwicker, J.G., Missiuna, C. and Boyd, L.A. (2009), "Neural correlates of Developmental Coordination Disorder: A review of hypotheses", *Journal of Child Neurology*, Vol. 24, No. 10, pp. 1273–1281.

35

NEURO/COGNITIVE AND SOCIOCULTURAL PERSPECTIVES ON LANGUAGE AND LITERACY DISABILITIES

Moving from parallel play to productive cooperation

C. Addison Stone

As many have noted (e.g., Kovorsky and Maxwell, 1997; Purcell-Gates *et al.*, 2004; Stone, 2004; Trent *et al.*, 1998), the history of scholarship and practice regarding language and literacy disabilities can be viewed as two parallel traditions—termed here the neuro/cognitive and sociocultural perspectives—working largely independently of each other. Although there has been increasing discussion in recent years regarding the value of integrating these perspectives (Stone, 2004), this is still largely a missed opportunity. Instead, as is evident in this volume, we have two rich traditions, which are engaged, in essence, in parallel play. My goal in this chapter is to sketch a principled approach to bringing these two traditions together in the service of a better understanding of individuals with language and literacy disabilities.

In the initial section, I provide a brief characterization of the two traditions, highlighting contrasting features and providing examples of work on language and literacy within each tradition. In the following section, I describe recent developments in theory and research that provide reasons to think that the time is ripe for an integration of the two traditions. I then provide an overview of an approach for achieving that integration, followed in the final section by a discussion of the implications of an integrated model, along with key questions that must be addressed as we strive to make such an integration feasible and fruitful.

Parallel perspectives on language and literacy disabilities

The two broad theoretical traditions have been identified with various labels, but here I will refer to them as the neuro/cognitive and sociocultural perspectives. Table 35.1 provides an overview of some of the key distinguishing features of the two perspectives. In the following paragraphs and in Table 35.1, I contrast these two perspectives, with an emphasis on their treatment of childhood language and literacy disabilities. In doing so, I have inevitably over-

Table 35.1 Some defining contrasts between alternative perspectives on language and literacy.

Neuro/Cognitive Perspective	Sociocultural Perspective
The individual as the unit of analysis	Social participation as the unit of analysis
Capability as skill	Capability as practice/activity
Learning as acquisition/internalization	Learning as participation/appropriation
Context as modifying or triggering	Context as constitutive
Language as a partially innate rule system	Language as routinized patterns of social communication
Literacy as a decontextualized symbol system for representing oral language	Literacy as a set of culturally situated social practices

simplified and sharpened the contrasts, but I hope that I have not done injustice to the core nature of the differences.[1] (For a more detailed discussion of the two perspectives and their views of language and literacy, see Stone, 2004; for more details regarding the perspectives' views of disabilities, see Stone and Learned, 2014.)

The neuro/cognitive perspective

Those working within the neuro/cognitive tradition tend to view language as involving a partially innate set of rules underlying performance. Although exposure to a well-formed native language is viewed as essential to normal language acquisition, emphasis is placed on innate constraints, on exposure to one's native language as a trigger for predetermined options, and as a moderator of the pace and completeness of acquisition, rather than as a source of the rules themselves. Thus, the focus is on the individual language learner, with context as a background factor. In contrast to language, literacy is viewed as a culturally defined symbol system that must be mastered through direct instruction and that involves discrete processes (e.g., phonological coding), which are themselves seen as semi-autonomous skills that are only partially determined by experiential factors.

As a consequence of these basic assumptions, language and/or literacy disabilities are viewed as rooted in innate (often genetically determined) structural or functional differences in the substrate supporting language processing and the learning of literacy systems. Social and educational experiences are seen as potential avenues to improved functioning but not as key sources of the atypical patterns of behavior evidenced by the individual.

We are indebted to the neuro/cognitive perspective for a detailed analysis of the complex cognitive and linguistic precursors of mature literacy skills. Another benefit of this perspective is its insights into the real-time processes involved in fluent literacy performance, as well as the related distinction between effortful and automatic processes. Flowing from these insights are valuable recommendations for interventions targeted at fostering a strategic approach to literacy as well as fluent component processes.

The sociocultural perspective

Although there is less agreement among those working within the sociocultural tradition regarding how to conceptualize language than there is within the neuro/cognitive tradition, there is a shared assumption that social and cultural factors play a greater formative role. Language tends to be viewed as a set of regularized social practices. It is acquired via participation in communication exchanges, from which the child appropriates patterns of speaking, including, for some (e.g., Ford *et al.*, 2003), the grammatical "rules" themselves. In this sense, social context serves far more than a facilitative or modifying role. Although some socioculturalists accept the view that some aspects of language (e.g., certain grammatical constructions) may be linked to a dedicated processing system, some do not, and even those who do place greater emphasis on the constitutive role of social/cultural experience in typical language development. In contrast to their somewhat disparate views regarding language, socioculturalists largely agree in their conception of literacy as a set of cultural practices that are independent of any dedicated processing system.[2]

When focusing on language and literacy disabilities, socioculturalists tend to downplay the existence of intrinsic limitations in functioning and to emphasize the social/cultural forces that play a role in atypical learning experiences—both in creating atypical patterns of functioning and in allowing the individual to integrate smoothly into society.

We are indebted to the sociocultural perspective for its emphasis on the inherently cultural nature of language and literacy practices. Flowing from this emphasis are guidelines for embedding interventions in meaningful tasks that foster motivation and identity as a reader or writer.

Cross-talk?

Although there are some individuals who argue that their perspective is the only productive approach to furthering our understanding of individuals with disabilities, or the only ethical approach to working with these individuals, the majority of scholars and practitioners acknowledge the utility of certain core features of the alternative perspective. Adherents of the neuro/cognitive perspective acknowledge the influence of context on behavior, for example. Similarly, adherents of the sociocultural/sociological perspective acknowledge the reality of certain underlying physical conditions that pose challenges to the mastery of typical communication systems. However, the majority of such acknowledgements constitute little more than lip service to the potential contributions of the other perspective.

Indeed, when one looks carefully at such acknowledgements, it becomes apparent that neither perspective fully appreciates the core contributions of the other perspective. Of perhaps even greater importance, neither side realizes that attempts at progress within their own perspective that do not incorporate key components of the other perspective run the risk of neglecting key aspects of an interlocking set of dynamics. It is this latter point that is the focus of my comments below.

What is each perspective in danger of neglecting? For the neuro/cognitive perspective, there is a risk of underestimating the formative power of context. Individuals working within this perspective routinely acknowledge that context is important. However, discussions of context typically consist of descriptions of situations in which contextual variation (e.g., exposure to environmental toxins, ineffective instructional routines, limited parental education, or non-Western cultural practices) leads simply to slower growth, inefficient functioning, or a less-rich knowledge base. The notion that contextual factors may actually alter the inherent structure or function of emerging language or literacy is seldom mentioned.

Similarly, those working within the sociocultural perspective often acknowledge the existence of biologically based differences in the structure or function of the child. However, their pictures of the capabilities of the individual and their views about appropriate approaches to prevention/intervention seldom incorporate such differences. As a result, their model of human (in)capability often seems overly idealistic.

Thus, there are issues of past practice within each perspective that have worked against more productive cross-talk among scholars and practitioners working on issues related to language and literacy disability. In addition, some scholars (e.g., Sfard, 1998) have argued that efforts at integration are doomed to fail because of the inherent conflicts in theoretical assumptions represented by the two perspectives (see Stone, 2004, for a brief review of these arguments). Although I appreciate the concerns expressed by these scholars, I tend to side with the more pragmatic voices in favor of integration (e.g., Bransford et al., 2006; Hacking, 1999; Larsen-Freeman, 2007; Pearson, 2004).

Despite past practical and theoretical barriers, there have been some isolated efforts at integration. I mention here two such efforts that stand out because of the richness of theoretical and empirical detail incorporated in the proposals. First, Purcell-Gates et al. (2004) provide a detailed argument for the affordances of an integrated model of print literacy development. In developing their model, they embrace the work on literacy from both the cognitive and sociocultural frameworks. Using the image of concentric circles, they argue that the cognitive and linguistic processes operating in literacy learning take place within the context of social and cultural practices, in a "transactional" dynamic.

Unfortunately, like the authors of most nested models, Purcell-Gates et al. provide only brief indications of how the set of nested dynamics is interrelated. At times, they appear to argue that the broader sociocultural frame (the outer circles in their nested image) serves merely as a background context within which the cognitive processes subserve literacy function. However, at other times, they seem to suggest a more transactional relationship in which newly acquired cognitive skills enable movement into new social spaces, and in which "what may appear to be purely cognitive skills in perception, recognition, and memory *turn out to be cognitive traces of socioculturally based community literacy practices*" (Purcell-Gates et al., 2004, p. 133, emphasis added). The model developed by Purcell-Gates et al. provides a useful way to keep both the cognitive and social in the same field of vision; however, a true integrative framework needs to become even more detailed regarding the interface of the two sets of dynamics.

In another extended proposal for the integration of perspectives, Waber (2010) focuses explicitly on the case of learning disabilities. She endorses recent emphasis on the role of cognitive efficiency (including attention and working memory) in the skill deficits evidenced by children with academic disabilities. However, she stresses the fact that an underlying inefficiency is only problematic within a particular social/institutional context. In her own words:

> From this more systemic perspective, the learning disability diagnosis is best understood *as a social construction that serves to correct for the inherent incompatibility between* normally occurring *biological heterogeneity and socially determined expectations.* It is not a problem of *disability* but of *adaptation.* In this developmental paradigm, the location of the problem similarly does not lie in a defect or disability in the child, but in the *interaction between the child and the world.* That is, the problem is located in the dynamic relationship between a particular child's complement of skills and the particular environment in which that child is developing. (p. 43)

Waber's emphasis on the interplay of cognitive processes and environmental expectations harkens back to earlier critiques of traditional views of "intrinsic, immutable" disabilities offered by theorists within the sociocultural tradition (e.g., Cole and Traupmann, 1981). This is an important argument, and one that is not often made in such detail by scholars steeped in the neuro/cognitive perspective. However, Waber's proposed framework shortchanges the complexities of social/cultural dynamics, and thus falls short of a true integration of perspectives.

Thus, there are limitations to each of these promising efforts at integration. I am optimistic, however, that it is possible over time to overcome such limitations; I also think that recent developments within each tradition make this a promising time to work toward a more productive integration. What we need is to take the dynamics stressed in both perspectives seriously, and to provide meaningful links between them. I consider possible openings for such integration in the next section, along with further discussion of the challenges to achieving this goal.

Is integration possible?

Arguably, one major candidate for skepticism regarding the feasibility of integrating the neuro/cognitive and sociocultural perspectives has been the seemingly wide gap in views regarding the neurological basis for many language and literacy skill deficits. Traditionally, scholars and practitioners within the neuro/cognitive perspective have emphasized the enduring nature of underlying neurological functions, while scholars within the sociocultural tradition have emphasized the seemingly infinite potential for change afforded by social/cultural experiences. Against this backdrop, it is encouraging to examine four recent developments regarding the neural basis of language and literacy acquisition.

First, and perhaps most importantly, within the neuro/cognitive tradition there is a growing acknowledgement of the *potential for practice-based changes in neural function* (and, perhaps, also neural structure). An increasing number of neurocognitivists are now emphasizing epigenesis and neural plasticity (e.g., Berninger and Richards, 2009; Huttenlocher, 2002; Karmiloff-Smith, 2012; Pennington, 2002; Ridley, 2003). As Ridley so succinctly phrased it:

> By far the most important discovery of recent years in brain science is that genes are at the mercy of actions as well as vice versa.... Senses, memory, and action all influence each other through genetic mechanisms. These genes are not just units of heredity—that description misses the point altogether. They are themselves exquisite mechanisms for translating experience into action.
>
> *(Ridley, 2003, p. 275)*

Consistent with Ridley's characterization, there is, in the subfield of neuroconstructivism, a growing number of critiques of the traditional view of genetic/innate unfolding as well as the fixed-locus views of language and cognitive development (Elman *et al.*, 1996; Karmiloff-Smith, 2012; Lewontin, 2000; Satel and Lilienfeld 2013; Zimmer, 2013).

A second and related development that holds promise for an integrated model is the growing evidence of *neural change in response to behavioral interventions* (Anguera *et al.*, 2013; Kandel, 2013; Lyon and Weiser, 2013; Shaywitz and Shaywitz, 2013). Third, there is evidence of *individual differences in neural plasticity*, or the potential for change, and of stress-related determinants of such differences (Belsky and Pluess, 2009; McEwen and Gianaros, 2011).[3] Finally, there is recent evidence that one hypothesized *neural signature of dyslexia (visual motion processing) is a result, not a cause of atypical reading patterns* (Olulade *et al.*, 2013).

This flurry of evidence regarding openness of the neural system to experience-induced change must be viewed against two cautions. First, there is considerable evidence that plasticity is more possible in higher cortical circuits than in lower-level (e.g., sensory or motor) circuits (Huttenlocher, 2002). Second, and related, there are continuing assumptions regarding the reality of lower-level intractable deficits and the limits of neural re-programming. Even with these important cautions, however, there is increasing evidence that we do not yet know what is possible. This sense of possibility opens space for acknowledgement of the formative influence of social/cultural practices in language and literacy functioning.

At the same time that those working within the neuro/cognitive tradition are recognizing the greater potential for neural change in response to targeted experiences, socioculturalists are increasingly open to acknowledging the reality of underlying neural bases for atypical functioning in individuals with academic disabilities. This openness is evident in the work of scholars in both the American (Cole, 2006) and British (Shakespeare, 2006) branches of sociocultural work on disabilities.

The developments outlined above give cause for thinking that a meaningful rapprochement may be possible. Indications of this "magic moment" are also evident in public discourse (e.g., Brooks, 2013; Lewontin, 2000; Satel and Lilienfeld, 2013) and in the creation of new university programs designed to foster collaboration across perspectives (e.g., the University of Michigan's Biosocial Methods Collaborative, http://record.umich.edu//articles/u-m-collaborative-sparks-integration-biological-and-social-data). Thus, the time may be ripe for integrating perspectives. Our challenge is to develop an integrated model that does justice to the insights of both traditions while being clear about the interface between the parallel sets of formative dynamics embodied in the two traditions.

A proposal for integration

What might a truly integrated model look like? A fully satisfying answer to this question is beyond the scope of this chapter. However, I hope to convey a general impression of how one might tackle this challenge. The key starting point is an acknowledgement that there are meaningful points of intersection between the two frameworks. Perhaps the most productive intersect is the acknowledgement of the neurological embodiment of all action, and the ensuing implications for neurological entrenchment following from repeated engagement in cultural routines (e.g., memory heuristics, preferred patterns of engagement with oral or written language). As a second step, one must accept certain basic premises from each framework. For example, from the neuro/cognitive framework, a given is the existence of circumscribed lower-level structural/functional differences, with potential cascading effects (Cole, 2006; Vygotsky, 1993). Working from the sociocultural framework, one must acknowledge the potentially powerful role of social/cultural practices in altering that cascade.

In Figure 35.1, I suggest one way to concretize this proposed integration. The figure contains a representation of essential tenets of each perspective, together with an indication of where those tenets intersect. From the cognitive perspective, I include the assumption of biologically-based variation in the neural substrate for language or literacy learning. Second, I include the notion of processes subserving one or more specific language or literacy skills that are "entrenched"—that is, well-engrained through frequent use. Third is the distinction between "effortful" (i.e., consciously applied) and "automatic" processes. A final feature is the importance placed by cognitively-oriented practitioners on explicit instruction oriented to the building of automatic skills.

From the sociocultural perspective, I again propose adding four features to an integrated model. First, the notion that all learning and performance takes place in specific activity settings; that is, the assumption that even seemingly neutral settings for learning (e.g., round-robin reading, vocabulary lessons) or assessment (e.g., oral reading, book reports, essay exams) are colored by cultural goals and implied courses for action. Second, we need the related but broader notion that language and literacy are productively conceptualized as a set of culturally embedded practices, with associated social/cultural valences or values. Included here is the idea that, in using specific practices, one adopts, explicitly or implicitly, a certain identity within a broader social frame, an identity that may have implications for future patterns of use or an individual's reactions to intervention efforts. The third feature from the sociocultural perspective is the notion of individual appropriation of cultural practices through (guided) participation in those practices. Finally, I would add an emphasis on approaches to intervention that are embedded in authentic task goals. Note that I include this feature as a complement to, rather than as a replacement to, the cognitivists' emphasis on explicit instruction.

Linking the elements from the two perspectives is the assumption that participation over time in repeated social practices results in the creation of activity-specific neural circuits or "functional systems" (Berninger and Richards, 2009; Luria, 1973). Such circuits take on the quasi-permanence of any neurally grounded action, and as such simultaneously form part of a set of social practices and a neural network. This linking assumption serves to weave the various other components of the two perspectives into a coherent whole.

What exactly am I advocating? I believe that the two perspectives CAN be brought together into an integrated framework, rather than existing in parallel communities of practice. Thus, neuro/cognitivists must acknowledge the complexity of the "black box" they call "context," as well as its potential power to genuinely shape, rather than merely moderate, linguistic and cognitive processes. Likewise, socioculturalists must acknowledge that at least some characteristics of atypical language and literacy practices are grounded in biology (i.e., genetic mutations or perinatal insults), and that they have potentially profound implications for participation in, and thus learning via, social practices. More generally, they must acknowledge that all language and

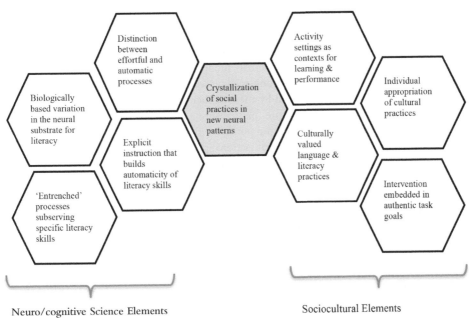

Figure 35.1 Key components of an integrated model of language/literacy disabilities.

Note. The four hexagons on the left represent features from the cognitive science perspective. The four hexagons on the right represent features from the sociocultural perspective. The central solid hexagon represents a key linking assertion. See text for details. (Adapted with permission from Stone and Learned, 2014).

literacy practices have a neural dimension, and that repeated practices can alter neural pathways and functioning. This does not mean that professionals within each tradition need to tackle all of each other's issues, but rather that they should design studies and interventions that are mindful of their colleagues' concerns, and that the implications they draw from their work remain mindful of the complete set of dynamics. This amounts to a movement from parallel play to something approximating cooperative play.

Implications of the proposed model

Fleshing out this sketch of an integrated model would require considerable work; however, I hope that I have managed to convey an impression of how one might proceed to undertake that work. Doing so would have broad implications. First, the model can serve as a framework guiding the future development of theory and research related to atypical patterns of language and literacy development. Although such examples are evident in the literacy and special education fields, the picture is different in the field of Speech–Language Pathology (SLP). To identify examples of recent work in SLP that takes an integrated perspective, or at least puts strong emphasis on evidence that experience influences basic processing, I undertook a hand search of the 2012 and 2013 issues of two leading journals: *Journal of Speech, Language, and Hearing Research* and *Language, Speech, and Hearing Services in the Schools*. Looking specifically at those articles focused on language, using a liberal criterion, I found eight candidates to consider. Here, I highlight two of those eight.

In a large-scale longitudinal study of verbal and nonverbal abilities in children with specific language impairment, Conti-Ramsden *et al.* (2012) found evidence that some children whose nonverbal skills were age-appropriate in the early years showed increasing evidence over time of nonverbal deficits alongside their language deficits. The authors interpreted these findings as consistent with the view that language difficulties alter engagement with the world, resulting in a continually evolving pattern of (dis)abilities. In another example, McGinty *et al.* (2012), working from what they term a "transactional" model of language development, hypothesized that the verbal participation in shared book-reading sessions of children with specific language impairment (SLI) would be influenced by their mother's level of language use, which in turn would influence the children's future participation. Although the study's results were disappointing, the authors emphasized the positive results from related studies and argued for the importance of further work from a transactional perspective.

A second implication of an integrated model is its potential to inform the design and delivery of support services for language and literacy development. Having a framework for an integrated perspective provides a principled basis for collaboration between medical/clinical and educational practitioners. In addition, it should enable a greater appreciation of the implications of alternative prevention/intervention programming. Although not focused on language or literacy, the recent study by Anguera *et al.* (2013) provides a good example of how a carefully crafted task environment can produce meaningful change in skills long thought to be immutable in an aging population. See also the theoretical examinations of intervention settings by Damico and Damico (1997) and Daniels (2001) for examples of how a framework that is sensitive to both intrinsic characteristics of the individual and the formative influence of social settings can yield interesting proposals for intervention paradigms. Examples such as these point to the possibility of designing interventions involving integrated socio-contextual modifications and neurologically-based training.

As we work toward a meaningful integration of perspectives, a number of key questions will arise, questions whose answers will eventually serve to make the integration more detailed and more useful. For example, we might ask:

- In positive responses to intervention (i.e., resulting in "normal neural signatures"), what is changing, and what is not? For example, Berninger and Swanson (2013) suggest that positive responses to intervention reflect changes in the individual's phenotype but an invariant and potentially resurfacing genotype. Is this the best way to conceptualize responses to intervention, or should we place more emphasis on changes in routine practices and their underlying changes in neural connectivity?
- What are key parameters of effective interventions, that is, interventions that result in new functional systems (e.g., amount of necessary practice, developmental timing, routine/varying nature, intensity)? It may be instructive here to consult particularly effective examples (e.g., Anguera *et al.*, 2013; Battro, 2000). A related question is what we should conclude from the existence of non-responders to particularly effective interventions regarding the limits of neural plasticity (Lyon and Weiser, 2013).
- If we identify, via longitudinal projects, examples of individuals at genetic risk for a specific disability but who show no overt or covert (e.g., neuroimaging) signs of a target phenotype, can we gain greater insight into the nature of supporting contextual (i.e., interpersonal or institutional) contributors to the positive outcome?

Questions such as these should contribute over time to a more nuanced understanding of the complex interplay among neuro/cognitive processes and sociocultural dynamics.

Notes

1 In actuality, what I am discussing here is two families of theories. Sociocultural theorists differ amongst themselves in terms of their skepticism about notions of knowledge representation, for example, or about the dynamics of learning and the existence of innate variation in human capabilities. Similarly, theorists from the neuro/cognitive perspective differ amongst themselves in terms of their insistence on neurologically real models of processing, and in terms of their views about the notion of innate, dedicated processing modules. However, members of each perspective have more in common with fellow members than with members of the competing perspective.
2 Although many socioculturalists use a concept of literacy that is considerably broader (e.g., Gee, 2011), for the purposes of the current discussion, I restrict my treatment to print literacy.
3 It is interesting to note that these authors stress that plasticity may work in both directions; that is, stress may limit the degree of plasticity, but reductions in stress may open opportunities for plasticity.

References

Anguera, J.A., Boccanfuso, J., Rintoul, J.L., Hashimi, O., Faraji, F., Janowich, J., *et al.*, (2013), "Video game training enhances cognitive control in older adults", *Nature*, Vol. 501, pp. 97–103. doi: 10.1038/nature12486.

Battro, A.M. (2000), *Half a Brain is Enough: The Story of Nico*, Cambridge, UK: Cambridge University Press.

Belsky, J. and Pluess, M. (2009), "The nature (and nurture?) of plasticity in early human development", *Perspectives on Psychological Science*, Vol. 4, pp. 345–351.

Berninger, V. and Richards, T. (2009), "Brain and learning", in Anderman, E.M. (Ed.-in-Chief), *Psychology of Classroom Learning: An Encyclopedia, Vol. 1*, Detroit, US: Macmillan Reference USA, pp. 15–22.

Berninger, V.W. and Swanson, H.L. (2013), "Diagnosing and treating specific learning disabilities in reference to the brain's working memory system", in Swanson, H.L., Harris, K.R. and Graham, S. (Eds.), *Handbook of Learning Disabilities, 2nd Ed.*, New York, NY: Guilford Press, pp. 307–325.

Bransford, J.D., Barron, B., Pea, R.D., Meltzoff, A., Kuhl, P., Bell, P., *et al.*, (2006), "Foundations and opportunities for an interdisciplinary science of learning", in Sawyer, R.K. (Ed.), *The Cambridge Handbook of the Learning Sciences*, New York: Cambridge University Press, pp. 19–34.

Brooks, D. (June 17, 2013), "Beyond the brain", *New York Times*. www.nytimes.com/2013/06/18/opinion/brooks-beyond-the-brain.html?_r=0

Cole, M. (2006), "Culture and cognitive development in phylogenetic, historical, and ontogenetic perspective", in Kuhn, D. and Siegler, R. (Eds.), *Handbook of Child Psychology, Vol. 2: Cognition, Perception, and Language* (Damon, W. and Lerner, R.M., Editors-in-Chief), New York: John Wiley, pp. 636–683.

Cole, M. and Traupmann, K. (1981), "Comparative cognitive research: Learning from a learning-disabled child", in Collins, W.W. (Ed.), *The Minnesota Symposium in Child Psychology, Vol. 14*, Hillsdale, NJ, US: Erlbaum, pp. 125–154.

Conti-Ramsden, G., St. Claire, M.C., Pickles, A. and Durkin, K. (2012), "Developmental trajectories of verbal and nonverbal skills in individuals with a history of specific language impairment: From childhood to adolescence", *Journal of Speech, Language, and Hearing Research*, Vol. 55, pp. 1716–1735.

Damico, J.S. and Damico, S.K. (1997), "The establishment of a dominant interpretive framework in language intervention", *Language, Speech, and Hearing Services in the Schools*, Vol. 28, pp. 288–296.

Daniels, H. (2001), *Vygotsky and Pedagogy*, New York: Routlege/Falmer.

Elman, J.L., Bates, E.A., Johnson, M.H., Karmiloff-Smith, A., Parisi, D. and Plunkett, K. (1996), *Rethinking innateness: A connectionist perspective on development*, Cambridge, MA, US: MIT Press.

Ford, C.E., Fox, B.A. and Thompson, S.A. (2003), "Social interaction and grammar", in Tomasello, M. (Ed.), *The New Psychology of Language: Cognitive and Functional Approaches to Language Structure*, Mahweh, NJ, US: Lawrence Erlbaum Associates, pp. 119–143.

Hacking, I. (1999), *The Social Construction of What?* Cambridge, MA, US: Harvard University Press.

Huttenlocher, P.R. (2002), *Neural Plasticity: The Effects of Environment on the Development of the Cerebral Cortex*, Cambridge, MA, US: Harvard University Press.

Kandel, E.R. (Sept. 6, 2013), "The new science of mind", *New York Times*.

Karmiloff-Smith, A. (2012), "From constructivism to neuroconstructivism: The activity-dependent structuring of the human brain", in Marti, E. and Rodriguez, C. (Eds.), *After Piaget*, New Brunswick, NJ, US: Transaction, pp. 1–14.

Kovorsky, D. and Maxwell, M. (1997), "Rethinking the context of language in the schools", *Journal of Speech, Language, and Hearing Services in the Schools*, Vol. 28, pp. 219–230.

Larsen-Freeman, D. (2007), "Reflecting on the cognitive-social debate in second language acquisition", *Modern Language Journal*, Vol. 91, pp. 773–787.

Lewontin, R. (2000), *It ain't Necessarily so: The Dream of the Human Genome and Other Illusions*, New York: New York Review Books.

Luria, A.R. (1973), *The Working Brain*, New York: Basic Books.

Lyon, G.R. and Weiser, B. (2013), "The state of the science in learning disabilities", in Swanson, H.L., Harris, K.R. and Graham, S. (Eds.), *Handbook of Learning Disabilities, 2nd Ed.*, New York: Guilford Press, pp. 118–144.

McEwen, B.S. and Gianaros, P.J. (2011), "Stress and allostatis-induced brain plasticity", *Annual Review of Medicine*, Vol. 62, pp. 431–445.

McGinty, A.S., Justice, L.M., Zucker, T.A., Gosse, C. and Skibbe, L.E., (2012), "Shared reading dynamics: Mothers' question use and the verbal participation of children with specific language impairment", *Journal of Speech, Language, and Hearing Research*, Vol. 55, pp. 1039–1052.

Olulade, O.A., Napoliello, E.M. and Eden, G.F. (2013), "Abnormal visual motion processing is not a cause of dyslexia", *Neuron*, Vol. 79, pp. 180–190.

Pearson, P.D. (2004), "The reading wars", *Educational Policy*, Vol. 18, pp. 216–252.

Pennington, B.F. (2002), "Genes and brain: Individual differences and human universals", in Johnson, M.H., Munakata, Y. and Gilmore, R.O. (Eds.), *Brain Development and Cognition: A Reader, 2nd Ed.*, Malden, MA, US: Blackwell Publishers, pp. 494–508.

Purcell-Gates, V., Jacobson, S. and Degener, E. (2004), *Print Literacy Development: Uniting Cognitive and Social Practice Theories*, Cambridge, MA, US: Harvard University Press.

Ridley, M. (2003), *The agile gene: How nature turns on nurture*, New York, NY: Harper.

Satel, S. and Lilienfeld, S.O. (2013), *Brainwashed: The Seductive Appeal of Mindless Neuroscience*, New York: Basic Books.

Sfard, A. (1998), "On two metaphors for learning and the dangers of choosing just one", *Educational Researcher*, Vol. 27, No. 2, pp. 4–13.

Shakespeare, T.W. (2006), *Disability Rights and Wrongs*, London: Routledge.

Shaywitz, S.E. and Shaywitz, B.A. (2013), "Making a hidden disability visible: What has been learned from neurobiological studies of dyslexia", in Swanson, H.L., Harris, K.R. and Graham, S. (Eds.), *Handbook of Learning Disabilities, 2nd Ed.,* New York: Guilford Press, pp. 643–657.

Stone, C.A. (2004), "Contemporary approaches to the study of language and literacy development: A call for the integration of perspectives", in Stone, C.A., Silliman, E.R., Ehren, B.J. and Wallach, G.P. (Eds.), *Handbook of Language and Literacy: Development and Disorders*, New York: Guilford Press, pp. 3–24.

Stone, C.A. and Learned, J.E. (2014), "Atypical language and literacy development: Toward an integrative framework", in Stone, C.A., Silliman, E.R., Ehren, B.J. and Apel, K. (Eds.), *Handbook of Language and Literacy: Development and Disorders—2nd Ed.*, New York: Guilford Press, pp. 5–25.

Trent, S.C., Artiles, A.J. and Englert, C.S. (1998), "From deficit thinking to social constructivism: A review of theory, research, and practice in special education", *Review of Research in Education*, Vol. 23, pp. 277–307.

Vygotsky, L. (1993), *The Collected Works of L.S. Vygotsky, Vol. 2: The Fundamentals of Defectology*, Rieber, R.W. and Carton, A.S., Eds., New York: Plenum Publishing.

Waber, D.P. (2010), *Rethinking Learning Disabilities: Understanding Children who Struggle in School*, New York: Guilford Press.

Zimmer, C. (September 23, 2013), "DNA doubletake", *New York Times*.

36

COMMUNICATION AS DISTRIBUTED COGNITION

Novel theoretical and methodological approaches to disruptions in social communication following acquired brain injury

Melissa C. Duff, Bilge Mutlu, Lindsey J. Byom and Lyn S. Turkstra

Communication as distributed, situated cognition

The distributed cognition framework (Hollan *et al.*, 2000; Hutchins, 1995; Salomon, 1993) aims to understand the organization of cognitive systems by analyzing the interactions among individuals, representational media (e.g., objects, artifacts), and the rich environments within which complex human activity is situated. Consistent with socio-cultural perspectives (Cole, 1996; Vygotsky, 1978; Wertsch, 1985), the distributed cognition framework argues that higher-order cognitive functions such as language develop through and are dynamically linked with our social interactions with people and the environment. A core theoretical principle of distributed cognition is that cognition, learning, and knowledge are not confined to the products of an isolated individual; rather, they are distributed across individuals, time, and the environment (Hutchins, 1995). Methodologically, the unit of analysis is not the individual performance on a particular task or a specific domain of cognition within the individual. Instead, the goal is to capture and understand the functional activities and social spaces in which complex behavior emerges and the full range of resources (human, cognitive, semiotic and material) that are deployed for interactional success. A distributed cognition perspective requires researchers and clinicians to develop tools for capturing the orchestration of systems and theories that account for how, when, and why such systems are called upon in the service of executing complex behavior.

The tenets of the distributed cognition framework fit particularly well with efforts to understand communication in social context. Indeed, researchers have used ethnographic methods to apply this framework to examine communicative activities, including analysis of verbal and nonverbal resources, the forms and functions of communication, and the dialogic trajectory of communication across functional, goal-directed activity (see Hutchins and Palen, 1997; Prior and Hengst, 2010; Rogers, 2006). While the distributed cognition framework has garnered considerable attention in cognitive science and psychology, it has received less attention in communication sciences and disorders. We argue that the distributed cognition framework provides a promising approach to the empirical study of communication and communication disorders, while paying special attention to the case of social communication problems in individuals with acquired brain injury (Duff *et al.*, 2012). In this chapter we: 1) outline the empirical and clinical challenges of studying and treating social communication problems in acquired brain injury and propose that the distributed cognition framework holds tremendous promise in meeting these challenges; 2) present a series of experimental protocols from our ongoing research program on social perception and communication in individuals with traumatic brain injury (TBI) that draws on the distributed cognition framework; and 3) offer preliminary data from individuals with TBI and neurologically intact individuals to demonstrate the feasibility of our protocols for capturing the complex communication disruptions in TBI within a distributed cognition framework.

Distributed cognition as a window into disrupted social communication in TBI

TBI is a pervasive public health issue affecting more than 1.7 million Americans annually (Faul *et al.*, 2010). Impairments in social behavior are a hallmark of moderate–severe TBI (Kelly *et al.*, 2008; McDonald *et al.*, 2008), and have deleterious effects on academic, vocational, and interpersonal pursuits (Coelho, 2007; Engberg and Teasdale, 2004). While TBI can result in a range of cognitive and behavioral disorders, the most common complaint, and perhaps the greatest obstacle to community re-integration and employment, is that persons with TBI have "odd" social behaviors, such as making inappropriate or irrelevant comments, monopolizing conversations, and generally appearing to be insensitive to the social needs of others (Struchen *et al.*, 2008). These are *social communication problems*. The term social communication problem differentiates the disruptions in *communication* (not language) in TBI observed in a variety of *social* contexts secondary to impairments in cognition (e.g., memory) from disruptions in language (not communication) observed in the aphasias secondary to impairments in the linguistic system (Heilman *et al.*, 1971).

Many studies have documented social communication problems in TBI and their impact on communication partners (e.g., Kelly *et al.*, 2008; Struchen *et al.*, 2008), yet there is little evidence that treatment of these problems results in improved communication in everyday interactions (Dahlberg *et al.*, 2007; McDonald *et al.*, 2008). One possible reason is that our treatments lack a robust set of theoretical and methodological tools for conceptualizing and analyzing social communication problems in the context of social interaction. For example, traditional approaches (see Cherney *et al.*, 1998) focus on the verbal productions of an individual performing isolated monologue discourse tasks in highly controlled settings, without considering how individuals communicate in multi-interlocutor interactions to negotiate functional activities situated in the social environment. Many current therapies focus on communication *performance* in treating social communication problems. They do so by re-teaching "appropriate" behaviors (e.g., training eye contact or turn taking) without considering how communication is shaped by the specific social context (i.e., the physical world, objects, people) in which these behaviors are situated, the time course over which behaviors arise, or the dynamic orchestration of underlying impairments that produce these behaviors. Thus, clinicians rely on decontextualized assessment protocols that fail to capture and account for the social and interactional nature of the deficits in TBI, and lack theoretically grounded treatments that can improve the social and communicative lives of individuals with TBI (Coelho, 2007; Hengst *et al.*, 2010; Snow and Douglas, 2000).

We have proposed that distributed cognition offers a unique lens and set of tools with which to approach the theoretical, methodological, and clinical challenges of social communication problems in TBI (Duff *et al.*, 2012). In an ongoing research program, we have assembled a protocol that embraces the tenets of distributed cognition to examine social perception and social communication in adults with TBI. There is growing evidence that the cause of impaired communication performance may be a failure to read social cues, i.e., impaired *social perception*. Social perception problems after TBI may range from failure to read basic nonverbal cues, such as gaze direction (Turkstra, 2005; Turkstra *et al.*, 2006), to errors perceiving complex social cues such as sarcasm (Martin-Rodriguez and Leon-Carrion, 2010). An understanding of social perception problems in adults with TBI is critical for clinical management: an individual with TBI may have excellent performance skills, but these skills are useless if the individual does not recognize when to use them in social context. To address this disconnect between basic research and clinical practice, we used the principles of distributed cognition to design a series of studies that systematically examined perception and use of social cues in dynamic social contexts in individuals with TBI.

Our approach combines eye-tracking, computational modeling, and fine-grained behavioral analysis to examine different types of social perception in social contexts ubiquitous throughout everyday communication. We *simulate* social cues in humanlike robots and create experimental scenarios in which participants interact with these humanlike representations (Figure 36.1[1]). Our paradigm enables the creation of precisely controlled, reliable, and ecologically valid social stimuli. We also capture social perception and communication in interactive situations "on-line" or in the moment. This paradigm offers greater experimental control than would the use of human confederates, because it allows for greater control over verbal and nonverbal cues provided by the confederate. It also achieves minimal variability in how cues are presented across experimental trials. Control of verbal and nonverbal cues is critical for behaviors such as eye gaze, which are highly proceduralized and difficult to control in humans. This paradigm offers stronger ecological validity than image- and video-based studies, as it allows us to present social cues to participants in dynamic, interactive situations and capture their responses using objective and behavioral measures. The overarching goal of this work is to identify impairments in social perception in context in individuals with TBI and relate those deficits to impairments in social communication. In the next section, we present components of our experimental protocol.

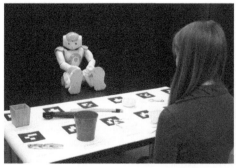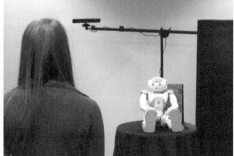

Figure 36.1 An experimenter demonstrating two experimental protocols that we have developed with humanlike robots involving precise manipulations in gaze cues. On the left is the Nonverbal Leakage Task, and on the right is the Interpersonal Intimacy Task.

Experimental protocols for studying distributed, situated social communication in TBI

The tasks described below address social perception of three types of cues: gaze cues, emotion cues from affect displays, and cues to intent and beliefs. Tasks were selected because of their importance in everyday communication and adherence to the tenets of distributed cognition. Specifically, empirical data from our group, literature on TBI, and our extended clinical experience in TBI suggest that these aspects of social perception are impaired in adults with TBI. Cues to be studied have direct links to widely used therapy methods for social communication problems, so results can translate directly into clinical trials. Performance can also be reliably measured using validated tools developed by the investigators and others, so results can be replicated. Finally, tasks were designed to differentiate problems in social perception from effects of impairments in nonsocial cognitive functions (e.g., executive functions) that typically are impaired after TBI and confound interpretation of poor performance on some types of social perception tasks (Leslie *et al.*, 2005; McKinnon and Moscovitch, 2007). Next, we present more detail on the three types of social perception cues used in our work, describe the tasks, and present preliminary data.

Perception of gaze

From a very early age, humans are sensitive to the eyes of others and use information from others' eyes to make inferences about mental states (see Frischen *et al.*, 2007 and Emery, 2000 for reviews). While individuals with TBI are described as having "poor eye contact" (Snow and Ponsford, 1995), studies of basic eye contact during conversations do not reveal systematic differences between individuals with TBI and typical peers (Turkstra, 2005; Turkstra *et al.*, 2006). It is possible that individuals with TBI look toward their partners' eyes during interactions, but fail to accurately interpret the meaning of their partners' gaze cues, and it is this interpretive failure that contributes to partner complaints of poor social communication skills in individuals with TBI. One way to test this hypothesis is to vary the nature of information implied by gaze cues, from simple gaze direction, to gaze direction as a cue to object location, to increased eye contact, as an attempt to reduce interpersonal distance. In this way, it is possible to differentiate impairments in basic gaze processes (e.g., lack of fixation on the partner's eyes) from impairments in use or function of gaze in dynamic social interactions.

A distributed cognition approach to studying communication argues for the examination of gaze across individuals and objects in the environment while a participant is engaged in a functional activity. Indeed, studying eye gaze in social interaction is critical in linking gaze behavior to communicative success or disruption. As Wilms and colleagues (2010) noted, experimental methods should combine real-time interactions between participants with social stimuli under experimental control. However, there are inherent methodological challenges associated with attempts to control eye-gaze behavior in human confederates while maintaining high experimental control across trials and participants. To address this methodological challenge, we built on prior work demonstrating that in interactive social behaviors, such as gaze, individuals interact with humanlike robots as they do with other humans (Fong *et al.*, 2003). Thus, our approach preserves the elements of social interaction across varied tasks while maintaining precise experimental control, by examining gaze using simulated social interaction tasks in which participants interact with a humanlike robot. A description of these tasks follows.

The Nonverbal Leakage Task

The Nonverbal Leakage Task, developed by Mutlu *et al.* (2009), is a variant of the 20-Questions Game that allows observation of how participants use leakage cues (quick gaze shifts that carry task-relevant information) produced by a humanlike robot (see Figure 36.1, left panel). In the game, the robot covertly selects an object from an array of 10 objects on a table, located between the robot and participant. The participant asks the robot questions that it can answer with "yes" or "no", in order to guess which object the robot has chosen (e.g., Is it made of wood?). In half the trials, along with verbal answers the robot will "leak" information via a brief gaze shift toward the target object. In the other trials, the robot looks straight ahead while answering questions. Healthy individuals are sensitive to this type of gaze cue, as they ask fewer questions and require less time to identify selected objects on the leakage cue trials than on trials with only verbal responses (Mutlu *et al.*, 2009). The Nonverbal Leakage Task allows us to determine if individuals with TBI use the gaze-based leakage cues to guide task performance and allows us to test our hypothesis that individuals with TBI do not use these subtle nonverbal cues in the context of social interaction. Preliminary data from an individual with TBI and a healthy counterpart lend early support for this prediction, as illustrated in Figure 36.2. The presence of the gaze-based leakage cues improved task performance in the healthy individual, while data from the individual with TBI show the opposite trend.

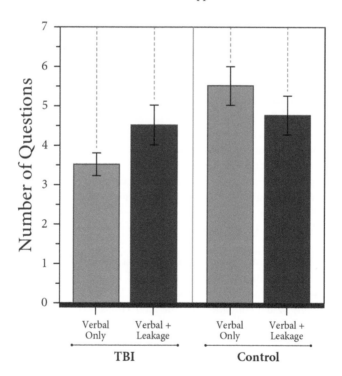

Figure 36.2 Preliminary data from an individual with TBI (left) and a healthy individual (right). The predicted effects of "leakage" gaze cues are visible as trends. The presence of gaze cues improves mentalizing ability in the healthy individual but not in the individual with TBI.

Interpersonal Intimacy Task

One key function of gaze cues is to regulate the level of intimacy among communication partners. Individuals adjust their social behavior in response to cues from their partners to achieve an interpersonal "equilibrium" (Argyle and Dean, 1965). For example, an interaction may be perceived as more intimate if the amount of eye contact between partners is increased. To re-establish equilibrium, partners may compensate by increasing their interpersonal distance (Patterson, 1973). A common complaint is that adults with TBI violate others' personal space. Related research has documented difficulty establishing an appropriate level of situational intimacy in individuals with TBI (Beer *et al.*, 2006; Byom and Turkstra, 2012).

While interpersonal distance has not been addressed empirically in TBI research, the general clinical notion has been that "close talking" is due to either a lack of inhibition or a lack of knowledge about personal space boundaries. We propose an alternative hypothesis: individuals with TBI fail to interpret increased gaze as an attempt to increase intimacy; thus, they do not modify their behavior accordingly. This hypothesis was tested within a simulated social interaction and the use of the Interpersonal Intimacy Task (Mumm and Mutlu, 2011) (Figure 36.3). In this task, participants are seated across from a humanlike robot and must get up and approach the robot to retrieve a word from a list placed behind the robot. During half of the trials, the robot maintains direct eye gaze with participants as they approach it, attempting to increase interpersonal intimacy. Our prediction is that, in contrast with the responses of typical individuals, the gaze behavior of the robot will not influence the behavior of the individuals with TBI.

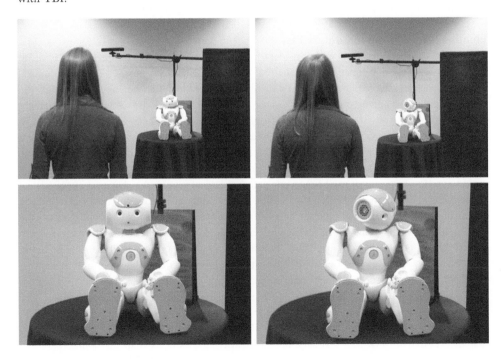

Figure 36.3 In the Interpersonal Intimacy Task, participants are asked to approach the robot to retrieve a number placed behind it. Across trials, the robot either maintains or avoids eye contact with the participant, while the distance that the participant maintains with the robot is automatically captured using video processing techniques. The images on the left illustrate the robot maintaining eye contact, and those on the right show the robot avoiding eye contact.

Perception of emotion in context

Facial expressions of emotion have been the subject of scientific study for over a century (Darwin, 1872; Ekman and Friesen, 1969). Research suggests that individuals are able to reliably categorize facial expressions into basic emotion categories such as happy and angry from an early age (Boyatzis *et al.*, 1993; Walker-Andrews, 1998). The bulk of this work has asked participants to make judgments of emotional states from only the face by relying exclusively on facial structure configuration (e.g., the corners of the mouth turned upward shows a happy emotion). Yet, a distributed cognition approach argues for understanding how information from the social and physical context shapes and interacts with core cognitive processes. Indeed, the interpretation of facial affect is highly influenced by contextual factors (Darwin, 1872; Barrett *et al.*, 2011).

Emotion identification deficits are common after TBI (Radice-Neumann *et al.*, 2007; Turkstra *et al.*, 2001). Consistent with the larger research base, tasks used to study emotional identification in TBI have required participants to make judgments based solely on the face of an actor. Consequently, considerably less is known about how physical, linguistic, and social context influence the perception and identification of facial emotion in TBI. On one hand, it is possible that individuals with TBI benefit from additional information available in context-rich stimuli. For example, in typical adults, interpretation of emotions is strongly influenced by verbal and nonverbal context (Barrett *et al.*, 2011). On the other hand, many adults with TBI have impairments in attending to and interpreting contextual information (Salmond *et al.*, 2006) and may be less sensitive to contextual factors in making their judgments.

Emotion Identification in Context Task

To analyze context effects on emotion identification, we used The Emotion Identification in Context (EIC) Task developed by Turkstra *et al.* (2014). The task is comprised of 60 emotionally evocative black and white photographs of individuals in daily life: 30 photographs display only the face of an individual and 30 photographs show an individual in a rich visual context. Photographs were chosen from the *LIFE* magazine photograph archives, and show emotionally evocative scenes. Participants view each photograph while their eye movements are monitored using a mobile eye-tracking device, and are asked to label the emotion that the target individual is feeling. As responses are open-ended rather than forced choice from a limited set of alternatives (the typical emotion recognition method), participants' responses represent a dynamic interaction of the stimulus, the participant's perceptual abilities, and his or her knowledge of the social world and people in it. We predicted that typical adults would be more likely to name basic emotions for the photographs showing only a face, and social emotions for the photographs showing faces in scenes. Social emotions combine basic emotions with mental-state inferences (e.g., guilt, embarrassment, jealousy), and one would expect those mental states to be supported by context information. EIC response accuracy is measured by comparing participants' answers to responses from a large group of typical adults. We also examine eye-gaze patterns to help understand how participants use information in the photographs to arrive at their answers (see Figure 36.4).

Preliminary data from an individual with TBI and a neurologically normal counterpart show that the adult with TBI was less accurate in identifying emotions than his counterpart (see Figure 36.5). More interestingly, we observed the individual with TBI attributing "social" emotions to 86 percent of the photographs, while the healthy individual attributed "social" emotions to 50 percent of the photographs. This finding indicates that the individual with TBI over-attributed social context to faces in photographs with no social context information. Analysis of gaze data is ongoing.

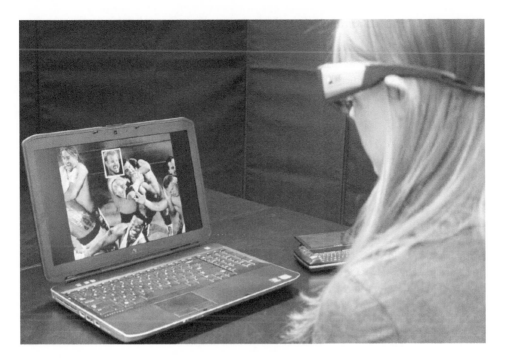

Figure 36.4 An experimenter demonstrating the Emotion Identification in Context (EIC) Task. In the protocol, participants are asked to identify the emotions felt by the target individual in a photograph while their eye movements are monitored using a mobile eye-tracking device.

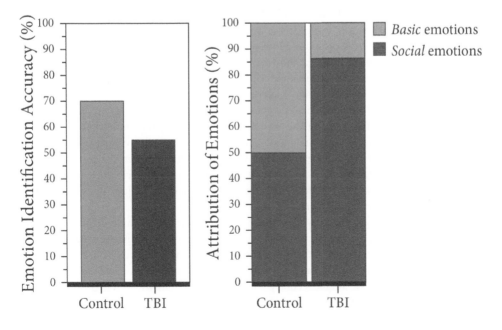

Figure 36.5 EIC Task: Preliminary data from a healthy individual and an individual with TBI.

Perception of intents and beliefs

In addition to the perception of gaze and affect cues, successful social interaction requires humans to use these cues to make inferences about the thoughts and feelings of others and to use such inferences to predict their behavior, i.e., we must have a "theory of mind (ToM)" (see chapters in this volume by Hutchins and Prelock; Longard and Moore). In many classic ToM tasks, participants are presented with a described or depicted social scenario from which they must answer questions about characters' mental states and future behaviors. For example, in the Strange Stories Task (Happé, 1994), participants hear short stories featuring pragmatic language acts, such as sarcasm, deception, or faux pas. Participants then are asked probe questions about story characters' mental states and behavior. Groups of participants with TBI have been reported to have impairments on similar tasks (see review in Martin-Rodriguez and Leon-Carrion, 2010), especially when required to make second-order ToM inferences (i.e., asking participants to infer what person A is thinking about person B). A concern about ToM tasks is that they impose cognitive demands beyond ToM. Most notably, second-order ToM tasks require participants to hold story information in mind while processing linguistically-complex probe questions that themselves have a high working memory load. Turkstra (2008) and others (Bibby and McDonald, 2005) have shown that domain-general cognitive demands affect how individuals with TBI perform on second-order ToM tasks. A further critique of traditional ToM tasks is that, while they describe a social scenario, they lack much of the dynamic contextual information available in real-world social interactions (Byom and Mutlu, 2013).

Video Social Inference Task

To investigate how individuals with TBI use dynamic social and contextual cues to make ToM inferences with controlled working memory demands Turkstra (2008) developed the Video Social Inference Task (VSIT), which was designed to broadly examine social cognition, of which ToM is an important component. Based on the format of The Awareness of Social Inference Test (TASIT; McDonald *et al.*, 2002), the VSIT is comprised of 20 paired video vignettes of adolescent actors engaged in actual social interactions (Figure 36.6). During each video vignette, actors display prosodic, affective, postural, and linguistic cues that are congruent with a particular pragmatic act (e.g., showing interest in one's partner). Participants must use these cues to make social inferences about characters' mental states. Each pair of vignettes is comprised of an initial interaction and a later interaction with the same actors. Following the first vignette in each pair, the participant is asked to make a social inference (e.g., Do they want to work together?). After viewing the second vignette, participants must explain the same character's behavior based on their mental-state inferences from the first vignette. Memory load is manipulated by inserting a 30-second delay with a distracter between the first and second vignettes in 10 of the vignette pairs. The delay was designed to move us closer to understanding the real-world demands of social interaction in which delays and distractions are routine aspects of turn taking and topic management.

Figure 36.7 illustrates preliminary data from a healthy individual and an individual with TBI from the ongoing study. Scores are reported for the first item of each pair, showing basic social inference with no memory manipulation, pairs with no 30-second delay and distracter, and pairs with a delay and distracter. Consistent with our prediction, the individual with TBI shows a more substantial decrease in task accuracy when working memory load is high (87.5 percent vs. 50 percent) than does the healthy individual (87.5 percent vs. 75 percent).

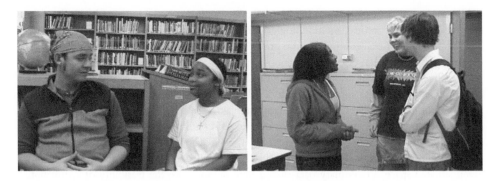

Figure 36.6 Stills from the video vignettes used in the Video Social Inference Task (VSIT).

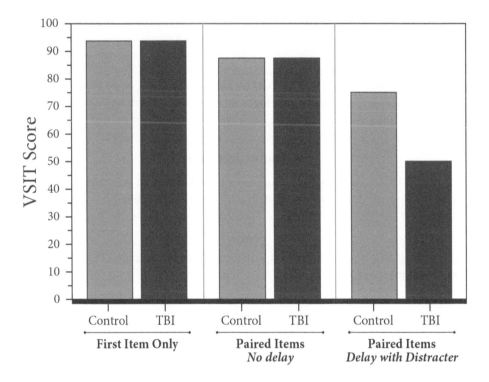

Figure 36.7 VSIT scores from a healthy individual and an individual with TBI from our preliminary data collection.

Summary and future clinical directions

Social communication problems are the most common complaint about individuals with TBI, and are potentially the greatest obstacle to achieving positive long-term outcomes for individuals with TBI and their caregivers. Although knowledge about social communication in TBI is growing, researchers and clinicians still face critical challenges to improving detection and treatment of social communication problems in this population.

413

We have argued that distributed cognition offers a unique perspective and set of tools for approaching the theoretical, methodological, and clinical challenges associated with capturing and understanding social communication problems in adults with TBI (Duff *et al.*, 2012). In this chapter, we presented a series of experimental protocols from our ongoing research program, which draw on the distributed cognition framework to study social perception and communication in social contexts in individuals with TBI. This framework, in contrast with more traditional approaches to studying communication in TBI, shifts the problem space and unit of analysis from the lone individual or the isolated cognitive process to the communicative activities in which complex behavior emerges. It also considers the full range of resources—social, cognitive, semiotic, and material—that individuals deploy to interact successfully in a given situated space. Preliminary data shared here demonstrate the feasibility of a distributed cognition approach to the empirical study of social communication problems in TBI.

The distributed cognition framework, embodied in the experimental procedures presented here, offers a deeper and more complete understanding of how individuals with TBI perceive dynamic social and environmental information across a range of social contexts. Distributed cognition views communication as a socially distributed and situated cognitive activity that is co-constructed among interlocutors and their social and physical environment. As such, it is uniquely suited to examining social communication in context. We believe that this novel theoretical and methodological approach will lead to new directions in the empirical study of social communication problems and in clinical decision-making and treatment planning for individuals with acquired brain injury.

Acknowledgements

Research presented in this chapter was supported by NICHD grant R01 HD071089, Social perception and social communication in adults with traumatic brain injury.

Note

1   All individuals in the figures of this chapter are members of our research team and gave permission for their photos to be used.

References

Argyle, M. and Dean, J. (1965), "Eye-contact, distance and affiliation", *Sociometry*, Vol. 36, No. 2, pp. 289–304.

Barrett, L., Mesquita, B. and Gendron, M. (2011), "Context in emotion perception", *Current Directions in Psychological Science*, Vol. 20, No. 5, pp. 286–298.

Beer, J.S., John, O.P., Scabini, D. and Knight, R.T. (2006), "Orbitofrontal cortex and social behavior: Integrating self-monitoring and emotion-cognition interactions", *Journal of Cognitive Neuroscience*, Vol. 18, No. 6, pp. 871–879.

Bibby, H. and McDonald, S. (2005), "Theory of mind after traumatic brain injury", *Neuropsychologia*, Vol. 43, No. 1, pp. 99–114.

Boyatzis, C.J., Chazan, E. and Ting, C.Z. (1993), "Preschool children's decoding of facial emotions", *Journal of Genetic Psychology*, Vol. 154, No. 3, pp. 375–382.

Byom, L.J. and Mutlu, B. (2013), "Theory of mind: Mechanisms, methods, and new directions", *Frontiers in Human Neuroscience*, Vol. 7, p. 413.

Byom, L.J. and Turkstra, L.S. (2012), "Effects of social cognitive demand on Theory of Mind in conversations of adults with traumatic brain injury", *International Journal of Language and Communication Disorders*, Vol. 47, No. 3, pp. 310–321.

Cherney, L.R., Coelho, C.A. and Shadden, B.B. (1998), *Analyzing Discourse in Communicatively Impaired Adults*, MD, US: Aspen Publishers.

Coelho, C.A. (2007), "Management of discourse deficits following traumatic brain injury: Progress, caveats, and needs", *Seminars in Speech and Language*, Vol. 28, pp. 122–135.

Cole, M. (1996), *Cultural Psychology*, Cambridge, MA, US: Harvard University Press.

Dahlberg, C.A., Cusick, C.P., Hawley, L.A., Newman, J.K., Morey, C.E., Harrison-Felix, C.L. and Whiteneck, G.G. (2007), "Treatment efficacy of social communication skills training after traumatic brain injury: A randomized treatment and deferred treatment controlled trial", *Archives of Physical Medicine and Rehabilitation*, Vol. 88, No. 12, pp. 1561–1573.

Darwin, C. (1872), *The Expression of the Emotions in Man and Animals (1st ed.)*, London: John Murray.

Duff, M.C., Mutlu, B., Byom, L. and Turkstra, L. (2012), "Beyond utterances: Distributed cognition as a framework for studying discourse in adults with acquired brain injury", *Seminars in Speech and Language*, Vol. 33, No. 1, pp. 44–54.

Ekman, P. and Friesen, W.V. (1969), "Nonverbal leakage and clues to deception", *Psychiatry*, Vol. 32, No. 1, 88–106.

Emery, N.J. (2000), "The eyes have it: The neuroethology, function, and evolution of social gaze", *Neuroscience and Behavioral Reviews*, Vol. 24, pp. 581–604.

Engberg, A.W. and Teasdale, T.W. (2004), "Psychosocial outcome following traumatic brain injury in adults: A long-term population-based follow-up", *Brain Injury*, Vol. 18, No. 6, pp. 533–545.

Faul, M., Xu, L., Wald, M.M. and Coronado, V.G. (2010), *Traumatic Brain Injury in the United States: Emergency Department Visits, Hospitalizations and Deaths 2002–2006*, Centers for Disease Control and Prevention, National Center for Injury Prevention and Control, Atlanta, GA, US.

Fong, T., Nourbakhsh, I. and Dautenhahn, K. (2003), "A survey of socially interactive robots", *Robotics and Autonomous Systems*, Vol. 42, No. 3, pp. 143–166.

Frischen, A., Bayliss, A.P. and Tipper, S.P. (2007), "Gaze cueing of attention: Visual attention, social cognition, and individual differences", *Psychological Bulletin*, Vol. 133, No. 4, pp. 694–724.

Happé, F. (1994), "An advanced test of theory of mind: Understanding of story characters' thoughts and feelings by able autistic, mentally handicapped, and normal children and adults", *Journal of Autism and Developmental Disorders*, Vol. 24, No. 2, pp. 129–154.

Heilman, K.M., Safran, A. and Geschwind, N. (1971), "Closed head trauma and aphasia", *Journal of Neurology, Neurosurgery and Psychiatry*, Vol. 34, pp. 265–269.

Hengst, J.A., Duff, M.C. and Dettmer, A. (2010), "Rethinking repetition in therapy: Repeated engagement as the social ground of learning", *Aphasiology*, Vol. 24, Nos. 6–8, pp. 887–901.

Hollan, J., Hutchins, E. and Kirsh, D. (2000), "Distributed cognition: Toward a new foundation for human-computer interaction research", *ACM Transactions on Computer-Human Interaction (TOCHI)*, Vol. 7, No. 2, pp. 174–196.

Hutchins, E. (1995), *Cognition in the Wild*, Cambridge, MA, US: Cambridge University Press.

Hutchins, E.L. and Palen, L. (1997), "Constructing meaning from space, gesture, and speech", in L.B. Resneck, R. Saljo, C. Pontecorvo, and B. Burge (1997), *Tools and Reasoning: Essays in Situated Cognition*, Vienna, Austria: Springer-Verlag, pp. 23–40.

Kelly, G., Brown, S., Todd, J. and Kremer, P. (2008), "Challenging behaviour profiles of people with acquired brain injury living in community settings", *Brain Injury*, Vol. 22, No. 6, pp. 457–470.

Leslie, A.M., German, T.P. and Polizzi, P. (2005), "Belief-desire reasoning as a process of selection", *Cognitive Psychology*, Vol. 50, No. 1, pp. 45–85.

Martin-Rodriguez, J.F. and Leon-Carrion, J. (2010), "Theory of mind deficits in patients with acquired brain injury: A quantitative review", *Neuropsychologia*, Vol. 48, No. 5, pp. 1181–1191.

McDonald, S., Flanagan, S. and Rollins, J. (2002), *The Awareness of Social Inference Test (TASIT)*, Austin, TX, US: Harcourt Assessment.

McDonald, S., Tate, R., Togher, L., Bornhofen, C., Long, E., Gertler, P. and Bowen, R. (2008), "Social skills treatment for people with severe, chronic acquired brain injuries: A multicenter trial", *Archives of Physical Medicine and Rehabilitation*, Vol. 89, No. 9, pp. 1648–1659.

McKinnon, M.C. and Moscovitch, M. (2007), "Domain-general contributions to social reasoning: Theory of mind and deontic reasoning re-explored", *Cognition*, Vol. 102, No. 2, pp. 179–218.

Mumm, J. and Mutlu, B. (2011), "Human-robot proxemics: Physical and psychological distancing in human-robot interaction", in *Proceedings of the 6th International Conference on Human-Robot Interaction (HRI 2011)*, ACM, New York, NY, pp. 331–338.

Mutlu, B., Yamaoka, F., Kanda, T., Ishiguro, H. and Hagita, N. (2009), "Nonverbal leakage in robots: Communication of intentions through seemingly unintentional behavior", *4th ACM/IEEE Conference on Human-Robot Interaction*. ACM, New York, NY, pp. 69–76.

Patterson, M. (1973), "Compensation in nonverbal immediacy behaviors: A review", *Sociometry*, Vol. 32, No. 2, pp. 237–252.

Prior, P.A. and Hengst, J.A. (2010), *Exploring Semiotic Remediation as Discourse Practice*, New York: Plagrave MacMillan.

Radice-Neumann, D., Zupan, B., Babbage, D.R. and Willer, B. (2007), "Overview of impaired facial affect recognition in persons with traumatic brain injury", *Brain Injury*, Vol. 21, No. 8, pp. 807–816.

Rogers, Y. (2006), "Distributed cognition and communication", in Brown, K. (Ed.), *The Encyclopedia of Language and Linguistics*, Oxford: Elsevier, pp. 181–202.

Salmond, C.H., Menon, D.K., Chatfield, D.A., Pickard, J.D. and Sahakian, B.J. (2006), "Changes over time in cognitive and structural profiles of head injury survivors", *Neuropsychologia*, Vol. 44, No. 10, 1995–1998.

Salomon, G. (1993), *Distributed Cognitions: Psychological and Educational Considerations*, New York: Cambridge University Press.

Snow, P. and Douglas, J.M. (2000), "Conceptual and methodological challenges in discourse assessment with TBI speakers: Towards an understanding", *Brain Injury*, Vol. 14, No. 5, pp. 397–415.

Snow, P. and Ponsford, J. (1995), "Assessing and managing changes in communication and interpersonal skills following TBI", in Ponsford, J. (Ed.), *Traumatic Brain Injury: Rehabilitation for Everyday Adaptive Living*, Hove, UK: Lawrence Erlbaum Associates, pp. 137–164.

Struchen, M.A., Pappadis, M.R., Mazzei, D.K., Clark, A.N., Davis, L.C. and Sander, A.M. (2008), "Perceptions of communication abilities for persons with traumatic brain injury: Validity of the La Trobe Communication Questionnaire", *Brain Injury*, Vol. 22, No. 12, pp. 940–951.

Turkstra, L.S. (2005), "Looking while listening and speaking: Eye-to-face gaze in adolescents with and without traumatic brain injury", *Journal of Speech, Language and Hearing Research*, Vol. 48, No. 6, pp. 1429–1441.

Turkstra, L.S. (2008), "Conversation-based assessment of social cognition in adults with traumatic brain injury", *Brain Injury*, Vol. 22, No. 5, pp. 397–409.

Turkstra, L., Brehm, S.E. and Montgomery, E.B.J. (2006), "Analysing conversational discourse after traumatic brain injury: Isn't it about time?", *Brain Impairment*, Vol. 7, No. 3, pp. 234–245.

Turkstra, L.S., McDonald, S. and DePompei, R. (2001), "Social information processing in adolescents: Data from normally developing adolescents and preliminary data from their peers with traumatic brain injury", *The Journal of Head Trauma Rehabilitation*, Vol. 16, No. 5, pp. 469–483.

Turkstra, L.S., Vandenheuvel, S. and Visscher, K. (2014), "Emotion identification in context", Presented at the 10th World Congress on Brain Injury. San Francisco: CA, US.

Vygotsky, L.S. (1978), *Mind In Society: The Development of Higher Psychological Processes*, Cambridge, MA, US: Harvard University Press.

Walker-Andrews, A.S. (1998), "Emotions and social development: Infants' recognition of emotions in others", *Pediatrics*, Vol. 102 (5 Suppl. E), pp. 1268–1271.

Wertsch, J.V. (1985), *Vygotsky and the Social Formation of Mind*, Cambridge, MA. US: Harvard University Press.

Wilms, M., Schilbach, L., Pfeiffer, U., Bente, G., Fink, G.R. and Vogeley, K. (2010), "It's in your eyes— Using gaze-contingent stimuli to create truly interactive paradigms for social cognitive and affective neuroscience", *Social Cognitive and Affective Neuroscience*, Vol. 5, No. 1, pp. 98–107.

INDEX